PDxMD

Hematology & Oncology

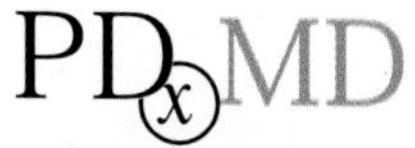

An Imprint of Elsevier Science

Philadelphia ■ St Louis ■ London ■ Sydney ■ New York ■ Toronto

ID Medical Conditions Series is dedicated to health and healing professionals everywhere. ...re privileged to be in your service and hope our efforts help you in your quest for better quality-of-life and optimized outcomes for all your patients.

PDxMD
An imprint of Elsevier Science

Publisher: Steven Merahn, MD
Project Managers: Caroline Barnett, Lucy Hamilton, Zak Knowles
Programmer: Narinder Chandi
Production: Aoibhe O'Shea – GMS UK, Alan Palfreyman – PTU
Designer: Jayne Jones
Layout: Alan Palfreyman, The Designers Collective Limited

NOTICE
Medicine is an ever-changing field. Standard safety precautions must be followed, but as new research and clinical experience broaden our knowledge, changes in treatment and drug therapy may become necessary or appropriate. Readers are advised to check the most current product information provided by the manufacturer of each drug to be administered to verify the recommended dose, the method and duration of administration, and contraindications. It is the responsibility of the licensed prescriber, relying on experience and knowledge of the patient, to determine dosages and the best treatment for each individual patient. Neither the publisher nor the editor assumes any liability for any injury and/or damage to persons or property arising from this publication.

All PDxMD contributors are participating in the activities of PDxMD in an individual capacity, and not as representatives of or on behalf of their individual affiliated hospitals, associations or institutions (where indicated herein), and their participation should not be taken as an endorsement of PDxMD by their individual affiliated hospitals, associations or institutions. Individual affiliated hospitals, associations or institutions are not responsible for the accuracy or availability of information on the product.

Printed in China by RDC Group

PDxMD
Elsevier Science
The Curtis Center
625 Walnut Street,
Philadelphia, PA 19106

The Publisher's policy is to use **paper manufactured from sustainable forests**

ISBN 1-932141-05-7

Contents

Introduction

Contents

Introduction

What is PDxMD?

PDxMD is a new, evidence-based primary care clinical information system designed to support your judgment with practical clinical information. The content is continuously updated by expert contributors with the latest on evaluation, diagnosis, management, outcomes and prevention – all designed for use at the point and time of care.

First and foremost, PDxMD is an electronic resource. This book gives you access to just a fraction of the content available on-line. At www.pdxmd.com, you will find:

- Over 1400 differential diagnoses for you to search for information according to your patient's chief complaint via a unique signs and symptoms matrix
- Information on more than 450 medical conditions and more than 750 drugs and other therapies, organised in condition-specific 'MediFiles'
- Patient information sheets on 300 topics for you to customize and hand to your patient during consultation

About This Book

The PDxMD Medical Conditions Series is a print version of the comprehensive approach offered on line. Concise information on medical conditions is systematically organized in a consistent MediFile format, our electronic equivalent of chapters.

Each MediFile covers summary information and background on each condition, and comprehensive information on diagnosis, treatment, outcomes, and prevention, and other resources, especially written and designed for use in practice. Each MediFile is organized identically to allow you to find information consistently and reliably for every condition. See the MediFile 'Road Map' inside the back cover for more information.

Ranging from epidemiology to risk assessment and reduction, from diagnostic evaluation and testing to therapeutic options, prognosis and outcomes - you'll find the information that you need is easier to locate with this methodical approach.

How to Use This Book

Find the MediFile for any specific medical condition in the Contents list. Familiarize yourself with the MediFile Road Map (see inside back cover) to rapidly find the precise information you require.

Information on drugs and tests are found within the MediFiles for the specific conditions. For an overview, see the 'Summary of options' sections under DIAGNOSIS and under TREATMENT in the relevant MediFile. Details of tests, drugs and other therapies then follow.

PDxMD believes that physician clinical judgment is central to appropriate diagnostic and therapeutic decision-making. The information is designed to support professional judgment and, accounting for individual patient differences, does not provide direct answers or force specific practices or policies.

How is PDxMD created?

PDxMD is created through Collaborative Authoring. This process allows medical information to be reviewed and synthesized from multiple sources – including but not limited to peer-reviewed articles, evidence databases, guidelines and position papers – and by multiple individuals. The information is organized around and integrated into a template that matches the needs of primary care physicians in practice.

Professional medical writers begin the process of reviewing and synthesizing information for PDxMD, working from core evidence databases and other expert resources and with the guidance of Editorial Advisory Board (EAB) members. This first draft is sent to a physician 'clinical reviewer', who works with the writer to make sure the information is accurate and properly organized. A second review by the physician clinical reviewer ensures that appropriate changes are in place.

After these first two levels of clinical review, the files are reviewed and edited by the relevant specialist member of the Editorial Advisory Board. A primary care member of the EAB, who has final sign-off authority, then conducts the final review and edit. Editorial checks are conducted between all review stages and, after primary care sign-off, a pharmacist double checks the drug recommendations prior to a final editorial review.

There are a minimum of three and as many as five physicians involved in each MediFile, and additional clinical reviewers and/or EAB members are added when appropriate (e.g., alternative/complementary medicine experts, or conditions requiring multi-disciplinary approaches). The contributor team for each MediFile is listed in the Resources section.

A complete list of Editorial Faculty and staff of PDxMD is provided below. All Editorial Faculty, and specifically the Editorial Advisory Board members, participate in PDxMD as individuals and not as representatives of, or on behalf of, their affiliated institutions or associations and any indication of their affiliation with a specific institution or association should not be taken as an endorsement of PDxMD or any participation of their institution or association with PDxMD.

Continuous Product Improvement

PDxMD is committed to continuous quality improvement and welcomes any comments, suggestions and feedback from the professional community. Please send any ideas or considerations regarding this volume or any other volume in the PDxMD series via e-mail to feedback.pdxmd@elsevier.com or to PDxMD, Elsevier Science, The Curtis Center, 625 Walnut Street, Philadelphia, PA 19106.

Introduction

Evidence-Based Medicine Policies

PDxMD is committed to providing available and up-to-date evidence for the diagnostic and therapeutic recommendations provided in our knowledge base. All MediFiles begin with a core set of evidence-based references from recognized sources. These are supplemented with extensive searches of the literature and reviews of reference books, peer-reviewed journals, association guidelines and position papers, among others.

Criteria for Evidence-Based Medicine

Evidence Sources

PDxMD has taken the best evidence currently available from the following:

Published Critically Evaluated Evidence

- Cochrane Systematic Reviews – respected throughout the world as one of the most rigorous searches of medical journals with highly structured systematic reviews and use of meta-analysis to produce reliable evidence
- Clinical Evidence – produced jointly by the British Medical Journal Publishing Group and the American College of Physicians–American Society of Internal Medicine. Clinical Evidence provides a concise account of the current state of knowledge on the treatment and prevention of many clinical conditions based on the search and appraisal of the available literature
- The National Guideline Clearinghouse – a comprehensive database of evidence-based clinical practice guidelines and related documents produced by the Agency for Healthcare Research and Quality in partnership with the American Medical Association and the American Association of Health Plans

Evidence Published in Peer-Reviewed Journals

- Association Guidelines and Position Papers

Where evidence exists that has not yet been critically reviewed by one of the sources listed above, for example randomized controlled trials and clinical cohort studies, the evidence is summarized briefly, categorized, and fully referenced.

Clinical Experience

While recognizing the importance of these evidence-based resources, PDxMD also highlights the importance of experience in clinical practice. Therefore, our Editorial Advisory Board also provide advice from their own clinical experience, within Clinical Pearl sections of the MediFiles and elsewhere. Contributing expert physicians are identified in the Resources section of every MediFile.

Evaluation of Evidence

PDxMD evaluates all cited evidence according to the AAFP Recommended Basic Model for Evaluating and Categorizing the Clinical Content of CME, based on the model used by the University of Michigan:

Level M Evidence from either:
Meta-analysis or
Multiple randomized controlled trials

Level P Evidence from either:
A well-designed prospective clinical trial or
Several prospective clinical cohort studies with consistent findings (without randomization)

Level S Evidence from studies other than clinical trials, such as:
Epidemiological studies
Physiological studies

References

The information provided by PDxMD is concise and action-oriented. As a result, our editorial policy is to cite only essential reference sources. References and evidence summaries are provided in four areas:

1. In the Diagnostic Decision section under Diagnosis
2. In the Guidelines and Evidence sections under Treatment
3. In the Outcomes section under Evidence
4. In the Key Reference Section under Resources

Where on-line references to the Cochrane Abstracts, BMJ Clinical Evidence and National Guideline Clearinghouse are cited in the text, the internet addresses of the home pages are given. The internet addresses of individual reports are not given.

When references are to association guidelines and position papers, the internet address of the association home page is generally provided. When possible, the internet address of the specific report is provided.

Editorial Faculty and Staff

Executive Committee

Editorial Board

Editorial Faculty and Staff

Editorial Faculty and Staff

Editorial Faculty and Staff

Gary M White, MD
Editorial Board, Dermatology Illustration
Associate Clinical Professor
Dept of Dermatology
University of California, San Diego
San Diego, CA

Basil J Zitelli, MD
Editorial Board, Pediatrics Illustration
Professor of Pediatrics
University of Pittsburgh School of Medicine
Children's Hospital of Pittsburgh
Pittsburgh PA

Clinical Reviewers

Januario E Castro, MD
Hematology/Oncology
Clinical Fellow, Division of Hematology-Oncology
Department of Medicine
University of California, San Diego
San Diego, CA

Naixi N Chen, MD
Hematology/Oncology
H Lee Moffitt Cancer Center and Research
Institute,, University of South Florida
Tampa, FL

Luciana G O Clark, MD
Hematology/Oncology
Blood and Marrow Transplant Program
H Lee Moffitt Cancer Center & Research
Institute,, University of South Florida
Tampa, FL

Otavio A Clark, MD
Hematology/Oncology
Blood and Marrow Transplant Program
H Lee Moffit Cancer Center & Research Institute
University of South Florida
Tampa, FL

Dwight Eichelberger, MD
Primary Care
Medical Director
Department of Primary Care
Ammonoosuc Community Health Services
Littleton, NH

Sandeep Garg, MD
Hematology/Oncology
Internal Medicine and Oncology
Providence Hospital and Medical Center
Farmington Hills, MI

Mary Jo Groves, MD
Primary Care
Director, Student Health Services
Department of Student Health Services
Wittenberg University
Springfield, OK

Dinesh S Rao, MD
Hematology/Oncology
Research Fellow
Department of Internal Medicine
University of Michigan
Ann Arbor, MI

Ted Turnquest, MD
Hematology/Oncology
H Lee Moffitt Cancer Center and Research
Institute
University of South Florida
Tampa, FL

Editorial Faculty and Staff

Writers

Lory E Baraz, MD
Jon M Berkowitz, MD
Kim S Berman
Patricia M Clark, MSN, RN, CS
Tony W B Crockett, BMBS, DRCOG, MRCGP
Anne E Dyson, MB BS
Kelly D Karpa, RPh, PhD, BSPharm
Fiona McCrimmon, MBBS, MRCGP
Beth E K Oliver, BSc Occupational Therapy
Mary E Selby, MB ChB, DRCOG, MRCGP
Colin R Tidy, MBBS, MRCGP, MRCP
Everetta M Woods
Tony M J Woolfson, MB BS, DM, MRCP

Staff

Management Team
Fiona Foley, Steven Merahn, MD, Daniel Pollock, Zak Knowles, Howard Croft, Tanya Thomas, Lucy Hamilton, Julie Volck, Bill Bruggemeyer, Andrea Ford

Editorial Team
Anne Dyson, Sadaf Hashmi, Debbie Goring, Louise Morrison, Ellen Haigh, Robert Whittle, Claire Champion, Caroline Barnett, Laurie Smith, Li Wan, Paul Mayhew, Carmen Jones, Fi Ward

Technical Team
Martin Miller, Narinder Chandi, Roy Patterson, Aaron McGrath, John Wylie, Sarah Craze, Cameron Sangster

We would also like to acknowledge the extraordinary contributions of the following individuals to the conceptualization and realization of PDxMD over the initial years of its growth and development:

Tim Hailstone, Jonathan Black, Alison Whitehouse, Jayne Harris, Angela Baggi, Sharon Bambaji, Sam Bedser, Layla van den Bergh, Stuart Boffey, Siobhan Egan, Helen Elder, Mark Mitchenall, Chris Moodie, Tony Pollard, Simon Seljeflot, Liz Southey, Tim Stentiford, Matthew Whyte

ACUTE LYMPHOCYTIC LEUKEMIA

SUMMARY INFORMATION

DESCRIPTION

- Acute lymphocytic leukemia (ALL) is a disease characterized by replacement of the bone marrow with abnormal lymphoblasts
- The usual presenting features are pallor and fatigue, bleeding and bruising, and fever and infection due to anemia, thrombocytopenia and leukopenia, respectively
- Hepatosplenomegaly and lymphadenopathy may be present at diagnosis
- Treatment is with intensive chemotherapy and radiotherapy which are given in three phases: induction of remission, intensification/central nervous system prophylaxis and maintenance
- Prognosis depends on a number of factors, including cell type and age at presentation
- Most patients will achieve remission; 80% of children are cured but only 30–40% of adults, due to higher frequency of adverse genetic abnormalities of leukemic lymphoblasts of adults
- This is improving as a result of newly developed therapies and information from clinical trials

URGENT ACTION

- Send complete blood count immediately
- Treat bacterial infections with broad-spectrum antibiotics if patient is febrile
- Refer to specialist without delay for full diagnosis and treatment

KEY! DON'T MISS!

- Severe anemia needing blood transfusion
- Severe thrombocytopenia needing platelet transfusion
- Severe infection needing immediate antibiotic treatment
- Specific symptoms of meningeal leukemia (headache, confusion, cranial nerve neuropathies) or hyperleukocytosis (headache, confusion, focal neurologic defects, dyspnea, and priapism) may also be present and mandate immediate intervention as an oncologic emergency

BACKGROUND

ICD9 CODE

204.0 Lymphoid leukemia.

SYNONYMS

- ALL
- Acute lymphoblastic leukemia
- Acute lymphoid leukemia

CARDINAL FEATURES

- Acute lymphocytic leukemia (ALL) is a malignant proliferation of abnormal immature lymphocytes in the bone marrow with possible dissemination into the blood, the central nervous system, and other organs
- It may be divided into different types by histologic, cytochemical, immunologic and cytogenetic studies of the abnormal cells. The French-American-British (FAB) Co-operative Study Group has classified ALL into three groups: L1 to L3. L2 is the most common subtype in adults. This typing is useful in defining prognosis and treatment
- One-third of all cases occur in adults
- Patients usually present with pallor and fatigue, bleeding and bruising, and fever and infection, due to anemia, thrombocytopenia, and leukopenia, respectively. Cytopenia results from replacement of the bone marrow with abnormal cells and consequent deficiencies of the normal blood elements
- Lymphadenopathy, hepatomegaly, and splenomegaly may also be present
- Treatment is with combination chemotherapy, cerebral irradiation, intrathecal chemotherapy and, in some cases, bone marrow transplantation
- Most patients will achieve a remission with induction therapy
- Cure rate is better than 60% in children but only one-third of adults survive this disease

CAUSES

Common causes

- Usually unknown
- Related to viral infections with HTLV-1 in cases of T cell ALL in Japan, the Caribbean, southern US, and some parts of Africa
- May be related in some cases to viral infections with Epstein-Barr virus
- Psoriasis has been associated with a higher risk of ALL in adults
- Environmental exposure: an increased risk is associated with exposure to industrial residues of paper and allied products, iron, steel, aluminum, and also with contamination of drinking water with trichloroethylene
- Smoking increases the risk three times

Contributory or predisposing factors

- Benzene and toluene are known causes of acute leukemia
- Radiation exposure is leukemogenic. Increased incidence of leukemia is proportional to the cumulative radiation dose to which a person has been exposed. It has been observed in atomic bomb survivors
- 5-fold increased risk has been observed in siblings

EPIDEMIOLOGY

Incidence and prevalence

- Worldwide:10–65 cases per million people
- Incidence is rising slowly in the US: approximately 3100 new cases annually, (17 cases per million people); 930 new cases diagnosed annually in individuals aged 20 years or over

Demographics

AGE

Incidence is relatively high through the teenage years, falls during the next two decades, and increases steadily beyond 45 years of age.

GENDER

Slightly more common in males (60:40).

RACE

- No specific preponderance in adults
- Poorer prognosis in African-Americans

GENETICS

- Association with Down syndrome (trisomy 21). The risk of developing acute leukemia in individuals with Down syndrome is nearly 20 times greater than would normally be expected
- Association with Philadelphia chromosome
- Association with some other chromosomal translocations (e.g. t9:22, t8:14, t4:11, q21:23). Leukemogenesis in young patients may occur *in utero*

GEOGRAPHY

HTLV-1 associated T cell ALL in Japan, the Caribbean, southern US, and some parts of Africa.

SOCIOECONOMIC STATUS

The possibility that viruses play a role in common ALL of childhood is suggested by epidemiologic data linking increased risk with higher socioeconomic status and other community characteristics that lead to delayed exposure to the usual infections of infancy.

DIFFERENTIAL DIAGNOSIS

The presenting features are nonspecific and related to anemia, neutropenia, thrombocytopenia, and infection.The differential diagnosis is therefore mainly with other disorders that involve the bone marrow.

Acute myelogenous leukemia

Acute myelogenous leukemia (AML) is a group of disorders characterized by replacement of the bone marrow with abnormal immature cells of the myeloid series. Patients usually present with anemia, thrombocytopenia, and neutropenia.

FEATURES

- May be indistinguishable on clinical grounds and requires specific pathologic tests
- Organomegaly and adenopathy may be present but are not very common
- Bone pain occurs in less than 20% of patients
- 13% of patients with AML have leukemic skin infiltration (the lesions are often violaceous and nodular and may precede the diagnosis)
- Greater than 30% blasts on aspirate or peripheral blood, Auer rods, and Phi bodies are considered pathognomonic of AML

Aplastic anemia

Aplastic anemia is a bone marrow failure leading to pancytopenia, either due to an acquired exposure or familial association.

FEATURES

- May be indistinguishable on clinical grounds. Requires specific pathologic tests
- Usually idiopathic, may be linked to marrow toxins (cytotoxic drugs, radiation), drug reaction (chloramphenicol, gold, sulfur compounds, carbamazepine), or a viral infection (hepatitis B virus, hepatitis C virus, cytomegalovirus, HIV, parvovirus)
- Onset is gradual, with fatigue and bleeding noted first; infection is a later problem
- No organomegaly occurs
- Complete blood count: normochromic-normocytic anemia, diminished number of platelets, reticulocyte count is zero, and a pancytopenia is present

Thrombocytopenic purpura

Thrombocytopenic purpura is one of the major causes of platelet destruction.

FEATURES

- May be indistinguishable on clinical grounds and requires specific pathologic tests
- It may present as bleeding (after aspirin or nonsteroidal anti-inflammatory drug (NSAID) use), menorrhagia, epistaxis, or purpuric rash following a viral infection
- The physical examination findings are otherwise normal (spleen usually may be slightly enlarged, no lymphadenopathy, hepatomegaly, or sternal tenderness is present)
- Mild fever is sometimes noted

Infectious mononucleosis

Infectious mononucleosis is a viral illness caused by Epstein-Barr virus (EBV), affecting mainly adolescents and young adults.

FEATURES

- Clinical features: malaise, headache, fever (40°C), pharyngitis, and lymphadenopathy (tonsillar/cervical lymph nodes may be quite enlarged, painful, and tender) lasting from one to several weeks
- Laboratory findings: relative or absolute lymphocytosis and positive serology (Paul-Bunnell)

Myelofibrosis

Myelofibrosis can be classified as primary (idiopathic) or secondary (chronic myeloid leukemia, cancers, vasculitis (lupus, rheumatoid arthritis)).

FEATURES

- May be indistinguishable on clinical grounds. Requires specific pathologic tests
- It is remarkable for pancytopenia despite extraordinarily large numbers of circulating hematopoietic progenitor cells

Multiple myeloma

Multiple myeloma is a neoplastic proliferation of a single clone of plasma cells producing a monoclonal immunoglobulin resulting in extensive skeletal destruction (osteolytic lesions, hypercalcemia, anemia) renal failure, recurrent bacterial infections, or hyperviscosity syndrome.

FEATURES

- Bone pain (particularly in the back or chest), usually induced by movement and that does not occur at night except with change of position, is present at diagnosis in more than two-thirds of patients
- The patient's height may be reduced because of vertebral collapse
- Pallor, weakness, and fatigue are common and often associated with anemia
- X-rays usually show characteristic lytic lesions
- Criteria for diagnosis: increased monoclonal plasma cells in bone marrow, monoclonal protein in serum or urine (Bence-Jones protein)

Secondary deposits from carcinomas

Secondary deposits may occur from, for example, carcinoma of breast, lung, prostate.

FEATURES

- Patients often have bone pain
- X-rays may show sclerotic or lytic lesions
- Differentiation from leukemia is readily accomplished with immunophenotypic analysis or electron microscopy

Systemic lupus erythematosus

Systemic lupus erythematosus (SLE) is a chronic multisystemic disease of autoimmune origin.

FEATURES

- Symptoms are nonspecific (e.g. fatigue, fever, weight loss) with fatigue being the chief complaint
- Myalgia, arthralgia, and arthritis occur at some point in nearly all patients
- Arthritis is usually symmetric and may include the small joints of the hands and feet, wrists, elbows, knees, and ankles
- The classic physical finding in SLE is the malar or butterfly rash
- Laboratory findings: antinuclear antibody (ANA) positive with titers of 1:1280 or greater serves as screening
- The presence of antibody to double-stranded (native) deoxyribonucleic acid (DNA) is pathognomonic for lupus

Leukemoid reaction to infection

May be indistinguishable on clinical grounds. Requires specific pathologic tests.

SIGNS & SYMPTOMS

Signs

There are no specific signs found in ALL. Physical signs are those of anemia, thrombocytopenia or organ infiltration.

- Pallor
- Bruising
- Ecchymoses/petechiae
- Purpuric rash
- Lymphadenopathy
- Hepatomegaly and/or splenomegaly, mediastinal mass
- Sternal tenderness
- Meningismus may indicate central nervous system (CNS) leukemic infiltration
- Leukemic infiltrates in the optic fundus appear as Roth's-like spots with flame hemorrhages
- Gingival enlargement

Symptoms

There are no specific symptoms of ALL. Symptoms are attributable to anemia, thrombocytopenia, organ involvement, metabolic disturbances, and infection secondary to leukopenia.

- Weakness and fatigue are the most common symptoms
- Shortness of breath
- Bleeding
- Weight loss
- Abdominal discomfort, if it represents hepatosplenomegaly
- Bone pain is more common in ALL than in AML and results from bone erosion or leukemic involvement of the periosteum
- Headaches, nausea, vomiting, blurred vision, or cranial nerve dysfunction, if CNS involvement present
- Renal colic or other urinary symptoms if urate output very high and deposits/stones are formed
- Fever, either secondary to infection or directly due to the disease process
- Involvement of testes as extramedullary site of relapse is not uncommon

ASSOCIATED DISORDERS

Down syndrome with Philadelphia chromosome.

KEY! DON'T MISS!

- Severe anemia needing blood transfusion
- Severe thrombocytopenia needing platelet transfusion
- Severe infection needing immediate antibiotic treatment
- Specific symptoms of meningeal leukemia (headache, confusion, cranial nerve neuropathies) or hyperleukocytosis (headache, confusion, focal neurologic defects, dyspnea, and priapism) may also be present and mandate immediate intervention as an oncologic emergency

CONSIDER CONSULT

- All patients should be referred for specialist investigation.

INVESTIGATION OF THE PATIENT

Direct questions to patient

- Q **Have you been feeling unwell?** Often a presenting symptom
- Q **Have you been weak, tired or short of breath?** May indicate anemia
- Q **Have you lost weight recently?** Weight loss may be a feature of ALL
- Q **Have you had nosebleeds, bruising, blood in the urine?** Can be due to thrombocytopenia
- Q **Have you had any aches and pains or abdominal discomfort?** May suggest bone involvement or hepatosplenomegaly
- Q **Have you developed any lumps in your neck, armpits, or groin?** Lymphadenopathy is common
- Q **Have you been hot and cold or shivering?** Fever is often present either from the disease process itself or caused by bacterial infections secondary to neutropenia
- Q **Have you noticed any changes in passing urine?** Deposition of uric acid crystals in the kidneys secondary to increased cell breakdown can affect renal function, causing nocturia, oliguria or renal colic if stones pass down the ureter
- Q **Have you experienced headaches or any mental changes?** These are often present if the CNS is involved

Contributory or predisposing factors

- Q **Have you been exposed to industrial solvents or unusual doses of radiation?** Said to be associated with exposure to certain toxins (e.g. benzene) and exposure to ionizing radiation.

Family history

- Q **Has anyone in your family ever been diagnosed with acute leukemia?** Five-fold increased risk has been observed in siblings.

Examination

- **Is the patient anemic?** Anemia may be a feature of ALL
- **Is the body temperature raised?** Fever is very common in ALL, even if there is no evidence of bacterial infection
- **Is there any evidence of abnormal bleeding?** Bruising, ecchymoses, purpura, hemorrhages in optic fundi often occur
- **Is there any abnormal lymphadenopathy?** Very common in ALL
- **Is the liver or spleen enlarged?** Very common in ALL

Summary of investigative tests

- Complete blood count should be performed in all patients, and may reveal anemia, thrombocytopenia, neutropenia or the presence of lymphoblasts in the peripheral blood
- Bone marrow examination (aspiration and biopsy) is normally performed by a specialist: the diagnosis of acute leukemia is established by bone marrow examination. More than 30% of blasts are needed in bone marrow to establish the diagnosis. A similar number of blasts in the peripheral blood film will also make the diagnosis. Cytochemistries and immunologic cell-surface markers should be evaluated in all cases of suspected ALL
- Serum urate should be requested routinely and particularly after induction chemotherapy because the level will increase as a result of tissue breakdown and this may cause tumor lysis syndrome
- Serum renal and liver function tests
- Serum phosphate and calcium, increased cell destruction is also responsible for hyperphosphatemia and hypocalcemia
- Urine examination and culture provide a good early indicator of urine infection or nephropathy
- Serum lactate dehydrogenase (LDH) can also be diagnostically helpful
- Standard workup for fever with blood culture, urine culture, and chest X-ray. Additional workup directed according to symptoms

- Lymph node biopsy. Normally performed by a specialist. May be useful if enlarged superficial nodes present, and may give an earlier diagnosis than bone marrow aspiration
- Chest X-ray may reveal enlarged hilar lymph nodes, infiltration or infection of the lungs
- Skeletal lesions can be demonstrated radiographically in more than 50% of patients. Look for 'leukemic lines' (transverse metaphysical radiolucent lines adjacent to the zone of provisional calcification at the end of long bones), generalized rarefaction of bones, cortical and trabecular osteolytic lesions, and periosteal new bone formation
- Abdominal ultrasound scanning or computerized (CAT) scanning will indicate the extent of involvement of liver, spleen and intra-abdominal lymph nodes. CAT scan may be used for staging and is usually requested by a specialist
- Lumbar puncture. Normally performed by a specialist. Indicated if there is meningismus or a suspicion of CNS involvement, or after bone marrow remission to assess whether there is remaining infiltration or involvement which is not clinically detectable. Fluid should be cultured routinely for acid-fast bacilli, fungi, and bacteria. Expect to find increased CSF pressure, elevated levels of CSF protein, and decreased glucose values
- Bone marrow aspirate and biopsy should be performed by a specialist; aspirate smears should be studied with a battery of cytochemical stains; separate specimens of marrow should be sent for cytogenetic, immunophenotypic, and molecular studies

DIAGNOSTIC DECISION

- The definitive diagnosis is made on the peripheral blood film and bone marrow examination
- ALL has been defined as an abnormal white cell count and differential, abnormal hemoglobin and platelet count, abnormal bone marrow with more than 30% lymphoblasts and signs and symptoms of the disease
- Different types of ALL are defined according to the characteristics of the abnormal cells. Morphologic features, cytochemistry, immunologic surface markers, and cytogenetics are all taken into account

CLINICAL PEARLS

- Once a diagnosis of leukemia is considered, the major issues in making the correct diagnosis of ALL are to distinguish non-neoplastic proliferations of lymphoid cells and to exclude myeloid leukemias
- Although physical findings related to extramedullary leukemic infiltration may be present at initial evaluation, they are rarely symptomatic

THE TESTS

Body fluids

COMPLETE BLOOD COUNT

Description

Venous blood sample.

Advantages/Disadvantages

Advantages:

- Quick and inexpensive
- May be diagnostic

Normal

- Hemoglobin: men, 13.6–17.7g/dL (8.4–11.0mmol/L; women, 12–15g/dL (7.4–9.3mmol/L)
- Platelets: 150–400x10^9/L
- Leukocytes: 4.5–10.5x10^9/L
- Neutrophils: 50–70%, 3.0–7.0x10^9/L
- Lymphocytes: 30–50%, 2.0–5.0x10^9/L

Abnormal

- A normochromic, normocytic anemia is often present
- 60% of patients with ALL have increased total leukocyte counts, 10% have counts $>100x10^9/L$
- 80% of patients have decreased neutrophil counts $<2x10^9/L$
- 90% of patients have reduced platelet counts $<150x10^9/L$

Cause of abnormal result

Replacement of bone marrow with rapidly proliferating abnormal lymphocytes.

PERIPHERAL BLOOD FILM

Description

- Venous blood sample
- Cells are examined microscopically for their morphology

Advantages/Disadvantages

Advantages:

- Results contribute specifically to diagnosis
- Quantifying abnormal blast cells can aid prognosis

Normal

Normal whole blood constituent cells only.

Abnormal

The presence of characteristic leukemic blast cells.

Cause of abnormal result

- Proliferation of a leukemic cell line which destroys normal bone marrow function
- Immature blast cells are released into the peripheral circulation and can be seen on blood film

SERUM LACTATE DEHYDROGENASE

Description

Venous blood sample.

Advantages/Disadvantages

Advantages:

- Inexpensive, rapid answer
- May be helpful diagnostically in that it is often raised in ALL

Disadvantage: nonspecific

Normal

50–150 IU/L.

Abnormal

>150 IU/L.

Cause of abnormal result

Increased leukemic cell turnover.

Drugs, disorders and other factors that may alter results

Any condition that leads to cell destruction or increased cell turnover can cause a rise in LDH, e.g. renal failure or myocardial infarction.

SERUM URATE

Description

Venous blood sample.

Advantages/Disadvantages

Advantages:

- Inexpensive, rapid answer
- Indicates a need for treatment if significantly raised

Normal

2–7mg/dL (120–420mcmol/L).

Abnormal

>7mg/dL (420mcmol/L).

Cause of abnormal result

Increased tissue breakdown. Uric acid is an end product of protein metabolism.

Drugs, disorders and other factors that may alter results

- Hyperuricemia may be precipitated by treatment of ALL with chemotherapy
- Some drugs can increase uric acid levels

SERUM CREATININE

Description

Venous blood sample.

Advantages/Disadvantages

Advantages:

- Inexpensive, rapid answer
- Reflects renal function accurately

Normal

0.6–1.2mg/dL (50–110mcmol/L).

Abnormal

>1.2mg/dL (110mmol/L).

Cause of abnormal result

Fall in glomerular filtration rate, often due to acute urate nephropathy.

Drugs, disorders and other factors that may alter results

- Renal failure from acute urate nephropathy may be precipitated by chemotherapy in ALL
- Many medications and medical conditions can affect renal function and raise creatinine levels

BLOOD CULTURE

Description

- Venous blood innoculated immediately into a liquid culture medium
- Two bottles of culture medium are used for aerobes and anaerobes

Advantages/Disadvantages

Advantages:

- May grow the bacteria causing infection in neutropenic patients
- Inexpensive
- Can test for antibiotic sensitivities

Disadvantages:
- 48h incubation usually needed
- Negative result does not exclude infection
- Risk of false-positive from contamination

Normal
No growth.

Abnormal
- Significant growth of infecting organism(s)
- May be more than one type of bacterium in profoundly neutropenic patients

Cause of abnormal result
Insufficient neutrophils to eliminate circulating bacteria.

Drugs, disorders and other factors that may alter results
- Contamination of the sample may lead to false-positives
- Contaminated intravenous lines can also affect results

URINE EXAMINATION/CULTURE
Description
Clean, preferably midstream, specimen of urine.

Advantages/Disadvantages
Advantages:
- Inexpensive, rapid answer for microscopy
- Good early indicator of urine infection or nephropathy

Disadvantage: Culture takes 48h

Normal
- Stick test – pH 4.5–8, protein absent, glucose absent, hemoglobin (or RBC) absent, leukocytes absent
- Microscopy – RBC 0–5/high-power field, leukocytes 0–5/high-power field, casts 0–4/low-power field, crystals absent
- Culture – no growth of bacteria

Abnormal
- Stick test – RBC, leukocytes, or significant protein indicate nephropathy or infection
- Microscopy – >5 RBC or leukocytes, >4 casts raise possibility of infection. Significant amounts of urate crystals indicate possible urate nephropathy
- Culture – significant (>100,000 organisms/mL) growth of bacteria suggests active urinary tract infection

Cause of abnormal result
- Direct effects on the kidney of infection or high urate concentrations
- Bacterial infection within the bladder

Drugs, disorders and other factors that may alter results
Contaminated or catheter specimens may give false-positive results.

Imaging

CHEST X-RAY

Description

Posterior/anterior/lateral X-ray films of the chest during inspiration.

Advantages/Disadvantages

Advantages:

- Inexpensive, rapid answer
- Will detect thymic masses, hilar lymph node enlargement, and pulmonary infiltrations

Normal

No masses or infiltrations.

Abnormal

Presence of abnormal masses or infiltrations.

Cause of abnormal result

Abnormal cell line infiltration of lymph nodes in the chest.

Drugs, disorders and other factors that may alter results

- Pre-existing lung or heart pathology may produce an enlarged hilum on the chest X-ray
- Other malignancies

ABDOMINAL ULTRASOUND SCAN

Description

Ultrasound scan of the abdomen.

Advantages/Disadvantages

Advantages:

- Useful in detecting hepatic or splenic enlargement, or the presence of intra-abdominal lymph nodes
- No exposure to ionizing radiation
- Inexpensive

Disadvantage: Requires skilled operator

Normal

- No organomegaly
- No lymphadenopathy

Abnormal

Presence of enlarged liver or spleen or abnormal lymph nodes.

Cause of abnormal result

- Abnormal cell infiltration into the liver and spleen causing organ enlargement
- Lymph node enlargement due to collection of abnormal lymphoid cells

Drugs, disorders and other factors that may alter results

- Alcohol abuse can lead to abdominal organomegaly
- Other malignancies and/or conditions
- Other infections such as glandular fever

TREATMENT

CONSIDER CONSULT

All patients should be referred to a specialist for treatment.

IMMEDIATE ACTION

- If an acute leukemia is suspected, a complete blood count should be sent immediately
- If the patient is febrile, panculture should be sent and broad-spectrum antibiotics started
- Preparations should be made to transfer the patient to a specialist unit for further treatment

PATIENT AND CAREGIVER ISSUES

Impact on career, dependants, family, friends

- This is a potentially fatal disorder and cure rates are lower for adults than in children
- The patient will be hospitalized immediately and will remain in hospital for the period of induction of remission. The time frame for this treatment is highly variable between patients but can be weeks to months and then 2–3 years of maintenance treatment

Patient or caregiver request

- Patients and their families may have assumptions about the prognosis of the disease which may be very different from the reality of the individual case
- It is very important to see that they are fully and truthfully informed of the prognosis and the possibilities for treatment

MANAGEMENT ISSUES

Goals

- Identify and treat acute infections
- Carry out the initial investigations
- Refer without delay for specialist diagnosis and treatment
- Recognize relapse/recurrence in those with diagnosed acute lymphocytic leukemia (ALL) and refer immediately to hospital

SUMMARY OF THERAPEUTIC OPTIONS

Choices

- All patients with ALL should be treated in a hospital setting under hematologist supervision. All patients should begin treatment with allopurinol, before starting chemotherapy in ALL
- The treatment of ALL is divided into stages: induction of remission, consolidation, central nervous system (CNS) prophylaxis, and maintenance
- Optimal induction therapy must include an anthracycline in addition to vincristine and prednisone with or without asparaginase. Once complete remission (CR) is achieved, consolidation treatment is essential to improve the duration of CR. Maintenance therapies generally include methotrexate, 6-mercaptopurine, vincristine, and prednisone
- The average length of treatment of ALL varies between 1.5 and 3 years
- Standard options for CNS prophylaxis: cranial irradiation plus intrathecal methotrexate, or high-dose systemic methotrexate and IT methotrexate without cranial irradiation, or IT chemotherapy alone. CNS prophylaxis should be given early rather than late in the postremission phase
- During the course of treatment the patient may require transfusions of blood and platelets as well as intravenous antibiotics
- Colony-stimulating factors given on completion of administration of the induction drugs may shorten the duration of neutropenia by 2–4 days and appear to lessen morbidity. Studies have shown that use of these factors is safe
- The use of hydration, alkalinization of urine, and allopurinol can prevent urate nephropathy
- Most patients relapse within 3 years, and very few relapses occur after 6 years

- ALL may relapse systemically or in sanctuary extramedullary sites (testicle or CNS). Patients who have isolated CNS relapse are treated with CNS irradiation plus intrathecal chemotherapy or with radiation to testes for testicular relapse. In half the cases, systemic relapse may be successfully treated with the agents used to induce the original remission. Recurrence is associated with a poor prognosis unless secondary remission can be achieved
- Bone marrow transplant (BMT) is not recommended during first CR for adults with ALL. Due to the poor prognosis of patients with relapsed ALL consideration should be given to BMT. Results of allogeneic BMT are most promising during the second CR for patients with ALL. For selected patients the long-term leukemia-free survival following BMT from a matched sibling donor is 20–30%
- Many forms of complementary therapy have been tried in ALL, and may be used as well as chemotherapy and radiotherapy

Clinical Pearls

Physical examination should carefully evaluate for intact neurologic status, clinical signs of disseminated intravascular coagulation, and occult infection.

Never

Never forget the possibility that a febrile patient with bacterial infection with abnormal smear might have an acute leukemia.

FOLLOW UP

Plan for review

- Frequency of review will depend on the stage of treatment and the clinical condition of the patient
- The patient will also require ongoing specialist follow up

Information for patient or caregiver

As accurate as possible a prognosis and a full discussion of the treatment possibilities is essential.

DRUGS AND OTHER THERAPIES: DETAILS

Drugs

ALLOPURINOL

Dose

- Regular dosage 300–600mg/day orally
- 600–800mg/day orally for 3 days associated with increase in the intake of fluids is recommended for prevention of uric acid nephropathy during aggressive chemotherapy

Efficacy

Reduces serum and urinary uric acid concentrations.

Risks/Benefits

Risks:

- Use caution in hepatic or renal impairment
- Treatment should be discontinued at first sign of allergic reaction, such as skin rash or other reaction
- Ensure adequate fluid intake during treatment

Benefit: prevents uric acid nephropathy secondary to tumor lysis

Side-effects and adverse reactions

- Central nervous system: drowsiness, headache
- Gastrointestinal: nausea, abdominal pain, peptic ulceration, cholestatic jaundice, diarrhea, liver failure
- Genitourinary: renal failure
- Musculoskeletal: athralgia, myopathy
- Skin: rash, alopecia, Stevens-Johnson syndrome

Interactions (other drugs)

■ Antacids ■ Azathioprine ■ Cyclophosphamide ■ Mercaptopurine ■ Oral anticoagulants ■ Theophylline ■ Angiotensin-converting enzyme (ACE) inhibitors

Contraindications

Patients who have developed a severe reaction to allopurinol should not be restarted on the drug.

Follow up plan

Allopurinol treatment should be discontinued when the potential for overproduction of uric acid is no longer present.

Radiation therapy

RADIOTHERAPY

Efficacy

- Efficient for CNS prophylaxis (although there are protocols based on chemotherapy only)
- Used as treatment of testicular relapse

Risks/Benefits

- Risk: in adults, testicular irradiation doses greater than 4–6Gy may result in persistent azoospermia
- Benefit: combined with chemotherapy provides EFS (event-free survival) of 53% in 4 years for testicular relapse

Follow up plan

Patient followed mainly by the hematologist/oncologist.

Chemotherapy

- Optimal induction therapy must include an anthracycline in addition to vincristine and prednisone with or without asparaginase. Once CR is achieved, consolidation treatment is essential to improve the duration of CR. Maintenance therapies generally include methotrexate, 6-mercaptopurine, vincristine, and prednisone
- Described below are three intensive regimens, selected from recent co-operative group reports, representing the current approach to the treatment of adult ALL. These three chemotherapy courses are always given under direct supervision of a hematologist in a hospital setting

CALGB PROTOCOL 9111

- Duration of therapy 24 months, divided into induction, consolidation (two courses), CNS therapy, late intensification (phase I/II)
- Maintenance with eight different chemotherapy drugs combined during the period

Efficacy

- Complete response rate: 82%
- 3-year disease-free survival: 40%
- 3-year overall survival: 43%

Risks/Benefits

Risks:

- Neutropenia with infections due to chemotherapy
- Tumor lysis syndrome

Benefits:

- Regression of signs and symptoms
- Improvement in wellbeing and prolonged survival

GMALL PROTOCOL 02/84

- Duration of therapy 30 months
- Induction (phase I/II), consolidation I, reinduction (phase I/II), consolidation II, maintenance

Efficacy

- Complete response rate: 75.4%
- 7-year disease-free survival: 39%
- 7-year overall survival: 36%

Risks/Benefits

Risks:

- Neutropenia with infections due to chemotherapy
- Tumor lysis syndrome

Benefits:

- Regression of signs and symptoms
- Improvement in wellbeing and increased survival

SWOG PROTOCOL 8001

- Duration of therapy 36 months
- Induction, consolidation (phase I/II), maintenance (phase I/II)

Efficacy

- Complete response rate: 68%
- 5-year overall survival: 26%

Risks/Benefits

Risks:

- Neutropenia with infections due to chemotherapy
- Tumor lysis syndrome

Benefits:

- Regression of signs and symptoms
- Improvement in wellbeing and increased survival

OUTCOMES

EFFICACY OF THERAPIES

Although acute lymphocytic leukemia (ALL) is a serious and potentially fatal disease, therapies are becoming more effective and clinical trials are defining the most effective forms of treatment.

PROGNOSIS

- Complete remission (CR) is the most important prognostic factor. A CR is defined as all of the following: bone marrow containing less than 5% blasts, resolution of cytopenias and organomegaly
- Around 50–85% of adults with ALL will achieve a successful remission and 30–40% of these are likely to survive 2 years. Further improvements in prognosis can be expected
- Not all patients have the same prognosis. Adverse prognostic factors include: age less than one year or more than 9 years, with the poorest prognosis in the elderly; WBC count greater than 50,000/mL in children, or 30,000/mL in adults; presence of t9;22, the Ph1 chromosome, which occurs in 10% of children and 30% of adults with ALL; presence of CNS leukemia, hepatosplenomegaly, lymphadenopathy or mediastinal mass; slow response to treatment
- FAB L3 subtype and B cell myeloid ALL have the worst prognosis. T cell ALL and CD10-negative B cell ALL have a poor prognosis

Clinical pearls

The sudden transfer of the intracellular contents and cellular breakdown products to the extravascular space can cause life-threatening elevations of uric acid, potassium, and phosphate in the so-called 'tumor lysis syndrome'. Thus patients presenting with acute leukemia should be routinely initiated on fluid support and allopurinol therapy in anticipation of rapid application of definitive chemotherapy.

COMPLICATIONS

- Treatment of leukemia is intrinsically linked with supportive management of the complications. Many of the complications occur initially in hospital, both as a consequence of the disease process as well as side-effects of chemotherapy
- The most common complication with ALL is recurrence which may involve the bone marrow or CNS/testes
- As survival from leukemia improves, complications arising as a result of the therapies are becoming apparent
- Treatment with cranial irradiation can lead to transient encephalopathy which occurs in up to 60% of patients. Symptoms include somnolence, headache, vomiting, and low-grade fever; it can be fatal in some patients. Leukoencephalopathy may develop in patients given large doses of intravenous methotrexate after brain irradiation. Neuropsychologic effects are more commonly seen in children
- Teniposide has been associated with the appearance of acute nonlymphocytic leukemias
- Avascular necrosis of bone may occur during treatment
- Anthracyclines are cardiotoxic and can lead to impairment of cardiac function

PREVENTION

- There are no obvious risk factors for acute lymphocytic leukemia (ALL)
- Ionizing radiation and chemical toxin exposure have been implicated, but the evidence is not good

RESOURCES

ASSOCIATIONS

The Leukemia and Lymphoma Society
1311 Mamaroneck Ave
White Plains, NY 10605
Tel: (914) 949-5213
Fax: (914) 949-6691
www.leukemia-lymphoma.org

Cancer Care
275 7th Ave
New York, NY 10001
Tel: (212) 221-3300
Fax: (212) 719-0263
E-mail: info@cancercare.org
www.cancercare.org

Association of Online Cancer Resources
www.acor.org

National Cancer Institute
Building 31, Room 10A31
31 Center Drive, MSC 2580
Bethesda, MD 20892-2580
www.nci.nih.gov

National Comprehensive Cancer Network
50 Huntingdon Pike, Suite 300
Rockledge, PA 19046
Tel: (215) 728-4788
Fax: (215) 728-3877
www.nccn.org

Information
For both the patient and PCP about specific chemotherapeutic drugs used in leukemia, at http://www.rxlist.com
Excellent source on radiotherapy from the National Cancer Institute, at http://cis.nci.nih.gov

KEY REFERENCES

- Adult Acute Lymphoblastic Leukemia (PDQ) From NCI CancerNet website: http://www.nci.nih.gov
- Ching-Hon P, Evans W. Acute lymphocytic leukemia. N Engl J Med 1998;339:605–18
- Gaynor J, Chapman D, Little C, et al. A cause-specific hazard rate analysis of prognostic factors among 199 adults with acute lymphoblastic leukemia: The Memorial Hospital experience since 1969. J Clin Oncol 1988;6:1014–30
- Green DL, Freeman AI, Sather HN, et al. Comparison of three methods of central nervous system prophylaxis in childhood acute lymphoblastic leukemia. Lancet 1980;1:1398–402
- Hoelzer D, Thiel E, Loffler H, et al. Prognostic factors in a multicenter study for the treatment of acute lymphoblastic leukemia in adults. Blood 1988;71:123–31

- Jankovic M, Brouwers P, Valsecchi MG, et al. Association of 1800 cGy cranial irradiation with intellectual function in children with acute lymphoblastic leukemia. Lancet 1994;344:224–7
- Nesbit ME Jr, Sather HN, Robison LL, et al. Presymptomatic central nervous system therapy in previously untreated childhood acute lymphoblastic leukemia. A report for Children's Cancer Study Group. Lancet 1981;1:461–6
- Pullen J, Boyett J, Shuster J, et al. Extended intrathecal chemotherapy trial for prevention of CNS relapse in good-risk and poor-risk patients with B-progenitor acute lymphoblastic leukemia. J Clin Oncol 1993;11:839–49
- Whitlock JA, Gaynon PS. Acute lymphocytic leukemia. In: Lee GR, ed. Wintrobe's Clinical Hematology. Philadelphia: Lippincott, Williams & Wilkins, 1999, p2241–71
- Zhang MJ, Hoelzer D, Horowitz MM, et al. Long term follow up of adults with acute lymphoblastic leukemia treated with chemotherapy or bone marrow transplantation. Ann Intern Med 1995;123:428–31

FAQS

Question 1

Do all patients with acute lymphocytic leukemia (ALL) need referral?

ANSWER 1

Because of the specialized treatment involved, including knowledge of specific chemotherapy protocols, newly diagnosed patients with ALL should be hospitalized and their care provided by a specialist.

Question 2

What are common presenting signs of the patient with ALL?

ANSWER 2

ALL patients classically present with pallor and fatigue. Other findings may include lymphadenopathy, bruising, and splenomegaly.

Question 3

Is the complete blood count (CBC) a useful screening test for ALL?

ANSWER 3

The CBC may be abnormal, especially if immature cells spill into the circulation. However, the only positive finding in the CBC occasionally is the presence of anemia. A relatively normal CBC, therefore, should not preclude the diagnosis of ALL in the presence of clinical suspicion.

Question 4

Are there hereditary or familial forms of ALL?

ANSWER 4

There is an association between ALL and trisomy 21. However, most cases of ALL occur in otherwise normal patients (and most trisomy 21 patients do not develop ALL).

CONTRIBUTORS

Randolph L Pearson, MD
Otavio A Clark, MD
Sandeep Garg, MD

ACUTE MYELOGENOUS LEUKEMIA

SUMMARY INFORMATION

DESCRIPTION

- Acute myelogenous leukemia is a group of disorders characterized by replacement of the bone marrow with abnormal immature cells of the myeloid series
- Patients usually present with anemia, thrombocytopenia, and neutropenia
- Treatment is with chemotherapy, bone marrow transplantation, and, in some cases, with radiotherapy to extramedullary sites
- Treatment consists of two stages: induction of remission and postremission
- Prognosis and details of treatment depend on a number of factors including cell type, number of circulating abnormal cells, and age
- Two-thirds of patients achieve complete remission and up to 25% may be cured
- New forms of treatment, including gene therapy, are being evaluated and offer exciting possibilities for the future

URGENT ACTION

- A complete blood count, serum electrolytes, creatinine, fibrinogen, and uric acid levels should be sent immediately and significant abnormalities treated
- If the patient is febrile, blood and urine cultures should be sent and broad-spectrum antibiotic therapy commenced
- If there is a very high white cell count and leukostasis, active rehydration and treatment with hydroxyurea (and radiotherapy if there is cerebral leukostasis) should be started if possible. A differentiation should be done for when to perform a strong rehydration and treatment with hydroxyurea (for the primary care physician, hydration is easier). Note that even with a high white cell count, the patient may be granulocytopenic and may need care to prevent/treat infections
- Preparations should be made to transfer the patient to a specialist unit for further treatment

KEY! DON'T MISS!

- Severe anemia, needing blood transfusion
- Severe thrombocytopenia, needing platelet transfusion
- Severe infection, needing immediate antibiotic treatment
- Cerebral leukostasis

ICD9 CODE

205.0 Acute myelogenous leukemia.

SYNONYMS

- Acute nonlymphoblastic leukemia (ANLL)
- Acute nonlymphocytic leukemia
- Acute myeloid leukemia (AML)

CARDINAL FEATURES

- AML is a malignant proliferation of abnormal immature cells of the myeloid series in the bone marrow and other organs
- It may be divided into a number of different types defined by the French-American-British (FAB) Co-operative Group, and this typing is most important in assessing prognosis and choosing treatment
- AML occurs more frequently in adults. The median age at presentation is 65 years
- Patients usually present with anemia, thrombocytopenia, and infections resulting from replacement of the bone marrow with abnormal cells and consequent deficiencies of the normal blood elements
- Lymphadenopathy, hepatomegaly, and splenomegaly may also be present
- Treatment is with combination chemotherapy, bone marrow transplantation, and, in some cases, radiotherapy to extramedullary deposits
- Treatment is divided into two stages: induction of remission and postremission
- Most patients will achieve a remission with induction therapy
- The prognosis is better with younger patients; overall, a cure rate of up to 25% may be expected

CAUSES

Common causes

- Previous chemotherapy (alkylating agents, topoisomerase II inhibitors)
- Other drugs (chloramphenicol, phenylbutazone causing marrow failure)
- Ionizing radiation (radiotherapy, exposure to nuclear weapons). The primary carcinogenic effect involves breaking DNA molecules. Risk correlates with radiation dosage and age at exposure (rapid peak early in life <15 years and rapid decline in those exposed at older ages)
- Toxins (benzene, rubber)
- Smoking: risk is two to three times higher in male smokers who have exceeded 20 pack-years

Contributory or predisposing factors

- Chromosomal abnormalities
- Other translocations, e.g. t(15;17), t(8;21)
- Marrow failure syndromes: Fanconi anemia, Shwachman-Diamond syndrome, familial aplastic anemia, drug-induced marrow failure
- Myeloproliferative disorders, e.g. myelofibrosis
- Myelodysplastic syndromes

EPIDEMIOLOGY

Incidence and prevalence

INCIDENCE

- 2.25 per 100,000 in the US
- Accounts for 80–90% of cases of acute leukemia in adults

Demographics

AGE

- Most patients 30–60 years; median age 65 years
- Incidence increases with age (fewer than one per 100,000 under 30 years, >17 per 100,000 at 75 years)

GENDER

Incidence is higher in males than in females.

RACE

- Higher prevalence in Eastern European Jews
- Lower in Oriental populations

GENETICS

- Some genetic syndromes are at greater risk to develop AML. Down syndrome (trisomy 21) patients are at a 20 times greater risk for acute leukemia. Others include Bloom's syndrome, neurofibromatosis, Klinefelter's syndrome, and Turner's syndrome
- Marrow failure syndromes are also at greater risk, such as Fanconi's anemia (about 9% increase in risk), Dyskeratosis congenita, Blackfan-Diamond's syndrome
- The risk of familial leukemia may be increased with consanguinity or inherited chromosomal instability syndromes (such as Fanconi's anemia). It is probably caused by a rare genetic predisposition within a family or a common environmental exposure

SOCIOECONOMIC STATUS

Incidence rates are greater in developed countries and in industrialized cities.

DIFFERENTIAL DIAGNOSIS

The presenting features are nonspecific and related to anemia, neutropenia, thrombocytopenia, and infection. The differential diagnosis is, therefore, with other disorders affecting the bone marrow.

Acute lymphocytic leukemia

Acute lymphocytic leukemia (ALL) is a malignant proliferation of abnormal immature lymphocytes in the bone marrow with possible dissemination into the blood, the central nervous system (CNS), and other organs.

FEATURES

- May be indistinguishable on clinical grounds
- The diagnosis is made on bone marrow examination

Leukemoid reactions

FEATURES

- May be indistinguishable on clinical grounds
- The diagnosis is made on bone marrow examination and serology

Myeloproliferative/myelodysplastic disorders

FEATURES

- May be indistinguishable on clinical grounds
- The diagnosis is made on bone marrow examination

Infiltrations of the bone marrow

FEATURES

- Usually by secondary deposits from other neoplasms
- The diagnosis is made on bone marrow examination

Autoimmune conditions

Examples include systemic lupus erythematosus and Felty's syndrome.

FEATURES

- May be indistinguishable on clinical grounds
- The diagnosis is made on bone marrow examination and serology

Viral infections

With Epstein-Barr or similar viruses.

FEATURES

- May be indistinguishable on clinical grounds
- The diagnosis is made on bone marrow examination and serology

SIGNS & SYMPTOMS

Signs

Generally, the physical signs are those of anemia, thrombocytopenia, or organ infiltration:

- Pallor
- Hemorrhagic signs – bruising, petechiae, ecchymoses, purpuric rash, epistaxis. These may be found in up to 50% of patients at diagnosis and correlate with the severity of thrombocytopenia
- Lymphadenopathy
- Hepatomegaly and/or splenomegaly

- Leukemia cutis (leukemic infiltration of the skin) occurs in some 10% of patients, more commonly in those with monocytic types. The lesions are violet in color and nodular in form
- Infiltration of the gums is also seen with acute monocytic leukemia
- Extramedullary spread may occur in the form of granulocytic sarcoma (also called myeloblastoma or chloroma).Tumors may appear greenish and are found in bone, soft tissues, lymph nodes, or skin

Symptoms

There are no symptoms specific to acute myelogenous leukemia (AML). Symptoms are attributable to anemia, thrombocytopenia, organ involvement, metabolic disturbances, and infection secondary to leukopenia:
- Weakness
- Shortness of breath
- Bleeding
- Weight loss (50% of patients)
- Abdominal discomfort
- Bone pain (20% of patients)
- Mental disturbances if CNS involvement present
- Renal colic or other urinary symptoms if urate output is very high and deposits/stones are formed (less common than in ALL)
- Fever, either secondary to infection or directly due to the disease process (presenting feature in 15–20% of patients)

KEY! DON'T MISS!

- Severe anemia, needing blood transfusion
- Severe thrombocytopenia, needing platelet transfusion
- Severe infection, needing immediate antibiotic treatment
- Cerebral leukostasis

CONSIDER CONSULT

Where there is a strong suspicion of acute leukemia, patients should be referred immediately to a specialist for full investigation.

INVESTIGATION OF THE PATIENT

Direct questions to patient

- Q **Have you been feeling unwell?** Often a presenting symptom
- Q **Have you been weak, tired, or short of breath?** May indicate anemia
- Q **Have you lost weight recently?** Not common, but may occur
- Q **Have you had nosebleeds, bruising, blood in the urine?** Can be due to thrombocytopenia or to disseminated intravascular coagulation (DIC), which is particularly common in acute promyelocytic leukemia
- Q **Have you had any aches and pains or abdominal discomfort?** May suggest bone involvement or hepatosplenomegaly
- Q **Have you developed any lumps in your neck, armpits, or groins?** Lymphadenopathy is not uncommon
- Q **Have you noticed any colored lumps in your skin?** These could indicate leukemia cutis
- Q **Have you been hot and cold, or shivering?** Fever is often present either from the disease process itself or caused by bacterial infections secondary to neutropenia
- Q **Have you noticed any changes in passing urine?** Deposition of uric acid crystals in the kidneys secondary to increased cell breakdown can affect renal function, causing nocturia, oliguria or renal colic if stones pass down the ureter
- Q **Have you experienced headaches or any mental changes?** These are often present if the CNS is involved

Contributory or predisposing factors

- Q **Have you ever been exposed to radiation in any form?** Exposure to radiation from reactors or nuclear weapons predisposes to certain malignancies, including leukemias
- Q **Have you received chemotherapy previously?** Previous treatment with topoisomerase II inhibitors may cause leukemia
- Q **Have you worked with rubber or industrial solvents?** These are both risk factors
- Q **Do you smoke, or have you smoked heavily in the past?** There may be an association between smoking and AML

Family history

- Q **Has anyone in your family ever had an acute leukemia?** There may be an increased familial incidence.

Examination

- **Is the patient anemic?**
- **Is the body temperature raised?** Fever is very common in AML, even if there is no evidence of bacterial infection
- **Is there any evidence of abnormal bleeding?** Bruising, ecchymoses, purpura, hemorrhages in optic fundi often occur
- **Is there any abnormal lymphadenopathy?** Common in AML
- **Is the liver or spleen enlarged?** Very common in AML
- **Is there swelling or sponginess of the gums?** Common in monocytic leukemia
- **Are there any purplish lumps in the skin?** May be leukemia cutis
- **Is there any mental disturbance?** May indicate cerebral leukostasis

Summary of investigative tests

- Complete blood count should be performed in all patients and may reveal anemia, thrombocytopenia, neutropenia, or the presence of abnormal blasts in the peripheral blood
- Serum lactate dehydrogenase (LDH) may be helpful in some circumstances
- Serum potassium may be abnormally high or low. Abnormal levels require treatment
- Serum urate should be requested routinely and particularly after induction chemotherapy, because the level will increase as a result of tissue breakdown and this may cause stone formation or acute renal failure
- Serum creatinine can be measured to assess renal function
- Plasma fibrinogen, fibrin split products, and coagulation factors will reveal whether there is DIC, which requires treatment
- Blood culture and urine tests and cultures should be taken in all febrile patients to confirm or exclude bacterial infection
- Lysozyme serum levels (raised levels may indicate the need to monitor kidney function and potassium as lysozyme causes proximal tubular damage)
- Lymph node biopsy – normally performed by a specialist. May be useful if enlarged superficial nodes present, and may give an earlier diagnosis than bone marrow aspiration
- Skin biopsy of any skin nodules. Normally performed by a specialist. May be leukemia cutis
- Chest X-ray may reveal enlarged hilar lymph nodes or interstitial infiltrates (pulmonary leukostasis) or infection of the lungs
- Abdominal ultrasound scanning or computerized (CAT) scanning will indicate the extent of involvement of liver, spleen, and intra-abdominal lymph nodes. Normally requested by a specialist for staging
- Bone marrow examination – normally performed by a specialist. Aspiration and biopsy may both be necessary to obtain cells for microscopic examination, cytochemistry, immunophenotyping, and cytogenetics. All this information is used to define prognosis and which forms of treatment will be used

- Lumbar puncture – normally performed by a specialist. Indicated if there is a suspicion of CNS involvement, or after bone marrow remission to assess whether there is remaining infiltration or involvement that is not clinically detectable. This is important in deciding which treatment will be used, either initially or after first remission

DIAGNOSTIC DECISION

- AML is usually suspected by a primary care physician (PCP) when abnormalities are seen on routine hemograms
- The clinical diagnosis of AML is often not difficult once it is considered
- Abnormal blasts are usually found in the peripheral blood, but bone marrow samples taken by aspiration or biopsy are needed for more detailed typing studies to define prognosis and to decide on treatment modalities
- AML has been defined as: an abnormal bone marrow with >30% abnormal blasts, signs and symptoms of the disease, abnormal white cell count and differential, abnormal hemoglobin and platelet counts, demonstration of pathognomonic Auer rods in bone marrow aspirates
- The classification used is that of the French-American-British (FAB) Co-operative Group, which goes from M0 to M7, depending upon the characteristics of the abnormal cells

CLINICAL PEARLS

- Radiation therapy is less leukemogenic than chemotherapy
- Hyperleukocytosis can alter laboratory data: falsely elevated platelet count (because white cell fragments are counted as platelets), pseudohypoxemia caused by oxygen consumption by leukemia cells, falsely prolonged coagulation tests, pseudohyperkalemia, and pseudohypoglycemia

THE TESTS

Body fluids

COMPLETE BLOOD COUNT

Description

Venous blood sample.

Advantages/Disadvantages

Advantages: inexpensive, rapid, and may be diagnostic

Normal

- Hemoglobin: men 14–18g/100mL, women 12–16g/100mL
- Platelets: 150–400x10^9/L
- Leukocytes: 4.5–10.5x10^9/L
- Neutrophils: 50–70%, 3.0–7.0x10^9/L
- Lymphocytes: 30–50%, 2.0–5.0x10^9/L

Abnormal

- A normochromic, normocytic anemia is often present
- White cell counts vary greatly: 50% of patients have raised counts, sometimes with blasts present; 20% have a total count of >100,000x10^9/L. High counts may cause leukostasis in the brain, lungs, and genitourinary tract. Blood vessels are blocked and urgent treatment is mandatory
- Thrombocytopenia is almost invariable, and may or may not be part of DIC
- Keep in mind the possibility of a false-positive result

SERUM LACTATE DEHYDROGENASE

Description

Venous blood sample.

Advantages/Disadvantages
Advantage: inexpensive, rapid result, useful for disease monitoring

Normal
50–150 IU/L.

Abnormal
- >150 IU/L
- Keep in mind the possibility of a false-positive result

Cause of abnormal result
- Increased turnover of leukemic cells, particularly in monocytic leukemias
- Seen less often than in ALL

SERUM LYSOZYME (MURAMIDASE)
Description
Venous blood sample.

Advantages/Disadvantages
Advantages:
- Relatively inexpensive, rapid
- Raised levels may indicate the need to monitor kidney function and potassium (lysozyme causes proximal tubular damage)

Normal
4–13mcg/mL.

Abnormal
- >13mcg/mL
- Keep in mind the possibility of a false-positive result

Cause of abnormal result
- Increased activity and number of leukemic myeloid cells
- Increased serum lysozyme activity is present in tuberculosis, sarcoidosis, megaloblastic anemias, acute bacterial infections, ulcerative colitis, regional enteritis, and Crohn's disease

SERUM POTASSIUM
Description
Venous blood sample.

Advantages/Disadvantages
Advantage: inexpensive, rapid, and can have important consequences if levels are abnormal.

Normal
3.5–5.5mEq/L (3.5–5.5mmol/L).

Abnormal
- May be low because of proximal tubular damage with increased lysozyme levels or uptake by leukemic cells
- May be high if there is rapid tumor lysis
- Keep in mind the possibility of a false-positive result

SERUM URATE

Description

Venous blood sample.

Advantages/Disadvantages

Advantage: inexpensive, rapid, requires treatment if significantly raised

Normal

2–7mg/100mL (120–420mcmol/L).

Abnormal

>7mg/100mL (420mcmol/L).

Cause of abnormal result

- Increased cell breakdown
- Urate is an end-product of protein metabolism
- Keep in mind the possibility of a false-positive result

SERUM CREATININE

Description

Venous blood sample.

Advantages/Disadvantages

Advantage: inexpensive, rapid result, reflects renal function accurately

Normal

0.6–1.2mg/100mL (50–110mcmol/L).

Abnormal

>110mg/100mL (110mcmol/L).

Cause of abnormal result

- Fall in glomerular filtration rate may be associated with hyperuricemia
- Keep in mind the possibility of a false-positive result

Drugs, disorders and other factors that may alter results

This may be caused by extensive breakdown of cells following treatment.

PLASMA FIBRINOGEN

Description

Venous blood sample.

Advantages/Disadvantages

Advantage: inexpensive, rapid, indicates need for treatment if low (DIC).

Normal

200–400mg/100mL (2.0–4.0g/L).

Abnormal

- <200mg/100mL (2.0g/L)
- Keep in mind the possibility of a false-positive result

Cause of abnormal result
Consumption of clotting factors in intravascular coagulation.

FIBRIN SPLIT PRODUCTS
Description
Venous blood sample.

Advantages/Disadvantages
Advantage: inexpensive, rapid answer, indicates need for treatment if high

Normal
<10.0mcg/mL.

Abnormal
- This test is not specific to AML but an abnormal result can contribute to the diagnosis. Detects problems in the coagulation system
- Keep in mind the possibility of a false-positive result

Cause of abnormal result
Breakdown of fibrinogen in disseminated intravascular coagulation.

COAGULATION FACTORS
Description
- Venous blood sample
- Various factors, e.g. factor V, factor VIII, may be involved

Advantages/Disadvantages
Advantages:
- Relatively inexpensive
- Levels may indicate a need for treatment

Normal
Values may vary between laboratories.

Abnormal
- Levels will be reduced if significant intravascular coagulation present
- Keep in mind the possibility of a false-positive result

Cause of abnormal result
Consumption of clotting factors in intravascular coagulation.

BLOOD CULTURE
Description
- Venous blood inoculated immediately into liquid culture medium
- Two bottles of culture medium used for aerobes and anaerobes

Advantages/Disadvantages
Advantages:
- Inexpensive
- Usually reveals the organism responsible for severe infections

Disadvantage: 48h incubation often needed

Normal
No bacterial growth.

Abnormal
- Significant growth of infecting organism(s)
- May be more than one type of bacterium in profoundly neutropenic patients
- Keep in mind the possibility of a false-positive result

Drugs, disorders and other factors that may alter results
Chemotherapy contributes to the neutropenia during treatment.

URINE TEST AND CULTURE
Description
Clean, preferably midstream specimen of urine.

Advantages/Disadvantages
Advantages:
- Inexpensive, rapid partial result from stick test and microscopy
- Good early indicator of nephropathy or infection

Disadvantage: 48h incubation needed for culture

Normal
- Stick test: pH 4.5–8, protein absent, glucose absent, hemoglobin (or red blood cells (RBC)) absent, leukocytes absent
- Microscopy: RBC 0–5/high power field, leukocytes 0–5/high power field, casts 0–4/low power field, crystals absent
- Culture: no growth of bacteria

Abnormal
- Stick test: RBC, leukocytes, or significant protein indicate nephropathy or infection
- Microscopy: >5 RBC or leukocytes, >4 casts raise possibility of infection. Significant amounts of urate crystals indicate possible urate nephropathy
- Culture: significant (>100,000 organisms/mL) growth of bacteria suggests active urinary tract infection
- Keep in mind the possibility of a false-positive result

Cause of abnormal result
Direct effects on the kidney of infection or high urate concentrations.

Biopsy
LYMPH NODE BIOPSY
Description
Removal of superficial lymph node under local anesthesia.

Advantages/Disadvantages
Advantage: simple to do, few complications, may be diagnostic

Normal
Normal architecture and cells.

Abnormal
Normal cells replaced with abnormal blasts.

SKIN BIOPSY

Description

Removal of skin nodule under local anesthesia.

Advantages/Disadvantages

Advantage: simple to do, few complications, may be diagnostic

Abnormal

Characteristic histologic appearance of leukemia cutis or of myeloblastic sarcoma.

Imaging

CHEST X-RAY

Advantages/Disadvantages

Advantage: inexpensive, immediate result, useful for comparisons.

Abnormal

- Presence of hilar lymph nodes and other abnormal masses
- Pulmonary infiltration

ABDOMINAL ULTRASOUND SCAN

Advantages/Disadvantages

Advantage: inexpensive, immediate result, no X-ray exposure.

Abnormal

May reveal hepatomegaly, splenomegaly, enlarged lymph nodes, or other abnormal masses or infiltrations.

CAT SCAN OF CHEST OR ABDOMEN

Advantages/Disadvantages

Advantage: high resolution, rapid result.

Disadvantages:

- Expensive
- Significant X-ray exposure

Abnormal

Will reveal hepatomegaly, splenomegaly, enlarged lymph nodes, or other abnormal masses or infiltrations if present.

Special tests

BONE MARROW ASPIRATION/BIOPSY

Description

Sample of bone marrow obtained in most cases by aspiration. Where the examination is difficult or the marrow is hypocellular, marrow biopsy may be required.

Advantages/Disadvantages

Advantage: essential to reach an accurate diagnosis and obtain sufficient tissue for typing by histologic, cytochemical, immunologic, and cytogenetic methods

Disadvantages:

- Marrow biopsy is unpleasant for the patient
- Requires a skilled practitioner to obtain the sample

Abnormal
Abnormalities depend on the type of ALL and the cellularity of the marrow.

Other tests

LUMBAR PUNCTURE

Description

- A sample of cerebrospinal fluid (CSF) is taken for diagnostic purposes
- Centrifugation may be required to concentrate the cells for analysis

Advantages/Disadvantages
Advantage: necessary if CNS involvement suspected; not needed otherwise – CNS involvement is uncommon in AML (unlike ALL, where it is very common)

Disadvantages:

- Unpleasant for the patient
- May cause post lumbar puncture headache
- Requires a skilled practitioner to perform the test

Abnormal
Presence of leukemic cells.

CONSIDER CONSULT

All patients should be referred to a specialist for treatment.

IMMEDIATE ACTION

- A complete blood count, electrolytes, creatinine, fibrinogen, and uric acid levels should be sent immediately, and significant abnormalities treated
- If the patient is febrile, blood and urine cultures should be sent and broad-spectrum antibiotic therapy commenced
- If there is a very high white cell count and leukostasis, active rehydration and treatment with hydroxyurea (and radiotherapy if there is cerebral leukostasis) should be started if possible
- Preparations should be made to transfer the patient to a specialist unit for further treatment

PATIENT AND CAREGIVER ISSUES

Impact on career, dependants, family, friends

- Acute myelogenous leukemia (AML) is a potentially fatal disorder and cure rates are lower with increasing age
- The patient will be hospitalized immediately and will be an inpatient for some time
- Plans must be made for the future, bearing in mind that frequent hospital attendance will be required

MANAGEMENT ISSUES

Goals

- Identify and treat acute infections
- Do initial investigations
- Institute urgent treatment (e.g. for cerebral leukostasis)
- Refer without delay for specialist diagnosis and further treatment

Management in special circumstances

SPECIAL PATIENT GROUPS

- AML does occur in pregnancy, although it is rare
- 85% present in the second and third trimesters, and treatment with chemotherapy and supportive care can result in a successful outcome for mother and baby
- The first trimester is more difficult because the chemotherapeutic agents are teratogenic, and therapeutic abortion is sometimes considered. Otherwise, supportive therapy is given until the second trimester

SUMMARY OF THERAPEUTIC OPTIONS

Choices

- The treatment of AML is divided into two stages: induction of remission and postremission consolidation or intensification. Longer-term maintenance treatment is no longer generally used
- For induction of remission, a combination of cytarabine and daunorubicin or idarubicin is normally the basis for treatment. Thioguanine and etoposide may be added
- Patients with acute promyelocytic (M3) leukemia respond to treatment with all-*trans* retinoic acid (ATRA), either alone or as part of combined induction therapy
- In patients with very high white cell counts, cerebral or pulmonary leukostasis may occur and this requires urgent treatment with intensive rehydration, high-dose hydroxyurea, and cranial irradiation if the cerebral circulation is involved
- Central nervous system (CNS) infiltration is much less common than in acute lymphocytic leukemia (ALL) and if present, should be treated with intrathecal cytarabine or methotrexate. Prophylactic treatment is not indicated in adults, although it may be in children
- Disseminated intravascular coagulation is common and may require treatment with heparin
- Postremission therapy is always required if a cure is intended

- Allogeneic bone marrow transplantation gives the lowest relapse rate, but HLA-matched sibling donors are normally required, and overall mortality is unaffected because of complications associated with the procedure itself
- Autologous bone marrow rescue is also a possibility, but possibly should be reserved for poor-risk patients and relapses
- Many forms of complementary therapy have been tried in AML, and may be used as well as standard medical treatments

Clinical pearls

Advances in therapy have changed the cure rates in AML from <20% in the 1960s to 40–70% for selected groups in the 1990s.

Never

- Never forget the possibility that a febrile patient with neutropenia may have an acute leukemia
- Never try to manage a patient with AML without the supervision of a hematologist

FOLLOW UP

Plan for review

- Frequency of review depends on the stage of treatment and the clinical condition of the patient
- The patient will also require ongoing care from a hematologist

Information for patient or caregiver

It is important to give full and truthful information to the patient's relatives or carers.

DRUGS AND OTHER THERAPIES: DETAILS

Drugs

CYTARABINE

Cytarabine (cytosine arabinoside) is an antineoplastic agent that inhibits DNA polymerase in leukemic cells.

Dose

- Dosage should be administered by a specialist
- Usually 75–100mg/m^2/day subcutaneously or by intravenous infusion
- Frequency and duration as defined by treatment schedule

Risks/Benefits

Risks:

- Specialist supervision required
- Platelet and leukocyte counts and bone marrow examinations must be carried out frequently
- Use caution when administering to patients with pre-existing drug-induced bone marrow suppression
- Use caution in renal or hepatic impairment
- Use caution when adminstering to breast-feeding mothers
- Risk of severe or fatal CNS, gastrointestinal, and pulmonary toxicity
- Risk of cardiomyopathy

Side-effects and adverse reactions

- Gastrointestinal: nausea, vomiting, anorexia, diarrhea, stomatitis
- Hematologic: anemia, leukopenia, thrombocytopenia, megaloblastosis
- Other: infections (viral, bacterial, fungal, parasitic, or saprophytic), cytarabine (Ara-C) syndrome (fever, myalgia, bone pain, occasionally chest pain, maculopapular rash, conjunctivitis and malaise)

Interactions (other drugs)

■ Digoxin dose may need to be adjusted when patient is receiving cytarabine ■ Gentamicin (efficacy of gentamicin may be affected)

Contraindications

■ Hypersensitivity to the drug ■ Pregnancy category D

Acceptability to patient

- May cause nausea and vomiting in higher doses
- May cause severe pulmonary or neurologic toxicity

DAUNORUBICIN

Daunorubicin is an anthracycline cytotoxic antibiotic obtained from a streptomyces mold.

Dose

- Dosage should be administered by a specialist
- 45mg/m^2/day (30mg/m^2/day if patient is over 60 years), given into a rapidly running intravenous infusion
- Frequency and duration as defined by treatment schedule

Risks/Benefits

Risks:

- Specialist supervision required
- Daunorubicin hydrochloride must be given into a rapidly flowing intravenous infusion. It must never be given by the intramuscular or subcutaneous route
- Risk of cardiac toxicity
- Severe myelosuppression will occur with treatment with therapeutic levels
- Dosage should be reduced in patients with renal or hepatic impairment
- Complete blood counts should be taken frequently
- Risks of hyperuricemia secondary to rapid lysis of leukemic cells

Side-effects and adverse reactions

- Cardiovascular system: cardiotoxicity
- Hematologic: myelosuppression
- Hypersensitivity: anaphylactoid reaction, fever, chills, skin rash
- Gastrointestinal: nausea, vomiting, diarrhea
- Skin: alopecia, tissue necrosis (if extravasation occurs during administration)

Interactions (other drugs)

None known.

Contraindications

■ Hypersensitivity to daunorubicin ■ Pregnancy category D

Acceptability to patient

May cause pericarditis or myocarditis.

Patient and caregiver information

Patient should report chest pain or shortness of breath.

IDARUBICIN

Idarubicin is a semisynthetic anthracycline antibiotic.

Dose
- Dosage should be administered by a specialist
- 12–15mg/m^2/day given over a short period into a rapidly running intravenous infusion
- Frequency and duration as defined by treatment schedule

Risks/Benefits
Risks:
- Specialist supervision required
- Idarubicin HCl should be given slowly into a freely flowing intravenous infusion. It must never be given intramuscularly or subcutaneously
- Risk of cardiac toxicity
- Severe myelosuppression will occur
- A dose reduction should be considered in patients with hepatic and/or renal impairment

Side-effects and adverse reactions
- Cardiovascular system: cardiac toxicity, congestive heart failure
- Central nervous system: headache, fever
- Gastrointestinal: nausea, vomiting, constipation, abdominal cramps, diarrhea
- Genitourinary: red-colored urine
- Hematoligc: thrombocytopenia, leukopenia
- Skin: alopecia, rash, mucositis
- Other: infection, mucositis

Interactions (other drugs)
None known.

Contraindications
■ Pregnancy category D or breast-feeding ■ Hypersensitivity to idarubicin ■ Bone marrow depression: should not be given to patients with pre-existing bone marrow suppression induced by previous drug therapy or radiotherapy (unless the benefit warrants the risk) ■ Congestive heart failure

Acceptability to patient
- May cause nausea and vomiting
- Potentially cardiotoxic

Patient and caregiver information
Patient should report shortness of breath or chest pain.

THIOGUANINE
Thioguanine is a purine analog that inhibits nucleic acid synthesis.

Dose
- Dosage should be administered by a specialist and depends on situation
- Up to 3mg/m^2/day orally
- Frequency and duration as defined by treatment schedule

Risks/Benefits
Risks:
- Specialist supervision required
- Use caution with renal and hepatic impairment
- Use caution when administering to breast-feeding mothers
- Bone marrow suppression is the common toxic effect

Side-effects and adverse reactions

- Gastrointestinal: nausea, vomiting, anorexia, stomatitis
- Hematologic: myelosuppression
- Metabolic: hyperuricemia
- Other: infection, immunosupression

Interactions (other drugs)

■ Mercaptopurine (cross-resistance) ■ Busulfan: hepatotoxicity, esophageal varices, and portal hypertension were reported in some patients receiving long-term therapy of thioguanine and busulfan concomitantly

Contraindications

■ Pregnancy category D ■ Hypersensitivity to thioguanine ■ Known resistance to this drug

Acceptability to patient

Generally well tolerated.

ETOPOSIDE

Etoposide is a semisynthetic derivative of podophyllotoxin.

Dose

- Dosage should be administered by a specialist
- 50–100mg/m^2/day slowly intravenously
- Frequency and duration as defined by treatment schedule

Risks/Benefits

Risks:

- Specialist supervision required
- Patients being treated with etoposide must be frequently observed for myelosuppression
- Risk of anaphylactic reaction manifested by chills, fever, tachycardia, bronchospasm, dyspnea, and hypotension

Side-effects and adverse reactions

- Gastrointestinal: nausea, vomiting, abdominal pain, anorexia, stomatitis
- Hematologic: anemia, thrombocytopenia, leukopenia
- Skin: alopecia, hair loss

Interactions (other drugs)

Cyclosporine (may cause increased levels of etoposide as well as increased etoposide toxicity).

Contraindications

■ Hypersentivity to etoposide ■ Pregnancy category D ■ Safety and efficacy in children have not been established

Acceptability to patient

May cause nausea and vomiting.

ALL-*TRANS* RETINOIC ACID

All-*trans* retinoic acid (ATRA) is a retinoid that induces maturation of immature cells in acute promyelocytic leukemia (APL).

Dose

- Dosage should be administered by a specialist
- 45mg/m^2/day orally
- Given during induction and for 30 days after remission achieved

Risks/Benefits

Risks:

- Risk of retinoic acid-APL (RA-APL) Syndrome in patients with APL treated with tretinoin
- Risk of evolving leukocytosis
- Risk of pseudotumor cerebri
- Up to 60% of patients develop hypercholesterolemia and/or hypertriglyceridemia
- May elevate liver function test results
- Use caution when administering to children

Side-effects and adverse reactions

- Central nervous system: headache, fever, weakness, fatigue
- Eyes, ears, nose, and throat: visual disturbances, ocular disorders
- Gastrointestinal: nausea, vomiting
- Musculoskeletal: bone pain
- Skin: skin/mucous membrane dryness, rash, mucositis, pruritis, sweating, alopecia
- Patients with APL: hemorrhage, infections, gastrointestinal hemorrhage, disseminated intravascular coagulation, pneumonia, septicemia, and cerebral hemorrhage

Interactions (other drugs)

Inducers or inhibitors of the hepatic P-450 system.

Contraindications

- **Known hypersensitivity to retinoids or to parabens (preservatives in the gelatin capsule)**
- **Patients without the t(15;17) translocation should be considered for alternative treatment**
- **Pregnancy category D** ■ **Breast-feeding**

Acceptability to patient

May cause headaches, fever, fatigue.

Patient and caregiver information

- Highly teratogenic
- Effective contraception essential

HYDROXYUREA

Hydroxyurea is an antineoplastic agent that inhibits DNA synthesis.

Dose

- Dosage should be administered by a specialist
- Up to 80mg/kg daily orally
- Duration as defined by treatment schedule

Risks/Benefits

Risks:

- Specialist supervision required
- Use caution with renal impairment
- Use caution when administering to breast-feeding mothers
- AIDS patients: fatal and nonfatal pancreatitis have occurred in HIV-infected patients during therapy with hydroxyurea and didanosine, with or without stavudine
- Usually requires the concomitant administration of allopurinol to avoid hyperuricemia
- Weekly hematologic monitoring required

Side-effects and adverse reactions

- Central nervous system: drowsiness, headache, dizziness, disorientation, hallucinations, convulsions (all rare)
- Gastrointestinal: stomatitis, anorexia, nausea, vomiting, diarrhea, constipation
- Hematologic: neutropenia
- Skin: maculopapular rash, skin ulceration, dermatomyositis-like skin changes, peripheral erythema, facial erythema, hyperpigmentation, atrophy of skin and nails, scaling and violet papules, alopecia
- Urinary: dysuria, temporary renal impairment
- Other: fever

Interactions (other drugs)

None known.

Contraindications

■ Hypersensitivity to hydroxyurea ■ Severe anemia ■ Safety and efficacy in children have not been established ■ Marked bone marrow suppression (leukopenia, under 2500 white blood cells (WBC); or thrombocytopenia under 100,000)

Acceptability to patient

Sometimes causes nausea and vomiting.

METHOTREXATE

Methotrexate is a potent antimetabolite used in CNS disease.

Dose

- Dosage should be administered by a specialist
- Usually 12mg with 50mg hydrocortisone intrathecally
- Frequency and duration as defined by treatment schedule

Risks/Benefits

Risks:

- Must be administered under specialist supervision
- Serious toxic reactions are possible, which may be fatal
- Only use with severe recalcitrant, disabling disease which is not adequately responsive to other forms of therapy
- The patient should be fully informed of the risks involved
- Closely monitor for bone marrow, liver, lung, and kidney toxicity
- Use caution with infection and bone marrow depression
- Use caution with peptic ulceration and ulcerative colitis
- Use caution with renal and hepatic impairment
- Use caution with the elderly

Side-effects and adverse reactions

- Central nervous system: headache, seizures, dizziness, drowsiness
- Eyes, ears, nose, and throat: visual disturbances, tinnitus
- Cardiovascular system: pericardial infusion
- Cental nervous system: fever
- Gastrointestinal: abdominal pain, diarrhea, hepatotoxicity, intestinal pneumonitis nausea, vomiting, stomatitis
- Genitourinary: renal failure, urinary retention, depression of and defective spermatogenensis, hematuria

- Hematologic: blood cell disorders
- Musculoskeletal: osteoporosis, muscle pain and wasting
- Respiratory: pulmonary fibrosis
- Skin: rashes, acne, dermatitis, alopecia, hyperpigmentation, vasculitis

Interactions (other drugs)

■ Aminoglycosides ■ Antimalarials ■ Binding resins ■ Chloramphenicol ■ Co-trimoxazole ■ Ethanol ■ Cyclosporin ■ Etretrinate ■ Live vaccines ■ Omeprazole ■ Sulfinpyrazon ■ Penicillins ■ Probenicid ■ Salicylates ■ Tetracycline ■ NSAIDS

Contraindications

■ Pre-existing profound bone marrow depression ■ Severe renal or hepatic impairment ■ Nursing mothers, pregnancy; conception should be avoided for 6 months after stopping ■ Hypersensitivity to the drug ■ Ascites or pleural effusion ■ Dehydration

Acceptability to patient

Lumbar puncture necessary.

Patient and caregiver information

Patients should be warned of the danger of toxic reactions.

Radiation therapy

RADIATION THERAPY

- Cranial irradiation is used as part of the treatment for cerebral leukostasis
- Cranial and spinal irradiation are given to treat CNS infiltration
- Radiotherapy to other areas of the body (e.g. spleen, bones) is used to help control local areas of leukemic infiltration
- Total body irradiation is necessary prior to bone marrow transplantation (BMT)

Efficacy

The treatment is effective locally in palliation of symptoms or for treating CNS infiltration.

Risks/Benefits

Risk: cerebral irradiation does adversely affect brain function in survivors, at least in children, and should only be given where the benefits outweigh the risks

Acceptability to patient

Radiotherapy has fewer side-effects than chemotherapy and may be well tolerated by the patient.

Other therapies

BONE MARROW TRANSPLANTATION

- Its benefits come from ablation of the diseased marrow and probably from a graft vs leukemia reaction
- BMT is valuable in the treatment of relapses and in poor-risk patients, where it may still achieve a cure
- Allogeneic BMT is very successful in terms of prevention of relapses. The quality of matching is critical. HLA-matched sibling donors are best, but are not always available
- The effectiveness in preventing relapses is balanced by the complications of the procedure itself, such as graft vs host reactions and pulmonary and hepatic toxicity
- Autologous BMT is less effective, but causes fewer complications. It may be best used in the treatment of relapses

Acceptability to patient

BMT is extremely unpleasant and demanding for the patient and the family. However, it is potentially life-saving.

OUTCOMES

PROGNOSIS

- Some 65% of adults with acute myelogenous leukemia will achieve successful remission and up to 25% may be cured
- Patients may be divided into good or poor prognostic groups according to various features at presentation
- Favorable factors include: age <45 years; absence of infection; white cell count <25,000/mm^3; normal serum lactate dehydrogenase; the presence of Auer rods in the leukemic cells and circulating eosinophils; French-American-British (FAB) typing of M2, M3, and M4; presence of CD34-, CD14-, and CD13 surface markers; negative HLA-DR status; and t(15;17), t(8;21), or inv(16) chromosomal abnormalities
- Adverse factors include age <2 or >60 years; previous hematologic disorders or chemotherapy; white cell count >100,000/mm^3; the presence of extramedullary or central nervous system disease; megaloblastic erythroid cells; cellular dysplasia; FAB typing of M0, M6, or M7; the presence of CD34+ or MDR-1 surface markers; two or more lymphoid surface markers; and -7, del(7(q), -5, del 5(q), or 11q23 chromosomal abnormalities or complex karyotype

Clinical pearls

Remission induction (initial therapy): anthracycline/cytarabine combination leads to disappearance of detectable leukemia in 70% of patients.

COMPLICATIONS

As survival from the leukemia improves, complications arising as a result of the therapies become more apparent.

- Treatment with cranial irradiation affects brain function and may predispose to nonleukemic brain tumors of various types
- Teniposide has been associated with the appearance of acute nonlymphocytic leukemias
- Avascular necrosis of bone may occur during treatment
- Anthracyclines are cardiotoxic and can lead to impairment of cardiac function
- Various endocrine disturbances may be seen secondary to damage of glandular tissues by chemotherapy and radiotherapy

RISK FACTORS

- Exposure to benzene, rubber, tobacco smoke, and ionizing radiation: all known risk factors
- Toxin exposure: adequate protective clothing should be worn by those working in industries where toxins are in use
- **Smoking:** has other dangers and is best avoided
- Exposure to therapeutic X-rays: should be kept to a minimum
- Working in nuclear industry: adequate protection is vital for those working in the nuclear industry

RESOURCES

ASSOCIATIONS

The Leukemia and Lymphoma Society Inc
1311 Mamaroneck Avenue
White Plains, NY 10605
Tel:(914) 949-5213
Fax: (914) 949-6691
www.leukemia-lymphoma.org

Cancer Care Inc
275 Seventh Avenue
New York, NY 10001
Tel: (212) 712-8080
Fax: (212) 712-8495
Email: info@cancercare.org
www.cancercare.org

Association of Online Cancer Resources
173 Duane Street, Suite 3A
New York, NY 10013–3334
Tel: (212) 226-5525
www.acor.org

National Cancer Institute
Building 31, Room 10A31
31 Center Drive, MSC 2580
Bethesda, MD 20892–2580
Tel: (800) 422-6237
Tel TTI: (800) 332-8615
www.cancer.gov/cancer_information/

National Comprehensive Cancer Network
50 Huntingdon Pike, Suite 200
Rockledge, PA 19046
Tel: (215) 728-4788
Fax: (215) 728-3877
E-mail: information@nccn.org
Provides practice guidelines and information for patients and doctors
www.nccn.org

National Institutes of Health (NIH) website
www.cancer.gov/cancer_information/

KEY REFERENCES

- American Society of Clinical Oncology. Recommendations for the use of hematopoetic colony-stimulating factors: evidence based clinical practice guidelines. J Clin Oncol 2000;18:3558–85
- Appelbaum FR. Allogeneic hematopoetic stem cell transplantation for acute leukemia. Semin Oncol 1997;24:114–23
- Bennett JM, Catovsky D, Daniel MT, et al. Proposed revised criteria for the classification of acute myeloid leukemia: a report of the French-American-British Cooperative Group. Ann Intern Med 1985;103:620–5
- Bortin MM, Horowitz MM, Gale RP, et al. Changing trends in allogeneic bone marrow transplantation for leukemia in the 1980s. JAMA 1992;268:607–12
- Cassileth PA, Lynch E, Hines JD, et al. Varying intensity of post-remission therapy in acute myelogenous leukemia. Blood 1992;79:1924–30
- Christensen NP. Allogeneic bone marrow transplantation in the treatment of acute adult leukemias. Hemat Oncol Clin N Am 1993;7:177–200
- Hertenstein B, Heil G, Heimpel H. Allogeneic bone marrow transplantation or chemotherapy for patients with acute myelogenous leukemia in first complete remission. Ann Hematol 1996;72:223–30
- Jankovic M, Brouwers P, Valsecchi MG, et al. Association of 1800 cGy cranial irradiation with intellectual function in children with acute lymphoblastic leukemia. Lancet 1994;344:224–7
- Kumar L. Leukemia. Management of relapse after allogeneic bone marrow transplantation. J Clin Oncol 1994;12:1710–17
- National Comprehensive Cancer Network (NCCN). Guidelines for the diagnosis and treatment of acute myelogenous leukemia. Oncology (Huntingd) 2000;14:53–61
- Preisler HD, Anderson K, Rai K, et al. The frequency of long-term remission in patients with acute myelogenous leukaemia treated with conventional maintenance chemotherapy. Brit J Haematol 1989;71:189–94
- Reiffer J, Gaspard MH, Maraninchi D, et al. Comparison of allogeneic and autologous bone marrow transplantation and chemotherapy in patients with acute myelogenous leukaemia in first remission. Br J Haematol 1989;72:57–63
- Takeshita A, Shibata Y, Shinjo K, et al. Successful treatment for relapse of acute promyelocytic leukemia with a new synthetic retinoid. Ann Internal Med 1996;124:893–6

FAQS

Question 1

Can a complete blood cell count be enough to diagnose acute myelogenous leukemia (AML)?

ANSWER 1

Yes, in many patients this simple test can give a prompt diagnosis of AML.

Question 2

Will a bone marrow biopsy always be required for diagnosis, classification, and staging purposes?

ANSWER 2

No, a sample of bone marrow obtained by aspiration only can be sufficient, but if the examination is difficult or the marrow is hypocellular, marrow biopsy may be required.

Question 3

What are the advantages and disadvantages of allogeneic and autologous transplantation?

ANSWER 3

Mainly, allogeneic bone marrow transplantation prevents more relapses, but autologous causes fewer complications.

CONTRIBUTORS

Randolph L Pearson, MD
Otavio A Clark, MD

APLASTIC ANEMIA

SUMMARY INFORMATION

DESCRIPTION

- Pancytopenia caused by bone marrow failure, either due to an acquired exposure or familial association
- Acquired aplastic anemia is associated with chemical and physical agents, viral infections, mycobacterial infections, and miscellaneous other causes
- Familial aplastic anemia is associated with Fanconi's constitutional pancytopenia, Shwachman-Diamond's syndrome (pancreatic deficiency in children), and a putative hereditary defect in cellular folate uptake
- The condition presents with skin pallor, ecchymosis, petechiae, and possible fever
- Treated with platelet and red blood cell transfusion, bone marrow transplantation, immunosuppressive therapy

URGENT ACTION

- Discontinue use of offending drugs or agents that appear to be causing the anemia
- Refer patient to hospital for possible platelet and red blood cell transfusions or bone marrow transplantation

ICD9 CODE
- 284.9 Aplastic anemia
- 284.8 Acquired aplastic anemia
- 284.0 Congenital aplastic anemia

SYNONYMS
- Refractory anemia
- Hypoplastic anemia

CARDINAL FEATURES
- The term 'aplastic anemia' encompasses a group of disorders that are characterized by pancytopenia caused by bone marrow failure (either due to an acquired exposure or familial association), anemia, and neutropenia
- Acquired aplastic anemia is associated with chemical and physical agents, viral infections, mycobacterial infections, and miscellaneous other causes
- Familial aplastic anemia is associated with Fanconi's constitutional pancytopenia, Shwachman-Diamond's syndrome (pancreatic deficiency in children), and a putative hereditary defect in cellular folate uptake
- The condition presents with skin pallor, ecchymosis, petechiae, and possible fever
- The diagnosis carries a 67% mortality rate within 6 months of onset, most commonly a consequence of infection (resulting from neutropenia) or bleeding
- Treated with platelet and red blood cell transfusion, bone marrow transplantation, immunosuppressive therapy

CAUSES
Common causes
- Viral infection (hepatitis, Epstein-Barr virus, HIV, dengue)
- Mycobacterial infection
- Autoimmune disease
- Chemical exposure (ionizing radiation, benzene, sulfur or nitrogen mustard and congeners, antimetabolites, antimitotic agents, certain antibiotics, inorganic arsenic, dichlorovinylcysteine, estrogens)

Rare causes
- Antimicrobial agents (chloramphenicol, organic arsenicals, quinacrine, penicillamine)
- Anticonvulsants (acetazolamide, carbamazepine, hydantoins, trimethadione)
- Antithyroid drugs
- Antidiabetic drugs
- Antihistamines
- Analgesics (phenylbutazone)
- Sedatives and tranquilizers
- Insecticides
- Gold compounds

Serious causes
- Viral infection (parvovirus B19, hepatitis, Epstein-Barr virus, HIV, dengue)
- Mycobacterial infection
- Autoimmune disease
- Chemical exposure (ionizing radiation, benzene, sulfur or nitrogen mustard and congeners, antimetabolites, antimitotic agents, certain antibiotics, inorganic arsenic, dichlorovinylcysteine, estrogens)

- Chemotherapeutic agents
- Antimicrobial agents (chloramphenicol, organic arsenicals, quinacrine)
- Anticonvulsants (hydantoins, trimethadione)
- Antithyroid drugs
- Antidiabetic drugs
- Antihistamines
- Analgesics (phenylbutazone)
- Sedatives and tranquilizers
- Insecticides
- Gold compounds

Contributory or predisposing factors

- Diabetes (due to antidiabetic drug trigger)
- Thyroid diseases (due to antithyroid drug trigger)
- Seizure disorders (due to anticonvulsant drug trigger)
- Bacterial infection (due to antimicrobial agent trigger)
- Cigarette smoking may be contributory

EPIDEMIOLOGY

Incidence and prevalence

INCIDENCE

0.002–0.009 cases/1000 patients.

Demographics

AGE

Overall, the condition occurs most often in individuals aged 60 years and over; there is another peak in those aged between 15 and 25 years.

GENDER

Data have shown no confirmed influence of gender in occurrence of aplastic anemia. However, some studies have suggested that females have higher mortality than males with this condition.

RACE

Data have shown no confirmed influence of race in occurrence of aplastic anemia.

GENETICS

Data have shown no confirmed influence of familial genetics in occurrence of aplastic anemia.

GEOGRAPHY

Data have shown that the condition is more frequent in Asia, with rates of 4 patients/million people seen in Bangkok and rural Thailand.

SOCIOECONOMIC STATUS

Data have shown no confirmed influence of socioeconomic status in occurrence of aplastic anemia. However, persons of lower socioeconomic status may be more likely to be exposed to hazardous chemicals in the workplace, which may lead to aplastic anemia.

DIFFERENTIAL DIAGNOSIS

Severe infection

Severe infection can cause a profound suppression of bone marrow function due to the elaboration of inflammatory cytokines and bacterial toxins.

FEATURES

- Red blood cell (RBC) count and hemoglobin are decreased
- In profound infection, even white blood cell (WBC) count may be decreased
- Platelet count may be increased in the early stages (acute-phase reaction)
- Presence of symptoms and signs suggesting infection and patient history can usually differentiate severe infection from aplastic anemia due to other causes

Bone marrow infiltration

Infiltration of the bone marrow with leukemic cells (e.g. plasma cells) can cause replacement of normal marrow cells and lead to anemia and pancytopenia.

FEATURES

- Pancytopenia may be present
- Bone marrow biopsy and/or aspirate will show the presence of abnormal cells in the bone marrow, and can lead to a definitive diagnosis

Hypoplastic acute lymphoblastic leukemia

Characterized by uncontrolled proliferation of abnormal, immature lymphocytes, and progenitor cells.

FEATURES

- Seen in children
- Purpura or easy bruising of skin
- Lymphoadenopathy or hepatosplenomegaly
- Fever, bone pain, oliguria, weakness, weight loss, mental status changes

Hypoplastic myelodysplastic syndrome

An acquired clonal disorder affecting the hematopoietic stem cells.

FEATURES

- Seen in adults
- Cytopenia with hypercellular bone marrow
- Morphologic abnormalities in hematopoietic cell lines
- Splenomegaly, skin pallor, mucosal bleeding, ecchymosis
- Fatigue
- Fever, infection, dyspnea common

Hypoplastic acute myeloid leukemia

Characterized by uncontrolled proliferation of primitive myeloid cells.

FEATURES

- Seen in adults
- Weakness or fatigue (due to anemias)
- Bleeding, petechiae, ecchymosis (due to thrombocytopenia)
- Infection and fever (due to neutropenia)
- Skin pallor, bruises
- Hepatosplenomegaly
- Peripheral lymphadenopathy

Hypersplenism
Characterized by splenomegaly, cytopenia, and compensatory hyperplastic bone marrow.

FEATURES
- Most often seen in patients with chronic liver disease and congestive splenomegaly
- Early satiety, abdominal pain, pleuritic pain (left upper quadrant)
- Cytopenias
- Splenic infarct

Hairy cell leukemia
A lymphoid neoplasm characterized by proliferation of mature B cells with prominent cytoplasmic projections.

FEATURES
- Splenomegaly
- Pallor, ecchymosis, evidence of infection
- Weakness, lethargy, fatigue

Paroxysmal nocturnal hemoglobinuria
A rare disorder with incidence about 2/million of population.

FEATURES
- Manifested either as pancytopenia (with low platelets in about 80% of patients) or intravascular hemolytic disorder, characterized as hemoglobinemia and hemoglobinuria
- May also present with thrombosis in unusual sites (e.g. hepatic venous thrombosis)

Vitamin B12/folate deficiency
Characterized by megaloblasts in the bone marrow (erythroblasts that have delayed nuclear maturation because of impaired DNA synthesis), usually with anemia, which may be severe.

FEATURES
- Mean corpuscular volume (MCV) is usually increased
- Serum vitamin B12 and/or folate levels decreased

SIGNS & SYMPTOMS
Signs
- Skin pallor, ecchymosis, petechiae, retinal hemorrhage
- Mouth and tongue ulcerations
- Possible audible systolic ejection murmur with profound anemia
- With congenital anemia: short stature or skeletal and nail abnormalities

Symptoms
Abnormal bleeding is the most common reason for a patient with aplastic anemia to come to medical attention. Other symptoms include:
- Fatigue
- Shortness of breath
- Angina
- Menorrhagia
- Easy bruising
- Epistaxis
- Fever
- Pharyngitis

CONSIDER CONSULT

- If aplastic anemia is suspected, refer patient to hematologist for bone marrow aspiration and biopsy
- To rule out splenomegaly, refer patient for abdominal sonogram or computed tomography (CT) scan
- To evaluate possible thymoma-associated RBC aplasia, refer patient for thymus CT scan

INVESTIGATION OF THE PATIENT

Direct questions to patient

- Q **Have you suffered any abnormal bleeding episodes recently?** Abnormal bleeding is the commonest reason for patients with aplastic anemia to present
- Q **How have you been feeling generally?** Fever, fatigue, shortness of breath, and angina are all documented symptoms of aplastic anemia
- Q **Does your throat feel inflamed or painful?** Pharyngitis may be caused by parvovirus B19 and other viral and bacterial agents that may cause aplastic anemia. Parvovirus B19 is typically associated with transient aplastic crisis, say in patients with hemolytic anemia or HIV, but is not associated with generalized bone marrow failure
- Q **Have you been bruising easily?** This is a documented symptom of aplastic anemia
- Q **What do you do for a living? What kind of chemicals are you exposed to in your workplace?** Toxin exposure (benzene, insecticides) is a common factor in aplastic anemia
- Q **What drugs are you currently taking and what medications have you been taking recently?** A large group of drugs has been documented to be a contributing factor in the development of aplastic anemia
- Q **What illnesses have you experienced recently?** Infections, including hepatitis C and HIV, have been found to trigger aplastic anemia
- Q **Are you pregnant?** Pregnancy can contribute to the development of aplastic anemia
- Q **Did either of your parents or any grandparents have anemia?** Fanconi's anemia is an inherited form of bone marrow failure disorder

Contributory or predisposing factors

- Q **What do you do for a living? What kind of chemicals are you exposed to in your workplace?** Toxin exposure (benzene, insecticides) is a common factor in aplastic anemia
- Q **What drugs are you currently taking and what medications have you been taking recently?** A large group of drugs has been documented to be a contributing factor in the development of aplastic anemia
- Q **What illnesses have you experienced and have you been hospitalized recently?** Infections, including hepatitis C, HIV, and some nosocomial infections, have been found to trigger aplastic anemia
- Q **Are you pregnant?** Pregnancy can contribute to the development of aplastic anemia
- Q **Did either of your parents or any grandparents have anemia?** Fanconi's anemia is an inherited form of bone marrow failure disorder

Family history

- Q **Did either of your parents or any grandparents have anemia?** Fanconi's anemia is an inherited form of aplastic anemia.

Examination

- **Examine the patient's skin:** pallor, ecchymosis, petechiae, and retinal hemorrhage are common physical signs of anemias
- **Examine patient's oral cavity:** mouth and tongue ulcers, along with pharyngitis, are common signs of anemias
- **Measure patient's body temperature:** due to associated infections, patients with aplastic anemia frequently have a fever
- **Listen to patient's heart sounds:** with profound anemia, an audible systolic ejection murmur can sometimes be heard

Summary of investigative tests

- Complete blood count (CBC) may reveal pancytopenia. Macrocytosis and toxic granulation of neutrophils may be present. Isolated cytopenias may be seen in early aplastic anemia
- Reticulocyte count will reveal reticulocytopenia
- Hepatitis C titer: because hepatitis C infection can be associated with aplastic anemia, this test is useful in the differential diagnosis
- Bone marrow examination (normally performed by a specialist) will reveal absence of or decrease in erythropoietic and myelopoietic precursor cells (often showing 100% fat)
- Abdominal sonogram or CT scan (normally performed by a specialist) may be conducted to rule out splenomegaly
- CT scan of thymus area (normally performed by a specialist) may be conducted to rule out thymoma-associated red blood cell aplasia

DIAGNOSTIC DECISION

The critical issue is to distinguish severe and very severe aplastic anemia from moderate aplastic anemia.

Severe and very severe aplastic anemia:

- Anemia with reticulocytopenia (<1% corrected reticulocyte count)
- Thrombocytopenia (platelets $<20x10^3/mm^3$ ($<20x10^9/L$))
- Neutropenia (neutrophils $<500/mm^3$ ($<0.5x10^9/L$))
- Hypoplastic bone marrow (<25% of hypocellularity or moderate hypocellularity with <30% of hematopoietic cells)
- Severe aplastic anemia is diagnosed if any two blood criteria and either marrow criterion is met. Very severe aplastic anemia is diagnosed as severe aplastic anemia plus ANC (absolute neutrophil count $<200/mm^3$ ($<0.2x10^9/L$))

Moderate aplastic anemia is defined as the failure to meet criteria for severe aplastic anemia but with at least two of three blood counts decreased:

- Reticulocyte count $<40x10^3/mm^3$ ($<40x10^9/L$)
- Platelets $<40x10^3/mm^3$ ($<40x10^9/L$)
- ANC $<1500/mm^3$ ($<1.5x10^9/L$)
- And hypocellular marrow biopsy

The following points are worthy of note:

- Aplastic anemia should be entertained as a diagnosis in cases of pancytopenia, as well as anemia
- Definitive diagnosis rests on a bone marrow biopsy showing hypocellularity, and an abnormal myeloid/erythroid ratio
- Common causes of anemia should be ruled out (e.g. iron deficiency, folate/B12 deficiency, alcoholism) before proceeding to a bone marrow biopsy

CLINICAL PEARLS

- In every patient with pancytopenia, rule out easily reversible causes of pancytopenia (such as vitamin B12/folate deficiency) and transient causes of aplasia (e.g. parvovirus B19, which is typically associated with transient aplastic crisis, e.g. in patients with hemolytic anemia or HIV, but not generalized bone marrow failure)
- Hepatitis associated with aplastic anemia is typically seronegative (i.e. non-A, non-B, non-G)
- Dry tap is usually not typical for aplastic anemia (usually indicates marrow infiltrative process)

THE TESTS

Body fluids

COMPLETE BLOOD COUNT

Description

Battery of tests consisting of WBC count, RBC count, hematocrit, hemoglobin, RBC indices (including platelet count), and WBC differential. A venous anticoagulated (EDTA) blood sample of 5mL or more is collected.

Advantages/Disadvantages

- Advantage: simple, single-sample specimen collection for all tests
- Disadvantage: if patient is uncomfortable with venipuncture, it may be difficult to obtain sample (may need to perform fingerstick instead)

Normal

- WBC count: 5000–10,000/mm^3 (5.0–10x10^9/L)
- RBC count: females, 4–5x10^6/mm^3 (4–5x10^{12}/L); males, 4.5–5.5x10^6/mm^3 (4.5–5.5x10^{12}/L)
- Hemoglobin: females, 12–16g/dL (120–160g/L); males, 14.0–17.4g/dL (140–174g/L)
- Hematocrit: 36–48% (females) or 42–42% (males)
- MCV: 84–96mcm^3 (84–96fL)
- Mean corpuscular hemoglobin concentration: 32–36g/dL (320–360g/L)
- Mean corpuscular hemoglobin: 28–34pg
- Platelets: 140–400x10^3/mm^3 (140–400x10^9/L)

WBC differential (values presented as percent of total cells seen):

- Segmented neutrophils: 50–62%
- Eosinophils: 1–4%
- Basophils: 0.5–1%
- Monocytes: 3–7%
- Lymphocytes: 25–40%
- Bands: 3–6%

Abnormal

- Pancytopenia: decreased numbers of all cell types
- RBCs may be nucleated
- Normochromic normocytic anemia

Cause of abnormal result

- Aplastic anemia
- Leukemia
- Viral infections
- Hypersplenism
- Bone marrow depression (caused by drugs, ionizing radiation, heavy metal intoxication)
- Myelodysplastic disorders
- Immune-associated neutropenia
- Iron-deficiency anemia

Drugs, disorders and other factors that may alter results

- Dehydration or overhydration
- Fat-laden meals may alter some results due to lipemia
- Stress can alter normal values

RETICULOCYTE COUNT

Description

This test is used to differentiate anemias caused by bone marrow failure from those caused by hemorrhage or hemolysis, to check the effectiveness of treatment of pernicious anemia, to assess recovery of bone marrow in aplastic anemia, and to determine the effects of radioactive substances. A single EDTA-anticoagulated venous blood sample is collected for this test.

Advantages/Disadvantages

- Advantage: simple, single test to differentiate anemias
- Disadvantage: not totally diagnostic for aplastic anemia

Normal

- Men: 0.5–1.5% of total erythrocytes
- Women: 0.5–2.5% of total erythrocytes
- Absolute count: 25–85x10^3/mm^3

Abnormal

- Men: <0.5 or >1.5% of total erythrocytes
- Women: <0.5 or >2.5% of total erythrocytes
- Absolute count: <25x10^3/mm^3 or >85x10^3/mm^3

Cause of abnormal result

Elevated levels seen:

- In hemolytic anemia
- After treatment of anemias

Decreased levels seen in:

- Untreated iron-deficiency anemia
- Aplastic anemia
- Untreated pernicious anemia
- Anemia of chronic disease
- Endocrine problems
- Bone marrow failure
- Myelodysplastic syndromes

Drugs, disorders and other factors that may alter results

- Alcoholism (decreased reticulocyte count)
- Patient undergoing radiation therapy (decreased reticulocyte count)
- Posthemorrhage (elevated reticulocyte count seen 3–4 days after the bleed)

HEPATITIS C TITER

Description

This test is used for differential diagnosis of viral hepatitis types. A single 5mL blood serum sample is collected using standard biohazard precautions. Antibodies to the hepatitis C virus are detected by immunoassay. Other, more sensitive and specific tests may be used to confirm this diagnosis (detection of hepatitis C RNA in the serum).

Advantages/Disadvantages

- Advantage: single test can determine presence of hepatitis C virus
- Disadvantage: nonspecificity can be a problem; does not provide definitive diagnosis of aplastic anemia, but useful in differential diagnosis

Normal

Negative titer.

Abnormal

Positive titer.

Cause of abnormal result

Hepatitis C viral infection.

Drugs, disorders and other factors that may alter results

Disorders in which there are circulating nonspecific antibodies, such as rheumatoid arthritis and systemic lupus erythematous, can yield nonspecific results for the hepatitis C antibody assay.

Biopsy

BONE MARROW ASPIRATION AND EXAMINATION

Description

Bone marrow aspirates are collected from the posterior iliac crest or sternum. This procedure is typically performed by a specialist.

Advantages/Disadvantages

- Advantage: one of the conclusive diagnostic tests for identification of aplastic anemia
- Disadvantage: patient may find procedure very uncomfortable, even with local anesthesia; complications can include bleeding and sternal fracture, infection of biopsy site

Normal

Erythroid cell:myeloid cell ratio will be 1:2 to 1:4.

Abnormal

Marrow should show marked decrease in RBC precursors, erythroid cell/myeloid cell ratio will be significantly less than 1:3.

Cause of abnormal result

- Multiple myeloma, plasma cell myeloma, macroglobulinemia
- Chronic or acute leukemias
- Anemia, including megaloblastic, macrocytic, and normocytic anemias
- Toxic states that produce bone marrow depression or destruction
- Neoplastic diseases (metastatic carcinoma, myeloproliferative, and lymphoproliferative diseases)
- Agranulocytosis
- Platelet dysfunction
- Histoplasmosis and tuberculosis
- Deficiency of body iron stores, microcytic anemia
- Lipid or glycogen storage disease

TREATMENT

CONSIDER CONSULT

Referral to hematologist for treatment program is recommended when diagnosis of aplastic anemia is suspected.

IMMEDIATE ACTION

- Discontinue any offending drugs or agents
- Evaluate patient for bone marrow transplant (refer to hematologist)
- If the patient's absolute neutrophil count is <500/mm^3 (<0.5x10^9/L), platelet count is <20x10^3/mm^3 (<20x10^9/L), or corrected reticulocyte count is <1%, then admission to hospital is necessary
- Note: corrected reticulocyte count is calculated by multiplying the reticulocyte count (%) by the patient hematocrit and dividing the result by an average normal hematocrit (47 for men and 42 for women)

PATIENT AND CAREGIVER ISSUES

Forensic and legal issues

If patient arrives at physician's office in a febrile or unconscious state, then treatment may need to be started without consent; referral to hospital may be needed without patient consent.

Impact on career, dependants, family, friends

- Patient may require bone marrow transplant, involving family members as possible donors (needing bone marrow aspiration to check for tissue match)
- Long-term patient monitoring may require extensive support from family/friends for follow up visits to primary care physician (PCP)
- Aggressive immunosuppressive treatments may require isolation of patient from carer, dependants, family, and friends due to possibility of infection

Patient or caregiver request

Once I discontinue the medication that is causing this condition, will I be cured? No, discontinuation of exposure to the causative agent does not cure aplastic anemia by itself. Patients will require extensive supportive therapy to resolve the anemia.

Health-seeking behavior

- **Have you been taking any over-the-counter (OTC) medications to treat your illness?** Some OTC medications such as antihistamines have been implicated in aplastic anemia
- **Did you discontinue or change any of your other medications when you started feeling the symptoms of this illness?** This may be important in cases of coexisting disease in which the patient may have stopped taking antiretroviral medications for HIV infection or medication for hepatitis C infection

MANAGEMENT ISSUES

Goals

- To return blood cell counts to normal range
- To resolve and prevent concomitant infections during treatment

Management in special circumstances

COEXISTING DISEASE

Patients being treated for hepatitis C virus infection or HIV infection may require additional referral consultations to ensure that disease management plans are aligned for all concomitant illnesses.

COEXISTING MEDICATION
Patients being treated for hepatitis C virus infection or HIV infection may require additional referral consultations to ensure that treatment regimens for those conditions are not creating more problems while also trying to treat the anemia.

SPECIAL PATIENT GROUPS
Pregnant women: immunosuppressive treatment regimens may be difficult to manage during pregnancy.

PATIENT SATISFACTION/LIFESTYLE PRIORITIES
Immunosuppressive therapy may make typical life activities difficult because patient may need to be isolated from others due to the high risk of infection.

SUMMARY OF THERAPEUTIC OPTIONS

Choices

- First choice of treatment is bone marrow transplantation (BMT) or immunosuppressive treatment using antithymocyte globulin, antilymphocyte globulin, and/or cyclosporine (this is an off-label indication) for patients who are not eligible for BMT (because of age or lack of a suitable donor)
- A supplementary treatment consists of platelet/red blood cell transfusion
- In addition to the above treatments, meticulous attention must be paid to the prevention of infections in these patients. Hand-washing, as well as precautions in the face of neutropenia (isolation, gown, and gloves) should be instituted in the care of these patients. Prompt treatment of infections is a must, and should include empirically instituted broad-spectrum antibiotics

Clinical pearls

The choice of treatment in young patients (<40 years old) who have fully compatible human leukocyte antigen (HLA) sibling donor is allo-transplant (based on the assessment of the probability of success and benefits/risks of allo-BMT vs immunosuppressive therapy). For older patients, treatment is more controversial, but most centers would transplant patients up to age of 50 (provided that the patient fully understands the benefits/risks of allo-BMT and has consented to it, of course).

Never

Avoid performing transfusion of blood products to patients who are candidates for bone marrow transplantation except in life-threatening situations – the benefits of transfusion in the acute setting may save the patient's life.

FOLLOW UP

Plan for review

The physician should plan on long-term patient monitoring, with periodic physical examinations and routine laboratory testing to screen for relapse.

Information for patient or caregiver

Patients should be aware that relapse can occur. Inform them of the possible early signs of recurrence of anemia, identify when they should return to the office for evaluation, and provide them with information regarding what other treatment options may be available if relapse occurs.

DRUGS AND OTHER THERAPIES: DETAILS

Drugs

ANTITHYMOCYTE GLOBULIN
Immunosuppressive therapy with this product has been shown to treat effectively those patients with moderate-to-severe aplastic anemia who are unsuitable for BMT.

Dose

This treatment should be administered by a specialist who is experienced in its use.

Efficacy

When administered with a regimen of supportive care, antithymocyte globulin may induce partial or complete hematologic remission.

Acceptability to patient

Acceptable, but intravenous dose administration may be uncomfortable for patient. Requires inhospital dose administration and follow up observation.

Follow up plan

Monitor patient's physical response to treatment, and evaluate for side-effects and adverse experiences with medication.

Patient and caregiver information

- Provide patient with detailed information regarding possible side-effects and adverse experiences they can expect
- Prepare patient for the need for isolation due to immunosuppressive effects of the drug

ANTILYMPHOCYTE GLOBULIN

Immunosuppressive therapy with this product has been shown to treat effectively those patients with moderate-to-severe aplastic anemia who are unsuitable for BMT.

Dose

This treatment should be administered by a specialist who is experienced in its use.

Efficacy

When administered with a regimen of supportive care, antilymphocyte globulin may induce partial or complete hematologic remission.

Acceptability to patient

- Acceptable, but intravenous dose administration may be uncomfortable for patient
- Requires inhospital dose administration and follow up observation

Follow up plan

Monitor patient's physical response to treatment, and evaluate for side-effects and adverse experiences with medication.

Patient and caregiver information

- Provide patient with detailed information regarding possible side-effects and adverse experiences they can expect
- Prepare patient for the need for isolation due to immunosuppressive effects of the drug

CYCLOSPORINE

Off-label indication.

Dose

This treatment should be administered by a specialist experienced in its use.

Efficacy

- Produces immunosuppression by inhibiting T-lymphocytes
- Also inhibits lymphokine production and release (including interleukin-2)
- Does not cause bone marrow suppression

Risks/Benefits

Risks:
- Increased susceptibility to infection and possible development of neoplasia
- Bacterial, fungal, viral, and protozoal infections often occur and can be fatal
- Avoid excessive sunlight
- Use caution in hypertension
- Use caution in children and the elderly
- Use caution in hepatic or biliary tract disease
- Recent vaccinations will be rendered inneffective

Benefits:
- Oral medication
- Can be continued at home with little difficulty
- Has no depressant effects on bone marrow

Side-effects and adverse reactions
- Cardiovascular system: hypertension
- Central nervous system: tremors, seizures, encephalopathy, confusion, depression, headache, dizziness, insomnia, paresthesias, fever
- Eyes, ears, eyes, nose, and throat: gingival hyperplasia
- Gastrointestinal: nausea, vomiting, diarrhea, elevated hepatic enzymes, hepatotoxicity, abdominal pain, gingivitis, stomatitis, anorexia, dyspepsia, flatulence
- Genitourinary: nephrotoxicity, hyperuricemia, menstrual irregularity, spermatogenesis inhibition, gynecomastia
- Hematologic: thrombotic thrombocytopenic purpura, leukopenia
- Metabolic: hyperkalemia, hypercholesterolemia, hypomagnesemia, hyperglycemia
- Musculoskeletal: arthralgia, fatigue, weakness, dysarthria, myalgia
- Skin: hirsuitism, acne, alopecia, rash, skin ulcers, flushing

Interactions (other drugs)

■ Antidiabetics (glipizide, glyburide, pioglitazone, troglitazone) ■ Androgens ■ Corticosteroids ■ Creatine ■ Allopurinol, colchicine ■ Bromocriptine ■ Immunosuppressives ■ Danazol ■ Antidepressants (fluoxetine, fluvoxamine, nefazodone, St John's wort) ■ Cisplatin ■ Warfarin ■ Estrogens ■ Methotrexate ■ Metoclopramide ■ Misoprostol ■ Modafinil ■ Tacrolimus ■ Orlistat ■ Mycophenolate ■ Neuromuscular blockers ■ Vinca alkaloids ■ Sirolimus ■ Nonsteroidal anti-inflammatory drugs ■ Rifampin ■ Other: Grapefruit juice (increases cyclosporine levels); food (decreases cyclosporine levels) ■ Omeprazole, rabeprazole ■ Drugs utilizing cytochrome P-450 to be metabolized ■ Antivirals (acyclovir, ganciclovir, antiretroviral protease inhibitors, foscarnet, nevirapine, delavirdine) ■ Antidysrhythmics (amiodarone, calcium channel blockers, digoxin) ■ Antihypertensives (angiotensin-converting enzyme (ACE) inhibitors, acetazolamide, carvedilol, clonidine, potassium-sparing diuretics) ■ Antibiotics (aminoglycosides, ceftriaxone, ciprofloxacin, clarithromycin, clindamycin, erythromycin, dalfopristin, quinupristin, imipenem; cilastatin, nafcillin, norfloxacin, polymyxin B, sulfamethoxazole; trimethoprim, troleandomycin, vancomycin, sulfonamides) ■ Antifungals (amphotericin B, bacitracin, fluconazole, itraconazole, ketoconazole, griseofulvin) ■ Anticonvulsants (carbamazepine, fosphenytoin, phenobarbital, phenytoin, primidone) ■ Antineoplastics (daunorubicin, doxorubicin, epirubicin, docetaxel, etoposide (VP-16), melphalan, mitoxantrone, paclitaxel) ■ Antilipemics (fenofibrate, statins, probucol)

Contraindications

■ Psoralens and Ultraviolet Application (PUVA: psoriasis patients are at increased risk of developing skin cancer with this treatment) ■ Rheumatoid arthritis ■ Renal impairment ■ Known polyoxyethylated castor oil hypersensitivity ■ Pregnancy and breast-feeding

Acceptability to patient

Acceptable, but side-effect profile and drug interactions may be problematic.

Follow up plan

Monitor patient's renal function (blood urea nitrogen, creatinine) and liver function, and evaluate circulating blood levels of drug (maintaining a 24-h trough level of 250–800ng/mL in whole blood or 50–300ng/mL in plasma should minimize side-effects and rejection events).

Patient and caregiver information

- Oral solution can be mixed with milk, chocolate milk, or orange juice to improve palatability
- Inform patient of possible side-effects and when to contact physician for dose modifications

Other therapies

BONE MARROW TRANSPLANTATION

- Allogeneic BMT is conducted to replace defective or missing marrow. In the case of the bone marrow failure that occurs in aplastic anemia, BMT replaces absent or abnormal stem cells with functional stem cells, allowing production of blood cells
- A potent immunosuppressive 'preparative' or 'conditioning' regimen is required prior to BMT (usually with cyclophosphamide and antithymocyte globulin)
- Patients older than 50 years or for whom a suitable bone marrow donor cannot be found may not be candidates for BMT

Efficacy

In patients younger than 50 years:

- Those with a matched related donor have a 70–90% chance of cure following BMT
- Those with a donor whose marrow nearly matches that of the patient (i.e. a one HLA-antigen mismatched related donor) have a 50% chance of cure following BMT
- Those with a matched unrelated donor have a 20–30% chance of cure following BMT

Risks/Benefits

Risks:

- It may not be possible to find a suitable bone marrow donor
- Graft-versus-host disease may occur following BMT
- The preparative immunosuppressive regimen predisposes patients to infections

Benefit: cure rates are high for those with a matched related donor

Acceptability to patient

- As the treatment may be curative, it may be highly acceptable to the patient if he/she has a matched related donor
- The downside is that, regardless of the quality of the match, the patient will have to receive a potent immunosuppressive cocktail prior to BMT. This means that the patient may have to be isolated from friends and family in order to prevent opportunistic infections, although visits are usually permitted if the friends/family comply with the procedures of the center, e.g. strict hand-washing, masks, no food

Follow up plan

Careful follow up, in conjunction with a hematologist, is a must to monitor for development of graft-versus-host disease.

PLATELET/RED CELL TRANSFUSION

- Red cells are often administered to patients with aplastic anemia. Anemia in itself is not necessarily an emergency, and transfusion is generally conducted when symptoms are not relieved by restriction of activity. However, bleeding associated with low platelet count requires transfusion as a matter of urgency, in order to prevent fatal hemorrhage
- Transfusion should not be from a close family member, because this may impact on BMT if that person is subsequently found to be a suitable marrow donor

Efficacy

- Effective in temporarily correcting anemia
- Reduces symptoms and prevents fatal hemorrhage associated with low platelets

Risks/Benefits

Risks:

- Alloimmunization (common in patients who have received repeated transfusions)
- Infection (due to agents that are infrequently present in blood products, including HIV, non-A/non-B hepatitis viruses, and hepatitis B virus)
- Graft-versus-host disease (rare)

Benefit: temporary correction of anemia

OUTCOMES

EFFICACY OF THERAPIES

- In the normal course of treatment of aplastic anemia, drug treatment (antithymocyte globulin, antilymphocyte globulin, cyclosporine) will be successful within 2–3 months
- Transfusion with red blood cells or platelets will produce a measurable increase in cell count shortly after injection, but resolution of symptoms will take 2–3 days to occur
- Bone marrow transplantation (BMT) is highly effective in resolving aplastic anemia, with symptom resolution apparent 14–21 days after the infusion of cells

Review period

Most patients will be referred to hematologist for overall treatment. Once patient returns to the care of the primary care physician, he/she should plan on long-term patient monitoring with periodic physical examinations and routine laboratory testing to screen for relapse.

PROGNOSIS

- Response to immunosuppressive therapy in aplastic anemia is independent of age, but increased mortality has been seen in older patients
- Patients who have received transfusions followed by BMT have an excellent probability of long-term survival and normal life if they had the transplants prior to the onset of transfusion-induced sensitization
- Age is a significant factor in the prognosis; graft-versus-host disease rate increases with age (>90% in patients older than 30 years of age)
- If patients receive BMT from human leukocyte antigen (HLA)-identical sibling, more than 70% of patients are long-term survivors and can be considered cured
- Patients with poor prognosis are those with 'severe aplastic anemia,' defined as absolute neutrophil count <500/mm^3 (<0.5x10^9/L), platelet count <20x10^3/mm^3 (<20x10^9/L), or corrected reticulocyte count <1%. In these patients, one-year survival without therapy is as low as 20%
- Note: corrected reticulocyte count is calculated by multiplying the reticulocyte count (%) by the patient hematocrit and dividing the result by an average normal hematocrit (47 for men and 42 for women)

Clinical pearls

Aplastic anemia is a medical emergency. The highest mortality is seen within first 4 months of the diagnosis. One-year mortality in untreated patients with severe aplastic anemia is as high as 80–90%.

COMPLICATIONS

Graft-versus-host disease can occur in patients receiving BMT who had already undergone transfusion therapy, with onset of transfusion-induced sensitization.

CONSIDER CONSULT

- If aplastic anemia recurs, then the patient should be referred back to hematologist for additional treatment
- If graft-versus-host disease occurs, the patient should be referred for additional evaluation and treatment

RISK FACTORS

- Toxin exposure: extended exposure to benzene, insecticides, or other known toxins has been found to increase the risk for aplastic anemia
- Ionizing irradiation: exposure to ionizing irradiation has been found to increase the risk for aplastic anemia
- Drug exposure: certain drugs can be common etiologic factors for development of aplastic anemia

MODIFY RISK FACTORS

Lifestyle and wellness

SEXUAL BEHAVIOR

Exposure to individuals with HIV or hepatitis C should be limited and precautions should be used to prevent infection.

ENVIRONMENT

- Exposure to benzene, insecticides, or other known toxins in the workplace or at home should be limited
- Exposure to ionizing irradiation in the workplace or at home should be limited

FAMILY HISTORY

Patients with a family history of Fanconi's anemia should be monitored for possible inheritance of the condition.

SCREENING

Due to low incidence of aplastic anemia, and the acquired form's association with drug/chemical exposure, screening the general population is not warranted.

PREVENT RECURRENCE

Reassess coexisting disease

- Patients who have been immunosuppressed for the treatment of other conditions (e.g. HIV or hepatitis C) may be at additional risk for relapse and should be monitored closely by the primary care physician (PCP)
- Patients who are now pregnant but have a history of aplastic anemia may be at additional risk for relapse during pregnancy; these patients should be monitored closely by the PCP

INTERACTION ALERT

Treatment for coexisting disease that may require any of the possible causative drug agents may lead to recurrence.

PATIENT SATISFACTION/LIFESTYLE PRIORITIES

Patients who have a history of aplastic anemia should use additional caution regarding exposure to toxins or infectious agents (HIV or hepatitis C) that may lead to possible recurrence.

RESOURCES

ASSOCIATIONS

Aplastic Anemia Foundation of America
PO Box 613
Annapolis, MD 21404
Tel: (800) 747-2820
www.aplastic.org

National Organization for Rare Disorders
PO Box 8923
New Fairfield, CT 06812–1783
Tel: (800) 999-6673
www.rarediseases.org

NIH/National Heart, Lung and Blood Institute Information Center
PO Box 30105
Bethesda, MD 20824–0105
E-mail: NHLBIinfo@rover.nhlbi.nih.gov
www.nhlbi.nih.gov

KEY REFERENCES

- Marsh J, Schrezenmeir H, Marin P, et al. Prospective randomized multicenter study comparing cyclosporin alone versus the combination of antithymocyte globulin and cyclosporin for treatment of patients with severe aplastic anemia: a report from the European Blood and Marrow Transplant (EBMT) Severe Aplastic Anemia Working Party. Blood 1999;93:2191–5. Medline
- Champlin RE, How WG, Feig SA, et al. Do androgens enhance the response to antithymocyte globulin in patients with aplastic anemia? A prospective randomized trial. Blood 1985;66:184–8. Medline
- Bacigalupo A, Bruno B, Saracco P, et al. Antilymphocyte globulin, cyclosporie, prednisolone, and granulocyte colony-stimulating factor for severe aplastic anemia: an update of the GITMO/EBMT study on 100 patients. Blood 2000;95:1931–4. Medline
- The College of American Pathologists Red Blood Cell Administration Practice Guideline Development Task Force. Practice parameters for the use of red blood cell transfusions. Arch Pathol Lab Med 1998;122:130–8 http://www.guidelines.gov/
- de-Medeiros CR, Ribeiro RC, Bittencourt MA, et al. Long-term outcome of 25 children and adolescents with severe aplastic anemia treated with antithymocyte globulin. Braz J Med Biol Res 2000;33:553–8. Medline
- Miller WJ, Branda RF, Flynn PJ, et al. Antithymocyte globulin treatment of severe aplastic anemia. Br J Haematol 1983;55:17–25. Medline
- Rothmann SA, Streeter RR, Bukowski RM, Hewlett JS. Treatment of severe aplastic anemia with antithymocyte globulin. Exp Hematol 1982;10:809–16. Medline

FAQS

Question 1

Is aplastic anemia the first diagnostic possibility in a patient with HIV who has a sudden drop in hemoglobin?

ANSWER 1

No. This is a classic presentation of parvovirus B19 infection, which should be immediately ruled out, as it is treatable condition (with high-dose immunoglobulin G).

Question 2

Can Fanconi's anemia be seen in a 30-year-old patient for the first time?

ANSWER 2

Although Fanconi's anemia is autosomal recessive inherited marrow failure disorder, which has typical clinical findings (e.g. microcephaly, thumb malformation), it is not uncommon that these phenotypic features are subtle and not recognized until late in the adulthood. The gold-standard test to diagnose Fanconi's anemia is to perform chromosome breakage analysis using clastogenic agents such as diepoxybutane or mitomycin C.

Question 3

Is the treatment for hepatitis-associated aplastic anemia different than that for the management of 'idiopathic aplastic anemia'?

ANSWER 3

No. Hepatitis-associated aplastic anemia seems to be equally responsive to immunosuppressive treatment.

Question 4

Is a complete normalization of complete blood count (CBC) after immunosuppressive treatment a rule?

ANSWER 4

No. Most patients will have some mild abnormality in CBC, even if they are considered 'cured'.

Question 5

What is the natural history of aplastic anemia treated with immunosuppressive treatment?

ANSWER 5

Late hematologic clonal disorders such as paroxysmal nocturnal hemoglobinuria or myelodysplasia/acute myelogenous leukemia are relatively common. Changes in CBC pattern or a clinical presentation should prompt evaluation for these disorders.

CONTRIBUTORS

Dwight Eichelberger, MD
Benjamin Djulbegovic MD, PhD
Dinesh S Rao, MD

BREAST CANCER

SUMMARY INFORMATION

DESCRIPTION

- Invasive carcinoma of breast – either ductal or lobular
- The most frequently diagnosed cancer in women in the US, and second most frequent cause of cancer death
- Lifetime risk of developing breast cancer is estimated at 1 in 8 for women
- Risk increases with age
- Etiology is complex; there are multiple risk factors
- Mammographic screening has been shown to reduce mortality from breast cancer for women aged 50–69
- Treatment consists of a combination of surgery, radiotherapy, chemotherapy, and hormonal therapy

KEY! DON'T MISS!

- Persistent mastalgia with no palpable mass warrants mammography
- Palpable mass that is not diagnostic on mammogram requires biopsy to rule out breast cancer
- Eczema or ulceration of the nipple – Paget's disease
- Family history of breast cancer in a concerned patient warrants referral to a specialist

ICD9 CODE
174.9 Malignant neoplasm female breast.

SYNONYMS
- Carcinoma of the breast
- Breast neoplasm
- Breast malignancy

CARDINAL FEATURES
- Breast cancer can either be in situ or invasive
- All carcinomas in situ are noninvasive histological types but have the potential to become invasive
- Close to 80% of invasive carcinomas are ductal adenocarcinomas, 8–15% are infiltrating lobular carcinomas
- Breast cancer is the most frequently diagnosed cancer in women in the US, and the second most frequent cause of cancer death (43,300 deaths per year in the US)
- Lifetime risk of developing breast cancer is estimated at 1 in 8 for women
- Fewer than 1% of all breast cancer cases occur in men
- Etiology is complex and there are multiple risk factors
- Genetics is implicated in 5–10% including the genes BRCA-1 and BRCA-2
- All patients with a discrete mass, nipple changes, or persistent mastalgia should be referred to a breast specialist
- Mammography screening has increased the diagnosis of breast cancers; 45% of breast cancers can be seen on mammography before they are palpable
- Treatment may require surgery, radiotherapy, chemotherapy, and hormonal therapy
- Palliative care enhances quality of life

EPIDEMIOLOGY
Incidence and prevalence
- Accounts for approximately 30% of all cancer diagnosed in the US
- Accounts for approximately 16% of all cancer deaths in American women
- There are approximately one million new cases annually, worldwide

INCIDENCE
- 175,000 patients develop breast cancer each year in the US
- There are 43,300 related deaths each year in the US
- The incidence of male breast cancer is about 2.5 per 100,000 population

Demographics
AGE

In the US, a woman's lifetime risk of developing breast cancer is estimated at 1 in 8 if she lives to be 110:
- More than half the risk is incurred after the age of 60
- One-third of the risk occurs after age 75

A more practical way to contemplate the risk is over periods of time: from birth, the chance of developing cancer by age 50 is 1 in 50 and the overall lifetime risk is approximately 1 in 8. The risks decrease with age in the absence of a previous diagnosis of breast cancer. For example:
- A 40-year-old woman has a 1 in 14 chance of developing breast cancer by age 70
- A 60-year-old woman has a 1 in 28 chance of developing breast cancer by age 70
- A 70-year-old woman has a 1 in 14 chance of ever developing breast cancer

Male breast cancer has a peak incidence 5–10 years later than that in women.

GENDER

- Breast cancer is 100 times more common in women than men
- Fewer than 1% of breast cancers occur in men

RACE

- Ashkenazi Jews have a higher incidence of mutations in the BRCA-1 and BRCA-2 genes
- The frequency of these two mutations is about 1 in 50 and they account for 25% of early-onset breast cancer, and up to 90% of families with multiple cases of both breast and ovarian cancer, among Ashkenazi Jews

GENETICS

Genetics is involved in 5–10% of cases of breast cancer:

- About 18,000 cases each year are associated with an obvious hereditary predisposition
- 200,000 breast cancer survivors in the US developed their primary cancers as a result of an hereditary predisposition, and remain at risk for secondary cancers
- Genetic involvement should be suspected if there are multiple cases of early-onset breast cancer within the family, if there is ovarian cancer alongside a family history of breast or ovarian cancer, if breast and ovarian cancer occur in the same woman, if there is bilateral breast cancer, or if there is Ashkenazi Jewish heritage

BRCA-1 and BRCA-2:

- These two genetic mutations are associated with a 50–85% risk of developing breast cancer
- BRCA-1 appears to be responsible for disease in 45% of families with multiple cases of breast cancer (only), and up to 90% of families with both breast and ovarian cancer
- Approximately 1 in 800 individuals in the general population may carry a pathogenic mutation in BRCA-1
- Men are at increased risk of colon and prostate cancer
- The BRCA-2 gene also increases the risk of ovarian cancer, but not as strongly as BRCA-1
- More information can be found at CancerNet – National Cancer Institute: Genetics, Causes, Risk Factors, Prevention

Klinefelter's disease: Men with this syndrome are at greater risk of breast cancer.

Family history:

- After gender and age, a positive family history is the strongest known predictive risk factor for breast cancer: one first-degree relative gives a relative risk of 1.5–2.0 (even higher if the relative had bilateral or premenopausal breast cancer); two first-degree relatives give a relative risk of 5.0
- Risk varies according to the age at which the affected relative was diagnosed: the younger that age, the greater the risk in relatives
- In most cases an extensive family history (more than four relatives in the same biological line affected) is not present

GEOGRAPHY

- The incidence of breast cancer increases when populations migrate from areas of low incidence of breast cancer to those with high incidence – indicating that environmental factors are important
- The highest rates are in Western countries (more than 100 cases per 100,000 women) and the lowest are in Asian countries (10–15 cases per 100,000 women)
- Within a country, rates can be greater in urban areas than rural
- Rates can be associated with religious and cultural differences (e.g. Mormons have a much lower breast cancer rate than the general population)

DIFFERENTIAL DIAGNOSIS

Fibrocystic breast disease

Nonmalignant breast lesions widespread in women over 20 years of age.

FEATURES

- Single most common disorder of the breast
- Accounts for more than half of all surgical operations on the female breast
- Unusual before adolescence: diagnosed frequently between the ages of 20 and 40 years; peaks at or just before the menopause; rarely develops after the menopause; premenopausal lesions may persist into later life
- Hormonal imbalance plays a role in fibrocystic breast disease: oral contraceptive use decreases the risk of fibrocystic changes; physical findings and symptoms may vary according to phase of menstrual cycle
- Exclusion of breast carcinoma by biopsy is indicated if mass, thickening, discharge, and pain are observed

Fibroadenoma

Fibroadenomas are benign tumors composed of both the stromal and epithelial elements of the breast. They are the second most common solid tumors in the breast (after carcinoma) and the most common tumors in women younger than 30 (accounting for 50% of breast biopsies in women >20 and 75% of breast biopsies in women <20 years).

FEATURES

- Firm, solitary tumors that may increase in size over several months of observation
- Usually solitary; multiple lesions seen in 10–15% of patients
- May be lobulated but slip easily under the examining fingers
- Mammography is of little help in distinguishing between cysts and fibroadenomas, but ultrasound will usually show the cavity of a cyst clearly
- There is a modest risk of subsequent carcinoma in women who have previously undergone treatment for fibroadenoma (about two times that in the general population)
- Fibroadenomas may recur
- A core needle biopsy to confirm the diagnosis may be performed, for example, on a patient in her teens or 20s who presents with a typical fibroadenoma on physical examination. If the lesion is typical it may be left in the breast, but if excision is recommended, cosmetic incisions around the areola are the proper choice

Hamartoma

A hamartoma is a benign nodule resulting from proliferation of the epithelium and stromal supporting tissue.

FEATURES

- Hamartomas are indistinguishable from fibroadenomas using physical examination, mammography, or gross inspection
- The hamartoma nodule is entirely benign, and removal is curative
- It occurs in postmenopausal women
- It does not recur
- Physical examination may reveal the nodule to be well-defined or indistinct, but soft and usually similar in texture to the surrounding breast tissue
- The classic (and diagnostic) mammographic appearance is a mass circumscribed by a thin radio-opaque capsule (seen if fat is present on both sides of the mass)

Adenoma

Adenoma, also known as mammary adenoma or tubular adenoma, is a cellular neoplasm of the ductules without the supporting stroma.

FEATURES
- During pregnancy and lactation, adenomas may increase in size
- Histologic examination will reveal secretory differentiation
- Malignancy is not a feature of tubular adenoma or lactating adenoma, but biopsy is required to establish the diagnosis

SIGNS & SYMPTOMS

Signs

- There may be no signs. Small breast cancers are increasingly found through mammography screening: 45% can be seen on mammography before they are palpable
- Nipple discharge: there is concern if this is unilateral, spontaneous, and bloody, emanates from one duct system alone, or occurs in a postmenopausal patient. However, nipple discharge is generally related to a benign condition and its most common cause is an intraductal papilloma (a benign condition treated by excision alone)
- Palpable breast lumps are detectable in 90% of patients and are the most common sign

Also:
- Skin and/or nipple retraction
- Eczematous ulcer of the nipple – see Paget's disease under Associated Disorders
- Skin edema/erythema
- Skin nodules
- Palpable lymphadenopathy in axilla and supraclavicular areas
- Lymphedema (Peau d'orange)
- In advanced disease there may be signs of pleural effusion, hepatomegaly, bone metastases

Symptoms

- Less commonly, patients may present with a history of pain and no mass
- Fixation of the mass to the chest wall or to overlying skin can lead to discomfort in advanced disease
- There may be bone pain due to metastasis in advanced disease

ASSOCIATED DISORDERS

Paget's disease:
- This is a cutaneous manifestation of underlying breast malignancy
- Presents as an eczematoid lesion (often weeping, red, and crusting in late presentation)
- Causes median delay in diagnosis of 6 months
- Occurs in approximately 1–4% of patients with breast cancer
- Is best treated with modified radical mastectomy and complete axillary dissection

KEY! DON'T MISS!

- Persistent mastalgia with no palpable mass warrants mammography
- Palpable mass that is not diagnostic on mammogram requires biopsy to rule out breast cancer
- Eczema or ulceration of the nipple – Paget's disease
- Family history of breast cancer in a concerned patient warrants referral to a specialist

CONSIDER CONSULT

Urgent referrals to a breast specialist should occur for the following:
- Breast lumps: any new palpable breast lump, asymmetrical nodularity that persists after menstruation, or any lump associated with nipple or skin changes

- Skin changes including peau d'orange and any new skin dimple
- Nipple changes: single duct discharge, blood-stained nipple discharge, nipple eczema suggestive of Paget's disease
- Persistent unilateral breast pain in postmenopausal women
- Breast mass that does not meet all three of the following radiologic criteria: size <15mm; up to 3 lobulations; >50% well-circumscribed in any radiologic view
- Family history of breast cancer in a concerned patient
- Abnormal serum prolactin or serum thyroid-stimulating hormone (TSH) levels warrant referral to an endocrinologist

INVESTIGATION OF THE PATIENT

Direct questions to patient

Q **Have you noticed a lump in your breast?** More than 80% of breast cancers are discovered as a lump by the patient. However, the patient may have noticed a lump in their breast for some time prior to presentation, especially if they have 'lumpy' breasts or are nervous to seek medical care

Q **Do you have breast pain?** Breast carcinoma can be pain-free, especially in the initial stages

Q **Do you have a personal history of breast cancer?** A previous history of breast cancer increases the risk

Q **Have you ever had a breast biopsy that showed hyperplasia?** Atypical hyperplasia increases the risk 4- to 5-fold compared to a control population. Atypia plus a family history of breast cancer increases the risk 11-fold compared to a control population

Q **Have you had a previous breast lump?** Fibrocystic disease and previous breast cancer increase the risk of future breast malignancies

Q **Have you noticed any skin changes around the nipple?** Retraction of the nipple or skin can be indicative of tumor. Paget's disease is a malignant disease presenting with a scaly, sore, eroding, bleeding ulcer of the nipple

Q **Have you lost weight?** This may imply metastatic disease

Q **Have you any back or bone pain?** Breast cancer can present with bone metastases, especially if the patient has not sought medical care for a persistent breast lump

Contributory or predisposing factors

Q **How old are you?** Risk of breast cancer increases substantially over age 50

Q **How old were you when you began menstruating?** Early menarche increases the risk of breast cancer by increasing breast exposure to estrogen

Q **Have you ever been pregnant?** Pregnancy before age 35 is associated with decreased risk. Nulliparity or pregnancy after age 35 is associated with increased risk

Q **Have you reached the menopause?** If so, determine age at menopause. Late menopause is also associated with increased risk of breast cancer by increasing breast exposure to estrogen

Q **Have you had a hysterectomy that included removal of your ovaries?** Oophorectomy before age 50 is associated with decreased risk

Q **Have you ever used hormone replacement therapy?** After 5 years of use, hormone replacement therapy increases the risk of breast cancer by 2–3%

Q **Have you ever taken oral contraceptives?** The combined pill is associated with a modest increase in risk; there are about five more cases of breast cancer per 100,000 among women using oral contraceptives

Family history

Q **Has anyone in your immediate family (sister, mother, daughter) ever had breast cancer?** Risk doubles if first-degree relative has breast cancer. Risk approaches 50% if family breast cancers have been diagnosed in premenopausal women, if breast cancers are bilateral and if they occur in multiple family members

- Q **Has anyone in your family had ovarian cancer?** Some genetic mutations in BRCA-1 and BRCA-2 increase the risk of breast and ovarian cancer
- Q **Are you descended from Ashkenazi Jewish people?** This particular group has a higher incidence of mutations in BRCA-1 and BRCA-2 and a corresponding increase in familial breast cancer

Examination

Breast examination should occur in a well lit room with the patient sitting upright, her arms above her head. Examination should first take place with the pectoral muscles tensed, and then with the patient's arms at her side. Indirect lighting should also be available, as this may reveal subtle skin changes.

- **Is there a dominant mass, asymmetry or skin change on visual inspection?** Breast cancer may present with skin changes
- **Is there any nipple retraction, inversion or excoriation of the superficial epidermis of the nipple?** Breast cancer may present with nipple alterations
- **Is there eczematous change or an ulcer of the nipple?** Paget's disease
- **Is there edema of the skin (Peau d'orange)?** This may indicate locally advanced disease
- **Is the skin erythematous with tenderness and warmth?** This may represent inflammatory breast cancer but is often mistaken for mastitis
- **Is there evidence of skin metastases?** Satellite nodules of the skin indicate local systemic spread of the cancer
- **Are there palpable axillary, supraclavicular lymph nodes?** These may be indicative of lymphatic spread of the carcinoma
- **Palpate both breasts while patient supine** – to ensure that there is no palpable breast mass
- **Examine each breast quadrant by pressing breast tissue against breast wall** – again, to ensure that there is no palpable breast mass
- **Palpate tissue beneath areola** – to check for breast tumor in this area

Summary of investigative tests

Investigations involve a triad of mammography, sonography, and fine-needle aspiration (FNA).

- Mammogram: detects 85% of breast cancers (15% cannot be visualized). A normal mammographic result does not rule out malignancy, but if there is a suspicious mass, biopsy must be performed. A mammogram can show abnormal breast tissue densities including masses, asymmetrical tissue distortion, skin thickening, axillary lymphadenopathy, nipple retraction, and microcalcifications. Used in screening or for evaluation of dominant mass felt on physical exam
- Sonogram (ultrasonography): used to differentiate between solid mass and cyst
- Fine needle aspiration (FNA): usually done after mammography to avoid possibility of hematoma that would confuse radiologic evaluation
- Core-cutting needle biopsy: used to obtain specimen readable by pathologist
- Stereotactic biopsy (normally performed by a specialist): used to evaluate nonpalpable masses and/or suspicious microcalcifications. Requires dedicated unit. Breast is held in place and target identified by computerized analysis of triangulated mammographic images
- Excisional or incisional biopsy (normally performed by a specialist): establishes diagnosis through complete or partial removal of mass
- Immunocytochemical assay (normally performed by a specialist): the breast tissue should be tested for presence or absence of ER/PR receptors and for overexpression of Her-2/neu receptor
- In women with intraductal and pathological stage I tumors, routine bone scanning, liver ultrasonography, and chest X-ray are not indicated

- In women with pathological stage II tumors, a postoperative bone scan is recommended as part of the baseline staging, but routine liver ultrasonography and chest X-ray are not indicated – although could be considered in patients with four or more positive lymph nodes
- In women with pathological stage III tumors, bone scanning, liver ultrasonography, and chest X-ray are all recommended postoperatively as part of the baseline staging
- In women for whom treatment options are restricted to tamoxifen or hormone therapy, or for whom no further treatment is indicated because of age or other factors, routine bone scanning, liver ultrasonography, and chest X-ray are not indicated as part of the baseline staging
- If no signs and symptoms suggest metastatic disease or complicating medical problems, the laboratory workup should include a complete blood count (CBC), measurement of renal and hepatic function and serum alkaline phosphatase levels, urinalysis, and an electrocardiogram (ECG)
- Currently no serum or plasma biomarkers have the sensitivity and specificity to justify their inclusion in the routine staging workup for patients with breast cancer
- Magnetic resonance imaging (MRI) and positron emission tomography (PET) scans may also prove useful

DIAGNOSTIC DECISION

- History focused on breast-related symptoms
- Risk assessment: a personal and family history (first-degree relatives) of breast cancer, or atypia noted on prior biopsies
- Physical examination: inspection and palpation of breasts in sitting and supine positions. Examination of nipple for Paget's disease
- Identification of palpable mass that is not dominant: note size, location, character, for follow up
- Identification of dominant palpable mass: aspirate mass using sterile technique with 18- to 25-gauge needle. Nonbloody aspirate and complete resolution of mass indicate simple cyst mass that does not resolve; bloody aspirate may indicate breast cancer
- Milky or bilateral nipple discharge: check serum prolactin and serum TSH levels
- Suspicious (heterogenous, linear, branching) microcalcifications on mammogram: stereotactic biopsy (if available) or open-excisional biopsy with confirmation of microcalcifications on specimen radiograph

The tumor-node-metastases (TNM) classification is used for clinical staging of breast tumors:

- Tis – cancer in situ
- T1 – <2cm
- T1mic – microinvasion 0.1cm or less in greatest dimension
- T1a – tumor more than 0.1cm but not more than 0.5cm in greatest dimension
- T1b – tumor more than 0.5cm but not more than 1.0cm in greatest dimension
- T1c – tumor more than 1.0cm but not more than 2.0cm in greatest dimension
- T2 – 2–5cm
- T3 – >5cm
- T4a – involvement of chest wall
- T4b – involvement of skin
- T4c – T4a + T4b
- T4d – inflammatory cancer
- N0 – no regional node metastases
- N1 – palpable ipsilateral axillary nodes
- N2 – fixed ipsilateral axillary nodes
- N3 – ipsilateral internal mammary node involvement
- M0 – no evidence of metastasis
- M1 – distant metastasis

- Stage I – T1N0M0
- Stage IIa – T0N1M0, T1N1M0, T2N0M0
- Stage IIb – T2N1M0, T3N0M0
- Stage IIIa – T0N2M0, T1N2M0, T2N2M0, T3N1M0, T3N2M0
- Stage IIIb – T4, any N, M0; any T, N3, M0
- Stage IV – any T, any N, M1

CLINICAL PEARLS

- Benign breast disease is common among American women, and its symptoms are the chief complaint for many women seeking treatment from their gynecologists
- In evaluating breast problems, it is critical to remember that mammography fails to detect 10–15% of all palpable malignant lesions

THE TESTS

Body fluids

COMPLETE BLOOD COUNT

Description

- Complete blood count is required to check overall health of patient
- Anemia may occur alongside breast cancer, especially where there is metastatic disease
- Cytopenia can occur due to bone marrow involvement

Advantages/Disadvantages

Advantages:

- Inexpensive
- Noninvasive
- Venous blood sample is simple to obtain

Abnormal

Hemoglobin <12g/dL.

Cause of abnormal result

- Anemia
- Could indicate disseminated breast cancer

Tests of function

LIVER FUNCTION TESTS

Description

- Liver function testing is needed in all breast cancer patients
- It can indicate liver metastases secondary to breast cancer
- Elevated alkaline phosphatase levels can indicate bone metastasis

Advantages/Disadvantages

Advantages:

- Inexpensive
- Noninvasive
- Venous blood sample is simple to obtain

Abnormal

- Elevated alanine aminotransferase >35U/L
- Elevated alkaline phosphatase >120U/L

Cause of abnormal result
- Liver disease
- Liver metastases secondary to breast cancer
- Bone metastasis

Drugs, disorders and other factors that may alter results
Alcohol can produce abnormal liver function test results.

Biopsy

FINE-NEEDLE ASPIRATION/FINE-NEEDLE ASPIRATION BIOPSY
Description
- Should only be performed by an experienced specialist
- Can help diagnose malignancy rapidly, avoiding undue delay in treatment
- Fluid or tissue specimen taken from dominant breast mass
- Cytological evaluation may be sufficient to confirm cancer but, if negative, needle or incisional biopsy is required as follow up

Advantages/Disadvantages
Advantages:
- Diagnostic and therapeutic for cystic masses
- Simple procedure that can be performed in the office
- Results aid rapid diagnosis, avoiding undue delay in treatment
- Accurate, provided skilled pathologist interprets
- Low morbidity
- Minimal patient discomfort
- Low cost

Disadvantages:
- Apparent simplicity of procedure leads to use by unskilled professionals
- Does requires experienced pathologist for accurate interpretation
- If negative result obtained, needle or incisional biopsy is required as follow up

Normal
- FNA: nonbloody fluid; mass disappears after aspiration
- FNA biopsy: normal breast epithelial cells

Abnormal
- FNA: bloody aspirate; mass does not resolve after aspiration
- FNA biopsy: atypical breast cells; acellular sample
- Falsely abnormal/normal results can occur

Cause of abnormal result
- Breast cancer
- Mass not in biopsy specimen

CORE-CUTTING NEEDLE BIOPSY
Description
- Core needle used to obtain biopsy specimen for pathologist interpretation
- Diagnostic of breast carcinoma
- Biopsy specimen can also be analyzed for estrogen and progesterone receptors

Advantages/Disadvantages

Advantages:

- Does not require specialized training of cytopathologist; any pathologist may interpret
- False-positives are rare
- Core needles are readily available, at low cost

Disadvantages:

- False-negative diagnoses may be slightly higher due to deflection into normal breast tissue of larger needle by mass
- Seeding of needle track with malignant cells is possible
- Spring-loaded, core-cutting needles are more costly

Normal

Normal breast tissue in specimen.

Abnormal

- Atypical breast tissue in specimen
- Falsely abnormal/normal results can occur

Cause of abnormal result

- Breast cancer
- Fibroadenoma
- Biopsy through radial scar

Imaging

MAMMOGRAM

Description

- Compression of the breast between radiographic plates
- Used for both screening and defining a diagnosed breast mass
- Used for stereotactic biopsies

Advantages/Disadvantages

Advantages:

- Can be used to diagnose breast abnormalities, including microcalcifications, at an early stage
- Two-view mammogram is cost-effective in screening for breast cancer
- Inexpensive and available in most settings
- Universal language for reporting exists: Breast Imaging and Reporting Data System (BI-RADS)
- X-ray exposure is low

Disadvantages:

- Mammography cannot be used in isolation to diagnose breast cancer
- False-negative rate may exceed 15%
- Utility dependent on technique used and experience of mammographer
- Negative result in patient with clinical picture suspicious for malignancy requires further follow up
- As a screening tool – the best interval for screening remains controversial – once- or twice-yearly – and the upper age limit is not established
- Breast compression may be painful

Normal

- No dominant masses
- No abnormal microcalcifications

Abnormal

- Mass present: spiculated mass is especially worrisome for breast cancer
- Subtle distortions in breast architecture
- 'Crab-like' lesions
- Ductal dilation
- Microcalcifications associated with mass
- Abnormal microcalcifications – linear, branching, heterogeneous – that may or may not be associated with the mass
- Keep in mind the possibility of a falsely abnormal result

Cause of abnormal result

- Fibrocystic disease
- Fibroadenoma
- Hamartoma
- Breast cancer

SONOGRAM

Description

- Use of ultrasound to distinguish characteristics of a breast mass
- Aids the workup of a breast mass
- Distinguishes solid from cystic masses
- Can aid in needle biopsy and/or aspiration

Advantages/Disadvantages

Advantages:

- Inexpensive, readily available
- Useful in guiding needle biopsy
- Distinguishes solid mass from cyst
- May reveal abscess

Disadvantages:

- Cannot distinguish benign solid mass from malignant solid mass
- Requires experienced ultrasonographer

Normal

No identifiable solid or cystic masses.

Abnormal

- Cyst
- Solid mass
- Keep in mind the possibility of a falsely abnormal result

Cause of abnormal result

- Fibrocystic disease
- Abscess
- Breast cancer
- Fibroadenoma
- Hamartoma

CHEST X-RAY

Description

- Used for the evaluation of metastatic disease
- Not necessary in all breast cancer patients

Advantages/Disadvantages

Advantages:

- Inexpensive
- Reliable and quick to perform
- Noninvasive
- Radiation dose relatively low

Abnormal

- Pleural effusion
- Nodules in the lung fields
- Bone abnormalities – lesions, fractures, and calcifications

Cause of abnormal result

- Lung disease
- Could be indicative of metastatic breast cancer

MAGNETIC RESONANCE IMAGING

Description

MRI scans can be useful in evaluating both local and metastatic disease. They are also useful in screening women with a hereditary risk of breast cancer.

Advantages/Disadvantages

Advantages:

- Excellent imaging technique for women with breast implants
- Identifies occult foci of disease when breast cancer has been diagnosed
- May be able to detect ductal carcinoma in situ (DCIS) extending away from primary tumor and allow planning for efficient local control
- Differentiates scar from breast cancer recurrence
- Can be useful in evaluating metastatic disease
- Shown to be more accurate than mammography in breast screening in women with a hereditary risk

Disadvantages:

- Requires dedicated breast coils
- Not always available
- Expensive, requiring experienced technician and radiologist to perform and report the scan
- Timing critical when using gadolinium enhancement to differentiate malignant from benign disease. If interval between injection and imaging too long, uptake of benign lesions may be enhanced

Abnormal

- Increased uptake of gadolinium in discrete lesion
- Keep in mind the possibility of a falsely abnormal result

Cause of abnormal result

- Benign lesion
- Breast cancer
- Metastatic disease

POSITRON EMISSION TOMOGRAPHY SCANNING

Description

- Uses fluorine 18-labeled glucose to detect increased metabolic activity associated with breast cancer
- Useful in the evaluation of metastatic disease

Advantages/Disadvantages

Advantages:

- Assesses breast, axilla, and possible metastatic spread throughout body
- May help differentiate low- and high-grade lesions for prognosis

Disadvantages:

- Requires highly specialized, expensive equipment not widely available
- Radioactive tracer difficult to produce. Must have cyclotron tracer excreted through kidneys (which may exclude use in elderly women)

Normal

No suspicious increase in metabolic activity seen in breast, axilla, or body.

Abnormal

- Areas of increased metabolic activity
- Keep in mind the possibility of a falsely abnormal result

Cause of abnormal result

- Primary breast cancer
- Metastatic breast cancer
- Infection

Drugs, disorders and other factors that may alter results

Intake of glucose immediately prior to this scan may cause a false-positive result in distant parts of the body.

BONE SCAN

Description

- Useful in the evaluation of metastatic disease
- Diagnostic of metastases to the bone

Advantages/Disadvantages

Disadvantages:

- Specialized technician needed to perform scan
- Radiologist needed to report scan
- Radiation dose to patient relatively high

Abnormal

Hot spots with increased uptake in the bone.

Cause of abnormal result

Metastatic bone disease.

Other tests

IMMUNOCYTOCHEMICAL ASSAYS

Description

Laboratory assays that determine the presence of the following markers in the biopsy material:

- Estrogen receptor
- Progesterone receptor
- HER2/NEU (fluorescence in situ hybridization)
- S-phase fraction (flow cytometry)
- Ki-67 protein

Advantages/Disadvantages

Advantages:

- Positivity of estrogen and progesterone receptors predicts response to adjuvant endocrine therapy
- Can be done in paraffin-embedded tissue

Disadvantages:

- Not all markers have a clear role in defining prognosis
- There may be variation in standard values between laboratories

Normal

- Varies according to test and laboratory
- Standard results of many tests can be found at www.aruplab.com

Abnormal

Standard results of many tests may be found at www.aruplab.com.

CONSIDER CONSULT

Refer:

- To a specialist breast surgeon for surgical excision of mass
- For evaluation and treatment with radiation therapy for local control
- For evaluation and treatment with chemotherapy

IMMEDIATE ACTION

- Spinal cord metastases can lead to cord compression – urgent radiotherapy is required
- Hypercalcemia needs urgent treatment with intravenous fluids and bisphosphonates
- Cerebral metastases can cause cerebral edema requiring urgent referral for intravenous dexamethasone and radiotherapy to the space-occupying lesions
- Pathological fractures will also need urgent referral

PATIENT AND CAREGIVER ISSUES

Forensic and legal issues

If patient consent unobtainable (e.g. due to mental status), guardian must give consent for treatment.

Impact on career, dependants, family, friends

Career impact:

- Job loss or demotion has been reported by breast cancer survivors
- Unwanted changes in job duties
- Problems with co-workers and employers: avoidance, decrease in communication
- Changes in attitude towards work due to decrease in physical stamina
- Concerns about health/life insurance

Family impact:

- Breast cancer diagnosis not associated with divorce if marriage previously stable
- 30% of patients will have persistent problems with body image which will affect sexual interest and sexual function
- The patient's mother, sisters, and daughters may have concerns about the genetic aspects of the disease
- Childcare may be a problem during treatment
- A mother undergoing treatment may seriously impact on her child

Impact on friends:

- Lack of physical stamina for social events with friends
- Avoidance by friends
- Anticipatory grief in friends

Patient or caregiver request

- **Will I die from my breast cancer?** Complying with the treatment regimen and close physician follow up give the best chance of success
- **Does the cancer require me to have my breast removed?** Not all women with breast cancer are candidates for mastectomy – breast-conserving surgery may be offered
- **Will I need further treatment after surgery?** It depends on the stage of the tumor and the patient's condition. In most cases, some type of treatment will follow surgery
- **Will I need chemotherapy?** Chemotherapy may be used to shrink the tumor preoperatively. Postoperatively, it may be used in cases of invasive breast cancer, depending on tumor size and lymph node involvement – and after full discussion with the oncologist
- **Are there any alternative treatments for breast cancer?** There is no evidence of the efficacy of alternative therapies

Health-seeking behavior

- **Are you using hormone replacement therapy?** Continued hormone replacement therapy is controversial in postmenopausal women, but recent studies show no significant increase in mortality from breast cancer. Risks, benefits, and controversies should be discussed with the individual patient before a decision to continue therapy is made
- **Do you practice sports?** Studies suggest that physical activity may be protective
- **Are you overweight?** Obesity may increase the risk of breast cancer (as well as other diseases)
- **Do you self-examine your breasts after every menstrual period?** Regular breast self-examination is useful – the woman will get to know her body and is more likely to detect changes when they appear
- **Do you have annual examinations with your physician?** Women in their 40s and older should be aware that a monthly breast self-examination is not a substitute for regularly scheduled screening mammograms and clinical breast examinations by a health professional

MANAGEMENT ISSUES

Goals

- Improve survival
- Prevent local or regional recurrence
- If metastatic disease present at diagnosis, delay progression of disease
- Maximize quality of life
- Support patient and their carers

Management in special circumstances

- Use of anthracycline-based chemotherapy in women with known heart disease requires careful monitoring of cardiac condition. If severe heart disease co-exists, anthracycline-based treatment is contraindicated
- Chemotherapeutic choices may be limited by kidney and liver dysfunction as most chemotherapy drugs are excreted by one of these routes
- Women >35 years are likely to become infertile through chemotherapy treatment; premenopausal women <35 have a 50% chance of infertility. Counseling on reproductive options is required

COEXISTING DISEASE

Coexisting cardiac conditions may limit choices for chemotherapy.

COEXISTING MEDICATION

- Over-the-counter (OTC) use of plant estrogens should be discouraged in women with estrogen receptor (ER)-positive breast cancer
- Hormone replacement therapy is contraindicated in patients with breast cancer, but studies have shown that it can be taken safely after 10 years of disease-free survival

SPECIAL PATIENT GROUPS

- It appears that women <40 years have a 50% risk of infertility following chemotherapy, and women >40 have a 90% risk of permanent amenorrhea and infertility following chemotherapy. Premenopausal women should be counseled regarding reproductive alternatives. Because pregnancy is not an option for women with iatrogenic menopause, alternatives such as in vitro fertilization and adoption need to be explored
- In 0.4–4.5% of cases, breast cancer is discovered during pregnancy. Detection is often delayed because of the physiologic changes of pregnancy and breast cancer is often misdiagnosed. The diagnostic delay and advanced stage at presentation account for poorer prognosis. Mastectomy is the treatment of choice
- The cancers that develop in older patients are as aggressive as those in younger patients and should be treated similarly

PATIENT SATISFACTION/LIFESTYLE PRIORITIES

- For women in full-time work, daily radiation therapy and/or chemotherapy schedules may interfere with work
- Fatigue related to chemotherapy and radiation therapy can be significant and also interfere with work/an active lifestyle
- Daily radiation therapy may be difficult if disability interferes with travel/transportation

SUMMARY OF THERAPEUTIC OPTIONS

Choices

Noninvasive disease

Lobular carcinoma in situ (LCIS):

- Is a premalignant lesion, but a marker that identifies women at increased risk of subsequent development of invasive breast cancer
- Is usually multicentric and frequently bilateral
- Most women can be managed without additional local therapy after biopsy
- There is no evidence that re-excision to obtain clear margins is required
- Tamoxifen has been shown to decrease the risk of developing breast cancer in women with LCIS and should be considered in the routine management
- Treatment options: observation after diagnostic biopsy; tamoxifen to decrease the incidence of subsequent breast cancers; ongoing breast cancer prevention trials, including a large clinical trial comparing risks and benefits of tamoxifen versus raloxifene in high-risk postmenopausal women; and bilateral prophylactic total mastectomy, without axillary node dissection

Ductal carcinoma in situ (DCIS):

- Noninvasive neoplasm of ductal origin (can progress to invasive cancer)
- With the increase in use of screening mammography, DCIS is more frequently diagnosed and now represents 30% of all malignant lesions
- Very few cases present as a palpable mass; 80% are diagnosed by mammography alone
- Treatment options: breast-conserving surgery and radiation therapy, with or without tamoxifen; total mastectomy with or without tamoxifen; breast-conserving surgery without radiation therapy
- Tamoxifen has been shown to significantly reduce the risk of invasive recurrence and has also been shown to reduce the risk of contralateral breast cancer by 50%
- The incidence of recurrent ipsilateral breast cancer was reduced with the addition of radiation to surgery

Early invasive disease

Stages I, II, and IIIa often require a multimodality approach to treatment.

Surgery:

- Breast-conserving surgery plus radiation therapy: all histologic subtypes may be treated this way; the rate of local recurrence is low and varies slightly according to the surgical technique used; radiation therapy is applied daily over a 5-week period
- Mastectomy plus reconstruction: the reconstruction may be immediate (at the time of surgery) or delayed; radiation therapy can be delivered after the surgery, but it may affect cosmesis and increase the incidence of capsular fibrosis, pain, or the need for implant removal
- Mastectomy alone
- Surgical staging of the axilla should also be performed: node status remains the most important predictor of outcome; at least 6–10 nodes, levels I–II should be removed; sentinel lymph node (SLN) biopsy does not yet substitute lymphadenectomy
- Survival is equivalent with any of these options as documented in randomized prospective trials
- Selection of a local therapeutic approach depends on the location and size of the lesion, analysis of the mammogram, breast size, and the patient's attitude toward preserving the breast

- The presence of multifocal disease in the breast or a history of collagen vascular disease are relative contraindications to breast-conserving therapy
- Large tumors (T2 lesions), positive axillary nodes, tumors with an extensive intraductal component, palpable tumors, and lobular histology benefit from wider margins

Adjuvant radiotherapy:

- Indicated for patients at highest risk of local recurrence: those with four or more positive axillary nodes, grossly evident extracapsular nodal extension, large primary tumors, close or positive margins of resection of the primary tumor (these parameters are currently being reviewed)
- Delays from 2–7 months in radiotherapy after surgery had no affect on the rate of local recurrence
- Late toxic effects of radiotherapy are uncommon but may include radiation pneumonitis, cardiac events, arm edema (increased risk in patients who received axillary dissection), brachial plexopathy (risk increased with higher radiation doses), risk of second malignancies (low risk, 0.2% for sarcomas)

Adjuvant hormonal therapy:

- Benefit of tamoxifen restricted to women with ER-positive or ER-unknown breast tumors
- Reductions in recurrence and mortality associated with 5 years of tamoxifen use are 47%
- A 50% decrease in contralateral breast cancer is seen with tamoxifen use, regardless of ER status
- Addition of chemotherapy to tamoxifen in postmenopausal women with ER-positive disease has a survival advantage
- The toxic effects of tamoxifen include an increased risk of endometrial cancer, deep venous thrombosis, and pulmonary emboli
- Ovarian ablation, using goserelin alone or with tamoxifen, is indicated for the management of advanced breast cancer in premenopausal and perimenopausal women
- Ablation improves survival in premenopausal women when compared to no treatment, but there is no benefit in adding ablation to chemotherapy
- The progestogen megestrol may be used as second- or third-line therapy
- Aromatase inhibitors such as anastrozole, letrozole, and exemestane may be more effective than progestogens. They are used in sequence with tamoxifen and progesterones in responsive patients

Adjuvant chemotherapy:

- Survival benefit (10-year survival rates) varies according to age: women aged less than 50 years have an absolute benefit of 7% if they have node-negative disease and 11% if they have node-positive disease; women aged 50–69 years have a 2% benefit if they have node-negative and 3% if they have node-positive disease
- Chemotherapy risks and side-effects include nausea and vomiting, myelosuppression, alopecia, mucositis, heart failure (if an anthracycline is used), thromboembolism, and premature menopause
- Patients who meet the following criteria do not need adjuvant chemotherapy: small primary tumors (<1cm); ER/PR +; tumor grade 1; negative axillary nodes

Inoperable stage IIIB or inflammatory breast cancers

- Neoadjuvant chemotherapy with anthracycline-based chemotherapy and/or taxane-based therapy is standard
- If the patient responds: total mastectomy with axillary dissection followed by postoperative radiotherapy to the chest wall and regional lymphatics is indicated; breast-conserving therapy can be considered; treatment is completed with chemotherapy and tamoxifen if receptors are positive

Stage IV

- The intentions of treatment are palliation of symptoms, improvement in quality of life, and prolonged survival
- Treatment is based on tamoxifen and chemotherapy
- Trastuzumab may be combined with chemotherapy if patient is HER2/NEU-positive
- Surgery and radiotherapy may be applicable in symptomatic metastasis
- Bisphosphonates (pamidronate) can be used to reduce skeletal morbidity in patients with bone metastases
- High-dose chemotherapy with stem cell support cannot be considered outside of a clinical trial

Local recurrence

- Patients may look forward to long-term survival with the appropriate therapy
- If there is local chest wall recurrence, surgery and/or radiation therapy (when feasible) may be curative

Analgesia

Acetaminophen, ibuprofen, codeine, and morphine can all be useful in relieving patients' pain.

Guidelines

Guideline Oversight Group. Breast cancer treatment. [1].

Clinical pearls

A patient's age should not be a determining factor in the selection of breast-conserving treatment vs mastectomy – in women aged 65 years or more, lumpectomy and radiation therapy produce survival and freedom-from-recurrence rates similar to those produced in younger women (those aged less than 65 years).

Never

- Never perform major surgery and adjuvant therapy without knowing the histology and staging of the breast cancer in question
- Never leave the patient in pain due to their breast cancer disease – always check that adequate pain relief has been given

FOLLOW UP

Careful follow up of breast cancer patients is needed, as recurrence may be treatable, with improved survival.

Plan for review

- Patients attending for chemotherapy and radiotherapy should be reviewed weekly to check treatment compliance and complications
- Adjuvant hormonal therapy will also require close follow up to monitor compliance and complications
- Periodic clinical review following successful completion of therapy is also necessary
- Annual mammography is necessary for all breast cancer patients
- Patients should be instructed in monthly breast self-examination technique

Information for patient or caregiver

- Patients require close follow up during and after completing treatment
- Patients need to be taught how to self-examine their breasts monthly

DRUGS AND OTHER THERAPIES: DETAILS

Drugs

TAMOXIFEN

- Antiestrogenic agent
- Used for both prophylaxis and treatment of breast cancer
- Useful for hormone-sensitive tumors

Dose

Adult oral dose: 20mg daily for 5 years.

Efficacy

Reduces the odds of recurrence by 47% and the odds of death by 26%. Also reduces the incidence of contralateral breast cancer by 47%.

Risks/Benefits

Risks:

- Use caution where there are menstrual irregularities or abnormal vaginal bleeding
- Use caution in leukopenia, neutropenia or thrombocytopenia, and in cataracts or visual disturbance

Side-effects and adverse reactions

- Cardiovascular system: thromboembolic events (deep vein thrombosis, pulmonary embolism or stroke)
- Central nervous system: headache, hot flashes
- Eyes, ears, nose, and throat: visual impairments, retinopathy, cataracts
- Gastrointestinal: nausea, vomiting, elevated hepatic enzymes, hepatic necrosis, cholestasis, hepatitis
- Genitourinary, women: endometrial cancer, amenorrhea, vaginal bleeding, menstrual irregularities, endometrial and uterine changes
- Genitourinary, men: changes in libido
- Hematologic: anemia, thrombocytopenia, leukopenia, neutropenia
- Metabolic: hypercalcemia, hyperlipidemia
- Musculoskeletal: bone pain

Interactions (other drugs)

■ Aminoglutethimide ■ Anticoagulants, NSAIDs, platelet inhibitors, thrombolytic agents ■ Antivirals ■ Benzodiazepines ■ Bromocriptine ■ Cyclosporine ■ Diltiazem ■ Nifedipine ■ Erythromycin

Contraindications

■ Pregnancy and breast-feeding ■ Avoid intramuscular injections in patients with a platelet count <50,000mm^3 ■ History of thromboembolic disorders (if tamoxifen is indicated for breast cancer prevention)

Evidence

- A systematic review compared adjuvant tamoxifen with placebo in patients with nonmetastatic breast cancer. Five years of treatment with tamoxifen had a similar effect on long-term survival and recurrence rates irrespective of age or menopausal status. Patients over 50 years old (usually postmenopausal) had a 29% reduced annual risk of recurrence with tamoxifen. Tamoxifen reduced the risk of death from any cause by 20% [2] *Level M*
- A greater reduction in the rate of recurrence was noted in patients with ER-positive tumors rather than ER-negative tumors after 5 years of tamoxifen treatment. Tamoxifen was also associated with a slightly greater reduction in the risk of 10-year recurrence in patients with node-positive compared with node-negative disease [2] *Level M*

- A systematic review and several randomized controlled trials (RCTs) have shown that 5 years of tamoxifen for nonmetastatic breast cancer is superior to shorter durations of treatment. There is no evidence that continuing treatment after 5 years is beneficial [3] *Level M*
- Two nonsystematic reviews (86 RCTs) of patients with metastatic breast cancer, unselected for ER status, found the overall objective response rate to tamoxifen was 34%. A further 20% achieved disease stabilization. The overall median duration of response was 12–18 months [4,5] *Level M*

Acceptability to patient
- Tamoxifen is known to produce a small increase in the risk of endometrial cancer and thromboembolic events
- Careful discussion with the patient of the risks vs the benefits is necessary
- Chemotherapy may have limiting side-effects such as nausea and vomiting

Follow up plan
- Careful patient follow up while on tamoxifen is needed
- The patient should be checked regularly for breast cancer disease recurrence

MEGESTROL
- Progesterone hormonal treatment
- Antineoplastic effects may result from suppressing luteinizing hormone by inhibition of pituitary function or by a local effect on cancerous cells

Dose

Adult oral dose: 40mg four times daily.

Efficacy
- Can be used in virtually any sequence with aromatase inhibitors and antiestrogens in responsive patients
- Objective responses are seen in 30% of all patients and 60% of estrogen-positive tumors

Risks/Benefits

Risks:
- Use caution in depression and in disorders that are influenced by fluid retention
- May mask onset of menopause

Benefits:
- Has a key role in improving survival rates of ER-positive breast cancer
- Can be taken orally
- Inexpensive and has few serious side-effects

Side-effects and adverse reactions
- Central nervous system: headache, insomnia, dizziness, depression
- Gastrointestinal: nausea, vomiting, diarrhea, weight gain
- Genitourinary: breast changes, hot flashes, amenorrhea, changes in cervical erosion
- Skin: rashes, urticaria, pruritus, alopecia, hirsuitism

Interactions (other drugs)

▪ Aminoglutethimide ▪ Antidiabetics ▪ Barbiturates and primidone ▪ Carbamazepine ▪ Cyclosporine ▪ Corticosteroids ▪ Coumarins ▪ Griseofulvin ▪ Lansoprazole ▪ Levacetylmethadol ▪ Nevirapine ▪ Oxcarbazepine ▪ Phenindione ▪ Phenytoin ▪ Rifampin ▪ Tacrolimus ▪ Topiramate ▪ Tretinoin

Contraindications

■ Thrombophlebitis ■ Thromboembolic disorders/cerebral hemorrhage ■ Breast cancer ■ Hepatic disease/dysfunction ■ Undiagnosed vaginal bleeding ■ Known or suspected pregnancy

Evidence

- A RCT (nonblinded) compared megestrol with tamoxifen in peri- or postmenopausal women with advanced or recurrent breast cancer. The women had not received prior hormonal therapy. The response rate was not significantly different between the groups, and there was no significant difference in survival. Cross-over response was seen following both treatments [6] *Level P*
- Progestins have been found to be as effective as tamoxifen as first-line hormonal therapy in metastatic breast cancer in RCTs, but they are not well tolerated. Women with bone pain or anorexia may benefit from progestins [7] *Level P*
- RCTs have shown that progestins are less effective than selective aromatase inhibitors when used as second-line hormonal therapy for women with metastatic breast cancer who have not responded to tamoxifen [7] *Level P*

Acceptability to patient

Few serious side-effects with oral dosing improves acceptability.

Follow up plan

The patient should be followed up closely to check for breast cancer disease recurrence.

Patient and caregiver information

The patient must not get pregnant when on this medication and good contraception is needed if the patient is fertile.

AROMATASE INHIBITORS

- Inhibit the enzymatic conversion of cholesterol-reducing estrogen leading to the blocking of the conversion of androgens to estrogens in the peripheral tissues
- Used to treat advanced cases pf postmenopausal breast cancer
- Used in sequence with tamoxifen and progesterones in responsive patients

Dose

Adult dosages:
Anastrozole: orally, 1g/day
Letrozole: orally, 2.5mg/day
Exemestane: orally, 25mg/day, after a meal

Efficacy

Can be used in virtually any sequence with antiestrogens and progesterones in responsive patients.

Risks/Benefits

Risks:

- Must be administered under specialist supervision
- Pregnancy must be excluded before starting treatment
- Use caution with hepatic impairment
- Exemestane should not be administered to premenopausal women
- Exemestane should not be coadministered with estrogen-containing agents

Benefits:
- Have a key role in improving survival rates in ER-positive breast cancer
- Objective responses are seen in 30% of all patients and 60% of estrogen-positive tumors
- Can be taken orally
- Inexpensive

Side-effects and adverse reactions
- Cardiovascular system: vasodilation, hypertension, hot flashes
- Central nervous system: dizziness, insomnia, depression, hypertonia, fatigue
- Gastrointestinal: abdominal pain, nausea, vomiting, diarrhea, anorexia
- Genitourinary: leukorrhea
- Musculoskeletal: asthenia, back pain, chest pain, pain, bone pain, arthralgia, breast pain
- Respiratory: cough, dyspnea, pharyngitis
- Skin: hair thinning, pruritus

Interactions (other drugs)
Anastrozole and exemestane: reactions catalyzed by cytochrome P-450 1A2, 2C8/9, and 3A4.

Contraindications
■ Exemestane should not be coadministered with estrogen-containing agents ■ Exemestane should not be administered to premenopausal women ■ Known hypersensitivity to treatment ■ Pregnancy and breast-feeding ■ Safety and efficacy in children not established

Evidence
- RCTs compared anastrozole with tamoxifen in postmenopausal patients with metastatic breast cancer. Anastrozole was found to be at least as effective as tamoxifen when used as first-line hormonal therapy [7] *Level P*
- RCTs have found that selective aromatase inhibitors are effective in the treatment of postmenopausal women with metastatic breast cancer who have progressed on first-line tamoxifen treatment or relapsed on adjuvant tamoxifen therapy. Anastrozole, letrozole, and exemestane prolong survival with minimal adverse effects [7] *Level P*
- Selective aromatase inhibitors are significantly more effective (and better tolerated) as second-line therapy than progestins and nonselective aromatase inhibitors, and are most effective in ER-positive women [7]
- A meta-analysis of patients with metastatic breast cancer compared second-line treatment with aromatase inhibitors vs megestrol. Aromatase inhibitors significantly prolonged survival compared with megestrol [8] *Level M*

Patient and caregiver information
- Liver function, complete blood counts (CBCs), and urea and electrolyte monitoring is necessary prior and during therapy
- Patients must seek medical care if they develop a temperature

GOSERELIN
- Used for hormonal treatment of metastatic breast disease in premenopausal women
- Chronic administration leads to sustained suppression of pituitary gonadotropins with subsequent suppression of serum estrogen
- Used to achieve a therapeutic postmenopausal state

Dose
Adult subcutaneous dose: 3.6mg implant into upper abdominal wall every 28 days.

Efficacy

Objective responses are seen in 30% of all patients and 60% of estrogen-positive tumors.

Risks/Benefits

- Risk: use caution in patients at risk of osteoporosis, patients with depression, and patients with hypertension
- Benefit: has a key role in improving survival rates of ER-positive metastatic breast cancer

Side-effects and adverse reactions

- Cardiovascular system: cerebrovascular accident, dysrhythmias, hot flashes, myocardial infarction
- Central nervous system: depression, anxiety, headaches, spinal cord compression
- Gastrointestinal: diarrhea, constipation, nausea, vomiting
- Genitourinary: decreased libido
- Skin: sweating, rash
- Miscellaneous: gynecomastia

Contraindications

Pregnancy.

Evidence

- Two RCTs found no significant difference in survival when gonadorelin analogs were compared with surgical ovariectomy or irradiation as first-line treatment in premenopausal patients with metastatic disease [9, 10] *Level P*
- A meta-analysis compared combination therapy with gonadorelin analogs plus tamoxifen vs a gonadorelin analog alone as first-line therapy in premenopausal patients with metastatic breast cancer. A significant improvement in progression-free survival and overall survival was found with combined hormonal therapy [11] *Level M*

RALOXIFENE

- Selective ER modulator
- Effective in preventing vertebral fractures in women at increased risk of osteoporosis
- Ongoing Study of Tamoxifen and Raloxifene (STAR) trial is comparing raloxifene with tamoxifen for chemoprevention

Dose

Adult oral dose: 60mg daily.

Efficacy

Reduces vertebral fractures and ER-positive breast cancer.

Risks/Benefits

Risks:

- Use caution in hepatic impairment and in patients with a history of breast cancer
- Also use caution with concurrent estrogen therapy

Side-effects and adverse reactions

- Eyes, ears, nose, and throat: sinusitis
- Hematologic: venous thromboembolism
- Gastrointestinal: nausea, vomiting, flatulence
- Genitourinary: infertility
- Metabolic: weight gain, decrease in total and LDL cholesterol and lipoprotein A
- Musculoskeletal: muscle cramps, myalgia
- Skin: hot flashes, peripheral edema, diaphoresis, maculopapular rash

Interactions (other drugs)

- Ampicillin ■ Cholestyramine ■ Warfarin

Contraindications

- Pregnancy and breast-feeding ■ Thromboembolism or history of thromboembolism
- Avoid when long periods of inactivity are required ■ Premenopausal women ■ Children

ACETAMINOPHEN

- Simple analgesia for breast cancer pain
- Can be used with other analgesic agents

Dose

Adult oral dose: 325–650mg four times daily.

Efficacy

- Effective analgesic, especially in combination with other analgesic agents
- Effective antipyretic agent

Risks/Benefits

Risks:

- Use caution in hepatic and renal impairment
- Overdose results in hepatic and renal damage, unless promptly treated
- Overdose may lead to multiorgan failure and may be fatal
- Accidental overdose can occur if OTC preparations containing acetaminophen are taken with prescribed drugs that contain acetaminophen

Benefits:

- Oral medication
- Inexpensive
- Few side-effects
- Nonsedating analgesic

Side-effects and adverse reactions

- Acetaminophen rarely causes side-effects when used intermittently
- Gastrointestinal: nausea, vomiting
- Hematologic: blood disorders
- Metabolic: acute hepatic and renal failure
- Skin: rashes
- Other: acute pancreatitis

Interactions (other drugs)

- Alcohol ■ Anticoagulants ■ Anticonvulsants ■ Isoniazid ■ Cholestyramine ■ Colestipol
- Domperidone ■ Metoclopromide

Contraindications

Known liver dysfunction.

Patient and caregiver information

Care needed to prevent inadvertent overdose, as acetaminophen present in many OTC medications.

IBUPROFEN

- Nonsteroidal anti-inflammatory agent (NSAID)
- Useful as analgesia for breast pain and bone pain
- Antipyretic properties

Dose

Adult oral dose: 200–800mg four times daily – not to exceed 3200mg daily.

Efficacy

- Effective analgesic agent especially for bone pain
- Effective antipyretic agent

Risks/Benefits

Risks:

- Use caution in the elderly
- Use caution in hepatic, renal and cardiac failure, and in bleeding disorders
- Can cause severe allergic reactions including hives, facial swelling, asthma, shock

Side-effects and adverse reactions

- Cardiovascular system: hypertension, peripheral edema
- Central nervous system: headache, dizziness, tinnitus
- Gastrointestinal: anorexia, nausea, dyspepsia, peptic ulceration, bleeding
- Genitourinary: nephrotoxicity
- Hematologic: blood cell disorders
- Hypersensitivity: rashes, bronchospasm, angioedema

Interactions (other drugs)

■ Aminoglycosides ■ Anticoagulants ■ Antihypertensives ■ Baclofen ■ Corticosteroids ■ Cyclosporine, tacrolimus ■ Digoxin ■ Diuretics ■ Lithium ■ Methotrexate ■ Warfarin ■ Phenylpropanolamine

Contraindications

■ Peptic ulceration ■ Hypersensitivity to any pain reliever or antipyretic (including NSAIDs) ■ Coagulation defects ■ Severe renal or hepatic disease

CODEINE

- Schedule II opiate derivative
- Used for mild to moderate pain
- Can be used in combination with other analgesic agents
- Can be given using the oral, intramuscular, or subcutaneous routes

Dose

Adult dose: 15–60mg every 4h.

Efficacy

- Rapid onset of action
- Effective for mild to moderate pain

Risks/Benefits

Risks:

- Use caution in the elderly
- Use caution in renal and hepatic disease, Addisons disease, and hypothyroidism

- Use caution in cases of recent head injury and in those who are pregnant or breast-feeding
- Use caution in patients with gastrointestinal disease, or cardiac disease
- There is a small risk of dependency – use caution in patients with a history of drug abuse

Side-effects and adverse reactions
- Cardiovascular system: bradycardia, tachycardia, palpitations, hypotension
- Central nervous system: headache, drowsiness, dizziness, dysphoria, addiction
- Gastrointestinal: nausea and vomiting, constipation, diarrhea, paralytic ileus, abdominal cramps
- Respiratory: respiratory depression
- Skin: rashes, urticaria

Interactions (other drugs)

■ Alcohol ■ Antidepressants (tricyclics and monoamine oxidase inhibitors) ■ Antipsychotics ■ Anxiolytics and hypnotics ■ Cimetidine ■ Ciprofloxacin ■ Domperidone ■ Ritonavir ■ Metoclopramide ■ Moclobemide

Contraindications

■ Severe pulmonary disease or respiratory failure ■ Children under one year of age ■ Colitis ■ Diarrhea secondary to poisoning or infectious diarrhea ■ Liver failure

MORPHINE
- Schedule II strong opioid
- Used for pain relief
- Can be given through the oral, subcutaneous, or intramuscular routes

Dose
- Adult oral dose: 4–30mg every 4h
- Adult intramuscular/subcutaneous dose: 4–15mg every 4h

Efficacy

Very effective for moderate to severe pain.

Risks/Benefits

Risks:
- Use caution in the elderly and patients under 18 years of age
- Use caution in hepatic and renal disease, hypothryoidism and Addison's disease, abdominal disorders, and prostatic hypertrophy
- Nausea may be aggravated, and morphine should therefore be given with an antiemetic

Side-effects and adverse reactions
- Cardiovascular system: bradycardia, tachycardia, palpitations, hypotension, hypertension, syncope
- Central nervous system: drowsiness, sedation, headache, vertigo, hallucinations, dysphoria, euphoria, mood changes, dependence, anxiety, restlessness
- Eyes, ears, nose, and throat: dry mouth, miosis, blurred vision
- Gastrointestinal: constipation, nausea, vomiting, abdominal pain, biliary spasm
- Genitourinary: urinary difficulties, decreased libido
- Respiratory: respiratory depression
- Skin: rashes, pruritus, urticaria, sweating, flushing

Interactions (other drugs)

■ Alcohol ■ Anticoagulants ■ Antidepressants (tricyclic) ■ Antihistamines ■ Cimetidine ■ Antihypertensives ■ Antipsychotics ■ Anxiolytics and Hypnotics ■ Opiate antagonists ■ Ciprofloxacin ■ Domperidone ■ Esmolol ■ Monoamine oxidase inhibitors ■ Rifamycins ■ Metoclopramide ■ Mexiletine ■ Moclobemide ■ Ritonavir

Contraindications

■ Heart failure secondary to chronic lung disease ■ Cardiac arrhythmias ■ Brain tumor ■ Acute alcoholism ■ Delerium tremens ■ Convulsive states ■ Respiratory depression ■ Hemorrhage ■ Acute asthma attack ■ Paralytic ileus ■ Injection in pheochromocytoma ■ Head injury or raised intracranial pressure

PAMIDRONATE

- Bisphosphonate used for malignant hypercalcemia
- Intravenous use of this agent has transformed the treatment of this complication
- In the presence of bone metastasis, intravenous pamidronate is given every 3–4 weeks

Dose

Adult intravenous dose is 90mg given over 2h for osteolytic bone metastasis and 60–90mg by intravenous infusion over 24h for hypercalcemia of malignancy.

Efficacy

- Very effective in the treatment of malignant hypercalcemia
- Can be used regularly for patients who are refractory to anticancer treatment

Risks/Benefits

Risk: use caution in renal dysfunction

Side-effects and adverse reactions

- Cardiovascular system: hypertension
- Central nervous system: headache, seizures
- Eyes, ears, nose, and throat: iritis
- Gastrointestinal: abdominal pain, anorexia, nausea, vomiting
- Metabolic: decrease in potassium, magnesium, and phosphate levels

Interactions (other drugs)

■ Aminoglycosides ■ Antacids ■ Calcium salts ■ Iron

Contraindications

Pregnancy and breast-feeding.

Evidence

- A systematic review compared bisphosphonates with placebo or no bisphosphonates in women with advanced breast cancer and clinically evident bone metastases. Patients were also receiving chemotherapy or hormonal therapy. The risk of developing a skeletal event was reduced, and the skeletal event rate was reduced. The time to a skeletal event was increased with bisphosphonates [12] *Level M*
- Bisphosphonates may reduce bone pain in women with bone metastases [12] *Level M*
- RCTs have found that pamidronate reduces skeletal complications in women with metastatic bone deposits. The median time to the first skeletal complication was prolonged, fewer women developed skeletal complications, and there was a significantly reduced requirement for radiotherapy to painful sites of bone lesions. There is no evidence of improved survival with bisphosphonates [13,14] *Level P*

DEXAMETHASONE
- Useful in cerebral metastases to reduce edema
- Used for initial treatment of cerebral metastases prior to radiotherapy

Dose
- Adult oral dose: 12–16mg daily
- Adult intravenous dose: 10mg loading and then 4mg every 6h

Efficacy
- Effective in reducing edema
- Improves patients' neurologic symptoms

Risks/Benefits

Risks:
- Overwhelming septicemia if patient has an infection
- Loss of control of blood glucose in those with diabetes
- Use caution in renal disease, esophagitis, peptic ulcer, and ulcerative colitis
- Use caution in cerebral malaria, latent tuberculosis, and AIDS

Side-effects and adverse reactions
- Side-effects are minimized by short duration of therapy
- Cardiovascular system: hypertension, thromboembolism
- Central nervous system: insomnia, euphoria, depression, psychosis
- Endocrine: adrenal suppression, impaired glucose tolerance, growth suppression in children
- Eyes, ears, nose, and throat: cataract, glaucoma, blurred vision
- Gastrointestinal: dyspepsia, peptic ulceration, esophagitis, oral candidiasis
- Musculoskeletal: proximal myopathy, osteoporosis
- Skin: delayed healing, acne, striae

Interactions (other drugs)

▪ Aminoglutethimide ▪ Antidiabetics ▪ Antilipemics ▪ Antivirals ▪ Oral contraceptives ▪ Barbiturates ▪ Cyclosporine ▪ Ephedrine ▪ Estrogens ▪ Isoniazid ▪ Ketoconazole ▪ Macrolide antibiotics ▪ NSAIDs ▪ Rifampin

Contraindications

▪ Avoid live virus vaccines in those receiving immunosuppressive doses ▪ Systemic infection ▪ Idiopathic thrombocytopenic purpura ▪ Lack of a definite diagnosis

Acceptability to patient
- Patients may not wish to take steroids due to the side-effects
- Dexamethasone is very effective at reducing neurologic symptoms, but compliance is important

Follow up plan
- Close follow up of the patient is required
- Radiotherapy will be needed once the neurologic symptoms are controlled, indicating reduction in edema

Patient and caregiver information
- Patients must be told that cerebral metastases can cause severe neurologic symptoms including fits
- Dexamethasone is very effective at reducing neurologic symptoms, but compliance is important
- Radiotherapy will be needed to prevent further neurologic complications

Surgical therapy

- Surgical removal of the tumor is indicated for breast cancer
- Survival rates for patients treated with simple mastectomy and radiation therapy are identical to those for radical modified mastectomy and radiation therapy
- Therefore, patient preference plays a major role in choice of treatment
- Breast-conserving surgery with radiation therapy generally gives good cosmetic results

BREAST-CONSERVING SURGERY

- Breast-conservation surgery may consist of excision of tumor with a 1cm margin of normal tissue – wide local excision
- More extensive surgery of a whole quadrant of breast may be indicated – quadrantectomy
- The wider the excision the lower the recurrence rate but the worse the cosmetic result
- There is no size limit for breast conservation surgery, but adequate excision of lesions over 5cm produces a poor cosmetic result
- Thus breast conservation surgery tends to be limited to lesions 5cm or less
- There is no age limit for breast conservation

Efficacy

Factors leading to poor cosmetic results include:

- Wider excisions
- Excision of any skin overlying the tumor – only dimpled or retracted skin should be excised
- Surgery performed outside of specialist breast units
- Clearance of axillary nodes
- Radiotherapy boosters to the tumor bed

Radiotherapy plus breast-conserving surgery achieves similar rates of survival and local recurrence as mastectomy.

Risks/Benefits

Risks:

- Breast cancer at excised margins
- Extensive in situ component
- Patient aged less than 35 years
- Lymphatic or vascular spread
- Higher grade histology/higher malignant potential

Evidence

- A systematic review compared breast-conserving surgery with mastectomy in patients who were potentially suitable for breast-conserving surgery. All patients received postoperative radiotherapy. There was no significant difference in risk of death over 10 years, or in rates of local recurrence between the groups [15] *Level M*
- Another systematic review (six RCTs) compared mastectomy with breast-conserving surgery. Meta-analysis of five trials found no significant difference in the risk of death at 10 years [16] *Level M*
- Radiotherapy reduces the risk of local recurrence when used after breast-conserving surgery. Radiotherapy plus breast-conserving surgery achieves similar rates of survival and local recurrence as mastectomy [3]

Acceptability to patient

- Breast-conserving surgery is far more acceptable to patients than mastectomy
- There are fewer problems with body image after breast-conserving surgery

Follow up plan

- Careful physical examination, CBC, and biochemistry profile every 4–6 months for 5 years, then every 12 months
- Mammography every 12 months
- Those patients on tamoxifen and with intact uteri need pelvic examination and a Pap smear every year
- Other diagnostic studies should be obtained as symptoms, physical findings, and blood chemistry studies dictate

MASTECTOMY

- Mastectomy should be reserved for tumors over 4cm, most central tumors and tumors, with more than one disease focus
- About one-third of localized breast cancers are unsuitable for breast conservation and require mastectomy
- The breast is removed from the chest wall muscles and is combined with axillary surgery
- There is no survival benefit for mastectomy compared to breast-conserving therapy in localized disease, providing that all local disease is excised
- Survival rates for patients treated with simple mastectomy and radiation therapy are identical to those for radical modified mastectomy and radiation
- Preoperative chemotherapy may shrink the tumor to enable surgery and avoid mastectomy
- Radiotherapy administered postoperatively reduces local recurrence

Efficacy

- There is no survival benefit derived from mastectomy compared to breast-conserving surgery for localized disease, providing that all local disease is excised
- Body image problems are more likely to occur with mastectomy, but breast reconstruction can follow mastectomy

Risks/Benefits

Risks:

- Mastectomy can lead to complications including seroma formation, infection, and flap necrosis
- Body image problems are more likely to follow mastectomy than breast-conserving surgery
- Mastectomy is linked to edema in the arm, sometimes severe

Evidence

- A systematic review compared supraradical mastectomy with radical mastectomy, radical with total mastectomy, and supraradical with total mastectomy in patients with operable, nonmetastatic breast cancer. There was no significant difference in the risk of death over 10 years [15] *Level M*
- The same systematic review found no significant difference in the risk of death over 10 years when radical and simple mastectomy and total and simple mastectomy were compared [15] *Level M*
- This systematic review also compared breast-conserving surgery with mastectomy in patients potentially suitable for breast-conserving surgery. All patients received postoperative radiotherapy. There was no significant difference in risk of death over 10 years, or in rates of local recurrence between the groups [15] *Level M*
- Another systematic review (six RCTs) compared mastectomy with breast-conserving therapy. Meta-analysis of five trials found no significant difference in the risk of death at 10 years [16] *Level M*

Acceptability to patient

Problems of body image occur with mastectomy.

Follow up plan

The patient should be reviewed every 6 months for the first 2 years and annually thereafter.

Patient and caregiver information

Support and counseling are needed for patients and their partners to overcome the psychological effects of mastectomy.

Radiation therapy

Radiation therapy is used after surgery as a local adjuvant treatment to destroy breast cancer cells that remain in the chest wall or regional lymph nodes. It is generally well tolerated and is the mainstay of treatment in locally advanced breast cancer as surgery (mastectomy) results in a high rate of local recurrence.

- Radiation therapy is given after completion of adjuvant chemotherapy (or after surgery if patient is not receiving adjuvant chemotherapy)
- Radiotherapy alone can lead to high rates of local remission in both the breast and axilla in locally advanced breast disease but can be even more successful if given in combination with appropriate systemic treatment
- Radiation therapy is used for palliation of metastatic disease including bony and cerebral metastases
- Radiotherapy can be used for DCIS to reduce the risk of recurrence

RADIOTHERAPY

- The course of radiotherapy will be dependent on its therapeutic use
- The course will be planned by the radiation oncologist
- Palpable tumor masses should receive treatment doses

Efficacy

- Radiotherapy prevents local recurrence of breast cancer
- Radiotherapy treats metastases of the bone, spinal cord, and brain

Risks/Benefits

Risks:

- Radiotherapy to the axilla can cause complications, including brachial plexopathy, reduced shoulder movement, and lymphedema
- Radiotherapy to the axilla cannot be repeated

Benefits:

- Radiotherapy to the axilla can reduce the recurrence rate of breast cancer
- Palliative radiotherapy can reduce bone pain

Evidence

There is evidence that radiotherapy given after breast-conserving surgery for DCIS reduces the risk of local recurrence and invasive carcinoma. There is no evidence of an effect on survival.

- A RCT compared radiotherapy with no radiotherapy after surgery for DCIS. There was no significant difference in survival at 8 years, but the risk of local recurrence was significantly reduced in patients treated with adjuvant radiotherapy [17] *Level P*
- Another RCT compared radiotherapy with no radiotherapy after surgery for DCIS. A significantly lower rate of recurrence of DCIS was noted in the radiotherapy group at median 4.25 years follow up. Local relapse-free survival was more likely for patients receiving radiotherapy at 4 years. There was a significant reduction in recurrence of invasive carcinoma [18] *Level P*

Radiotherapy reduces the risk of local recurrence when used after breast-conserving surgery. Radiotherapy plus breast-conserving surgery achieves similar rates of survival and local recurrence as mastectomy.

- A systematic review compared breast-conserving surgery plus radiotherapy versus surgery alone for the treatment of operable breast cancer. Radiotherapy-treated patients had a lower local relapse rate. There was no significant difference in 10-year survival [15] *Level M*
- Although the published trials do not report a difference in 10-year survival between breast-conserving therapy plus radiotherapy vs breast-conserving therapy alone, recent data released after the 5th Early Breast Cancer Trialists' Group meeting showed that there was a significant increase in survival in women receiving radiotherapy, when mortality from breast cancer was considered in absence of other causes of death [19]
- The review also compared breast-conserving surgery plus breast radiotherapy vs mastectomy (simple or modified radical) in women with invasive breast cancer. There was no difference in 10-year survival rates or local recurrences [15] *Level M*

Radiotherapy to the chest wall is effective in reducing the risk of mortality from breast cancer at 10 years, and reducing the risk of local recurrence when administered after mastectomy.

- A systematic review compared mastectomy alone vs mastectomy plus radiotherapy to the chest wall. Radiotherapy reduced local recurrence and slightly reduced breast cancer mortality. There was no significant difference in overall survival [15] *Level M*
- Subsequent RCTs of high risk patients receiving adjuvant chemotherapy after mastectomy compared radiation therapy to the chest wall and peripheral lymphatics with no radiotherapy. Radiotherapy reduced relative locoregional relapse rates. Overall, 10-year survival may be increased in patients treated with radiotherapy [19] *Level P*

Acceptability to patient

Patients may experience significant side-effects with radiotherapy and these must be fully discussed before consent is obtained.

Follow up plan

- Patients must be followed up carefully for complications of both breast cancer and radiotherapy
- Disease recurrence must be watched for, as further radiotherapy may be indicated

Patient and caregiver information

Patients may experience significant side-effects with radiotherapy and these must be fully discussed before consent is obtained.

Chemotherapy

- The use of chemotherapy in breast cancer is still undergoing evaluation
- At present it can be used preoperatively to shrink the tumor, postoperatively in axillary node-positive breast cancer or in patients with tumors >1cm, and in metastatic disease if required
- Chemotherapy has been shown to substantially improve long-term, relapse-free, and overall survival in both premenopausal and postmenopausal women

COMBINATION CHEMOTHERAPY

- The administration of polychemotherapy, i.e. *2 agents, is superior to single agents
- Cyclophosphamide and doxorubicin (AC), cyclophosphamide, methotrexate and 5-fluorouracil (CMF), or cyclophosphamide, doxorubicin and 5-fluorouracil (CAF), or cyclophosphamide, epirubicin and 5-fluorouracil (CEF), are the most commonly used chemoregimens in the adjuvant setting
- Regimens are given for 3–6 months (depending on the combination used)

- Anthracycline (doxorubicin, epirubicin)-based therapy results in a small but statistically significant improvement in survival over nonanthracycline-containing regimens
- After failing CMF or AC, sequential single agents can be tried. Drugs for end-stage disease are paclitaxel (Taxol), docetaxel (Taxotere), fluorouracil, methotrexate, vinorelbine, and gemcitabine

Efficacy

Efficacy is still being evaluated through chemotherapy trials. High-dose chemotherapy regimens with stem-cell support are being evaluated in patients in high-risk primary breast cancer.

Risks/Benefits

Risks:

- Use caution with infection and bone marrow depression
- Use caution with peptic ulceration and ulcerative colitis, and with renal and hepatic impairment
- Use caution in the elderly and in pregnancy
- Acute side-effects include nausea, vomiting, mucositis, fatigue, alopecia, and myelosuppression

Evidence

- Four RCTs found no difference in survival when neoadjuvant chemotherapy was compared with adjuvant chemotherapy in patients with primary operable breast cancer [3] *Level M*
- Neoadjuvant chemotherapy has been found to reduce the rate of required mastectomy in RCTs of patients with nonmetastatic breast cancer. The RCTs did not find a significantly higher local recurrence rate associated with neoadjuvant chemotherapy compared with adjuvant chemotherapy [3] *Level P*
- No significant difference has been found between different regimens of chemotherapy used in the neoadjuvant setting [3] *Level M*
- A systematic review compared prolonged adjuvant combination chemotherapy with no chemotherapy in patients with nonmetastatic breast cancer. Recurrence rates were significantly lower in patients receiving chemotherapy, and death from all causes was reduced in the chemotherapy group [20] *Level M*
- A systematic review found that adjuvant polychemotherapy typically produces an absolute improvement in 10-year survival of approx. 7–11% in women with early breast cancer aged under 50 years at presentation. Patients aged 50–69 had an improvement of approx. 2–3% [21] *Level M*
- First-line chemotherapy in patients with metastatic breast cancer has been found to be associated with an objective tumor response in 40–60% of women. Median response duration was 6–12 months, irrespective of menopausal or ER status. Complete remission may be achieved in a small proportion of women [7]

Acceptability to patient

Patients find it difficult to cope with the side-effects, especially the alopecia and vomiting. Support and patient counseling is needed to maximize treatment compliance.

Follow up plan

- Close follow up for treatment side-effects is needed
- Follow up for breast cancer recurrence is needed

Patient and caregiver information

- Patients must be informed about the side-effects of chemotherapy before consent is obtained
- Patients find it difficult to cope with the side-effects, especially the alopecia and vomiting
- Support and patient counseling is needed to maximize treatment compliance

LIFESTYLE

- Eating fruits and vegetables, even in very modest amounts, reduces the risk of breast cancer – although the benefits accrue with increasing portions
- Obesity is linked to breast cancer due to the peripheral conversion of estrogens in the adipose tissue leading to higher circulating levels
- Drinking alcohol is associated with an increased risk of breast cancer
- Folate supplementation of at least 600mcg may protect women who consume at least one alcoholic drink daily
- Cigarette smoking was postulated to protect against breast cancer due to its antiestrogenic effect. Recent evidence has shown that women who have smoked for more than 30 years increase their risk of developing breast cancer and at an earlier age
- Physical exercise has a protective effect against developing breast cancer
- Stress is not associated with breast cancer
- Breast-feeding: Some case-control studies suggest that there is a small protective effect of breast-feeding against the development of breast cancer

OUTCOMES

EFFICACY OF THERAPIES

- Localized breast cancer can be treated with breast-conserving surgery in two-thirds of cases
- Mastectomy confers no survival benefit over breast-conserving therapy combined with radiation therapy
- Radiotherapy reduces local disease recurrence

Evidence

Nonmetastatic breast cancer:

- Adjuvant tamoxifen in patients over 50 years old (usually postmenopausal) with nonmetastatic breast cancer reduces the annual risk of recurrence by 29%. Tamoxifen reduces the risk of death from any cause by 20% [2] *Level M*
- Five years of tamoxifen for non-metastatic breast cancer is superior to shorter durations of treatment. There is no evidence that continuing treatment after 5 years is beneficial [3] *Level M*
- Breast-conserving surgery and mastectomy have been compared in patients who were potentially suitable for breast-conserving surgery. All patients received post-operative radiotherapy. There was no significant difference in risk of death over 10 years, or in rates of local recurrence between the groups [15] *Level M*
- There is evidence that radiotherapy given after breast-conserving surgery for ductal carcinoma in situ (DCIS) reduces the risk of local recurrence and invasive carcinoma. There is no evidence of an effect on survival [3] *Level P*
- Radiotherapy reduces the risk of local recurrence when used after breast-conserving surgery. Radiotherapy plus breast-conserving surgery achieves similar rates of survival and local recurrence as mastectomy [15] *Level M*
- Radiotherapy to the chest wall is effective in reducing the risk of mortality from breast cancer at 10 years, and reducing the risk of local recurrence when administered after mastectomy [3] *Level M*
- There is no difference between neoadjuvant chemotherapy and adjuvant chemotherapy in terms of survival in patients with primary operable breast cancer. Neoadjuvant chemotherapy can reduce mastectomy rates [3] *Level M*
- A systematic review found that adjuvant polychemotherapy typically produces an absolute improvement in 10-year survival of approx. 7–11% in women with early breast cancer aged under 50 years at presentation. Patients aged 50–69 had an improvement of approx. 2–3% [21] *Level M*

Metastatic breast cancer:

- Progestins have been found to be as effective as tamoxifen as first-line hormonal therapy in metastatic breast cancer [7] *Level P*
- Anastrozole has been found to be at least as effective as tamoxifen when used as first-line hormonal therapy in postmenopausal patients with metastatic breast cancer [7] *Level P*
- Selective aromatase inhibitors are effective in the treatment of postmenopausal women with metastatic breast cancer who have progressed on first-line tamoxifen treatment or relapsed on adjuvant tamoxifen therapy. Anastrozole, letrozole, and exemestane prolong survival with minimal adverse effects [7] *Level P*
- A significant improvement in progression-free survival and overall survival was found with combined hormonal therapy (gonadorelin analogs plus tamoxifen) as first-line therapy in patients with metastatic breast cancer [11] *Level M*
- Bisphosphonates reduce the risk of developing a skeletal event, and the skeletal event rate in women with advanced breast cancer and clinically evident bone metastases. The time to a skeletal event was increased with bisphosphonates [12] *Level M*

- First-line chemotherapy in patients with metastatic breast cancer has been found to be associated with an objective tumor response in 40–60% of women. Median response duration was 6–12 months irrespective of menopausal or estrogen receptor status. Complete remission may be achieved in a small proportion of women [7]

Review period
Six months.

PROGNOSIS
Prognosis after curative surgery depends on the following:
- Size of the tumor
- Extent of nodal metastases. More than four lymph nodes involved is a bad prognostic sign
- Adverse histology of tumor: 90% 10-year survival if tumor <1cm with node-negative disease; 15% 10-year disease-free survival rate if more than four node metastases and no systemic adjuvant therapy is given

Therapeutic failure
- Radiotherapy, chemotherapy, and hormonal therapy can be used in treatment of relapsed or metastatic breast cancer
- Referral to an oncologist is essential to co-ordinate therapies

Recurrence
- Radiotherapy, chemotherapy, and hormonal therapy can be used in treatment of relapsed or metastatic breast cancer
- Referral to an oncologist is essential to co-ordinate therapies

Deterioration
Referral to an oncologist is essential to co-ordinate therapies.

Terminal illness
- Palliation should be undertaken by a palliative specialist
- Pain relief is essential
- Good palliation ensures the patient remains symptom-free in terminal disease

COMPLICATIONS
Complications of breast cancer include:
- Metastases, mainly to the bone, brain, lung, liver, and contralateral breast
- Malignant hypercalcemia, bone pain, and pathological fractures
- Cerebral edema and cord compression leading to neurologic signs
- Pleural effusions and liver failure
- Marrow infiltration
- Pain from the breast cancer and the metastases
- Anorexia, dysphagia, vomiting, constipation, dyspnea, and cough due to metastases

CONSIDER CONSULT
Referral:
- To an oncologist is essential for all breast cancer patients to co-ordinate care
- To a palliative specialist is required for all patients with terminal disease

PREVENTION

- Some rare familiar forms of breast cancer are linked to BRCA-1/BRCA-2 genes, so genetic counseling and investigation should be performed in families with a high incidence of breast cancer
- Over 50% of women with breast cancer have no identifiable major risk factor, indicating that the search for the etiology of breast cancer in the vast majority of clinical situations is largely incomplete
- Oral contraceptives containing estrogen lead to a small increase in risk of developing breast cancer – about five more cases per 100,000 women
- Postmenopausal estrogen replacement therapy appears to increase the risk modestly, especially after 10–20 years of use
- Genetics is implicated in up to 10% of cases
- Radiation exposure is implicated in development of breast cancer
- Diet may play a role in causing or promoting the growth of breast cancers but conclusive evidence is lacking about particular diets (e.g. high-fat diet)
- Eating even very modest amounts of fruit and vegetables reduces the risk of breast cancer – the benefits accrue with the amount ingested
- Obesity is linked to breast cancer due to the peripheral conversion of estrogens in the adipose tissue leading to higher circulating levels
- There is an association between drinking alcohol and an increased risk of breast cancer
- Folate supplementation of at least 600mcg may protect women who consume at least one alcoholic drink daily
- Cigarette smoking was postulated to protect against breast cancer due to its antiestrogenic effect. Recent evidence has shown that women who have smoked for more than 30 years increase their risk of developing breast cancer and at an earlier age
- Radiation exposure is cited as a contributory factor for breast cancer
- The excess of breast cancer cases among airline flight personnel has been linked to increased levels of ionizing radiation during flights
- Physical exercise has a protective effect against developing breast cancer
- Stress is not associated with breast cancer
- The incidence of breast cancer increases when populations migrate from areas of low incidence of breast cancer to those with a high incidence, indicating that environmental factors are important

MODIFY RISK FACTORS

- Diet may play a role in causing or promoting the growth of breast cancers but conclusive evidence is lacking about particular diets (e.g. high-fat diet)
- Eating fruit and vegetables reduces the risk of breast cancer
- Obesity is linked to breast cancer due to the peripheral conversion of estrogens in the adipose tissue leading to higher circulating levels
- Drinking alcohol increases the risk of breast cancer, but folate supplementation of at least 600mcg may protect women who consume at least one alcoholic drink per day
- Cigarette smoking was once postulated to protect against breast cancer due to its antiestrogenic effect. Recent evidence has shown that women who have smoked for more than 30 years increase their risk of developing breast cancer and at an earlier age
- Radiation exposure is cited as a contributory factor for breast cancer
- Airline flight personnel have a significant excess of breast cancer cases which has been linked to increased ionizing radiation during flights
- Physical exercise has a protective effect
- Stress is not associated with breast cancer
- The incidence of breast cancer increases when populations migrate from areas of low incidence of breast cancer to those with a high incidence, indicating that environmental factors are important

Lifestyle and wellness

TOBACCO

Tobacco is linked to breast cancer and women should not smoke if they wish to prevent it.

ALCOHOL AND DRUGS

Alcohol is linked to breast cancer and limiting alcohol intake should help prevent it.

DIET

Eating fresh fruit and vegetables is beneficial in preventing breast cancer.

PHYSICAL ACTIVITY

Physical exercise has a protective effect against developing breast cancer.

ENVIRONMENT

The incidence of breast cancer increases when populations migrate from areas of low incidence of breast cancer to those with a high incidence, indicating that environmental factors are important.

FAMILY HISTORY

- Genetics is implicated in 5–10% of cases
- Families at high risk have been identified
- BRCA-1, BRCA-2 genetic mutations are associated with high risk of developing breast cancer
- A family history of breast cancer in a first-degree relative triples a woman's risk of developing the disease
- This risk is even higher if a first-degree relative had bilateral or premenopausal breast cancer
- Women with multiple first-degree relatives developing breast cancer may have six times the risk of the general population
- Genetic modification is not possible, so careful screening is necessary
- Prophylactic mastectomies have occurred in patients with a very high risk of breast cancer
- It is also recognized that breast cancer is more prevalent in families who have had previous breast cancer and that approximately 5% of breast cancers cluster very tightly in what appears to be a hereditary fashion

DRUG HISTORY

- Oral contraceptives containing estrogen lead to a small increase in risk of developing breast cancer – about five more cases per 100,000 women – and should be avoided if women already carry an increased risk of developing breast cancer
- Postmenopausal estrogen replacement therapy appears to increase the risk modestly, especially after 10–20 years of use, and should be avoided in women at increased risk
- Medications containing phytoestrogen are linked to breast cancer and should be avoided

CHEMOPROPHYLAXIS

- The Breast Cancer Prevention Trial in North America involving more than 13,000 patients showed that the incidence of breast cancer was reduced by 49% when tamoxifen was given prophylactically to women at high risk of developing breast cancer for 55 months
- The Multiple Outcomes of Raloxifene Evaluation (MORE) study of nearly 8000 postmenopausal patients with osteoporosis at low to average risk of developing breast cancer showed a 76% reduction in the risk of invasive breast cancer after 3 years

SCREENING

The National Comprehensive Cancer Network (NCCN) Practice Guidelines for Breast Cancer Screening include the following:

- Women aged 20–39 years – should undergo physical breast examination every 1–3 years and be encouraged to self-examine breasts
- Women 40 years and older – should undergo physical breast examination annually and be encouraged to attend screening mammography and to self-examine breasts
- Women at high risk due to prior thoracic irradiation – should undergo annual mammography and physical breast examination every 6 months and regularly self-examine
- High-risk women – the NCCN has developed the Gail model to assess individual risk levels and then determine the screening required
- Women with a genetic predisposition – should undergo annual mammography and 6-monthly physical examinations from the age of 25 years
- Women with lobular carcinoma in situ – should undergo annual mammography and physical examination

The cost-efficacy is not fully established, but death may be prevented in one woman in every 1000 undergoing mammography.

PREVENT RECURRENCE

- Careful follow up
- Use of chemoprophylaxis including tamoxifen and raloxifene – trials are underway

Reassess coexisting disease

- Fibrocystic breast disease patients with ductal or lobular hyperplasia are at increased risk of developing breast cancer and careful follow up of these patients is required
- Klinefelter's syndrome is the only known risk factor for male breast cancer and Klinefelter's patients should have careful follow up for signs of breast cancer

ASSOCIATIONS

National Comprehensive Cancer Network
50 Huntingdon Pike, Suite 200
Rockledge PA 19046
Telephone: (215) 728-4788
Fax: (215) 728-3877
email: information@nccn.org
www.nccn.org

SHARE
Self-help for Women with Breast Cancer
19 W 44th Street, No 415
New York, NY 10036-5902
www.sharecancersupport.org

Y-ME
National Organization of Breast Cancer Information and Support
18220 Harwood Ave
Homewood, IL 80430
www.y-me.org

KEY REFERENCES

- Clare SE, Morrow M. Management of the palpable breast mass. In. Diseases of the Breast, 2nd edn. JR Harris, Ed. Philadelphia: Lippincott, Williams & Wilkins; 2000, pp 38–41
- Inglehart JD, Kaelin DM. Diseases of the breast. In Sabiston Book of Surgery. The Biological Basis of Modern Surgical Practice, 16th edn. CM Townsend, RD Beauchamp, BM Evers, KL Mattox, Eds. Philadelphia: WB Saunders; 2001. pp 560–4
- Institute for Clinical Systems Improvement. Diagnosis of breast disease, 2001
- Foster RS. Techniques of diagnosis of palpable breast masses. In. Diseases of the Breast, 2nd edn. JR Harris, Ed. Philadelphia: Lippincott, Williams & Wilkins; 2000, p95–100
- Venta LA. Image-guided biopsy of non-palpable breast lesions. In Diseases of the Breast, 2nd edn. JR Harris, Ed. Philadelphia: Lippincott, Williams & Wilkins; 2000, p149–64
- Kopans DB. Imaging analysis of breast lesions. In Diseases of the Breast, 2nd edn. JR Harris, Ed. Philadelphia: Lippincott, Williams & Wilkins; 2000, p123–47
- Maunsell E, Brisson C, Dubois L, Lauzier S, Fraser A. Work problems after breast cancer: an exploratory qualitative study. Psychooncology 1999:8:467–73
- Ganz PA, Coscarelli A, Fred C, et al. Breast cancer survivors: psychosocial concerns and quality of life. Breast Cancer Res Treat 1996;38:183–9
- Dorval M, Maunsell E, Taylor-Brown J, Kilpatrick M. Marital stability after breast cancer. J Natl Cancer Inst 1999; 91: 54–9
- Hassey-Dow K and Kalinawski BH. Nursing care in patient management of quality of life. In Diseases of the Breast, 2nd edn. JR Harris, ed. Philadelphia: Lippincott, Williams & Wilkins, 2000, p985–99
- Natrajan P, Saumakis K, Gambrell RD. Estrogen replacement therapy in women with previous breast cancer. Am J Obstet Gyn 1999; 181: 288–95
- Fisher B, Costantino JP, Wickerham DL, et al. Tamoxifen for the prevention of breast cancer: report of the National Surgical Adjuvant Breast and Bowel Project P-1 study. J Natl Cancer Inst 1998;90:1371–88
- Early Breast Trialists' Collaborative group. Tamoxifen for early breast cancer: an overview of the randomised trials. Lancet 1998;351:1451–67

Evidence references and guidelines

1 Guideline Oversight Group. Breast cancer treatment. Bloomington (MN): Institute for Clinical Systems Improvement (ICSI); 2000. Available at the National Guidelines Clearinghouse

2 Early Breast Cancer Trialists' Collaborative Group. Tamoxifen for early breast cancer: an overview of the randomized trials. Lancet 1998;351:1451–67. Reviewed in: Clinical Evidence 2001;6: 1353–80

3 Dixon MJ, Rodger A, Johnston S, Gregory K. Breast cancer: non-metastatic; Women's health. In: Clinical Evidence 2001;6:1353–80 London: BMJ Publishing Group

4 Jackson IM, Litherland S, Wakeling AE. Tamoxifen and other antiestrogens. In: Powels TJ, Smith IE, eds. Medical Management of Breast Cancer. London: Martin Dunitz, 1991:51–9. Reviewed in: Clinical Evidence 2001;6:1331–52

5 Arafah BM, Pearson OH. Endocrine treatment of advanced breast cancer. In: Jordan VC, ed. Estrogen/antiestrogen action and breast cancer therapy. Madison: University of Wisconsin Press, 1986:417–429. Reviewed in: Clinical Evidence 2001;6:1331–1352

6 Stuart NS, Warwick J, Blackledge GR, et al. A randomised phase III cross-over study of tamoxifen versus megestrol acetate in advanced and recurrent breast cancer. Eur J Cancer 1996;32A:1888–92. Medline

7 Johnston S, Stebbing J. Breast cancer: metastatic. In: Clinical Evidence 2001;6:1331–52. London: BMJ Publishing Group

8 Messori A, Cattel F, Trippoli S, Vaiani M. Survival in patients with metastatic breast cancer: analysis of randomized studies comparing oral aromatase inhibitors versus megestrol. Anticancer Drugs 2000;11:701–6. Medline

9 Taylor CW, Green S, Dalton WS, et al. Multicenter randomized clinical trial of goserelin versus surgical ovariectomy in premenopausal patients with receptor-positive metastatic breast cancer: an intergroup study. J Clin Oncol 1998;16:994–9. Reviewed in: Clinical Evidence 2001;6:1331–52

10 Boccardo F, Rubagotti A, Perotta A, et al. Ovarian ablation versus goserelin with or without tamoxifen in pre-perimenopausal patients with advanced breast cancer: results of a multicentric Italian study. Ann Oncol 1994;5:337–42. Reviewed in: Clinical Evidence 2001;6:1331–52

11 Klijn JGN, Blamey RW, Boccardo F, et al. Combined tamoxifen and luteneising hormone (LHRH) agonist versus LHRH agonist alone in premenopausal advanced breast cancer; a meta-analysis of four randomized trials. J Clin Oncol 2001;19:343–353. Reviewed in: Clinical Evidence 2001;6:1331–1352

12 Pavlakis N, Stockler M. Bisphosphonates in breast cancer (Cochrane Review). In: The Cochrane Library, 1, 2002. Oxford: Update Software.

13 Hortobagyi GN, Theriault RL, Porter L, et al. Efficacy of pamidronate in reducing skeletal complications in patients with breast cancer and lytic bone metastases. N Engl J Med 1996;335:1785–91. Reviewed in: Clinical Evidence 2001;6:1331–52

14 Theriault RL, Lipton A, Hortobagyi GN. Pamidronate reduces skeletal morbidity in women with advanced breast cancer and lytic bone lesions; a randomised placebo controlled trial. J Clin Oncol 1999;17:846–54. Reviewed in: Clinical Evidence 2001;6:1331–52

15 Early Breast Cancer Trialists' Collaborative Group. Effects of radiotherapy and surgery in early breast cancer: an overview of the randomised trials. N Engl J Med 1995;333:1444–55. Reviewed in: Clinical Evidence 2001;6:1353–80

16 Morris AD, Morris RD, Wilson JF, et al. Breast-conserving therapy versus mastectomy in early stage breast cancer: a meta-analysis of 10 year survival. Cancer J Sci Am 1997;3:6–12. Reviewed in: Clinical Evidence 2001;6:1353–80

17 Fisher B, Dignam J, Wolmark N, et al. Lumpectomy and radiation therapy for the treatment of intraductal breast cancer: findings of the National Surgical Adjuvant Breast and Bowel Project B-17. J Clin Oncol 1998;16:441–52. Reviewed in: Clinical Evidence 2001;6:1353–80

18 Julien JP, Bijker N, Fentimen IS, et al. Radiotherapy in breast-conserving treatment for ductal carcinoma in situ; first results of EORTC randomized phase III trial 10853. Lancet 2000;355:528–33. Reviewed in: Clinical Evidence 2001;6:1353–80.

19 Dixon MJ, Rodger A, Johnston S, Gregory K. Breast cancer: non-metastatic: women's health. In: Clinical Evidence 2001;6:1353–80 London: BMJ Publishing Group

20 Early Breast Cancer Trialists' Collaborative Group. Polychemotherapy for early breast cancer: an overview of the randomized trials. Lancet 1998;352:930–42. Reviewed in: Clinical Evidence 2001;6:1353–80

21 Early Breast Cancer Trialists' Collaborative Group. Multi-agent chemotherapy for early breast cancer (Cochrane Review). In: The Cochrane Library, 1, 2002. Oxford: Update Software.

FAQS

Question 1

What does being an altered BRCA-1 and BRCA-2 carrier mean to the patient?

ANSWER 1

- Their lifetime susceptibility to breast and ovarian cancers is substantially elevated
- They have an increased risk of developing breast cancer at a younger age (before menopause)
- Women in the general population have a 12% chance of developing breast cancer, while women with an altered BRCA-1 or BRCA-2 gene have a 50–85% chance (500–850 per 1000)
- Women in the general population have a 1.5% chance of developing ovarian cancer, while women with an altered BRCA-1 gene have a 5–40% chance, and women with an altered BRCA-2 gene have a 10–20% chance

Question 2

Which patients have to receive adjuvant therapy?

ANSWER 2

Decisions must be made on an individual basis, taking into account the following prognostic factors:

- Size
- Lymph node involvement
- Hormone receptor status
- Histologic grade
- Proliferation rate
- Oncogene activation

Menopausal status (whether or not the patient has gone through the menopause), her general health, and her personal preference are also important. The final decision must be made in consultation with an oncologist.

Question 3

How long is the adjuvant treatment?

ANSWER 3

That depends on the stage of the tumor. We commonly recommend chemotherapy for 6 months (generally one cycle every 3–4 weeks), radiotherapy 5 days a week for 5 weeks, and hormonal therapy (oral tamoxifen) every day for 5 years.

CONTRIBUTORS

Gordon H Baustian, MD
Luciana G O Clark, MD
Sandeep Garg, MD

CARCINOID SYNDROME

SUMMARY INFORMATION

DESCRIPTION

- Symptom complex characterized by paroxysmal vasomotor disturbances, diarrhea, bronchospasm, and cutaneous flushing
- Symptoms caused by the action of amines and peptides (serotonin, bradykinin, histamine) produced by tumors arising from neuroendocrine cells
- Cardiac valvular lesions (tricuspid incompetence and pulmonary stenosis) often result from the presence of these tumors
- Most carcinoid tumors that produce carcinoid syndrome originate in the intestine, and the syndrome usually does not appear until there is extensive metastasis by the carcinoid to the liver
- The syndrome may occur without liver metastasis, especially when the primary site is the ovary
- One- to two-thirds of patients develop liver metastases without carcinoid syndrome

URGENT ACTION

Urgent hospital referral for carcinoid crisis:

- When the tumor outgrows its blood supply and large amounts of mediators are released
- During surgical manipulation
- If symptoms worsen dramatically and may be life-threatening

Crisis is treated with high-dose octreotide and management of fluid balance (central line may be needed).

KEY! DON'T MISS!

- Carcinoid is rare but not as rare as is perceived and so easily missed
- The diagnosis should always be considered in a patient with flushing who does not respond to intervention for the perceived etiology, e.g. menopause

ICD9 CODE
259.2 Carcinoid syndrome.

SYNONYMS
- Thorson-Bioerck syndrome
- Argentaffinoma syndrome
- Flush syndrome
- Cassidy-Scholte syndrome

CARDINAL FEATURES
- A symptom complex characterized by paroxysmal vasomotor disturbances, diarrhea, bronchospasm, and cutaneous flushing
- Carcinoid syndrome may cause cardiac valvular lesions, most commonly leading to tricuspid incompetence and pulmonary stenosis
- Caused by the action of amines and peptides (serotonin, bradykinin, histamine) produced by tumors arising from neuroendocrine cells
- Carcinoid tumors are found in the: appendix (40%); small bowel (20%); rectum (15%); esophagus, stomach, colon (10%); ovary, biliary tract, and pancreas (3%)
- The occurrence and severity of the syndrome are directly related to tumor bulk in an area that drains into the systemic circulation
- In patients with hepatic metastasis, the syndrome is common and will almost always occur, at least biochemically, if involvement of the liver can be detected clinically
- The syndrome may occur without liver metastasis, especially when the primary site is the extraintestinal
- In one- to two-thirds of patients, liver metastases develop without the carcinoid syndrome
- Carcinoid arising in foregut derivatives (bronchus, stomach, pancreas, duodenum, biliary tract) may produce carcinoid syndrome and may be associated with the multiple endocrine neoplasia type I (MEN-I) syndrome (with parathyroid, pituitary, and pancreatic islet cell tumors)
- Treatment includes somatostatin analogs, surgical resection of tumors, hepatic vein embolization, and chemotherapy

CAUSES
Common causes
- The main causes are the carcinoid tumors, which can be found in the: appendix (40%); small bowel (20%); rectum (15%); esophagus, stomach, colon (10%); ovary, biliary tract, pancreas (3%); bronchus (3.5%)
- Most tumors leading to carcinoid syndrome originate in the intestine, and the syndrome usually does not appear until there is metastasis by carcinoid to the liver
- The syndrome may occur without liver metastasis, especially when the primary site is extraintestinal
- In one- to two-thirds of patients, liver metastases develop without carcinoid syndrome

EPIDEMIOLOGY
Incidence and prevalence
INCIDENCE
- Clinical disease: 7–13 cases per one million
- Autopsy: 6500 per one million
- About 5–10% of patients with carcinoid tumors develop symptoms of carcinoid syndrome

FREQUENCY
Carcinoid tumors are found incidentally in 0.5–0.75% of autopsies.

Demographics

AGE

Peak age incidence depends on location of tumor:

- Appendiceal tumors diagnosed at average age 36 years
- Nonappendiceal tumors typically diagnosed in the 40–60 years age group

GENDER

There is no sexual predominance.

GENETICS

- Generally thought to be sporadic
- There is increased incidence among first-degree relatives of patients with carcinoid
- Carcinoids of the bronchus, stomach, and duodenum may occur in association with MEN-I

DIFFERENTIAL DIAGNOSIS

The following differential diagnoses can mimic carcinoid syndrome.

Idiopathic flushing

FEATURES

- Normal 5-hydroxyindoleacetic acid (5-HIAA) excretion
- More often in younger females, usually not associated with other classic carcinoid symptoms such as diarrhea and hypotension
- With the carcinoid syndrome, patients turn red – they do not just feel warm all over; the exception is in African-Americans, in whom conjunctival injection may be the sole manifestation of flushing

Ingestion of certain foods and medications

There is usually a clear history of ingestion of the causative substance. Flushing occurs as a consequence; alcohol is a particularly common agent leading to flushing.

FEATURES

Flushing can occur with the following drugs:

- Diltiazem
- Nifedipine
- Nicotinic acid
- Levodopa
- Bromocriptine
- Thyrotropin-releasing hormone
- Amyl nitrite

Flushing can occur with the following foods:

- Ingestion of monosodium glutamate (Chinese restaurant syndrome)
- Ingestion of hot drinks
- Alcohol

Menopause

Hot flushes are a common symptom of the menopause.

FEATURES

- Women of menopausal age find that their menstruation becomes less frequent
- Elevated follicle-stimulating hormone (FSH) and luteinizing hormone (LH)
- Normal 5-HIAA

VIPoma

Vasoactive intestinal peptide – pancreatic islet cell tumor (islet D1 cell).

FEATURES

- Diarrhea
- Hypokalemia
- Hypochlorhydria

Medullary carcinoma of thyroid

Arise from parafollicular (C) cells of thyroid.

FEATURES
- Thyroid nodule
- Watery diarrhea
- Flushing (less marked than in carcinoid syndrome)

SIGNS & SYMPTOMS
Signs
- Flushing
- Heart valve defects, especially tricuspid regurgitation and pulmonary stenosis
- A mass in the abdomen
- Liver metastases are palpable in over 50% of cases

Flushing may be associated with dizziness, tachycardia, and hypotension and can be precipitated by anything that changes vascular tone. There are different types of flush.
Midgut flush:
- Usually associated with carcinoids of the ileum
- Appears like a mild sunburn involving the face, neck, and upper trunk
- Lasts for only seconds or minutes
- It is not terribly troublesome to the patient, who may feel a little warm
- Patients may develop facial telangiectasia concentrated over the Malar regions

Foregut flush:
- More intense than the midgut variety
- Usually associated with gastric or pulmonary carcinoids
- Frequently associated with conjunctival injection and facial edema
- Patients may take on a constant red or cyanotic hue and they may develop more persistent facial edema, producing a leonine appearance

Histamine variety:
- Identified with gastric carcinoids
- Generalized, spreading erythematous blotches and wheals, which will clear centrally
- These lesions are very pruritic and most distressing to the patient

Symptoms
Gastrointestinal tract carcinoid tumors have nonspecific clinical symptoms. The most common symptoms are:
- Abdominal pain
- Nausea and vomiting
- Weight loss
- Gastrointestinal blood loss

Symptoms of carcinoid syndrome include:
- Diarrhea (>70%) – often associated with abdominal bloating and audible peristaltic rushes. Uncommonly, may be exceedingly profuse, associated with life-threatening fluid and electrolyte losses. It is difficult to discern whether it is caused by the tumor per se or by mechanical factors (small bowel obstruction or surgery). Transit times are 2-fold faster in small bowel and 6-fold faster in colon in these patients
- Intermittent bronchospasm (25%) – severe dyspnea and wheezing
- Abdominal pain
- Intermittent intestinal obstruction
- Gastrointestinal bleeding

Carcinoid crisis (carcinoid crisis is often a terminal event):

- Observed in patients who have intense 'foregut' syndromes or greatly elevated 5-HIAA levels (=200mg/day (1046mcmol/day)); may occur spontaneously or may be precipitated by physically stressful situations, particularly the induction of anesthesia or during or soon after a course of chemotherapy
- Intense generalized flush that does not resolve spontaneously and may persist for hours or days
- Severe exacerbation of diarrhea associated with abdominal pain
- Mild light-headedness or vertigo
- Somnolence to deep coma
- Tachycardia
- Rhythm irregularity
- Hypertension
- Severe hypotension
- Sharp increase in 5-HIAA excretion (not all patients)

Carcinoid heart disease:

- Development of plaque-like thickenings on the endocardium of the heart valve leaflets, atria, and ventricles in about 20% of patients
- Patients almost always have a long history of the syndrome, averaging 6 years
- Usually have very high levels of 5-HIAA (mean value 270mg/24h)
- Pathology of carcinoid heart disease is restricted to the endocardium and subendocardium, preserving the deeper architecture of the valve
- Presents the characteristic murmurs of the respective valves involved
- Most common functional impairment will be right-sided heart failure
- Treatment is relieve of fluid retention and even valve surgery

ASSOCIATED DISORDERS

- Carcinoid arising in foregut derivatives (bronchus, stomach, pancreas, duodenum, biliary tract) may produce carcinoid syndrome and may be associated with the multiple endocrine neoplasia type I (MEN-I) syndrome (with parathyroid, pituitary, and pancreatic islet cell tumors)
- May be associated with pernicious anemia due to excessive gastrin stimulation

KEY! DON'T MISS!

- Carcinoid is rare but not as rare as is perceived and so easily missed
- The diagnosis should always be considered in a patient with flushing who does not respond to intervention for the perceived etiology, e.g. menopause

CONSIDER CONSULT

The primary care physician can perform the assessment of 5-HIAA levels; however, evaluation of the origin of carcinoid syndrome will require referral to a specialist.

INVESTIGATION OF THE PATIENT

Direct questions to patient

- Q **Have you experienced abdominal pain, nausea and vomiting, weight loss, or gastrointestinal blood loss?** Gastrointestinal tract carcinoid tumors have a nonspecific clinical presentation and all these can occur
- Q **Have you noticed your skin flushing, especially red-purple flushes in the face, spreading to the neck and upper trunk?** Cutaneous flushing occurs in 75–90% of patients
- Q **Have you had episodes of severe diarrhea associated with abdominal bloating and audible bowel sounds?** Diarrhea occurs in >70% of patients with carcinoid syndrome

- Q **Have you experienced wheezing and shortness of breath?** Intermittent bronchospasm occurs in 25% of patients
- Q **Have you suffered from episodes of severe abdominal pain, vomiting and constipation, and/or gastrointestinal blood loss or melena?** All can occur in carcinoid syndrome

Family history

- Q **Have any close relatives had a history of flushing and diarrhea, or been diagnosed as having carcinoid syndrome?** There is possibly an increased risk in first-degree relatives.

Examination

- **On examination of the face, is there evidence of telangiectasia?** Often present in carcinoid syndrome
- **On examination of the heart, are any murmurs present, especially suggestive of tricuspid regurgitation or pulmonary stenosis?** The right side of the heart is most commonly affected
- **On examination of the abdomen, are there any masses or hepatomegaly?** The primary tumor and liver metastases are palpable in >50% of patients

Summary of investigative tests

- Investigations should be aimed at detecting the site of the carcinoid tumor so that it can be resected
- No international staging system exists for carcinoid tumors
- The diagnostic hallmark is an increased 24-h urinary excretion of 5-HIAA, a metabolite of serotonin (5-hydroxytryptamine)
- Endoscopy is normally used to detect gastric, duodenal, intestinal, and colon carcinoid
- Imaging studies to detect the primary carcinoid tumor and metastases
- Chest X-ray is useful to detect bronchial carcinoids
- Assessment of the extent and localization of both primary and metastatic tumor is aided by computerized tomography (CT) of the abdomen and chest
- Angiography can be used to detect intestinal and hepatic carcinoid
- Octreotide scintigraphy, normally performed by a specialist, localizes the primary tumor and recurrences with accuracy
- Once the tumor site has been identified, biopsy of the tumor should be performed
- Echocardiography and monitoring for right-sided congestive heart failure is recommended in patients with unresectable disease

DIAGNOSTIC DECISION

No accepted, published guideline found.

CLINICAL PEARLS

- Serotonin is synthesized by the tumor from tryptophan and metabolized to 5-HIAA, which appears in the urine and is used to monitor the course of carcinoid syndrome
- Although there is a clear and direct relationship between urine 5-HIAA levels and the incidence and severity of the syndrome, this is not an invariable correlation
- The symptoms of the syndrome vary in frequency. Flushing is most frequent, followed by diarrhea, heart disease, and bronchoconstriction

THE TESTS

Body fluids

24-H URINARY EXCRETION OF 5-HYDROXYINDOLEACETIC ACID

Description

- 5-HIAA is a metabolite of serotonin (5-hydroxytryptamine), which is increased in carcinoid syndrome
- This metabolite is excreted in the urine

- At a set time, the patient should empty the bladder completely and this sample discarded
- The patient should then collect all urine passed in 24h
- At the end of the 24h, the bladder should be emptied and this sample added to the collection

Advantages/Disadvantages

Advantages:

- Simple and safe
- Noninvasive

Disadvantages:

- Sample collections may be inconvenient for the patient
- Dietary advice is necessary to avoid false-positive

Normal

Normal range urine 5-HIAA is 2–8mg/day (10–40mcmol/day).

Abnormal

24h urinary excretion of >9mg 5-HIAA.

Cause of abnormal result

- When dietary 5-hydroxyindoles are excluded, 24-h urinary excretion of >25mg 5-HIAA daily is diagnostic of carcinoid
- Elevation in the range of 9–25mg may be seen with carcinoid syndrome, nontropical sprue, or acute intestinal obstruction
- Ingestion of walnuts, pecans, butternuts, bananas, pineapples, and tomatoes
- If the 24-h level is 20mg/day (104mcmol/day) or higher, the test is positive, regardless of dietary intake

Drugs, disorders and other factors that may alter results

- Bananas and walnuts contain enough serotonin to produce abnormally elevated urinary excretion of 5-HIAA after their ingestion
- False elevations are also seen after ingestion of pineapples, eggplant, and avocados, as well as certain medications (acetaminophen, caffeine, guaifenesin, reserpine)

Biopsy

PERCUTANEOUS BIOPSY

Description

- The aim is to collect a sample of the lesion for histology
- The biopsy can be done percutaneously
- If the biopsy method is unsuccessful the patient should be put forward for laparoscopy

Advantages/Disadvantages

Advantages:

- Minimally invasive to obtain biopsy material
- Patient not requiring a general anesthetic
- Diagnostic for carcinoid
- Histologic grading of the carcinoid
- Treatment methods can be defined

Disadvantage: biopsy material can be limited, making histologic analysis difficult

Abnormal

Carcinoid tumor has the following histologic features:

- Uniform small cells arranged in nests with surrounding fibrous stroma
- Cellular cytoplasm is pink and stippled
- Small round nuclei with nucleoli
- Mitoses are infrequent

Cause of abnormal result

Carcinoid.

Imaging

CHEST X-RAY

Description

- A chest X-ray is abnormal in about 75% of patients with a pulmonary carcinoid tumor
- It will enable the detection of the site of the lesions within the lungs

Advantages/Disadvantages

Advantages:

- Noninvasive
- Inexpensive
- Low radiation dose given to patient

Abnormal

- Lobar atelectasis or obstructive pneumonia with proximally located carcinoid
- In the periphery is a well-demarcated, round, or ovoid radiopaque mass with sharp notched margins
- Hilar adenopathy is uncommon

Cause of abnormal result

Carcinoid tumors.

Drugs, disorders and other factors that may alter results

Other causes of coin lesions in the lung include:

- Malignancy
- Abscesses
- Granuloma
- Arteriovenous malformation
- Foreign body

COMPUTERIZED TOMOGRAPHY

Description

- CT scan may be used to detect the primary tumor and metastases
- It allows for the assessment of tumor disease in the bowel wall and mesentery, lymph nodes, and liver

Advantages/Disadvantages

Advantages:

- Simple, safe, and noninvasive
- Useful to detect liver metastases

Disadvantage: not sensitive in detecting the primary carcinoid if within the bowel

Abnormal

Stellate or curvilinear mesentery fibrosis radiating from lesion with distorted bowel loops; irregular hypodense metastatic lesions in the liver.

Cause of abnormal result

Carcinoid tumor and metastases.

ENDOSCOPY

Description

- Diagnostic endoscopy can be helpful in carcinoid tumor
- Upper endoscopy is useful for diagnosing lesions in the gastric and duodenal sites
- Colonoscopy is useful for detecting tumor lesions in the colon and rectum
- Biopsies of the tumor lesions can be taken to confirm diagnosis

Advantages/Disadvantages

Advantages:

- Diagnostic for carcinoid if lesions are biopsied
- Minimally invasive requiring no anesthetic

Disadvantages:

- Patients can find procedure unpleasant
- Specialist procedure with potentially serious complications

Abnormal

Lesions detected for biopsy.

Cause of abnormal result

- Carcinoid syndrome
- Other malignant disease

ANGIOGRAPHY

Description

Angiography can be used to detect lesions due to hepatic or intestinal carcinoid.

Advantages/Disadvantages

Advantages:

- Detects occult tumors
- Aids in defining management of disease
- Procedure not requiring anesthetic

Disadvantages:

- Invasive and requiring specialist expertise
- Not diagnostic

Abnormal

Lesions identified.

Cause of abnormal result

- Carcinoid syndrome
- Other malignant disease

OCTREOTRIDE SCINTIGRAPHY

Description

- Scanning with radiolabeled octreotride identifies sites of primary and metastatic tumor in about two-thirds of cases
- It is a diagnostic tool for carcinoid syndrome
- It has high specificity and sensitivity for carcinoid lesions
- The development of a 72-h half-life allows for three scans to be performed at 24-h intervals

Advantages/Disadvantages

Advantages:

- It is a diagnostic tool for carcinoid syndrome
- It has high specificity and sensitivity
- A positive test indicates a good response to treatment with octreotide

Disadvantage: 2% of cases will have false-negative scans.

Abnormal

Positive imaging of tumor.

Cause of abnormal result

- Carcinoid syndrome
- Other neuroendocrine tumors

ECHOCARDIOGRAPHY

Description

- Detects anatomy and function of the heart
- Uses ultrasound imagery
- Useful to detecting abnormalities in the cardiac anatomy and cycle

Advantages/Disadvantages

- Advantage: simple, safe, and noninvasive
- Disadvantage: specialist required to report the findings of the procedure

Abnormal

- Plaque-like thickening of endocardium of valvular cusps and cardiac chambers
- Endocardial fibrosis, predominantly involving endocardium, chordae, and valves
- The fibrosing process tends to produce incompetence of tricuspid valve and stenosis of the smaller pulmonary orifice
- Occurs primarily on right side of heart leading to right-sided congestive heart failure

Cause of abnormal result

- Carcinoid lesion can be causal of these changes.

CONSIDER CONSULT

Development of an appropriate management plan will require referral to a specialist.

IMMEDIATE ACTION

Urgent hospital treatment for carcinoid crisis is required with high-dose octreotide and management of fluid balance (central line may be needed).

PATIENT AND CAREGIVER ISSUES

Patient or caregiver request

- **What is carcinoid syndrome?** The patient will not know much about carcinoid syndrome as it is a rare condition. Full explanation of the cause, significance, and available treatments will be necessary
- **Is carcinoid disease malignant?** Not all carcinoid disease is malignant and this must be stressed to the patient

Health-seeking behavior

- **Have you sought medical advice?** The patient may well have already sought medical advice for nonspecific symptoms such as weight loss, abdominal pain, and diarrhea
- **Are you aware of the possible effects of the carcinoid tumor?** It is important to explain the nonspecific nature of effects of the carcinoid tumor before the carcinoid syndrome develops
- **Do any foods seem to trigger flushing?** The patient may have found that flushing is triggered by certain foods and avoidance of these foods is part of their symptom management

MANAGEMENT ISSUES

Goals

- Curative resection of the tumor is the prime goal
- Palliation of nonresectable hepatic metastases includes medical and surgical interventions
- Alleviation of symptoms, e.g. flushing, diarrhea through medication

SUMMARY OF THERAPEUTIC OPTIONS

Choices

- The aim is to surgically resect the carcinoid tumor to achieve cure in localized disease
- Metastatic disease may require no treatment if symptoms are not seriously interfering with quality of life and if the tumor is not exhibiting a biologically aggressive growth pattern
- Antiproliferative medical strategies to control the growth of metastatic carcinoid tumors include long-acting somatostatin analogs octreotide or lanreotide. However, the success rate is <50%
- Concerted strategy of removal of the primary tumor, reduction in tumor bulk, and the administration of octreotide can lead to considerable amelioration of symptoms and complications
- Palliative surgery can enable prolonged asymptomatic periods even with metastases present
- Percutaneous embolization of the hepatic arterial supply to the most involved hepatic lobe sometimes can reduce inoperable hepatic metastases; the procedure carries a high risk of complications

Control of clinical manifestations:

- The patient should avoid alcohol to prevent flushing
- Long-acting somatostatin analogs octreotide or lanreotide are the most effective treatments for flushing and diarrhea (lanreotide should be administered by a specialist)
- Diarrhea usually responds to diphenoxylate with atropine
- In patients with histamine-secreting gastric carcinoids, blockade of both H_1 and H_2 histamine receptors markedly ameliorates flushing, e.g. diphenhydramine 25–50mg four times daily and ranitidine 150mg twice daily
- Bronchospasm can be treated with both aminophylline and/or albuterol

- Niacin supplements may be useful to prevent pellagra as the tumor uses dietary tryptophan for serotonin synthesis and results in nutritional deficiency in some patients

Cytotoxic chemotherapy:
- There is no effective chemotherapy regimen for carcinoid tumors – most oncologists use a combination of 5-fluorouracil and streptozocin for advanced, progressive, and nonresectable carcinoid tumors
- Results are poor and the benefits may not counterbalance its toxicity

Clinical pearls
- There is no reason to tell patients to avoid serotonin-containing foods (walnuts, pecans, butternuts, bananas, pineapples, and tomatoes) unless they are collecting urine for a 5-hydroxyindoleacetic acid (5-HIAA) assay. These foods do not produce any significant aggravation of the syndrome
- 40–50% of patients with small intestine and proximal colon tumors experience the syndrome. The disorder is less frequent in patients with bronchial carcinoids, is rare with appendiceal carcinoids, and does not occur in patients with rectal carcinoids, even with advanced-stage tumors and metastases
- The carcinoid syndrome is a manifestation of late-stage disease. Two-thirds of the patients had physical signs of cancer when they presented with the syndrome – an enlarged liver or an abdominal mass

Never
- Surgical manipulation of the tumor can lead to a carcinoid crisis
- Therefore, full intensive care facilities are required during and after surgical resection

FOLLOW UP
Will depend on clinical context of symptoms, tumor origin, and presence of metastases.

Plan for review
Monitor effect of treatment on presence and severity of symptoms, and effect on quality of life – adjust treatment accordingly. Further management may be required for further spread of metastases.

Information for patient or caregiver
- Full discussion of prognosis and need for regular review to ensure optimum control of the disease
- Discuss features of carcinoid crisis and the need for urgent medical assistance

DRUGS AND OTHER THERAPIES: DETAILS
Drugs
OCTREOTIDE
- Long-acting analog of somatostatin
- Drug of choice to control diarrhea and flushing

Dose
- Regular octreotide: during the first 2 weeks of therapy, 100–600mcg/day subcutaneously in two to four divided doses (mean daily dosage is 300mcg)
- Experience with doses above 750mcg/day is limited
- A new long-acting octreotide given as a depot every 3 months is available. Patients should begin with regular octreotide injections given subcutaneously (as described above) for at least 2 weeks. Patients who tolerate the drug may be switched to the long-acting preparation. Initial dosage of octreotide long-acting preparation is 20mg given by the intramuscular route intragluteally at 4-week intervals for 2 months. Patients should continue to receive regular

octreotide for at least 2 weeks in the same dosage they were taking before the switch. After 2 months of a 20mg dosage of octreotide long-lasting preparation, dosage may be increased to 30mg every 4 weeks if symptoms are not adequately controlled. For patients who respond well the dosage can be lowered to 10mg octreotide long-lasting preparation

Efficacy

- Disappearance or improvement in flushes occurred in 68% (17 of 25) on octreotide
- Disappearance or improvement of diarrhea in 50% (11 of 22) on octreotide
- This is frequently associated with a reduction in urinary 5-HIAA excretion

Risks/Benefits

Risks:

- Single doses of octreotide acetate have been shown to inhibit gallbladder contractility and decrease bile secretion
- Octreotide acetate alters the balance between the counter-regulatory hormones, insulin, glucagon, and growth hormone, which may result in hypoglycemia or hyperglycemia
- Octreotide acetate may alter absorption of dietary fats in some patients
- In patients with severe renal failure requiring dialysis, the half-life of octreotide acetate may be increased, necessitating adjustment of the maintenance dosage

Benefits:

- Markedly improves the flushing and diarrhea in most patients with carcinoid syndrome
- A considerable improvement in quality of life may be achieved
- About 5% of patients achieve tumor regression
- Can prevent or treat carcinoid crises that accompany the massive release of mediators that sometimes occurs during operative procedures and tumor necrosis

Side-effects and adverse reactions

- Cardiovascular system: sinus bradycardia, conduction abnormalities, and dysrhythmias
- Central nervous system: fatigue, dizziness, headache, and weakness
- Gastrointestinal: nausea, vomiting, diarrhea, distension, flatulence, and pancreatitis
- Metabolic: hyperglycemia, hypoglycemia, hypothyroidism, and goiter
- Musculoskeletal: myalgia and Bell's palsy
- Skin: alopecia and local pain on injection

Interactions (other drugs)

Patients taking insulin, oral hypoglycemic agents, beta-blockers, calcium channel blockers, or agents to control fluid and electrolyte balance will require dose adjustments of these treatments.

Contraindications

- Pregnancy
- Breast-feeding
- Gall bladder disease
- Diabetes mellitus

Acceptability to patient

Patients may find three injections daily unacceptable.

Follow up plan

- Careful follow up to check that the carcinoid symptoms are being treated effectively
- Patient compliance may be limited by the need for injections

Patient and caregiver information

- Instruction in sterile subcutaneous injection technique
- For prolonged storage, ampoules and multidose vials should be stored in the refrigerator at 2–8°C (35.6–46.4°F)
- The solution can be allowed to come to room temperature prior to administration

LANREOTIDE

Long-acting analog of somatostatin.

Dose

Dosage ahould be decided by a specialist.

Efficacy

- Disappearance or improvement in flushes occurred in 53.8%
- Disappearance or improvement of diarrhea in 45.4%
- This is frequently associated with a reduction in urinary 5-HIAA excretion

Risks/Benefits

Benefits:

- Markedly improves the flushing and diarrhea in most patients with carcinoid syndrome
- A considerable improvement in quality of life may be achieved
- About 5% of patients achieve tumor regression
- Can prevent or treat carcinoid crises that accompany the massive release of mediators that sometimes occurs during operative procedures and tumor necrosis

Evidence

- Lanreotide is effective and safe in patients with gastrointestinal neuroendocrine tumors and hormone-related symptoms [1]
- Slow-release lanreotide treatment in endocrine gastrointestinal tumors has been demonstrated to be effective [2]
- Lanreotide was found to be effective and well tolerated in the treatment of carcinoid [3]

Acceptability to patient

Injections once every 10 days improves acceptability to patients.

Follow up plan

Follow up will depend on the clinical context.

Patient and caregiver information

Instruction in sterile subcutaneous injection technique.

DIPHENOXYLATE WITH ATROPINE

Used to control diarrhea.

Dose

- Adult oral dose: 5mg four times daily
- Should be accompanied by appropriate fluid and electrolyte therapy, when indicated

Efficacy

Only partially effective in reducing diarrhea.

Risks/Benefits

Risks:

- Classified as a Schedule V controlled substance by federal law
- Dosage recommendations must be strictly adhered to
- Risk of addiction
- Use extreme caution in patients with advanced hepatorenal disease and in all patients with abnormal liver function as hepatic coma may be precipitated
- Concurrent use of diphenoxylate hydrochloride atropine sulfate with monoamine oxidase inhibitors (MAOIs) may precipitate hypertensive crisis

- Diphenoxylate hydrochloride may potentiate the action of barbiturates, tranquilizers, and alcohol. Therefore, the patient should be closely observed when any of these are used concomitantly
- Use caution when administering to nursing mothers

Benefits:
- Safe
- Inexpensive

Side-effects and adverse reactions
- Cardiovascular system: tachycardia, flushing, These effects may occur, especially in children
- Central nervous system: euphoria, depression, malaise/lethargy, confusion, sedation/drowsiness, dizziness, restlessness, headache, hyperthermia
- Gastrointestinal system: toxic megacolon, paralytic ileus, pancreatitis, vomiting, nausea, anorexia, abdominal discomfort
- Genitourinary: urinary retention
- Hypersensitivity: allergic: anaphylaxis, angioneurotic edema, urticaria, swelling of the gums, pruritus
- Other: numbness of extremities
- Skin: dryness of the skin and mucous membranes

Interactions (other drugs)
■ Alcohol ■ Barbiturates ■ Tranquilizers ■ MAOIs

Contraindications
■ Known hypersensitivity to diphenoxylate or atropine ■ Obstructive jaundice ■ Diarrhea associated with pseudomembranous enterocolitis or enterotoxin-producing bacteria ■ Pregnancy category C ■ Not recommended in children under 2 years of age

Acceptability to patient
Fatigue may be a problem.

Patient and caregiver information
May cause fatigue, especially in combination with alcohol or tranquilizers.

DIPHENHYDRAMINE
- Antihistamine to control flushing symptoms
- Available over-the-counter (OTC)

Dose
- Dosage should be individualized
- Adult oral dose: 15–50mg every 4h
- Maximum 400mg/day

Efficacy
Useful in controlling flushing.

Risks/Benefits
Risks:
- Use caution in hepatic and renal disease
- Use caution in hypertension, cardiovascular disease, hyperthyroidism
- May cause drowsiness

Benefit: safe, inexpensive medication

Side-effects and adverse reactions
- Cardiovascular system: palpitations, tachycardia
- Central nervous system: sedation, dizziness, drowsiness
- Eyes, ears, nose, and throat: blurred vision, dry nose and throat
- Gastrointestinal: constipation, nausea, vomiting, dry mouth
- Genitourinary: urinary difficulties
- Hematologic: bone marrow suppression, hemolytic anemia
- Respiratory: increased secretions, wheezing

Interactions (other drugs)
Anticholinergics (may enhance central nervous effects of anticholinergics).

Contraindications
- **Narrow-angle glaucoma**
- **Bladder neck obstruction**

Acceptability to patient
May cause drowsiness and interfere with activities.

Patient and caregiver information
- Avoid driving or other hazardous activities if drowsiness occurs
- Avoid use of alcohol or other central nervous system depressants while taking drug

RANITIDINE
Competitive and reversible blocker of histamine H_2 receptors.

Dose
Adult oral dose: 150mg twice daily.

Efficacy
Effective in treating itching, flushing, and urticaria.

Risks/Benefits
Risks:
- Use caution with renal and hepatic disease
- Use caution with gastric malignancy and immunocompromised patients
- Use caution with the elderly

Benefits:
- Safe
- Inexpensive
- Well tolerated
- Effective

Side-effects and adverse reactions
- Cardiovascular system: atrioventricular block, palpatations
- Central nervous system: dizziness, vertigo
- Gastrointestinal: abdominal pain, constipation, diarrhea, hepatitis, pancreatitis
- Hematologic: granulocytopenia, leukopenia, thrombocytopenia
- Musculoskeletal: arthralgia, myalgia
- Skin: alopecia, erythema multiforme, rash

Interactions (other drugs)

■ Cephalosporins ■ Calcium channel blockers ■ Enoxacin ■ Glipizide ■ Ketoconazole

Contraindications

■ Known hypersensitivity to the drug ■ Pregnancy and breast-feeding

Acceptability to patient

Very well tolerated.

Patient and caregiver information

Stagger doses of ranitidine and antacids.

AMINOPHYLLINE

Useful if the patient has symptomatic wheezing.

Dose

- Adult initial oral dose: 16mg/kg/24h or 400mg/24h (whichever is less) of theophylline in divided doses at 6–8h intervals
- The above dosage may be increased in approx. 25% increments at 3-day intervals as long as the drug is tolerated
- Reduce dose to 2.5mg/kg every 8h in older patients, patients with heart failure, or cor pulmonale

Risks/Benefits

Risks:

- Many dose-related side-effects
- Many drug interactions
- Inferior to albuterol as a bronchodilator
- Use caution in cardiac disorders, hepatic disease, and history of peptic ulcer

Benefit: useful to improve breathing in wheezing patients

Side-effects and adverse reactions

- Cardiovascular system: circulatory failure, hypotension, palpitations, ventricular arrhythmias
- Central nervous system: dizziness, headache
- Gastrointestinal: nausea, vomiting, diarrhea
- Metabolism: hyperglycemia
- Respiratory: tachypnea
- Skin: alopecia, urticaria

Interactions (other drugs)

■ Adenosine ■ Beta-blockers ■ Anticonvulsants ■ Calcium channel blockers ■ Antibiotics (especially enoxacin) ■ Interferon ■ Lithium

Contraindications

Underlying seizure disorder.

Acceptability to patient

Gastrointestinal upset may be a problem.

Follow up plan

Careful follow up with blood levels of theophylline to prevent toxicity.

Patient and caregiver information

- Avoid large amounts of caffeine-containing products
- Notify clinician if nausea, vomiting, insomnia, jitteriness, headache, rash, palpitations occur

ALBUTEROL

Reliever medication for symptomatic wheezing.

Dose

Adult inhaled dose: one to two puffs of inhaler every 4–6h as needed.

Risks/Benefits

Risks:

- Tolerance may occur with prolonged use
- Concomitant use with other sympathomimetics is not recommended; however, inhaled beta-2 agonists can be used cautiously with oral forms
- Use caution in cardiac disease, hypokalemia, and hyperglycemia
- Use caution in pregnancy or breast-feeding
- Inhaled solution is less likely to produce side-effects

Benefits:

- Fast-acting relief of bronchospasm
- Can be administered through a nebulizer

Side-effects and adverse reactions

- Cardiovascular system: palpitations, sinus tachycardia, hypertension
- Central nervous system: anxiety, tremor, headache, insomnia, dizziness, nightmares, hyperkinesia
- Eyes, ears, nose, and throat: cough, throat irritation, epistaxis, bronchospasm, hoarseness, congestion
- Gastrointestinal: nausea, vomiting, dyspepsia, abdominal pain
- Metabolic: hyperglycemia, hypokalemia
- Musculoskeletal: cramps
- Skin: rash, urticaria, angioedema

Interactions (other drugs)

- Beta-blockers
- Sympathomimetics
- Thyroid hormones
- Tricyclic antidepressants
- MAOIs
- Diuretics

Contraindications

- Diabetes mellitus
- Hyperthyroidism
- Cardiac arrythmias
- Children under 12 years
- Hypersensitivity to sympathomimetics
- Ischemic heart disease
- Hypertension
- Seizures

Acceptability to patient

Fast acting, well tolerated.

Follow up plan

Careful follow up to check on symptom relief and inhaler technique.

Patient and caregiver information

See clinician if needing four or more inhalations per day on a regular basis.

NIACIN

- Dietary tryptophan is diverted by the tumor to form serotonin
- Niacin and an adequate protein intake is required to prevent pellagra

Dose

Niacin deficiency: adult oral dose 10–20mg/day; maximum 100mg/day.

Efficacy

Deficiency and clinical features of pellagra resolve with niacin.

Risks/Benefits

Risks:

- Cases of severe hepatic toxicity, including fulminant hepatic necrosis, have occurred in patients who have substituted sustained-release (modified-release, timed-release) nicotinic acid products for immediate-release (crystalline) nicotinic acid at equivalent doses
- Nicotinic acid should be used with caution in patients who consume substantial quantities of alcohol and/or have a past history of liver disease

Benefits:

- Effective and well tolerated
- Inexpensive

Side-effects and adverse reactions

- Cardiovascular system: orthostatic hypotension and syncope, angina, palpitations, sinus tachycardia
- Central nervous system: headache, dizziness, fatigue
- Eyes, ears, nose, and throat: cough
- Gastrointestinal: nausea, vomiting, diarrhea, constipation, abdominal pain
- Genitourinary: renal damage, impotence
- Hematologic: neutropenia, agranulocytosis, aplastic and hemolytic anemia, pancytopenia, thrombocytopenia
- Metabolic: hyperkalemia, hyponatremia
- Skin: angioedema, maculopapular rash

Interactions (other drugs)

▪ Allopurinol ▪ Azathioprine ▪ Insulin ▪ Iron ▪ Lithium ▪ Potassium ▪ Sodium ▪ Heparin ▪ Nonsteroidal anti-inflammatory drugs ▪ Antihypertensives (loop and potassium-sparing diuretics, prazosin, terazosin, doxazosin) ▪ Trimethoprim

Contraindications

▪ Pregnancy ▪ Angioedema ▪ Hypotension ▪ Children

Acceptability to patient

Flushing may be a problem with the medication – lessened with gradual titration of dose.

Follow up plan

Compliance needs to be checked to prevent pellagra.

Patient and caregiver information

- Take with meals and two glasses of water
- Avoid alcohol and hot beverages (may increase flushing)

Surgical therapy

- Surgery will be the only curative mode of treatment
- Debulking the tumor as a palliative procedure is effective
- Palliation can allow for long periods of asymptomatic disease

SURGICAL RESECTION

Efficacy

- Early diagnosis of carcinoid syndrome has led to complete surgical cure of a few patients with tumors arising in ovarian or testicular teratomas or in the bronchus. Although surgery offers the only chance of cure, most patients with carcinoid syndrome have metastasis and therefore are not cured by the surgery
- Palliative resection can allow for long asymptomatic periods as the tumor can be slow-growing
- In selected patients, palliative resection can be achieved by surgical debulking of tumor, including hemihepatectomy for unilobar metastases, excision of large superficial hepatic metastases, and removal of the primary tumor together with regional lymph nodes containing metastases

Risks/Benefits

Risks:

- Surgical manipulation of the tumor can cause severe vasomotor abnormalities and bronchospasm (carcinoid crisis)
- Intensive care facilities may be needed if a carcinoid crisis occurs

Acceptability to patient

- May produce cure
- Even palliative tumor reduction can lead to alleviation of symptoms

Follow up plan

Patients need careful follow up as further palliative surgery may be indicated.

Patient and caregiver information

- Full explanation of risks of surgical intervention
- Prospects of successful outcome and prognosis with and without surgery should be discussed
- Full informed consent should be obtained from the patient prior to surgery

Chemotherapy

Reserved for patients with metastatic disease associated with debilitating symptoms.

5-FLUOROURACIL

Efficacy

Response rates of 30% when used in combination with streptozocin are quoted for chemotherapy of metastatic carcinoids.

Risks/Benefits

Risks:

- Fluorouracil is a cytotoxic drug with frequent side-effects such as oral ulcers and diarrhea
- Patients should be carefully supervised, as therapeutic response is unlikely to occur without some evidence of toxicity

Acceptability to patient

Side-effects may make the treatment intolerable for the patient.

Follow up plan

The patient should be followed up intensively and therapy may need to be withheld when one of the following signs of toxicity appears:

- Stomatitis or esophagopharyngitis, at the first visible sign
- Leukopenia (WBC under 3500/mm^3) or a neutrophil count <1500/mm^3
- Frequent vomiting
- Severe diarrhea
- Gastrointestinal ulceration and bleeding
- Thrombocytopenia (platelets under 100,000/mm^3)
- Hemorrhage from any site

Patient and caregiver information

- Patients should be informed of expected toxic effects, especially oral manifestations
- Patients should be alerted to the possibility of alopecia and that it is usually a transient effect

STREPTOZOCIN

Efficacy

Response rates of 40% when used in combination with doxorubicin are quoted for chemotherapy of metastatic carcinoid.

Risks/Benefits

- Risk: patients must be monitored closely, particularly for evidence of renal, hepatic, and hematopoietic toxicity
- Benefit: tumor regression may be seen in up to 40% of patients, and a small but significant survival advantage has been observed

Acceptability to patient

Side-effects may make the treatment intolerable for the patient.

Follow up plan

The patient should be followed up intensively and therapy stopped if major side-effects occur.

Patient and caregiver information

- Confusion, lethargy, and depression may occur
- There may be a potential risk in driving or using complex machinery

Other therapies

PERCUTANEOUS EMBOLIZATION OF HEPATIC ARTERY

- As the blood supply of hepatic metastases is largely arterial, percutaneous embolization of the hepatic arterial supply to the most involved hepatic lobe sometimes can reduce inoperable hepatic metastases; the procedure carries a high risk of complications
- Chemoembolization is a technique combining intra-arterial chemotherapy with obstruction of the arterial blood flow to tumors via embolization of small particles, e.g. gel foam powder into the tumor vasculature
- Blocking the arterial system will produce ischemic necrosis of the tumors. Tumors receive 100% of their blood supply from the arterial system compared with normal liver, which receives 25% of its supply via the arterial system. Therefore, the normal liver should recover from embolization, whereas the tumor should not

Efficacy

In one study, survival analyses showed a median survival of 80 months and a 5-year survival rate of 60% from the performance of embolization on patients with midgut carcinoid tumors.

Risks/Benefits

Benefit: embolization has been shown to improve survival and quality of life, whether performed early or late in the disease process.

Acceptability to patient

Relatively simple procedure may have dramatic effect on quality of life and survival.

Follow up plan

- Patient will need close monitoring after the procedure
- Medication, e.g. somatostatin analogs, is usually continued

Patient and caregiver information

Full explanation of the procedure and prognosis with and without the procedure undertaken should be provided.

LIFESTYLE

Abstinence from alcohol will often alleviate problems with cutaneous flushing.

ACCEPTABILITY TO PATIENT

- Alcohol is potentially addictive, leading to poor compliance
- Compliance is improved when flushing becomes less symptomatic

EFFICACY OF THERAPIES

- Early diagnosis of the carcinoid syndrome has led to complete surgical cure of a few patients with tumors arising in ovarian or testicular teratomas or in the bronchus
- The success of antiproliferative medical therapies to control the growth of metastatic carcinoid tumors with long-acting somatostatin analogs octreotide or lanreotide is <50%
- Carcinoid tumors grow slowly; therefore, even if the tumor cannot be totally resected, effective reduction in tumor mass can ameliorate morbidity and improve the quality of life
- Cure is only rarely achieved in patients with carcinoid tumors, specifically those with limited nonmetastatic disease
- Tumor progression is very slow and patients may survive for years, so both medical and surgical therapy should be used for symptom palliation

PROGNOSIS

- Depends on site, size, and stage of the carcinoid tumor
- Localized disease has a 5-year survival of about 95%
- Carcinoid tumor with lymph node involvement has 5-year survival of about 65%
- Two-thirds of carcinoid syndrome patients have metastatic disease with a 5-year survival of 18%
- The tendency for metastatic spread correlates with tumor size and is substantially higher in lesions larger than 2.0cm
- Median survival if metastases are present is 38 months but may be much longer (up to 20 years)
- Carcinoid tumors of appendix and rectum have low malignancy potential and rarely produce carcinoid syndrome
- 5-year survival is excellent for carcinoids of appendix (86%) and rectum (72%), but far worse in cases of small intestine (55%), gastric (49%), and colonic carcinoids (42%)
- Surgically treated patients with carcinoid tumor have an overall favorable 83% 5-year survival rate
- Cardiac involvement has implications for prognosis. Patients without cardiac involvement in one series had a 68% 3-year survival, whereas those with cardiac lesions had only a 31% survival over the same interval

Clinical pearls

- Partial resection of hepatic metastases, which would be contraindicated in metastatic colon cancer, is accepted in the treatment of carcinoid tumors and carcinoid syndrome as providing much longer survival, decreasing tumor burden, and improving patient wellbeing
- Probably the most important point to emphasize with regard to the carcinoid syndrome is that just because patients are flushing does not mean they are going to be dead tomorrow. Flushing per se does not justify an immediate rush to aggressive intervention

Therapeutic failure

- Patients with carcinoid tumors metastatic to liver have been considered more likely to benefit from liver transplantation than patients with liver metastases of other malignancies
- Patients with unresected hepatic metastases from gastrointestinal neuroendocrine tumors have 5-year survival rates of between 13% and 43%
- It has been suggested that even with recurrence of neuroendocrine tumors after liver transplantation, their indolent behavior may permit relatively long-term survival in around 50% of patients

Recurrence

Chemotherapy:

- Combination chemotherapy is used in advanced metastatic disease
- More research is required for combination of chemotherapy with other treatments, e.g. hepatic artery embolization to establish treatment options for patients with advanced disease

Surgical resection or debulking procedure:
Palliative tumor debulking can lead to long asymptomatic periods.

Deterioration

The patient will need specialist review to establish appropriate further management. This management may include one or more of the following:

- Somatotropin analog with interferon
- Surgical debulking procedure
- Hepatic artery embolization
- Chemotherapy

Terminal illness

- The patient may suffer a great deal from abdominal pain, nausea and anorexia, and weakness during the terminal stages of the illness
- The patient may require opiate analgesia and antiemetic therapy either orally, by injection, or by infusion
- Fluid intake may become problematic and the patient may require intensive nursing care

COMPLICATIONS

Carcinoid crisis:

- Tumor outgrows its blood supply and large amounts of mediators are released
- Symptoms worsen dramatically and may be life-threatening
- May also occur during surgical manipulation
- The crisis is treated with high-dose octreotide and management of fluid balance (central line may be needed)

Carcinoid heart disease:

- Rare form of valvular heart disease, develops in 50–60% of patients with carcinoid syndrome
- Right heart disease is severe in 25% of patients with cardiac involvement
- The severity of cardiac damage appears to be proportional to the urine levels of 5-hydroxyindoleacetic levels
- Left-sided cardiac involvement is rarely seen except in patients with bronchial carcinoids or right-to-left intracardiac shunts
- The heart can also be affected by direct invasion of tumor and by high output cardiac failure

Pellagra – due to lack of nicotinic acid:

- Occurs in some patients with carcinoid because the tumor uses dietary tryptophan for serotonin synthesis and results in nutritional deficiency
- The classic triad of features is diarrhea, dermatitis, and dementia

CONSIDER CONSULT

Assessment of any clinical deterioration will require referral to a specialist.

PREVENTION

There are no preventive measures for carcinoid syndrome.

RESOURCES

ASSOCIATIONS

National Carcinoid Support Group Inc
#146, 6666 Odana Road
Madison, WI 53719–1012
http://members.aol.com/thencsg/

The Carcinoid Cancer Foundation Inc
1751 York Avenue
New York, NY 10128
Tel: (888) 722-3132 or (212) 722-3132
Fax: (914) 683-5919
E-mail: webmaster@carcinoid.org
www.carcinoid.org

KEY REFERENCES

- Strasberg Z, Hyland J, Salem S, et al. The role of angiography in the management of intestinal carcinoid. Angiology 1975;26:573–83
- Goldstein HM, Miller M. Angiographic evaluation of carcinoid tumors of small intestine: the value of ephinephrine. Radiology 1975;115:23–8
- Arnold R. Medical treatment of metastasizing carcinoid tumors. World J Surg 1996;20:203–7
- Rougier P, Mitry E. Chemotherapy in the treatment of neuroendocrine malignant tumors. Digestion 2000;62(Suppl 1):73–8
- O'Toole D, Ducreux M, Bommelaer G, et al. Treatment of carcinoid syndrome: a prospective crossover evaluation of lanreotide versus octreotide in terms of efficacy, patient acceptability, and tolerance. Cancer 2000;88:770–6
- Eriksson BK, Larsson EG, Skogseid BM, et al. Liver embolizations of patients with malignant neuroendocrine gastrointestinal tumors. Cancer 1998;83:2293–301
- Shebani KO, Souba WW, Finkelstein DM, et al. Prognosis and survival in patients with gastrointestinal tract carcinoid tumors. Ann Surg 1999;229:815–21; discussion 822–3
- Chen H, Hardacre JM, Uzar A, et al. Isolated liver metastases from neuroendocrine tumors: does resection prolong survival? J Am Coll Surg 1998;187:88–92
- Ladur AI, Zolotukhin SE, Timoshuk VA. Palliative resection of the small intestine for primary multiple malignant carcinoid tumor can improve the quality of life of the patient [in Russian]. Klin Khir 1998;5:45
- Memon MA, Nelson H. Gastrointestinal carcinoid tumors: current management strategies. Dis Colon Rectum 1997;40:1101–18
- Shebani KO, Souba WW, Finkelstein DM, et al. Prognosis and survival in patients with gastrointestinal tract carcinoid tumors. Ann Surg 1999;229:815–21
- Martin JK, Moertel CG, Adson MA. Surgical treatment of functioning metastatic carcinoid tumors. Arch Surg 1983;118:537–42
- Thompson GB, van Heerden JA, Martin JK, et al. Carcinoid tumors of the gastrointestinal tract: presentation, management and prognosis. Surgery 1985;98:1054–63
- Schupak KD, Wallnet KE. The role of radiation therapy in the treatment of locally unresectable or metastatic carcinoid tumors. Int J Radiat Oncol Biol Phys 1993;20:439
- Moertel CG, Sauer WG, Doekerry MG, Baggentoss AH. Life history of the carcinoid tumor of the small intestines. Cancer 1961;14:901
- Engstrom PF, Lavin PT, Folsch E. Streptozotocin plus fluorouracil versus doxorubicin therapy for metastatic carcinoid tumors. J Clin Oncol 1984;2:1255–9
- Hailer DG, Schutt A, Dayal Y, et al. Chemotherapy for metastatic carcinoid tumor: an ECOG phase II-III trial. Proc Am Soc Clin Oncol 1990;9:102
- Godwin JD. Carcinoid tumors: an analysis of 2837 cases. Cancer 1975;36:560–9
- Westergaard T, Frisch M. Carcinoid tumors in Denmark 1978–1989 and the risk of development of new cancers [in Danish]. Ugeskr Laeger 1996;158:3153–5

Evidence references

1 Wymenge AN, Eriksson B, Salmela PI, et al. Efficacy and safety of prolonged-release lanreotide in patients with gastrointestinal neuroendocrine tumors and hormone-related symptoms. J Clin Oncol 1999;17:1111

2 Tomassetti P., Migliori M, Gullo L. Slow-release lanreotide treatment in endocrine gastrointestinal tumors. Am J Gastroenterol 1998;93:1468–71

3 O'Toole D, Ducreux M, Bommelaer G, et al. Treatment of carcinoid syndrome: a prospective crossover evaluation of lanreotide versus octreotide in terms of efficacy, patient acceptability, and tolerance. Cancer 2000;88:770–6

FAQS

Question 1

What is the role of surgery in the treatment of carcinoid tumors and carcinoid syndrome?

ANSWER 1

Surgery has an important role in the management of carcinoid tumors. Resection of the primary tumor and of nodal metastases is primary therapy. Complications of recurrent or residual carcinoid may benefit from surgical intervention. Pain or physiologic abnormalities secondary to partial bowel obstruction may be greatly relieved by palliative surgical resection or bypass, or both. Palliative resection of hepatic metastases is appropriate to decrease tumor burden and improve patient wellbeing, and it results in much longer survival.

Question 2

Is radiotherapy a good option in the treatment of carcinoid tumors and carcinoid syndrome?

ANSWER 2

Radiotherapy is rarely used to treat carcinoid tumors or carcinoid syndrome. Patients frequently have extensive hepatic metastases and the dose-limiting toxicity of hepatic radiation limits its usefulness. Radiation therapy is useful for palliative treatment of bone metastases, and it should be considered in patients who require local control and palliation.

Question 3

What is the indication for chemotherapy in carcinoid tumors or carcinoid syndrome?

ANSWER 3

Antineoplastic therapy may be called for in patients whose cancers are aggressive, with progressive liver metastases, signs of partial or impending complete intestinal obstruction, or severe symptoms of carcinoid syndrome uncontrollable by other methods. Because no highly effective chemotherapy regimen is available, it is clear that patients should be carefully selected. Less toxic and more effective palliative therapies for carcinoid syndrome should always be used initially, reserving chemotherapy for those patients who are significantly disabled by unresponsive hormonally related symptoms or those with refractory symptoms due to tumor bulk.

Question 4

What is the prognosis for carcinoid tumors?

ANSWER 4

Carcinoid tumors usually grow slowly, so patients may live for many years, and the overall prognosis and survival rate is generally favorable. It varies accordingly to the site of the tumor: for appendiceal carcinoids, the 5-year survival rate is approx. 99%. Patients with rectal and lung carcinoids also have a favorable prognosis, with 5-year survival rates between 80% and 90%.

Those with carcinoids in the small intestine have a 5-year survival rate of approx. 50%. The extent of metastasis at the time of diagnosis is also a key point in defining prognosis. For example, rectal carcinoids with only local invasion are associated with a >90% 5-year survival rate, which decreases to approx. 45% in the presence of regional metastasis and to about 10% if distant metastases are present at diagnosis.

CONTRIBUTORS

Mary Jo Groves, MD
Luciana G O Clark, MD
Naixi N Chen, MD

CHRONIC LYMPHOCYTIC LEUKEMIA

SUMMARY INFORMATION

DESCRIPTION

- Chronic lymphocytic leukemia (CLL) is characterized by an accumulation of abnormal lymphoid cells of mature appearance in the bone marrow, lymph nodes, spleen, and peripheral blood
- It is the most common leukemia in the West, and affects an elderly population with a median age of 65 years at presentation
- It is often discovered by chance when blood tests done for other reasons reveal a high lymphocyte count, but it may present as more advanced disease with anemia, thrombocytopenia, lymphadenopathy, and hepatosplenomegaly
- Many patients with CLL have an unchanged life-expectancy and require monitoring rather than treatment
- Standard treatment is with chemotherapy and radiotherapy
- Most patients go into partial or total remission, but the effects of treatment on survival are as yet disappointing
- More modern approaches using biologic response modifiers, monoclonal antibodies, and bone marrow transplantation are being evaluated

URGENT ACTION

- Urgent action is sometimes required in patients with a high tumor burden who may experience airway obstruction caused by tracheal compression
- If the peripheral lymphocyte count is very high, neurologic manifestations can occur as a result of sludging in the cerebral arteries
- Infections associated with leukopenia may be life-threatening and also require immediate treatment (e.g. herpes zoster, *Pneumocystis carinii* infections, and *Candida albicans* infections)

KEY! DON'T MISS!

CLL is suggested by:

- Sustained peripheral blood lymphocyte count >10,000/mm^3 (10x10^9/L), with most of the cells being mature-appearing lymphocytes
- Bone marrow aspirate showing >30% lymphocytes
- Peripheral blood lymphocytes identified as monoclonal B cells

ICD9 CODE

204.1 Chronic lymphocytic leukemia.

SYNONYMS

CLL.

CARDINAL FEATURES

- Chronic lymphocytic leukemia (CLL) is a malignant proliferation and accumulation of abnormal, mature-appearing cells of the lymphoid series in the bone marrow, peripheral blood, lymph nodes, liver, and spleen and, occasionally, in other organs
- CLL may originate in T or B cells
- CLL is the most common leukemia in the western world (mostly the B cell type), and affects adults and the elderly (men twice as frequently as women)
- It is commonly discovered as an incidental finding on blood counts done for routine medical examinations or for other reasons
- Some patients present with weakness or tiredness, or with painless lymphadenopathy and hepatosplenomegaly if the disease is more advanced
- Blood tests usually show a high lymphocyte count, and the bone marrow is replaced to a variable degree with abnormal lymphocytes
- Chromosomal abnormalities are very common in the malignant cells
- Some patients are anemic, owing to bone marrow replacement or autoimmune hemolysis
- Patients may also have thrombocytopenia, hypogammaglobulinemia, and other immune disturbances
- The disease can be divided by the Rai or Binet staging systems into low-, medium-, and high-risk groups according to the results of blood tests and the number of sites involved
- CLL is not curable
- Patients in the low-risk groups have a life-expectancy equal to people of the same age without the disease; they should not be treated but should be carefully monitored, as the disease may progress to a form that does need treatment
- Some with more advanced disease should also not be treated if the condition is not progressive
- Treatment is usually with chemotherapy. Radiotherapy to local sites or the spleen may be helpful
- Splenectomy may be performed if there is painful splenomegaly or if the patient has autoimmune hemolytic anemia
- Treatments under evaluation include biologic response modifiers, monoclonal antibodies against components of the leukemic cells, and bone marrow transplantation
- Many patients achieve some form of remission, but treatments do not generally prolong survival
- The disease may transform into prolymphocytic leukemia, diffuse large-cell lymphoma, acute leukemia, or multiple myeloma, and patients undergoing these transformations generally have a poor prognosis

CAUSES

Common causes

- No single cause has been identified
- Unrelated to previous radiation exposure, chemicals, or drugs
- More common in farmers and in rubber and asbestos workers

Contributory or predisposing factors

Increased familial incidcence.

EPIDEMIOLOGY

Incidence and prevalence

INCIDENCE

- Current projected annual incidence estimates vary from as few as 7300 to approx. 12,500 new cases in the US
- Incidence appears to be decreasing, in part because of the more accurate distinction among the various CLLs

Demographics

AGE

Highest incidence in those aged 50–55 years.

GENDER

Males:female ratio 2:1 (relative frequency 1.3–2.6).

RACE

- T cell CLL is more common in Asian races, B cell CLL in Western races
- CLL accounts for 28.8% of all leukemias in Caucasians and 26.1% in African-Americans
- Occurs more commonly in Jewish people of Russian or eastern European ancestry

GENETICS

- Increased familial incidence. Also, within families, more frequent appearance of related disorders including immunoglobulin deficiencies and autoimmune disorders
- There appears to be genetic anticipation, whereby incidence increases in successive generations of a family
- Most common clonal abnormalities are trisomy 12 (17%), structural abnormalities of chromosome 13 (13%), and chromosome 14 (10%)

GEOGRAPHY

- B cell CLL is far more common than the T cell type in the US, making up at least 95% of cases
- In Asia, and Asian populations, the T cell type is more frequent

DIFFERENTIAL DIAGNOSIS

- Clinical diagnosis of chronic lymphocytic leukemia (CLL) is usually not difficult
- Essential to exclude: infectious diseases (mononucleosis) and a group of related hematologic disorders in which the differentiation is important because of variations in prognosis and optimal methods of treatment (hairy cell leukemia, prolymphocytic leukemia, nonHodgkin's lymphoma, and Waldenstrom's macroglobulinemia)
- CLL transforms into some of these other conditions in 15% of cases

Infectious mononucleosis

Infectious mononuculeosis is a viral illness caused by Epstein-Barr virus (EBV), affecting mainly adolescents and young adults.

FEATURES

- Malaise
- Headache
- Fever (40°C/104°F)
- Pharyngitis
- Lymphadenopathy (tonsillar and cervical lymph nodes may be quite enlarged, painful, and tender) lasting from one to several weeks
- Laboratory findings: relative or absolute lymphocytosis and positive serology (Paul-Bunnell)

Hairy cell leukemia

Lymphoid neoplasm characterized by the proliferation of mature B cells with prominent cytoplasmic projections ('hairy cells').

FEATURES

- Splenomegaly in 90% of patients
- Hepatomegaly in one-third of patients
- Varying degrees of leukopenia (occasionally leukocytosis) and/or pancytopenia
- Bone marrow usually fibrotic and infiltrated by an atypical cell with prominent cytoplasmic projections ('hairy cells')
- Bone marrow biopsies required for diagnosis and evaluation of the degree of hairy cell infiltration
- Cytologic appearance of the malignant cells, and the appearance and distribution of the infiltrates in the bone marrow, spleen, and lymph nodes distinguish this disorder from CLL

Prolymphocytic leukemia

Chronic variety of leukemia, marked by large numbers of circulating lymphocytes, predominantly prolymphocytes.

FEATURES

- Massive splenomegaly
- Lymphadenopathy in 40% of patients
- Skin infiltration in 20% of patients
- White cell count is often >100,000/mL ($100x10^9$/L)
- Cells tend to be larger than in CLL and the lymphocyte counts higher
- Prognosis is poor, with a median survival of 7 months

Leukemic phase of nonHodgkin's lymphoma

NonHodgkin's lymphoma is a heterogenous group of malignancies of the lymphoreticular system.

FEATURES

- Consists of various slightly different disorders, including the leukemic phases of mantle cell lymphoma, follicular lymphoma, and large cell lymphoma
- Differentiation is made on cell morphology and presence or absence of various surface markers
- Lymphadenopathy usually much more pronounced than in CLL

Waldenstrom's macroglobulinemia

A plasma cell dyscrasia.

FEATURES

- Monoclonal proliferation of plasma cells and B lymphocytes that produce immunoglobulin M (IgM)
- Diagnosis is made on the basis of typical symptoms and physical findings, presence of an IgM M protein in the serum, and lymphoplasma cell proliferation in the bone marrow
- Symptoms: weakness, fatigue, oronasal bleeding, weight loss, and visual or neurologic disturbances

Many clinical manifestations result from hyperviscosity syndrome:

- Diffuse bleeding (epistaxis, purpura, oozing from the oromucosa)
- Visual disturbances (blurring or loss of vision, retinal hemorrhages, exudates)
- Neurologic conditions (dizziness, headache, vertigo, nystagmus, hearing loss, ataxia, paresthesias, somnolence, and even coma)
- Cardiovascular disorders (hypervolemia, congestive heart failure)

SIGNS & SYMPTOMS

Signs

- Often few clinical signs in CLL as up to 60% of patients are diagnosed in an asymptomatic stage from a complete blood count (CBC) done for unrelated reasons
- Physical examination is normal at presentation in 20–30% of patients
- Lymphadenopathy or hepatosplenomegaly is present in 40–50% of patients

Signs that may be present include:

- Lymphadenopathy, which is nontender, painless, and mobile (often cervical or supraclavicular)
- Splenomegaly (mild-to-moderate enlargement)
- Hepatomegaly
- Anemia (uncommon at presentation)
- Ecchymoses and bruising (uncommon at presentation)
- Acute swelling and redness of joints (septic arthritis secondary to neutropenia)
- Less common manifestations: infiltration of tonsils (7.7%), abdominal masses caused by mesenteric or retroperitoneal lymphadenopathy (2%), and skin infiltration (2%)

Symptoms

- There are no symptoms specific to CLL
- Symptoms are attributable to anemia, thrombocytopenia, organ involvement, and infection secondary to leukopenia

Symptoms that may be present include:

- Weakness
- Tiredness
- Shortness of breath
- Bleeding

- Weight loss
- Abdominal discomfort
- Bone and joint pains
- Fever, usually secondary to infection (only rarely directly due to disease process)

KEY! DON'T MISS!

CLL is suggested by:

- Sustained peripheral blood lymphocyte count >10,000/mm^3 (10x10^9/L), with most of the cells being mature-appearing lymphocytes
- Bone marrow aspirate showing >30% lymphocytes
- Peripheral blood lymphocytes identified as monoclonal B cells

CONSIDER CONSULT

Refer to a specialist for full investigation if CLL is suspected.

INVESTIGATION OF THE PATIENT

Direct questions to patient

- Q **Have you been feeling unwell?** Often a presenting symptom
- Q **Have you been weak, tired, or short of breath?** May indicate anemia
- Q **Have you lost weight recently?** Not common, but may occur
- Q **Have you had nosebleeds, bruising, blood in the urine?** Can be due to thrombocytopenia
- Q **Have you had any aches and pains or abdominal discomfort?** May suggest bone involvement or hepatosplenomegaly
- Q **Have you developed any lumps in your neck, armpits, or groin?** Lymphadenopathy is common
- Q **Have you been hot and cold or shivering?** Fever, when present, is usually due to bacterial infections secondary to neutropenia and hypogammaglobulinemia
- Q **Have you had any swollen joints?** Septic arthritis may occur secondary to neutropenia

Contributory or predisposing factors

- Q **Have you worked on a farm, or with rubber or industrial solvents?** These are known risk factors.

Family history

- Q **Has anyone in your family ever had leukemia?** There is an increased familial incidence
- Q **Has anyone in your family had an autoimmune disease or other blood disorder?** There is an increased familial incidence of immunoglobulin deficiencies and various autoimmune disorders

Examination

- **Is the patient anemic?**
- **Is body temperature raised?** Fever is not common in CLL, except when there is secondary bacterial infection
- **Is there any evidence of abnormal bleeding?** Bruising, ecchymoses, and purpura may occur as a result of thrombocytopenia
- **Is there any abnormal lymphadenopathy?** Common in CLL. Often in the neck or supraclavicular regions
- **Is the liver or spleen enlarged?** Very common in CLL

Summary of investigative tests

- CBC with microscopic examination of the smear may reveal anemia, thrombocytopenia, reticulocytosis, or neutropenia; there will be an absolute lymphocytosis in the peripheral blood
- Serum lactate dehydrogenase (LDH) may be helpful diagnostically in some circumstances, as it is usually increased if there is a large tumor burden

- Serum urate should be requested routinely and particularly after chemotherapy because level will increase as a result of tissue breakdown and this can cause renal tract stone formation or acute renal failure
- Liver enzymes, aspartate transaminase (AST), and alanine transaminase (ALT) are useful if hepatic involvement is suspected
- Serum creatinine can be measured to assess renal function
- Serum proteins and electrophoresis will reveal whether globulins are raised and whether there is a monoclonal band
- Serum immuglobulins will define which type of immunoglobulin, if any, is being expressed
- Immunophenotyping of peripheral blood lymphocytes is essential to make a detailed diagnosis. This will often be ordered by a specialist, but can also be ordered from a primary care practice
- Serum beta-2-microglobulin is a very useful prognostic factor
- Blood culture and urine stick test, microscopy, and culture should be taken in all febrile patients to confirm or exclude bacterial infection
- Lymph node biopsy: may be useful if enlarged superficial nodes present, and may give an earlier diagnosis of a related disorder than bone marrow aspiration (normally performed by a specialist)
- Chest X-ray may reveal enlarged hilar lymph nodes or infiltration or infection of the lungs
- Abdominal ultrasound scanning will indicate extent of involvement of liver, spleen, and intra-abdominal lymph nodes
- Computed tomography scanning of chest or abdomen can also be used to show hepatomegaly, splenomegaly, enlarged lymph nodes, or other abnormal masses or infiltrations
- Bone marrow examination: aspiration and biopsy may both be necessary to obtain cells for microscopic examination, cytochemistry, immunophenotyping, and cytogenetics. This information is helpful in defining the prognosis and what forms of treatment will be used (normally performed by a specialist)

DIAGNOSTIC DECISION

The clinical diagnosis of CLL is often not difficult. It is diagnosed on the finding of an absolute increase in lymphocytes and/or bone marrow infiltration coupled with the characteristic features of morphology and immunophenotype used to define prognosis and to decide on treatment modalities. There are two current definitions of CLL.

The International Chronic Lymphocytic Leukemia Workshop diagnostic criteria ([1] are:

- Criterion 1: sustained peripheral blood lymphocyte count >10,000/mm^3 (10x10^9/L), with most of the cells being mature-appearing lymphocytes
- Criterion 2: bone marrow aspirate showing >30% lymphocytes
- Criterion 3: peripheral blood lymphocytes identified as monoclonal B cells
- Diagnosis of CLL is made if criterion 1 and either criterion 2 or 3 are present. If peripheral blood lymphocyte count is <10,000/mm^3 (10x10^9/L), then both criterion 2 and 3 must be present

The National Cancer Institute-sponsored CLL Working Group [2] requires:

- A peripheral blood lymphocyte count of >5000/mm^3 (5x10^9/L), with <55% of cells being atypical. The cells should be CD5-positive and may carry the B cell-specific surface antigens CD19, CD20, and CD24
- Of marrow nucleated cells, >30% must be CLL lymphocytes

Staging:
There is no universally accepted staging for CLL. The two main systems in use are outlined below.

Rai staging system [3] divides CLL into five stages:

- Stage 0: lymphocyte count >5000/mm^3 (5x10^9/L) (for >4 weeks); no lymphadenopathy, hepatosplenomegaly, anemia, or thrombocytopenia
- Stage I: lymphocyte count >5000/mm^3 (5x10^9/L) with lymphadenopathy; no hepatosplenomegaly, anemia, or thrombocytopenia
- Stage II: lymphocyte count >5000/mm^3 (5x10^9/L) with either hepatomegaly or splenomegaly, with or without lymphadenopathy
- Stage III: lymphocyte count >5000/mm^3 (5x10^9/L) and anemia (hemoglobin <11g/dL), with or without lymphadenopathy, hepatomegaly, splenomegaly
- Stage IV: lymphocyte count >5000/mm^3 (5x10^9/L) and thrombocytopenia (platelets <100,000/mm^3 (100x10^9/L)), with or without lymphadenopathy, hepatomegaly, splenomegaly, anemia
- A simplified version of this system – low risk (stage 0), intermediate risk (stages I and II), and high risk (stages III and IV) – is now generally accepted and is helpful in making decisions regarding treatment

Binet staging system [4] divides CLL into three stages:

- Clinical stage A: no anemia or thrombocytopenia; fewer than three areas of lymphoid involvement (possible areas are the cervical, axillary, and inguinal lymph nodes and the spleen) (Rai stages 0–II)
- Clinical stage B: no anemia or thrombocytopenia; three or more areas of lymphoid involvement (Rai stages I and II)
- Clinical stage C: anemia and/or thrombocytopenia, regardless of the number of areas of lymphoid involvement (Rai stages III and IV)

The International Workshop on Chronic Lymphocytic Leukemia has recommended combining the two systems to ensure inclusion of the Rai Stage 0 patients. This new system has the stages A(0), A(I), A(II); B(I), B(II); and C(III), C(IV).

The NCI Working Group has suggested standard guidelines for eligibility, response, and toxicity to be used in future trials.

THE TESTS

Body fluids

COMPLETE BLOOD COUNT

Description

Venous blood sample.

Advantages/Disadvantages

Advantage: inexpensive, rapid, and may be diagnostic

Normal

- Hemoglobin: men 14–18g/dL, women 12–16g/dL
- Platelets: 150,000–400,000/mm^3 (150–400x10^9/L)
- Leukocytes: 4500–10,500/mm^3 (4.5–10.5x10^9/L)
- Neutrophils: 50–70%, 3000–7000/mm^3 (3.0–7.0x10^9/L)
- Lymphocytes: 30–50%, 2000–5000/mm^3 (2.0–5.0x10^9/L)

Abnormal

- Anemia is often present in more advanced CLL. This may be due to marrow failure with replacement by leukemic cells, but the anemia can also be aplastic or autoimmune (hemolytic)

- Lymphocyte counts vary greatly. The absolute lymphocyte count must be >5000/mm^3 (>5.0x10^9/L) by any definition, and can rise to as high as 1,000,000/mm^3 (1000x10^9/L). The French-American-British classification system divides CLL into typical (<90% small lymphocytes), CLL-prolymphocytic (11–54% prolymphocytes), and atypical (varying morphology, <10% prolymphocytes)
- Thrombocytopenia is often present in more advanced disease, and like the anemia can be due to marrow replacement or to autoimmune destruction of cells
- Examination of the blood film will show reticulocytes if autoimmune hemolytic anemia is present

SERUM LACTATE DEHYDROGENASE

Description

Venous blood sample.

Advantages/Disadvantages

Advantage: inexpensive, rapid answer

Normal

50–150 IU/L.

Abnormal

>150 IU/L.

Cause of abnormal result

LDH is usually increased if there is a large tumor burden.

SERUM URATE

Description

Venous blood sample.

Advantages/Disadvantages

Advantages:
- Inexpensive, rapid
- If significantly raised, indicates that treatment is required

Normal

2–7mg/dL (120–420mcmol/L).

Abnormal

>7mg/dL (>420mcmol/L)

Cause of abnormal result
- Increased cell breakdown, often after treatment
- Urate is an end-product of protein metabolism

ASPARTATE TRANSAMINASE, ALANINE AMINOTRANSFERASE

Description

Venous blood sample.

Advantages/Disadvantages

Advantage: inexpensive, rapid answer

Normal
ALT and AST: 50–150 IU/L.

Abnormal
ALT and AST: >150 IU/L.

Cause of abnormal result
Raised level may indicate liver involvement.

SERUM CREATININE
Description
Venous blood sample.

Advantages/Disadvantages
Advantages:
- Inexpensive, rapid result
- Reflects renal function accurately

Normal
0.6–1.2mg/dL (50–110mcmol/L).

Abnormal
>110mg/dL (>110mcmol/L).

Cause of abnormal result
Decrease in glomerular filtration rate may be associated with hyperuricemia.

Drugs, disorders and other factors that may alter results
An abnormal result may be caused by extensive breakdown of cells following treatment.

SERUM PROTEINS AND ELECTROPHORESIS
Description
Venous blood sample.

Advantages/Disadvantages
Advantage: inexpensive

Normal
- Total protein: 6–8g/dL (60–80g/L)
- Albumin: 4.0–5.5g/dL (40–55g/L)
- Globulin: 1.2–3.0g/dL (12–30g/L)

Electrophoresis:
- Albumin: 4.0–5.5g/dL (40–55g/L)
- Alpha-1-globulin: 0.2–0.4g/dL (2–4g/L)
- Alpha-2-globulin: 0.6–1.0g/dL (6–10g/L)
- Beta-globulin: 0.6–1.0g/dL (6–10g/L)
- Gamma-globulin: 0.7–1.3g/dL (7–13g/L)

Abnormal
- Wide range of abnormalities are possible
- Albumin level may be low in any ill patient, particularly if infection is present
- Alpha-2-globulin may be raised in patients with infections

- Gamma-globulin level may be low since many patients with CLL have depressed immune function
- Gamma-globulin level may be raised and there may be a discrete monoclonal band visible in patients with macroglobulinemia

SERUM IMMUNOGLOBULINS

Description

Venous blood sample.

Advantages/Disadvantages

Advantage: inexpensive.

Normal

- IgA: 1.4–3.5mg/mL (1.4–3.5g/L)
- IgG: 8–16mg/mL (8–16g/L)
- IgM: 0.5–2.0mg/mL (0.5–2.0g/L)

Abnormal

- In immunocompromised patients all the results may be low
- In Waldenstrom's macroglobulinemia or multiple myeloma, the paraprotein is usually IgM
- In patients with CLL who have a paraprotein, it is not usually IgM; decreased levels of IgG is the most common finding

IMMUNOPHENOTYPING OF LYMPHOCYTES

Description

Venous blood sample.

Advantages/Disadvantages

- Advantage: essential to distinguish CLL from other disorders with chronic lymphocytosis
- Disadvantage: needs specialist interpretation

Normal

No abnormal lymphocytosis.

Abnormal

- CLL is characterized by lymphocytes that are positive for B cell markers, the most important of which is CD5. CLL cells are also negative for all T cell markers
- Conditions characterized by CD5-chronic lymphocytosis should not be considered as CLL; these must be further investigated by a specialist

SERUM BETA-2-MICROGLOBULIN

Description

Venous blood sample.

Advantages/Disadvantages

Advantage: marker of lymphocyte activation and/or destruction

Normal

0–0.22mg/dL (0–2.2mg/L).

Abnormal

>0.22mg/dL (>2.2mg/L).

BLOOD CULTURE

Description

- Venous blood inoculated immediately into liquid culture medium
- Two bottles of culture medium often used for each sample

Advantages/Disadvantages

Advantages:

- Inexpensive
- Usually reveals bacterium responsible for severe infections

Disadvantage: 48h incubation often needed

Normal

No bacterial growth.

Abnormal

- Significant growth of infecting organism(s)
- May be more than one type of bacterium in profoundly neutropenic patients

Drugs, disorders and other factors that may alter results

Chemotherapy contributes to the neutropenia during treatment.

URINE STICK TEST, MICROSCOPY, AND CULTURE

Description

Clean, preferably midstream, specimen of urine.

Advantages/Disadvantages

Advantages:

- Inexpensive, rapid partial answer from stick test and microscopy
- Good early indicator of nephropathy or infection

Disadvantage: 48h incubation needed for culture

Normal

- Stick test: pH 4.5–8, protein absent, glucose absent, hemoglobin (or red blood cells (RBCs)) absent, leukocytes absent
- Microscopy: RBCs 0–5/high-power field; leukocytes 0–5/high-power field; casts 0–4/low-power field; crystals absent
- Culture: no growth of bacteria

Abnormal

- Stick test: presence of RBCs, leukocytes, or significant protein indicate nephropathy or infection
- Microscopy: >5 RBCs, >5 leukocytes, or >4 casts raise possibility of infection; significant amounts of urate crystals indicate possible urate nephropathy
- Culture: significant growth of bacteria (>100,000 organisms/mL) suggests active urinary tract infection

Cause of abnormal result

Direct effects on kidney of infection or high urate concentrations.

Biopsy

LYMPH NODE BIOPSY

Description

Removal of superficial lymph node under local anesthesia.

Advantages/Disadvantages

Advantages:

- Simple to do, few complications
- Not necessary to diagnose CLL, but may point to lymphoma or Richter's syndrome

Normal

Normal lymph node architecture and normal cells.

Abnormal

Replacement or infiltration with abnormal cells may point to lymphoma or Richter's syndrome.

BONE MARROW ASPIRATION/BIOPSY

Description

- Sample of bone marrow obtained in most cases by aspiration
- Where examination is difficult or marrow is hypocellular, marrow biopsy may be required

Advantages/Disadvantages

- Advantage: whereas a bone marrow aspirate and biopsy are rarely required to confirm diagnosis of CLL, they may provide prognostic information and are valuable for assessing response to therapy
- Disadvantage: marrow biopsy is unpleasant for patient

Abnormal

Infiltration by at least 30% lymphocytes.

Imaging

CHEST X-RAY

Advantages/Disadvantages

Advantage: inexpensive, immediate result.

Normal
Clear pulmonary fields with no masses or infiltrates.

Abnormal
Presence of hilar lymph nodes in 5% of patients with CLL.

ABDOMINAL ULTRASOUND SCAN
Advantages/Disadvantages
Advantages:
- Inexpensive, immediate result
- No X-ray exposure

Abnormal
May reveal hepatomegaly, splenomegaly, enlarged lymph nodes, or other abnormal masses or infiltrations.

COMPUTED TOMOGRAPHY SCAN OF CHEST OR ABDOMEN
Advantages/Disadvantages
Advantage: high resolution, rapid result

Disadvantages:
- Expensive
- Significant X-ray exposure

Normal
Absence of masses or organomegalies.

Abnormal
May reveal hepatomegaly, splenomegaly, enlarged lymph nodes, or other abnormal masses or infiltrations.

TREATMENT

CONSIDER CONSULT

Although not all patients need treatment, refer all patients to a specialist with a view to full consideration of treatment if appropriate.

IMMEDIATE ACTION

Conditions requiring immediate treatment are airway obstruction, cerebral leukostasis, and severe infection.

PATIENT AND CAREGIVER ISSUES

Impact on career, dependants, family, friends

Impact very much depends on extent and stage of disease. Patients with indolent chronic lymphocytic leukemia (CLL) may die of other causes and therefore may not need therapy for the CLL. Others may progress to aggressive and unresponsive syndromes such as Richter's syndrome.

MANAGEMENT ISSUES

Goals

- To obtain a full and detailed diagnosis so that correct decisions may be made regarding treatment
- To alleviate symptoms and to prolong life

SUMMARY OF THERAPEUTIC OPTIONS

Choices

General principles:

- The most important decision in the management of CLL is whether to treat at all
- Benefits of treatment must be carefully considered as there is a significant group of patients who do not benefit from treatment
- Patients with stable low-risk smoldering CLL or Binet stage A disease do not require therapy, and survival may actually be shortened with chemotherapy because of treatment-related complications

In those patients for whom treatment is warranted, the following principles apply:

- Patients with intermediate-risk CLL (Binet group B with progressive disease or uncomfortable organ enlargement) or high-risk CLL (Binet group C) who have had no previous treatment, are usually treated with front-line therapy (usually fludarabine or chlorambucil, or possibly with cyclophosphamide). Such therapy would generally be given under the supervision of a specialist
- For patients who do not respond to fludarabine, chlorambucil, or cyclophosphamide alone, or who relapse, treatment with combination chemotherapy such as CHOP (cyclophosphamide, doxorubicin, vincristine, and prednisone) or radiotherapy; other possibilities are the newer nucleoside analogs cladribine (CdA, 2-chlorodeoxyadenosine) or pentostatin (dCF, 2-deoxycoformycin). All these patients should be entered into clinical trials, as the results of all the present treatments are relatively disappointing
- Normally, corticosteroids (e.g. prednisone) should be avoided, as they do not prolong survival and make infection more likely. They can, however, be helpful where patient develops an autoimmune hemolytic anemia or thrombocytopenia
- Patients with extensive disease may experience massive cell breakdown when first treated, and when this is anticipated, generous quantities of intravenous fluids and prophylactic allopurinol should be given to avoid the development of uric acid nephropathy
- Injections of gamma-globulin can reduce rate of intercurrent infections in patients with compromised immunity, but they do not prolong survival

- Prophylactic antibiotics, antifungal agents, and antiviral agents also have a place in immunocompromised patients
- Radiotherapy is normally only used as a local therapy to reduce tumor mass, but some patients with extensive disease benefit from more generalized treatment or from splenic irradiation
- Splenectomy may be considered if there is painful splenomegaly or evidence of hypersplenism
- Transfusions of red cells, white cells, or platelets may be required during treatment if the number of normal cells falls to critically low levels
- Bone marrow transplantation has been tried recently in a small number of patients with advanced disease. Remissions have been observed, but it is too early to assess the duration of remission or survival
- Granulocyte macrophage-colony stimulating factor (GM-CSF) has been shown to increase the neutrophil count and allow higher doses of chemotherapy to be given, but the clinical results of this are not yet clear

FOLLOW UP

Plan for review

Frequency of review depends on stage of treatment and clinical condition of patient.

Information for patient or caregiver

It is important to give full and truthful information to patient's relatives or caregivers.

DRUGS AND OTHER THERAPIES: DETAILS

Drugs

PREDNISONE

- A semisynthetic corticosteroid
- Normally, corticosteroids should be avoided, as they do not prolong survival and make infection more likely. They can, however, be helpful where patient develops an autoimmune hemolytic anemia or thrombocytopenia

Dose

- 30–60mg/day orally (dosage should be individualized)
- Frequency and duration as defined by treatment schedule

Risks/Benefits

Risks:

- Use caution in congestive heart failure, diabetes mellitus, renal disease
- Use caution in the elderly
- Use caution in glaucoma
- Use caution in ulcerative colitis, peptic ulcer
- Prednisone taken in doses >7.5mg for a period of 3 weeks or longer may lead to clinically relevant suppression of the pituitary-adrenal axis

Side-effects and adverse reactions

- Side-effects are minimized by short duration of therapy
- Cardiovascular system: hypertension, thromboembolism
- Central nervous system: insomnia, euphoria, depression, psychosis, seizures
- Endocrine: adrenal suppression, impaired glucose tolerance, growth suppression in children
- Eyes, ears, nose, and throat: cataract, glaucoma, blurred vision
- Gastrointestinal: dyspepsia, peptic ulceration, esophagitis, oral candidiasis
- Musculoskeletal: proximal myopathy, osteoporosis
- Skin: delayed healing, acne, striae, fragile skin

Interactions (other drugs)

■ Aminoglutethimide (increased clearance of prednisone) ■ Diuretics (effects inhibited) ■ Cardiac glycosides (toxicity increased) ■ Barbiturates (increased clearance of prednisone) ■ Antihypertensives (effects inhibited) ■ Antidiabetics (hypoglycemic effect inhibited) ■ Cholestyramine, colestipol (may reduce absorption of corticosteroids) ■ Ketoconazole ■ Clarithromycin, erythromycin, troleandomycin (may enhance steroid effect) ■ Cyclosporine (may increase levels of both drugs; may cause seizures) ■ Isoniazid (reduced plasma levels of isoniazid) ■ Nonsteroidal anti-inflammatory drugs (increased risks of bleeeding) ■ Oral contraceptives (enhanced effects of corticosteroids) ■ Rifampin (may inhibit hepatic clearance of prednisone) ■ Salicylates (increased clearance of salicylates) ■ Warfarin (alters clotting time)

Contraindications

■ Systemic infection ■ Avoid live virus vaccines in those receiving immunosuppressive doses ■ History of tuberculosis ■ Cushing's syndrome ■ Recent myocardial infarction

Acceptability to patient

May cause heartburn, nausea, and vomiting, which may limit acceptability.

ALLOPURINOL

Inhibits conversion of hypoxanthine into uric acid.

Dose

- 300mg/day orally
- Given during initial phase of treatment together with intravenous fluid if there is a large tumor burden

Risks/Benefits

Risks:

- Ensure adequate fluid intake during treatment
- Use caution in hepatic or renal impairment
- Treatment should be discontinued at first sign of allergic reaction, such as skin rash or other reaction

Side-effects and adverse reactions

- Central nervous system: drowsiness, headache
- Gastrointestinal: nausea, abdominal pain, peptic ulceration, cholestatic jaundice, diarrhea, liver failure
- Genitourinary: renal failure
- Musculoskeletal: athralgia, myopathy
- Skin: rashes, alopecia, Stevens-Johnson syndrome

Interactions (other drugs)

■ Angiotensin-converting enzyme (ACE) inhibitors ■ Antacids ■ Azathioprine ■ Theophylline ■ Cyclophosphamide ■ Mercaptopurine ■ Oral anticoagulants

Contraindications

Patients who have developed a severe reaction to allopurinol should not be restarted on the drug.

Acceptability to patient

Generally well tolerated.

GAMMA-GLOBULIN

Human gamma-globulin extracted by fractionation of blood.

Dose

- 250–400mg/kg intravenously every 3–4 weeks
- An initial loading dose of at least 200mg/kg at more frequent intervals, proceeding to 100–200mg/kg at 3-week intervals once a therapeutic plasma level has been established, can be used. However, treatment must be individualized for each patient due to variation among patients in catabolic rate of immunoglobulin (Ig) G

Risks/Benefits

Risks:

- Use caution in patients with a history of prior systemic allergic reactions following the administration of human immunoglobulin preparations
- If anaphylactic or severe anaphylactoid reactions occur, discontinue infusion immediately. Epinephrine should be available for the treatment of any acute anaphylactoid reactions

Side-effects and adverse reactions

- Central nervous system: headache, pyrexia, chills
- Gastrointestinal: hypotension, nausea
- Musculoskeletal: backache, myalgia
- Skin: flushing
- Patients previously sensitized to certain antigens, most commonly IgA, may be at risk of immediate anaphylactoid and hypersensitivity reactions

Interactions (other drugs)

May interfere with response by pediatric patients to live viral vaccines such as measles, mumps, and rubella.

Contraindications

- History of anaphylactic or severe systemic response to immunoglobulin intramuscular or intravenous preparations
- Should not be given to persons with isolated IgA deficiency

Acceptability to patient

Well tolerated.

Surgical therapy

SPLENECTOMY

- Splenectomy is usually considered when patients have autoimmune hemolytic anemia or thrombocytopenia, or when hypersplenism does not resolve with chemotherapy
- May also be useful in patients with painful splenomegaly

Risks/Benefits

Risk: carries all the usual risks of anethesia and abdominal surgery

Benefits:

- May improve hematologic profile, with increased hemoglobin level and platelet count
- May be beneficial for patients with hypersplenism that does not respond to chemotherapy
- May be useful for treating painful splenomegaly

Acceptability to patient

Varies. Some patients may be reluctant to undergo surgery that is not curative and that may not improve survival. Other patients may feel that the possible benefits to quality of life outweigh the risks.

Follow up plan

Usual postoperative follow up is required, as well as repeat complete blood counts.

Radiation therapy

RADIATION THERAPY

- Radiation therapy has been used extensively in CLL. Treatment can be given to the spleen, liver, mediastinum, lymph nodes, and any other affected areas
- Total body irradiation is necessary before bone marrow transplantation

Efficacy

Effective locally and significantly reduces tumor mass.

Acceptability to patient

Radiation therapy is not pleasant for patients and may make them feel unwell.

Chemotherapy

FLUDARABINE

- A nucleoside analog
- 25mg/m^2/day intravenously
- Given for 3–5 days monthly to best response plus an additional 2 months
- Not to exceed one year of treatment, because of concerns of cumulative myelotoxicity

Risks/Benefits

Risks:

- Fludarabine phosphate for injection should be administered under supervision of a qualified physician experienced in the use of antineoplastic therapy
- Severe bone marrow suppression, notably anemia, thrombocytopenia, and neutropenia, have been reported
- Patients undergoing therapy should be closely observed for signs of hematologic and nonhematologic toxicity
- Use of fludarabine phosphate in combination with pentostatin is not recommended due to risk of severe pulmonary toxicity

Side-effects and adverse reactions

- Central nervous system: fever, chills, malaise, fatigue
- Gastrointestinal: nausea, vomiting, anorexia
- Hematologic: myelosuppression (neutropenia, thrombocytopenia and anemia)
- Musculoskeletal: weakness
- Other: infection

Contraindications

■ Pediatric patients ■ Hypersensitivity to this drug or its components ■ Pregnancy, breast-feeding

Acceptability to patient

Nausea and vomiting may limit acceptability.

CHLORAMBUCIL

- Synthetic alkylating agent of the nitrogen mustard type
- 0.1mg/kg/day orally or 0.4mg/kg every 4 weeks
- Duration defined by clinical response

Risks/Benefits

Risks:

- Should only be administered under specialist supervision
- Chlorambucil can severely suppress bone marrow function
- Chlorambucil is a carcinogen in humans
- Should not be given to patients with conditions other than CLL or malignant lymphomas
- Chlorambucil should not be given at full dosages before 4 weeks after a full course of radiation therapy or chemotherapy
- Children with nephrotic syndrome and patients receiving high-pulse doses of chlorambucil may have an increased risk of seizures
- Persistently low neutrophil and platelet counts or peripheral lymphocytosis suggest bone marrow infiltration

Side-effects and adverse reactions

- Central nervous system: tremors, muscular twitching, myoclonia, confusion, agitation, ataxia, flaccid paresis, and hallucinations
- Gastrointestinal: nausea, vomiting, diarrhea, oral ulceration
- Metabolic: bone marrow suppression
- Skin: urticaria, angioneurotic edema
- Other: pulmonary fibrosis, hepatotoxicity and jaundice, drug fever, peripheral neuropathy, interstitial pneumonia, sterile cystitis, infertility, leukemia, and secondary malignancies

Contraindications

▪ Pregnancy category D ▪ Breast-feeding ▪ Safety and efficacy in pediatric patients have not been established

Acceptability to patient

Nausea and vomiting may limit acceptability.

CYCLOPHOSPHAMIDE

- Antineoplastic alkylating agent
- 1–5mg/kg/day orally or 10–15mg/kg intravenously every 10 days
- Dosages must be adjusted in accord with evidence of antitumor activity and/or leukopenia
- Duration of treatment defined by clinical response

Risks/Benefits

Risk: use caution when administering with radiation therapy

Side-effects and adverse reactions

- Cardiovascular system: cardiotoxicity (at high doses)
- Central nervous system: dizziness, headache
- Gastrointestinal: nausea, vomiting, diarrhea
- Genitourinary: amenorrhea, azoospermia, ovarian fibrosis, sterility, hematuria, hemorrhagic cystitis, neoplasms
- Hematologic: leukopenia, myelosuppression, panycytopenia, thrombocytopenia
- Metabolic: bone marrow supression
- Respiratory: fibrosis
- Skin: alopecia, dermatitis

Interactions

■ Allopurinol (increased cyclophosphamide toxicity) ■ Clozapine (may cause agranulocytosis) ■ Digoxin (decreased digoxin absorption from tablet form) ■ Pentostatin (increased toxicity with high-dose cyclophosphamide) ■ Phenytoin (reduced absorption of phenytoin) ■ Succinylcholine (prolonged neuromuscular blockade) ■ Suxemethonium (enhanced effect of suxemethonium) ■ Warfarin (inhibits hypoprothrombinemic response to warfarin)

Contraindications

■ Serious infections, including chicken pox and herpes zoster ■ Myelosuppression

Acceptability to patient

May cause a painful hemorrhagic cystitis (but this may be prevented with vigorous hydration and/or use of uroprotectants).

Patient and caregiver information

Patient should report dysuria or hematuria.

DOXORUBICIN

- Cytotoxic anthracycline antibiotic obtained from a streptomyces mold
- When used in combination with other chemotherapy drugs, most commonly used dosage of doxorubicin is 40–60mg/m^2 given as a single intravenous injection every 21–28 days
- Most commonly used dose schedule when used as a single agent is 60–75mg/m^2 as a single intravenous injection administered at 21-day intervals
- Maximum 450mg/m^2 (above this, risk of cardiac insufficiency increases markedly)

Risks/Benefits

Risks:

- Must be administered under specialist supervision
- Typically causes nausea, vomiting, tiredness, fall in white cell count, hair loss, and neuropathy
- Special attention must be given to cardiotoxicity induced by doxorubicin
- Cardiomyopathy and/or congestive heart failure may be encountered several months or years after discontinuation of doxorubicin therapy

Side-effects and adverse reactions

- Cardiovascular system: cardiotoxicity, phlebosclerosis
- Central nervous system: acute nausea and vomiting, mucositis, peripheral neurotoxicity
- Eyes, ears, nose, and throat: conjunctivitis, lacrimation
- Hematologic: secondary acute myeloid leukemia
- Hypersensitivity reactions: fever, chills, urticaria
- Genitourinary: red coloration to the urine for 1–2 days after administration
- Skin: severe cellulitis, vesication, tissue necrosis

Interactions

■ Paclitaxel ■ Progesterone ■ Verapamil ■ Cyclosporine

Contraindications

■ Marked myelosuppression induced by previous treatment with other antitumor agents or radiotherapy ■ Previous treatment with complete cumulative doses of doxorubicin, daunorubicin, idarubicin, and/or other anthracyclines and anthracenes ■ Breast-feeding ■ Pregnancy category D

Acceptability to patient

Nausea, vomiting, and other side-effects may limit acceptability.

Patient and caregiver information

Patient must report chest pain or shortness of breath.

VINCRISTINE

- Antineoplastic alkaloid obtained from the periwinkle plant
- Adults: usual dosage is 1.4mg/m^2. A 50% reduction in dose is recommended for patients with a direct serum bilirubin value >3mg/100mL
- Child: 2mg/m^2. For children weighing 10kg or less, starting dose should be 0.05mg/kg, administered once a week
- Drug is administered intravenously at weekly intervals

Risks/Benefits

Risks:

- Preparation is for intravenous use only. It should be administered by individuals experienced in administration of vincristine sulfate
- Risk of acute uric acid nephropathy
- Acute shortness of breath and severe bronchospasm have been reported
- Care must be taken to avoid contamination of the eye with concentrations of vincristine sulfate used clinically

Side-effects and adverse reactions

- Central nervous system: neuritic pain
- Eyes, ears, nose, and throat: blurred or double vision
- Gastrointestinal: constipation
- Central nervous system: headache, paresthesias
- Skin: alopecia
- Other: peripheral neuropathyleukopenia

Interactions

- May interact with oral or intravenous administration of phenytoin (may reduce blood levels of the anticonvulsant)

Contraindications

- Patients with the demyelinating form of Charcot-Marie-Tooth syndrome
- Breast-feeding
- Pregnancy category D

Acceptability to patient

Can cause severe neurologic side-effects, including paresthesias, neuritic pain, and motor disturbances, which may limit acceptability.

Patient and caregiver information

Patients should be warned of possible side-effects.

OUTCOMES

EFFICACY OF THERAPIES

- Single-drug therapy produces improvements in about half of patients with low-risk disease
- Combinations are superior in terms of response rate but do not improve overall survival
- Other forms of treatment are helpful in specific circumstances, and more modern agents and new approaches are undergoing clinical evaluation

Review period

Depends on clinical circumstances, but most patients require long-term review, and patients with intermediate- and high-risk disease (Binet group B with progressive disease or uncomfortable organ enlargement, or Binet group C) generally require long-term active treatment.

PROGNOSIS

- Patients with Binet group A disease, which is often discovered as an incidental finding when a complete blood count has been done for some other reason, have a median survival of >10 years untreated
- Patients with Binet group B disease with involvement of at least three sites have a median survival of 7 years
- Patients with Binet group C disease with anemia and thrombocytopenia survive for a median of 2 years
- Favorable prognostic factors include female sex, smaller cells with an absence of nucleoli, lymphocyte doubling time of >12 months, nodular or interstitial patterns in the bone marrow, normal karyotype or single chromosomal abnormality, and sensitivity to treatment with chlorambucil
- Unfavorable factors include presence of cleaved lymphocytes, surface marker patterns CD5-FMC7+, CD23-, CD13+ or CD11b+, elevated serum beta-2-microglobulin levels, diffuse marrow infiltration or a packed marrow, trisomy 12 or abnormalities of 14q, and a high percentage of cells in metaphase
- In general, patients with abnormal karyotypes have a worse prognosis than those with normal cytogenetics, and the prognosis is worst for those with multiple clonal abnormalities
- In 15% of patients, transformations occur into promyelocytic leukemia, diffuse large-cell lymphoma (Richter's syndrome), or acute leukemia. In promyelocytic leukemia arising in this way, the cells have many of the characteristics of chronic lymphocytic leukemia (CLL) cells, including the presence of CD5 surface antigen, which is different from the same clinical entity when it arises de novo. Richter's syndrome comprises increasing lymphadenopathy with splenomegaly, fever, and weight loss. Acute leukemias are rare, but do develop from CLL. All of these developments carry a poor prognosis
- Multiple myeloma is seen occasionally, almost invariably from a different clone of cells from the CLL clone, but clonal transformation can also occur in CLL itself
- Carcinomas may be more common in CLL patients, but this could be a result of the therapeutic agents used rather than part of the disease itself

Clinical pearls

- The majority of patients with CLL develop hypogammaglobulinemia, which is more common in the advanced stages of the disease and which worsens as the disease progresses, contributing to a marked susceptibility to severe, life-threatening infections
- In 10–15% of patients, CLL evolves into a more aggressive lymphoproliferative disease, the most common being Richter's syndrome, which occurs in about 5% of patients; features are lymphadenopathy, hepatosplenomegaly, fever, abdominal pain, weight loss, and progressive anemia and thrombocytopenia, and the median survival is 4–5 months

CONSIDER CONSULT

Refer patients whose CLL evolves into more aggressive disease.

RISK FACTORS

Known risk factors include exposure to rubber and asbestos.

MODIFY RISK FACTORS

Adequate protective clothing should be worn by those working in industries that involve rubber or asbestos.

RESOURCES

ASSOCIATIONS

The Leukemia and Lymphoma Society Inc
1311 Mamaroneck Avenue
White Plains, NY 10605
Tel: (914) 949-5213
Fax: (914) 949-6691
www.leukemia-lymphoma.org

Cancer Care Inc
275 7th Avenue
New York, NY 10001
Tel: (212) 221-3300
Fax: (212) 719-0263
E-mail: info@cancercare.org
www.cancercare.org

Association of Online Cancer Resources Website
173 Duane Street, Suite 3A
New York NY 10013-3334
Tel: (212) 226-5525
www.acor.org

National Cancer Institute
Building 31, Room 10A31
31 Center Drive, MSC 2580
Bethesda, MD 20892–2580
Tel: 1-800-4-CANCER (1-800-422-6237)
www.nci.nih.gov

National Comprehensive Cancer Network
50 Huntingdon Pike, Suite 200
Rockledge, Pennsylvania 19046
Tel: (215) 728-4788 or (888) 909-6226 (patient information service)
Fax: (215) 728-3877
E-mail: information@nccn.org
www.nccn.org

KEY REFERENCES

- American Society of Clinical Oncology. Recommendations for the use of hematopoetic colony-stimulating factors: evidence-based clinical practice guidelines. J Clin Oncol 2000;18:3558–85
- Bennett JM, Catovsky D, Daniel MT, et al. Proposals for the classification of chronic (mature) B and T lymphoid leukaemias. J Clin Pathol 1989;42:567–84

- Cancer Care Ontario Practice Guidelines Initiative. Fludarabine in intermediate and high risk chronic lymphocytic leukemia. Hamilton (ON): Cancer Care Ontario, 1999. Available online at the: National Guideline Clearinghouse
- Catovsky D, Fooks J, Richards S. The Medical Research Council CLL trials 1 and 2. Nouv Rev Fr Haematol 1988;30:423
- Dighiero G, Travade P, Chevret S, et al. B-cell chronic lymphocytic leukemia: Present status and future directions. Blood 1991;78:1901–14
- French Co-operative Group on CLL, Johnson S, Smith AG, et al. Multicentre prospective randomised trial of fludarabine versus cyclophosphamide, doxorubicin, and prednisone (CAP) for treatment of advanced-stage chronic lymphocytic leukaemia. Lancet 1996;347:1432–8
- Johnson RE. Total irradiation of chronic lymphocytic leukemia. Cancer 1979;5:59–64

Guidelines

1 International Workshop on chronic lymphocytic leukemia. Chronic lymphocytic leukemia: recommendations for diagnosis, staging and response criteria. Ann Intern Med 1989;110:236–8
2 Cheson BD, Bennett JM, Grever M, et al. National Cancer Institute-sponsored Working Group guidelines for chronic lymphocytic leukemia: revised guidelines for diagnosis and treatment. Blood 1996;87:4990–7
3 Rai KR, Sawitsky A, Cronkite EP, et al. Clinical staging of chronic lymphocytic leukemia. Blood 1975;46:219–34
4 Binet JL, Auquier A, Dighiero G, et al. A new prognostic classification of chronic lymphocytic leukemia derived from a multivariate survival analysis. Cancer 1981;48:198–206

FAQS

Question 1

What is the best way to decide which patients with chronic lymphocytic leukemia need treatment and which do not?

ANSWER 1

- The ability to identify patients who may need treatment has improved with the use of Rai and Binet classifications, e.g. patients who have Rai stage 0 disease at diagnosis have an approximately 60% or greater chance of surviving for 20 years with no treatment at all
- Consensus of opinion is to reserve treatment for patients who actually need it (i.e. those presenting with symptoms of bone marrow failure – anemia, thrombocytopenia; uncomfortable lymph node enlargement; or symptomatic splenomegaly). Some authorities suggest therapy for patients with a white cell count >100,000/mm^3 (100x10^9/L)

Question 2

How best and how often should patients be monitored for progression or changes?

ANSWER 2

There are no standard interval or follow-up schemes. Most physicians follow up every 1–3 months depending on prognostic factors and individual characteristics.

CONTRIBUTORS

Gordon H Baustian, MD
Otavio A Clark, MD
Dinesh S Rao, MD

CHRONIC MYELOGENOUS LEUKEMIA

SUMMARY INFORMATION

DESCRIPTION

- Chronic myelogenous leukemia (CML) is a malignant myeloproliferative disorder of hematopoietic stem cells in the bone marrow
- The natural history is progression from a chronic phase with no or few symptoms that may last 3–5 years
- There then follows an accelerated myeloproliferative phase manifested by worsening anemia and poor response to therapy. This phase may last up to 12 months
- Finally, there is a short terminal blastic or acute transformation stage characterized by elevated numbers of blast cells and multiple complications such as sepsis and bleeding. This stage may last only a few months
- CML is a clonal disorder and the leukemic cells of 95% of patients will have a distinctive cytogenetic abnormality, the Philadelphia chromosome
- The Philadelphia chromosome is formed by a reciprocal translocation between the long arms of chromosomes 9 and 22
- Rare patients do not present with the Philadelphia chromosome and these patients have a worse prognosis
- This mutation results in the production of an abnormal tyrosine kinase related to the disordered myelopoiesis found in CML

URGENT ACTION

- Refer any patient whose blood count is consistent with a diagnosis of CML
- Organize a complete blood count in any patient whose symptoms suggest CML as a possible diagnosis
- If a blast crisis is confirmed in any patient, refer to a specialist immediately
- Remember that a blast crisis can occasionally occur in patients whose chronic phase of CML has been previously asymptomatic and therefore undiagnosed

ICD9 CODE

201.1 Chronic myelogenous leukemia.

SYNONYMS

- CML
- Chronic myeloid leukemia
- Chronic granulocytic leukemia

CARDINAL FEATURES

- A malignant clonal disorder of hematopoietic stem cells that results in an increase in myeloid cells as well as platelets in the peripheral blood and marked myeloid hyperplasia in the bone marrow
- 40% of patients are asymptomatic and the diagnosis is found on an abnormal blood count
- In the remaining patients, most present with fatigue, anorexia, and weight loss
- Approx. 50% of patients have palpable splenomegaly
- The natural history is progression from a benign chronic phase to a rapidly fatal blast crisis within 3–5 years
- The blast crisis is often preceded by an accelerated phase characterized by a rapidly rising white blood cell count
- Approx. 95% of patients with chronic myelogenous leukemia (CML) have the Philadelphia chromosome, which is demonstrable in all hematopoietic precursors and which appears in all bone marrow-derived cells

CAUSES

Common causes

The strong association of CML with the Philadelphia chromosome strongly implicates the chromosomal abnormality as a cause of CML.

Rare causes

Most patients do not present with any risk factors, but radiation exposure has been implicated:

- Exposure to ^{32}P
- Exposure to radiation from atomic bombs (e.g. survivors from Hiroshima and Nagasaki or incidental exposure of people from nuclear bomb testing)
- Exposure to therapeutic radiation

Serious causes

The Philadelphia chromosome is present in over 95% of patients with CML:

- Philadelphia chromosome results from a reciprocal translocation between the long arms of chromosome 9 and chromosome 22; a segment of the c-abl gene from chromosome 9q34 is transposed onto the bcr gene on chromosome 22q11 creating a hybrid BCR-ABL gene. There is evidence of a direct link between the expression of the hybrid BCR-ABL gene and malignant proliferation of hematopoietic progenitor cells
- This abnormality results in the production of an abnormal tyrosine kinase related to the disordered myelopoiesis found in CML
- It was the first chromosomal abnormality to be associated with a specific neoplastic disorder

EPIDEMIOLOGY

Incidence and prevalence

INCIDENCE

Approx. 0.18/1000 patients.

FREQUENCY

- CML represents 15% of adult leukemias and 2–3% of childhood leukemias
- 4500 cases/year in the US
- 400 cases/year in the UK

Demographics

AGE

- More common in middle age and the elderly but can occur in all age groups, including children
- Median age for all cases of CML at presentation is 53 years
- Median age for patients who are Philadelphia chromosome-positive is 40–45 years
- Median age for patients who are Philadelphia chromosome-negative is 60–65 years

GENDER

CML occurs more frequently in males than in females (male:female ratio is 1.3:1).

RACE

CML is not significantly more common in any race.

GENETICS

- Strong association with the presence of Philadelphia chromosome
- This is a new mutation arising in patients rather than an inherited abnormality

DIFFERENTIAL DIAGNOSIS

Leukemoid reaction

Peripheral blood picture resembling that of leukemia or indistinguishable from it on the basis of morphologic appearance alone, with leukocytosis of varying degrees and increased numbers of immature cells in circulation.

FEATURES

- Extreme elevation of white cell count ((WBC) >50,000/mm^3 (>50x10^9/L)) composed of mainly mature cells; there is usually no basophilia
- Causes include infection, severe inflammatory diseases, and cancer
- Measurement of leukocyte alkaline phosphatase levels may distinguish this disorder from chronic myelogenous leukemia ((CML) the levels are high in leukemoid reaction and low in CML)
- Absence of Philadelphia chromosome

Idiopathic myelofibrosis

Idiopathic myelofibrosis is a rare entity characterized by marrow fibrosis, myeloid metaplasia with extramedullary hematopoiesis, and splenomegaly. The diagnosis is only made when the potential causes have been ruled out. These include CML, polycythemia vera, Hodgkin's disease, cancer metastatic to the marrow (e.g. breast and prostate cancers), infections, and hairy cell leukemia.

FEATURES

- Blood smear evaluation reveals tear-shaped red blood cells, nucleated red blood cells, and early granulocytic forms including promyelocytes
- Bone marrow examination may be required

Polycythemia vera

Polycythemia vera is the most common myeloproliferative syndrome. It is associated with low erythropoietin levels (other causes of increased red cell mass such as erythrocytosis are associated with high levels). Repeated phlebotomy may be required. 20% of patients develop myelofibrosis, <5% develop acute leukemia.

FEATURES

- Splenomegaly
- An increase in red cell mass and clinical manifestations related to increased blood viscosity – neurologic (tinnitus, vertigo, headache, visual disturbances) or thromboses (myocardial infarction, stroke, peripheral vascular disease) – may be present
- Erythrocytosis and thrombocytosis are also commonly present
- Absence of Philadelphia chromosome

Essential thrombocythemia

Usually noted as an incidental finding on routine blood counts; treatment is only required if there are symptoms or signs of complications (bleeding or thromboses). Diagnosis is one of exclusion of the other causes of thrombocythemia (CML, iron deficiency, splenectomy, malignancy, infection, myelodysplasia, polycythemia vera).

FEATURES

- Platelet count >500,000/mm^3 (>500x10^9/L)
- Usually asymptomatic
- May cause migraine headache, transient ischemic attacks, thromboses, or bleeding
- Absence of Philadelphia chromosome

Acute myelogenous leukemia

The distinction between chronic and acute myelogenous leukemia is usually made by peripheral blood examination, history, and bone marrow examination.

FEATURES

- Initial symptoms have usually been present for <3 months
- Clinically, anemia may cause pallor, fatigue, weakness, palpitations, and dyspnea on exertion
- Thrombocytopenia leads to spontaneous bleeding and bruising
- There is often cachexia, anorexia, and fever
- Bacterial and fungal superinfection are common and may be occult
- Hepatosplenomegaly occurs in about 33% of cases
- Leukemic meningitis may occur with headache, nausea, seizures, cranial nerve palsies, and papilledema
- WBC counts may be low, normal, or markedly elevated
- Metabolic abnormalities include hyponatremia, hypokalemia, hyperuricemia, and elevated lactic dehydrogenase (LDH) levels

SIGNS & SYMPTOMS

Signs

- Splenomegaly: the spleen may be only slightly enlarged or enormous, filling the abdomen. It is impalpable in about 10% of patients with chronic myelogenous leukemia
- Anemia
- Purpura
- Swollen or bleeding gums

Transition from the chronic phase to the accelerated and blastic phases results in:

- Increasing splenomegaly
- Hepatomegaly
- Worsening anemia
- Progressive leukocytosis especially increased basophilia, thrombocytosis, or thrombocytopenia
- Fractures of axial and long bones or vertebral collapse from destructive bone lesions
- Thromboses
- Hemorrhages, including retinal hemorrhages
- More rarely, meningeal spread leading to cranial nerve palsies
- With extreme elevations in WBC counts: priapism, mental state changes, and focal neurologic changes
- Acute gout secondary to rapid cell turnover and cell lysis

Symptoms

About 50% of patients in the chronic phase remain asymptomatic until the accelerated or blastic stages, and about 20% of patients are asymptomatic at diagnosis.

Common symptoms include:

- Fatigue and generalized weakness
- Abdominal discomfort and pain, premature satiety secondary to splenomegaly
- Weight loss
- Excessive sweating

Transition from the chronic phase to the accelerated and blastic phases can occur over a period of one year or more, or it may appear abruptly (blast crisis). May be asymptomatic, or it may result in:

- Increasing, often painful, splenomegaly
- Bone pains

- Fever
- Malaise
- Bleeding tendency

CONSIDER CONSULT

- Whenever a peripheral blood count shows an elevated white cell count of 25,000/mm^3 (25x10^9/L) or above
- All patients should be referred to a hematologist for an expert opinion and for bone marrow sampling, unless the primary care physician (PCP) has the facilities and expertise
- When the evaluation of a patient with high white cell count revels a low level of leukocyte alkaline phosphatase

INVESTIGATION OF THE PATIENT

Direct questions to patient

- Q **Have you been feeling inappropriately tired recently?** Fatigue that is of recent onset and that is sustained and predictable may indicate anemia
- Q **Do your gums bleed, or do you seem to bruise more easily lately?** Bleeding diatheses may be due to low platelet counts
- Q **Do you have difficulty in breathing on exertion recently?** Anemia commonly causes dyspnea on exertion
- Q **Have you been having any abdominal pains or abdominal distension recently?** Splenomegaly can cause both nonspecific abdominal pains and abdominal distension
- Q **Have you been feeling full after only a small amount to eat or drink?** Premature satiety can occur secondary to splenomegaly
- Q **Have you had recurrent fevers or any recent weight loss?** Both are nonspecific findings in CML
- Q **Have you recently starting suffering from hives or itching?** Increased basophils in the peripheral blood can raise blood histamine levels, resulting in pruritus and hives

Examination

- **Examine the skin and mucous membranes.** There may be pallor indicating anemia, swollen or bleeding gums indicating infiltrates, or thrombocytopenia or hives indicating excess blood histamine
- **Examine the lymph nodes.** The lymph nodes are not usually enlarged or tender in CML; if they are, consider alternative diagnoses
- **Examine the abdomen. Is there any splenomegaly?** About 90% of patients with CML will have splenomegaly, which can be massive
- **Is there any hepatomegaly?** This may be present in the accelerated or blast phases of CML
- **Examine the bones, especially the spine.** Spinal collapse and long bone fractures can occur as a consequence of CML
- **Examine the nervous system, especially the cranial nerves and optic fundi.** Leukemic meningitis can occur as a complication of CML

Summary of investigative tests

- Complete blood count is necessary for the diagnosis of CML. Anemia, thrombocytopenia, and elevated white cell counts all occur
- Bone marrow biopsy or aspirate are also essential, and should be considered in patients with suspicion of leukemias
- Leukocyte alkaline phosphatase levels are used to distinguish CML from leukemoid reactions, a low level being suggestive of CML
- Serum chemistry: uric acid and LDH levels may be elevated secondary to increased cell turnover

- Blood group and human leukocyte antigen (HLA) typing: examination of venous blood taken from a cuffed sample from the patient and siblings will establish possible bone marrow transplant candidates if needed
- The Philadelphia chromosome is present in bone marrow cells in over 90% of patients with CML. Its presence usually confirms the diagnosis of CML
- Confirmation of the presence of the Philadelphia chromosome should always be sought, generally by a specialist, using either polymerase chain reaction (PCR) or by fluorescence in situ hybridization (FISH) of bone marrow cells. These techniques allow the identification of specific regions of DNA or RNA in a cell. One of the products of the Philadelphia chromosome is BCR-ABL, which is a constitutionally activated tyrosine kinase, an enzyme present in virtually all cases of CML throughout the course of the disease

DIAGNOSTIC DECISION

The diagnosis of CML requires specific peripheral blood findings and specific bone marrow findings.

Peripheral blood findings:

- Elevated white cell count (usually >25,000/mm^3 (>25x10^9/L))
- Elevated platelet count (in about 50% of cases)
- Basophilia can be present
- Reduced leukocyte alkaline phosphatase activity
- All stages of granulocyte differentiation visible on peripheral smear

Bone marrow findings:

- Hypercellularity
- Reduced fat content
- Increased ratio of myeloid to erythroid cells
- Increased number of megakaryocytes
- Blasts and promyelocytes constitute <10% of all cells at chronic phase

CLINICAL PEARLS

Many patients with high white cell counts will prove to have a leukemoid reaction, not CML. Measurement of leukocyte alkaline phosphatase levels is very helpful in distinguishing these entities. A high level of leukocyte alkaline phosphatase combined with a reduced white cell count is very suggestive of CML.

THE TESTS

Body fluids

COMPLETE BLOOD COUNT

Description

- Microscopic examination of venous blood taken from a cuffed sample
- Initial examination is by autoanalyzer; subsequent examination should be done by a specialist hematologist

Advantages/Disadvantages

Advantages:

- Essential for diagnosis
- Easy to obtain
- Inexpensive

Normal

- Total white cell count: <12,000/mm^3 (<12x10^9/L)
- Hemoglobin: >12g/dL (>120g/L)
- Platelet count: 150–400x10^3/mm^3 (150–400x10^9/L)

Abnormal

- Total white cell counts of >25,000/mm^3 (>25x10^9/L) are usually found in CML; the total white cell count can exceed 100,000/mm^3 (100x10^9/L)
- All stages of granulocyte degeneration can be seen
- The diversity of circulating WBCs, from blasts to mature neutrophils, renders the peripheral blood film remarkably similar in appearance to a typical bone marrow aspirate
- Basophilia of 10–15% of the total white cell count is usually found in CML
- During the chronic phase, peripheral blast cells do not exceed 10%
- As the disease progresses to the accelerated phase, there is progressive leukocytosis, with >10% blasts, 20–30% promyelocytes, and 10–20% basophils in peripheral blood
- The blastic stage is characterized by >30% blasts in the peripheral blood
- Mild anemia is present in most cases of CML and its severity increases as the disease progresses
- Elevated platelet counts of up to 1000x10^3/mm^3 (1000x10^9/L) occur in 50% of patients with chronic myelogenous leukemia
- As the disease progresses, the platelet count falls and thrombocytopenia (often severe) occurs

Cause of abnormal result

Malignant myeloproliferation of hematopoietic stem cells in the bone marrow.

LEUKOCYTE ALKALINE PHOSPHATASE

Description

Microscopic examination of venous blood taken from a cuffed sample.

Advantages/Disadvantages

Advantages:

- The level of leukocyte alkaline phosphatase is low in CML and high in leukemoid reaction
- It is very useful in distinguishing CML from leukemoid reactions

Normal

13–100 (33–188U).

Abnormal

Values outside the normal range.

Drugs, disorders and other factors that may alter results

- The leukocyte alkaline phosphatase score can be increased by concomitant infection or corticosteroid therapy
- It is also raised during the accelerated and blast stages of CML

PHILADELPHIA CHROMOSOME

Description

- Microscopic examination of venous blood taken from a cuffed sample or from a bone marrow aspirate

- A shortened chromosome 22 caused by a translocation mutation between the long arms of chromosomes 9 and 22 – t(9:22)
- Its effects include the transmission of oncogenic signals to hematopoietic stem cells, which gain the ability to be independent of cytokines for growth, and which also appear to be protected from apoptosis
- The Philadelphia chromosome appears in all cells in the bone marrow and peripheral blood
- Its presence can be demonstrated by PCRs
- The Philadelphia chromosome is more apparent in marrow metaphases than peripheral blood metaphases
- Also found in patients with acute lymphoid leukemia

Advantages/Disadvantages

Advantages:

- About 95% of patients with CML are positive for Philadelphia chromosome
- The presence of the Philadelphia chromosome strongly confirms the diagnosis of CML in combination with findings of peripheral blood and bone marrow features

Disadvantage: the absence of the Philadelphia chromosome does not completely rule out a possible diagnosis of CML

SERUM CHEMISTRY (URIC ACID, LACTATE DEHYDROGENASE)

Description

Venous blood sample.

Advantages/Disadvantages

- Advantage: simple, readily available tests
- Disadvantage: nonspecific

Normal

- Uric acid: 2–7mg/dL (120–140mcmol/L)
- LDH: 50–150U/L (0.82–2.66mckat/L)

Abnormal

Values outside the normal range.

Cause of abnormal result

Increased cell turnover.

Drugs, disorders and other factors that may alter results

- Uric acid levels may be elevated in renal failure, gout, chemotherapy, radiotherapy
- Uric acid levels may be decreased during treatment with allopurinol, high-dose aspirin, warfarin, corticosteroids, alcoholism, liver disease, dietary deficiency of proteins or purines, syndrome of inappropriate antidiuretic hormone secretion, Wilson's disease, hemochromatosis
- LDH levels may be elevated in myocardial infarction, various hematologic abnormalities, muscle trauma, seizures, acute pancreatitis, muscular dystrophies, hypothyroidism

BLOOD GROUP AND HUMAN LEUKOCYTE ANTIGEN TYPING

Description

- Examination of venous blood taken from a cuffed sample from the patient and siblings will establish possible bone marrow transplant candidates if needed
- Ethical considerations must be taken into account, particularly when testing well siblings, to ensure that fully informed consent is given
- Testing implies that a suitable donor candidate will be willing to donate, and testing of well relatives should only be done on this basis

Drugs, disorders and other factors that may alter results

- Possible donors should also be tested for hepatitis B and C, cytomegalovirus, and HIV, after informed full consent
- Be aware that siblings who are unsuitable matches, for whatever reason, may feel guilt

Biopsy

BONE MARROW BIOPSY OR ASPIRATE

Description

- An invasive procedure requiring local anesthesia
- Usually taken from the sternum or pelvis
- Assesses cellularity, fibrosis, and cytogenetics

Advantages/Disadvantages

Advantage: together with peripheral blood film changes, provides confirmation of the diagnosis

Disadvantages:

- An invasive procedure with low risks of infection and hemorrhage
- Unpleasant for the patient

Abnormal

Chronic phase:

- Hypercellularity (>75%) with myeloid hyperplasia (myeloid:erythroid ratio between 10:1 and 30:1)
- Less than 10% blasts

Accelerated phase:

- >10% blasts
- 20–30% blasts plus promyelocytes
- >10–20% basophils with or without eosinophils

Blast phase:

- Morphologic changes are very similar to those of acute leukemia
- >30% blasts

TREATMENT

CONSIDER CONSULT

- Whenever a blood smear confirms or suggests the diagnosis of chronic myelogenous leukemia (CML)
- Immediately if the blood film suggests acute leukemia
- Immediately if there is evidence from a complete blood count (CBC) of an accelerated or blast phase
- At initial diagnosis, consideration should be given to referring younger patients (aged <60 years) to centers exploring potentially curative therapy with bone marrow transplantation (BMT) or experimental therapies
- Consideration should be given to referral to specialist centers with proven expertise
- For patients who may be suitable candidates for BMT, consider referral to centers with experience and expertise in such transplants

IMMEDIATE ACTION

Patients in the following categories should be urgently assessed in a specialist center:

- Any patient whose blood film suggests that the blastic stage has been reached
- Any patient with CML (at any stage) with unexplained fever, malaise, or acute illness
- Any patient with chronic myelogenous leukemia (at any stage) with severe infection or a seemingly trivial infection that is not responding to appropriate therapy
- Consider urgent leukapheresis if there is hyperleukocytosis (white cell count $>300,000/mm^3$; $>300 \times 10^9/L$). Such high counts are associated with leukostasis syndrome (vaso-occlusive events resulting in central nervous system or pulmonary infarction or hemorrhage)

PATIENT AND CAREGIVER ISSUES

Impact on career, dependants, family, friends

- CML usually consists of a chronic phase lasting 2–4 years; patients may feel well during this phase but will be aware that the blast stage can occur suddenly at any time
- There is therefore considerable stress on the patient, family, and friends, as well as significant impact on any long-term planning, such as employment
- Regular blood tests will be needed, at set intervals of weeks or months as well as in response to any changes in symptomatology, as the progression from the chronic to accelerated stages may well be asymptomatic
- Patients and caregivers will need to know what changes and symptoms are potentially important and when to seek immediate medical help

MANAGEMENT ISSUES

Goals

- To achieve a long-term remission
- To prolong survival for as long as possible
- To ensure the best possible quality of life at all times
- To provide symptomatic and supportive care when active therapy is no longer likely to be effective
- In advanced CML, the goal is to re-establish the chronic phase with the hope of later BMT

Management in special circumstances

COEXISTING DISEASE

Because BMT carries considerable risks of mortality and morbidity, it is less suitable for elderly or infirm patients or for patients with severe concomitant diseases such as chronic obstructive pulmonary disease, ischemic heart disease, or diabetes.

SPECIAL PATIENT GROUPS

The prognosis of CML is best in children and young adults.

PATIENT SATISFACTION/LIFESTYLE PRIORITIES

- In younger patients, the priority is for long-term remission
- In older age groups or in patients with other disabilities, the priority is for the maximum quantity of the best quality of life, rather than cure
- Patients with other severe disorders or elderly patients have an unacceptably high mortality and morbidity from BMT

SUMMARY OF THERAPEUTIC OPTIONS

Choices

Treatment options:

- Allogeneic BMT: matched related donor BMT offers the potential of long-term remission and is therefore the treatment of choice, especially in younger patients, despite its acute morbidity and mortality; matched unrelated donor BMT is an option reserved for patients for whom no suitable related donor is available, and this transplant is associated with a high level of mortality
- Interferon alfa-2b is the treatment of choice for all patients who are not receiving or are awaiting BMT, and for those whom a transplant has failed to cure. It is effective in diminishing the numbers of deaths, prolonging survival, and in causing the disappearance of the Philadelphia chromosome
- Cytarabine is a potent cytotoxic that can be used with interferon alfa to increase the cytogenetic response; it has hematologic responses that are similar to those of interferon alone. Cytarabine is also used by itself in the accelerated phase and blastic phase of CML; its dosage and administration should be organized by a specialist who is experienced in the use of this drug
- Hydroxyurea is the treatment of choice for hematologic control in patients in the chronic phase of CML who are awaiting BMT, or as sole therapy in patients who are not candidates for BMT and who cannot tolerate interferon alfa-2b
- Busulfan has now been superceded by hydroxyurea
- Imatinib mesylate is a specific tyrosine kinase inhibitor. It is a new drug with a specific inhibitory action against tyrosine kinase. It has recently been approved by the US Food and Drug Administration (FDA) and brings hope to many patients with CML, owing to the dramatic effects that have been seen with its use. It has been evaluated in many clinical trials, alone and in combination with other drugs
- Splenectomy does not alter the course or prognosis of CML, but it may be undertaken for symptomatic relief of abdominal pain and distension
- Adoptive immunotherapy using donor lymphocyte infusions is used in patients who relapse after allogeneic transplantation; this is a specialist procedure
- Allopurinol is used in the treatment of hyperuricemia that develops in CML. Is also used concomitantly with hydroxyurea
- Radiation can be used to treat painful lesions that can occur, especially painful bony lesions; radiation is also used in patients who are submitted to transplant

Factors to be considered in choosing treatment:

- Age of the patient
- Stage of the disease
- Availability of matching bone marrow donor

Treatment in the chronic phase:

- Treatment should be initiated as soon as the diagnosis is established
- Average overall duration of therapy is 3 years
- In many patients, treatment can be administered intermittently
- Potentially curative treatment consists of high-dose chemotherapy and total body irradiation followed by BMT; however, patients aged over 60 years are more likely to die of complications and suffer from serious side-effects and so are not usually considered for this option but receive chemotherapy and interferon
- If BMT is not an option, interferon alfa with or without chemotherapy is the treatment of choice
- If there is a cytogenic response to interferon, it should be continued
- If there is no or little cytogenic response, patients should be referred for enrolment in a suitable clinical trial of experimental therapy in a reputable center
- An alternative is to use the tyrosine kinase inhibitor imatinib mesylate, a new drug that has been shown to cause remission in many patients with CML and has been used alone or in combinations with other drugs
- Hydroxyurea is used in the management of CML to reduce the numbers of leukemic cells in the circulation

Treatment in the accelerated phase:

- Chemotherapy (hydroxyurea) produces the best results, although with shorter remission periods than in the chronic phase
- Interferon can also be used but it is not as effective as when given in the chronic phase
- BMT is not very effective at this stage

Treatment in the blast phase:

- The blast phase of CML resembles the acute leukemias; two-thirds of cases resemble acute myeloid leukemia (AML) and one-third resemble acute lymphoid leukemia (ALL)
- The AML-like CML responds to cytarabine in high doses
- The ALL-like CML responds to a combination of vincristine, prednisone, and doxorubicin
- Treatment with the tyrosine kinase inhibitor imatinib mesylate has been used as the treatment of choice
- BMT is not very successful at this stage, with long-term survival rates of about 10%, but autologous BMT (harvested during the chronic phase) may return the patient to the chronic phase, extending survival time
- Intensive chemotherapy with radiotherapy followed by reinfusion of marrow or peripheral blood (or both) collected and frozen during the chronic phase may be tried

At all stages:

- Supportive therapy
- Leukopheresis and splenectomy may relieve symptoms without prolonging survival
- Splenectomy has not been shown to increase survival time, delay conversion to the blast phase, or provide augmentation to chemotherapy
- Radiation therapy may be used to treat extramedullary granulocytic tumors

Clinical pearls

Many patients ask about the new drug imatinib mesylate and about cure. We cannot talk about cure yet, but there are long-term remissions with imatinib mesylate, which is a new drug that was recently approved for use in CML. It induces long-term remission and has a low side-effect profile. It is the drug of choice for many patients.

FOLLOW UP

All patients who have ever had a diagnosis of CML should be followed for life in order to assess wellbeing and ensure that the disease has not relapsed.

Follow up should include:

- A careful history: fatigue, tiredness, bruising, bleeding, dyspnea, abdominal pain, fever, weight loss, pruritus, and bony pain
- A careful examination: pallor, bruising, splenomegaly, hepatomegaly, bone tenderness
- Investigations: CBC and, if indicated, bone marrow examinations

Plan for review

Once in remission, review monthly for 12 months, then every 3–6 months when well.

Information for patient or caregiver

- Report any new symptoms or recurrence of symptoms immediately
- Seek medical attention for every acute infection, even if seemingly trivial, especially in the early stages of remission

DRUGS AND OTHER THERAPIES: DETAILS

Drugs

HYDROXYUREA

- A cytotoxic agent that reduces the number of hematopoietic cells in circulation
- Also known as hydroxycarbamide
- Can be given orally
- Relatively well tolerated

Dose

This drug should be administered by a physician who is experienced in its use. Recommended doses are:

- Can be given at 20–30mg/kg/day in a single daily dose until the white cell count falls to below 10,000/mm^3 ($10x10^9$/L), then decrease to 20mg/kg/day to maintain the white cell count of 5000–20,000/mm^3 ($5–20x10^9$/L), BMT is carried out, or other therapy instigated
- Therapy should be stopped if the white cell count falls below 2500/mm^3 ($2.5x10^9$/L)

Efficacy

More effective and less toxic than busulphan.

Risks/Benefits

Risks:

- Caution in pregnancy and in male or female patients who are contemplating conception
- Usually requires the concomitant administration of allopurinol to avoid hyperuricemia
- Weekly hematologic monitoring required

Benefits:

- Well tolerated and effective as first-line therapy
- Can also be used before more curative therapy or as monotherapy in cases where no other therapy is planned or possible
- Inexpensive

Side-effects and adverse reactions

- Central nervous system: drowsiness, headache, dizziness, disorientation, hallucinations, convulsions (all rare)

- Gastrointestinal: stomatitis, anorexia, nausea, vomiting, diarrhea, constipation
- Geniturinary: urinary – dysuria, temporary renal impairment
- Hematologic: myelosuppression (especially anemia, leukopenia)
- Skin: maculopapular rash, skin ulceration, dermatomyositis-like skin changes, peripheral erythema, facial erythema, hyperpigmentation, atrophy of skin and nails, scaling, and violet papules

Contraindications

■ Hypersensitivity to hydroxyurea ■ Safety and efficacy in children have not been established ■ Severe anemia ■ Marked bone marrow suppression (leukopenia, under 2500 white blood cells; or thrombocytopenia under 100,000/mm^3)

Acceptability to patient

- Usually well tolerated
- An acceptable controller of symptoms for most patients

Follow up plan

Careful monitoring with frequent CBCs is needed until the desired white cell counts are achieved or toxicity occurs.

Patient and caregiver information

Patients should be warned of the possible side-effects, especially on the skin, and of immunosuppression. They should be advised to seek medical attention early with any symptoms of fever, sore throat, malaise, or cough.

BUSULFAN

- Busulfan is as effective as hydroxyurea in reducing leukemic cell count, but inferior to hydroxyurea in terms of medial survival time and bone marrow toxicity of treated patients
- Has greater toxicity than hydroxyurea and is associated with an increased risk of complications when used before BMT. For these reasons it is now seldom used

Dose

4–8mg/day until the white cell count falls to 20,000/mm^3 (20x10^9/L), then stopped.

Efficacy

Busulfan is effective in lowering white cell counts and can be used as initial therapy before BMT.

Risks/Benefits

Risks:

- Specialist supervision required
- Must be diluted prior to use
- Will cause severe myelosuppression
- Risk of developing hepatic veno-occlusive disease
- Risk of bronchopulmonary dysplasia with pulmonary fibrosis
- Risk of cellular dysplasia
- Use caution in patients with a history of a seizure disorder or head trauma, or who are receiving other potentially epileptogenic drugs
- Use caution with breast-feeding mothers

Side-effects and adverse reactions

- Cardiovascular system: tachycardia, thrombosis, hypertension, vasodilation
- Central nervous system: headache, fever, asthenia, chills, anxiety, insomnia, dizziness, depression

- Gastrointestinal: nausea, stomatitis, vomiting, anorexia, abdominal pain, dyspepsia, constipation, dry mouth, rectal disorder, abdominal enlargement
- Metabolic: hypomagnesemia, hypokalemia, hyperglycemia, hypocalcemia, hyperbilirubinemia, edema, SGPT elevation, creatinine increased
- Musculoskeletal: pain, chest pain, back pain
- Respiratory: rhinitis, lung disorder, cough, epistaxis, dyspnea
- Skin: pain at injection site, rash, pruritus

Interactions (other drugs)

- Itraconazole (decreases busulfan clearance) ■ Phenytoin (increases busulfan clearance)
- Acetaminophen (may decrease busulfan clearance)

Contraindications

- Hypersensitivity to any component of treatment ■ Pregnancy category D
- The safety and efficacy of busulfan in children have not been established

Acceptability to patient

Low: it is less effective than hydroxyurea and has greater toxicity.

IMATINIB MESYLATE

- A tyrosine kinase inhibitor
- The Philadelphia chromosome produces a constitutionally activated tyrosine kinase enzyme, BCR-ABL
- The enzyme is present in nearly all cases of CML throughout the course of the disease
- Inhibition of the enzyme leads to hematologic and cytologic responses. The specific inhibitor of the BCR-ABL tyrosine kinase is imatinib mesylate

Dose

- This drug should be administered by a physician who is experienced in its use
- Recommended dose in chronic phase: 400mg/day
- Recommended dose in blast crisis or accelerated phase: 600mg/day
- Should be taken with food and a large glass of water to minimize this problem

Efficacy

Effective therapy for patients with Philadelphia chromosome-positive CML in chronic and blast crisis stages.

Risks/Benefits

Risks:

- Specialist supervision required
- Women of childbearing potential should be advised to avoid becoming pregnant
- Risk of edema and occasionally serious fluid retention
- Risk of severe hepatoxicity
- CBCs should be performed weekly for the first month, biweekly for the second month, and periodically thereafter

Benefit: well tolerated and is likely to become the first-line therapy for patients with CML who are Philadelphia chromosome-positive

Side-effects and adverse reactions

- Cardiovascular system: cerebral hemorrhage
- Central nervous system: headache, fatigue

- Gastrointestinal: nausea, vomiting, diarrhea, hemorrhage, weight increase, abdominal pain, constipation
- Metabolic: fluid retention
- Musculoskeletal: pain, arthralgia, myalgia
- Respiratory: dyspepsia, dyspnea
- Skin: rash

Interactions (other drugs)

■ Inhibitors of the cytochrome P-450 (CYP) 3A4 family (e.g. ketoconazole, itraconazole, erythromycin, clarithromycin) ■ Inducers of CYP3A4 (e.g. dexamethasone, phenytoin, carbamazepine, rifampicin, phenobarbital, or St John's wort) ■ Warfarin ■ CYP3A4 substrates that have a narrow therapeutic window (e.g. cyclosporine or pimozide)

Contraindications

■ Hypersensitivity to any component of treatment ■ Pregnancy category D ■ Breast-feeding ■ The safety and efficacy of imatinib mesylate in children have not been established

Acceptability to patient

High, because it is effective and well tolerated, although it is expensive.

INTERFERON ALFA-2B

- The current first-line treatment for patients who are not being considered for BMT
- Can induce hematologic and cytogenetic remissions
- Not curative
- At diagnosis it is difficult to predict which patients will benefit from interferon alfa. Even patients with poor prognostic features (age, splenomegaly, thrombocytosis, and high blast and basophil counts) may achieve a major cytogenetic response
- Consequently, all eligible patients should be offered the option of interferon alfa therapy
- Interferon is poorly tolerated if started in the presence of elevated white cell counts, and it should be initiated only after hydroxyurea has been used to lower the white cell count. Hydroxyurea should be continued during the initial phase of interferon alfa therapy to prevent rebound leukocytosis and to minimize associated toxicities
- There are trials of interferon plus imatinib mesylate (STI-571, Gleevec) in progress

Dose

- The optimal dose and duration of treatment have not yet been determined
- This drug should be administered by a physician who is experienced in its use

Efficacy

If there is a major cytogenetic response, with overall survival rates of about 80% at 5 years.

Risks/Benefits

Risks:

- Relatively toxic, with flu-like symptoms (headache, fatigue, fever, myalgia, arthralgia) in >50% of patients
- Use caution in seizure disorders
- Use caution in cardiac or pulmonary disease, diabetes mellitus
- Use caution in the elderly
- Use caution in renal or hepatic disease, thyroid disease
- Use caution in dental disease, psoriasis
- Use caution in pregnancy and breast-feeding
- Adverse effects are generally dose related

Benefit: long-term cytogenetic remission is possible, although long-term survival benefits are unclear

Side-effects and adverse reactions

- Cardiovascular system: chest pain, hypertension, edema, arrhythmias, myocardial infarction, cardiomyopathy
- Central nervous system: depression, suicidal ideation, dizziness, anxiety, confusion, paresthesias, insomnia, seizures, coma, flu-like symptoms
- Eyes, ears, nose, and throat: retinal hemorrhage, visual impairment
- Gastrointestinal: nausea, vomiting, diarrhea, weight loss, abdominal pain, taste disturbances, raised liver enzymes, gastrointestinal bleeding
- Hematologic: blood dyscrasias
- Metabolic: hyperthyroidism, hypothyroidism, hyperglycemia
- Skin: injection site reaction, rash, alopecia, pruritus, exacerbation of psoriasis, dry skin
- Respiratory: cough, dyspnea, sinusitis

Interactions (other drugs)

■ Aldesleukin ■ Aminophylline, theophylline ■ Antineoplastic agents ■ Zidovudine

Contraindications

■ Benzyl alcohol hypersensitivity ■ History of depression or severe psychiatric disorders ■ *Escherichia coli* protein hypersensitivity ■ History of hepatitis, autoimmune disease ■ Neonates, children under one year ■ Immunosuppression ■ Visceral AIDS-related Kaposi's sarcoma associated with rapidly progressive disease ■ Patients with platelet counts of $<50,000/mm^3$ ($50x10^9/L$) should not be administered interferon alfa-2b, recombinant for injection intramuscularly, but instead by subcutaneous administration ■ Women of childbearing age (unless undertaking contraceptive measures)

Acceptability to patient

Acceptability to patient may be limited by:

- Daily subcutaneous injections
- The many side-effects
- The high cost

Follow up plan

- Interferon alfa therapy should continue for 2–3 years after achievement of a complete cytogenetic remission and then be stopped
- Therapy should be resumed in cases of cytogenetic relapse
- Careful follow up for life is needed in all cases, with hematologic and cytogenetic analyses
- Thyroid function should be monitored every 6 months
- Discontinue therapy if the patient has suicidal tendencies, parkinsonism, or autoimmune hemolytic anemia

Patient and caregiver information

The initial malaise and influenza-like symptoms are often transitory so patient should persevere for as long as the side-effects can be tolerated.

ALLOPURINOL

- A xanthine oxidase inhibitor that reduces uric acid synthesis
- Used as adjunct therapy in CML to reduce the hyperuricemia that occurs secondary to increased cell turnover and lysis
- The hyperuricemia may increase when the leukemia is being actively treated

Dose

Injection:

- Adult: 200–400mg/m^2/day (maximum 600mg/day)
- Child: starting dose 200mg/m^2/day

Oral:

- Adult: 200–600mg/day, depending on severity; dose not to exceed 800mg/day
- Child 6–10 years of age: 300mg/day; child under 6 years:150mg/day. The response is evaluated after approx. 48h of therapy and a dosage adjustment is made if necessary

Efficacy

Very high.

Risks/Benefits

Risks:

- Caution in pregnancy and lactation
- Use caution in hepatic or renal impairment
- Treatment should be discontinued at first sign of allergic reaction, such as skin rash or other reaction
- Ensure adequate fluid intake during treatment

Benefit: well tolerated and effective

Side-effects and adverse reactions

- Central nervous system: drowsiness, headache
- Gastrointestinal: nausea, abdominal pain, peptic ulceration, cholestatic jaundice, diarrhea, liver failure
- Genitourinary: renal failure
- Musculoskeletal: athralgia, myopathy
- Skin: rashes, alopecia, Stevens-Johnson syndrome

Interactions (other drugs)

■ Angiotensin-converting enzyme (ACE) inhibitors ■ Antacids ■ Oral anticoagulants ■ Azathioprine ■ Cyclophosphamide ■ Mercaptopurine ■ Theophylline

Contraindications

Patients who have developed a severe reaction to allopurinol should not be restarted on the drug.

Acceptability to patient

Well accepted.

Surgical therapy

ALLOGENEIC BONE MARROW TRANSPLANT

- BMT carries risks of significant morbidity and mortality and is therefore usually considered only for otherwise healthy patients aged 60 years or less (some specialists will consider patients up to 70 years, some only up to 50 years)
- BMT is carried out in the chronic phase after hydroxyurea therapy and immediately after high-dose chemotherapy with total body irradiation
- Best results are from human leukocyte antigen (HLA)-identical sibling donor marrow. Only 30% of patients will have such a donor
- For the 70% of patients who do not have an HLA-identical sibling donor, alternatives include matched unrelated donor BMT, 1-antigen mismatched sibling transplant and haplo-identical (2- or 3- mismatched sibling) BMT

- Sternal trephining is usually carried out under general anesthesia and pelvic trephining is usually carried out under spinal anesthesia – recipient marrow is given immediately after harvesting by intravenous infusion

Efficacy
- The only potentially curative treatment modality for CML
- Best performed in the chronic phase of CML, especially within one year of diagnosis
- Percentage of patients who are disease-free at 5 years after receiving allogeneic bone marrow grafts from matched related donor: chronic phase 70%; accelerated phase 40%; blastic phase 15%
- The overall 5-year disease-free rate for patients receiving allogeneic bone marrow grafts from matched unrelated donor is 50%

Risks/Benefits
Risks:
- The considerable benefits must be weighed against the serious risks from transplant procedure, with transplant-related mortality of 20–40%
- Immediate effects: bone marrow failure; hemorrhage; infection (local and generalized); drug toxicity, especially from total body irradiation (gastrointestinal, parotitis, pancreatitis) or secondary to pancytopenia from the cytotoxic agents
- Early effects (weeks): graft failure or rejection; sepsis, generalized and local (bacterial, fungal, or viral); graft-versus-host disease, including rashes, diarrhea, and liver problems; interstitial pneumonitis; relapse of CML
- Late effects: chronic graft-versus-host disease; relapse of CML; infections
- Long-term effects: cataracts; sterility; growth retardation in children; increased tendency of further neoplastic diseases; donor marrow is harvested by trephining and aspiration – the risks to the donor include pain, bleeding, and infection

Acceptability to patient
- Acceptable to patients who are willing to risk the morbidity and mortality statistics for the best chance of cure
- Some patients may prefer to be treated with interferon alfa or imatinib mesylate initially

Follow up plan
- All patients should be carefully followed for life
- Patients should have chromosomal analyses every 6 months for 2 years followed by yearly cytogenetic analysis

Patient and caregiver information
- Patients need hospitalization during and after the procedure, on a strict isolation ward, until post-transplant blood indices return towards normal
- Until this time, patients are at grave risk of infection
- Transplantation of bone marrow is not always successful, and there are immediate, early, late, and lifelong risks

SPLENECTOMY

Efficacy
Splenectomy does not alter the course or prognosis of CML and does not increase survival times.

Risks/Benefits
Risks: there are small perioperative risks from the general anesthesia, sepsis, and hemorrhage

Acceptability to patient
Only acceptable in patients who are suffering severe symptoms from their splenomegaly.

Follow up plan

Patients need immunization against *Streptococcus pneumoniae*, *Haemophilus influenzae*, and hepatitis, and need to take lifelong penicillin prophylaxis.

Patient and caregiver information

- The procedure is for symptomatic relief only
- There is a lifelong increased susceptibility to infections, especially pneumococcal infections

Radiation therapy

RADIOTHERAPY

In the management of CML, radiotherapy can be used:

- Systemically (whole body irradiation) at high doses to establish bone marrow ablation after chemotherapy and immediately before BMT
- Locally for symptomatic relief of bone or nerve symptoms arising from local accumulation of leukemic masses

Efficacy

A necessary prerequisite to BMT.

Acceptability to patient

- High, because it offers hope of cure in combination with transplant
- If used locally, also high, because it provides symptom relief

EFFICACY OF THERAPIES

- Overall, therapy for chronic myelogenous leukemia (CML) has altered the prognosis from an universally fatal disease. Long-term remissions and occasionally cure are obtained with current therapy
- Even if cure is not possible, prolongation of life and reduction of symptoms is usual

Review period

- All patients should have lifelong, regular reviews following treatment. Initial review should be weekly for 8 weeks, then monthly for 12 months, and then every 3–6 months
- Reviews should include history (fatigue, abdominal pain, dyspnea, fever, pruritus) and examination (splenomegaly, lymphadenopathy, pallor, bleeding)
- Hematologic and cytogenetic analyses should also be included
- These analyses should take place every 6 months for 2 years, then yearly

PROGNOSIS

Median survival rates for patients with CML:

- Overall, 5–7 years, with 50–60% of patients alive at 5 years and over 30% alive at 10 years after diagnosis
- 4–6 years (range 1–10 years) for patients who are Philadelphia chromosome-positive
- About 18 months for patients who are Philadelphia chromosome-negative
- Increased splenomegaly, male sex, elevated serum lactate dehydrogenase, a high proportion of marrow or peripheral blasts and/or basophils, and anemia are all associated with poorer prognosis
- Children who are Philadelphia chromosome-positive have the best overall prognosis
- CML inevitably transforms and becomes refractory to therapy with hydroxyurea. It then enters the accelerated phase and within 3–18 months, 75% of patients enter the blast phase, which causes death within 3–6 months

Clinical pearls

The use of imatinib mesylate (STI-571, Gleevec) has the potential to revolutionize the treatment of CML. Many studies in different settings and using different combinations of drugs are currently being conducted.

Therapeutic failure

Successive treatments can be offered to patients with therapeutic failure, but the effects after a first failure look to be low. The use of imatinib mesylate (STI-571, Gleevec) is being tested and may prove to be helpful.

Recurrence

- If there is any suspicion of relapse, patients should be referred back to the specialist or center who treated them previously
- Relapse rates after allogeneic bone marrow transplantation range from 10% in the chronic phase to 80% in the accelerated phase

Prognosis is less gloomy than in the past because there are now several salvage therapies:

- Second transplants: the longer the relapse-free interval after the first transplant, the more likely a second transplant will be successful (relapse probability of 77% in patients whose disease relapsed within 6 months, and 59% if relapse was over 6 months)
- Interferon alfa may induce long-lasting cytogenetic remissions in 20–40% of patients who have a cytogenetic relapse in the chronic phase following an allogeneic bone marrow transplant
- Donor lymphocyte infusions are used as salvage immunotherapy for patients who relapse after an allogeneic bone marrow transplant. There is considerable mortality and morbidity from such therapy

Terminal illness

- Pain relief: consider opiates or radiotherapy for bone or localized nerve pain
- Anemia: consider blood transfusions for symptomatic relief
- Sepsis: antibiotics and leukocyte transfusions if appropriate
- Bleeding: platelet or whole blood transfusions

CONSIDER CONSULT

- Immediately, if there is any clinical, hematologic, or cytogenetic evidence, or suspicion of relapse or recurrence
- If there is unexplained fever, malaise, or splenomegaly

PREVENTION

Prevention of chronic myelogenous leukemia (CML) is difficult because most cases do not occur as a result of exposure to any known risk factors.

RISK FACTORS

- Radiation: exposure to radiation, especially from nuclear tests or explosions, or from ^{32}P, slightly increases the rates of CML
- Cigarette smoking: CML is among the many types of neoplastic disorders whose rates are higher in smokers; however, the excess risk from cigarette smoking is small

MODIFY RISK FACTORS

- Stop, or never start, smoking
- Minimal exposure to ionizing radiation, including medical X-rays

SCREENING

CML is not a suitable condition for screening.

RESOURCES

ASSOCIATIONS

The Leukemia and Lymphoma Society
1311 Mamarcheck Avenue
White Plains, NY 10605–5221
Tel: (914) 949-5213 or (800) 955-4572
Fax: (914) 949-6691
www.leukemia-lymphoma.org

National Marrow Donor ProgramÆ (NMDP)
3433 Broadway Street, NE, Suite 500
Minneapolis, MN 55413
Tel: (612) 627-5800
Toll-free: (800) MARROW 2 (800-627-7692)
Office of Patient Advocacy, tel: 1-888-999-6743
www.marrow.org

National Cancer Information Service
Public Information Office
Building 31, Room 10A03
32 Center Road, MSC 2580
Bethesda, MD 20892–2580
Tel: (800) A-CANCER
www.cancer.gov

American Cancer Society
1599 Clifton Road NE
Atlanta, GA 30329–4257
Tel: (404) 320-3333 or (800) ACS-2345
www.cancer.org

National Comprehensive Cancer Network
50 Huntingdon Drive, Suite 200
Rockledge, PA 19046
Tel: (215) 728-4788 or (888) 909-NCCN
Fax: (215) 728-3877
E-mail: information@nccn.org
www.nccn.org

KEY REFERENCES

- NCCN Practice guidelines for chronic myelogenous leukemia. Version 2000, revised 1 June 2000. National Comprehensive Cancer Network
- Chronic myelogenous leukemia, 2000 www.cancer.gov
- Sawyers CL. Chronic myeloid leukemia [review article]. N Engl J Med 1999;340:1330–8
- Goldman J. Management of chronic myeloid leukemia. www.haem.net/clinical/clinical013.asp
- www.leukemia.org
- McClave PB, Beatty P, Ash R, Hows JM. Bone marrow transplantation of chronic myelogenous leukemia: an overview of determinants of survival. Semin Hematol 1990;27:23–30
- Allan NC, Richards SM, Shepherd PC, et al. UK Medical Research Council randomised multicentre trial of interferon alpha for chronic myeloid leukemia: improved survival irrespective of cytogenetic response. Lancet 1995;345:1392–7
- Guilhot F, Chastang C, Michallet M, et al. Interferon alfa-2b combined with cytarabine versus interferon alone in chronic myelogenous leukemia. N Engl J Med 1997;337:223–9

- Pigneux A, Devergie A, Pochitaloff M, et al. Recombinant alpha-interferon as a treatment for chronic myelogenous leukemia in relapse after allogeneic bone marrow transplantation: a report from the Societe Francaise de Greffe de Meolle. Bone Marrow Transplant 1995;15:819–24
- Mackinnon S, Papadopoulos EB, Carabasi MH, et al. Adoptive immunotherapy evaluating escalating doses of donor leukocytes for relapse of chronic myelogenous leukemia after bone marrow transplantation: separation of graft-versus-leukemic responses from graft-versus-host disease. Blood 1995;86:1261–8
- Druker BJ, Talpaz M, Resta DJ, et al. Efficacy and safety of a specific inhibitor of the BCR-ABL tyrosine kinase in chronic myeloid leukemia. N Engl J Med 2001;344:1031–7
- Druker BJ, Sawyers CL, Kantarjian MD, et al. Activity of a specific inhibitor of the BCR-ABL tyrosine kinase in the blast crisis of chronic myeloid leukemia and acute lymphoblastic leukemia with the Philadelphia chromosome. N Engl J Med 2001;344:1038–42
- Goldman JM. Tyrosine-kinase inhibition in treatment of chronic myeloid leukemia. Lancet 2000;355:1031–2

FAQS

Question 1

Should a patient with high leukocyte count always be referred to a specialist?

ANSWER 1

No. If the levels are <50,000/mm^3 (<50x10^9/L), are falling, or the leukocyte phosphatase is high, the patient can be followed and re-evaluated before being referred.

Question 2

Can the new drug imatinib mesylate (STI-571, Gleevec) replace transplantation?

ANSWER 2

There is an expectation that this will occur, but as yet there is no solid evidence to support it. Some patients and physicians feel comfortable with this uncertainty and choose to try the drug first.

Question 3

What should a primary care physician do when confronted with a very high leukocyte count?

ANSWER 3

Refer the patient to a specialized center as soon as possible to avoid the complications that such a condition can cause.

Question 4

Is a bone marrow biopsy always required in the evaluation of patients with chronic myelogenous leukemia?

ANSWER 4

No. An aspirate of bone marrow can replace the biopsy in most cases.

Question 5

What are the chances that a patient with chronic myelogenous leukemia can achieve cure?

ANSWER 5

About 30–50% of those who are transplanted survive 5 years or longer and are considered cured; however, not many patients are suitable for transplantation, the mortality related to transplant is high (30%), and matched sibling donors are not available to all patients.

CONTRIBUTORS

Kathleen M O'Hanlon, MD
Otavio A Clark, MD
Naixi N Chen, MD

COLONIC NEOPLASM

SUMMARY INFORMATION

DESCRIPTION

- Malignant or premalignant tumors arising from the colonic mucosa
- Adenocarcinoma is the histologic type in 98% of colonic neoplasms
- Most adenocarcinomas arise from adenomatous polyps
- Colorectal carcinoma is the third commonest cancer in both sexes in the US
- Carcinoid tumors are rare neoplastic tumors of the colon
- Clinical features depend on the site of the tumor
- The definitive treatment for cure is resection
- Adjuvant chemotherapy or radiotherapy may be indicated for colorectal carcinoma according the site, stage, and location of the tumor

URGENT ACTION

- Refer to the emergency department in the case of acute obstruction or perforation
- Refer for immediate transfusion in the case of severe anemia

KEY! DON'T MISS!

- Synchronous colorectal carcinoma may be present in 5% of patients. The entire bowel should be investigated with colonoscopy in patients who are diagnosed with colonic neoplasm
- Patients presenting with iron-deficiency anemia (with the possible exception of a premenopausal, multiparous women) should be investigated for colorectal carcinoma

ICD9 CODE

154.0 Colorectal cancer.

SYNONYMS

- Colorectal carcinoma
- Colonic adenocarcinoma
- Bowel cancer

CARDINAL FEATURES

- Colorectal carcinoma is the third commonest cancer in the US in both men and women
- It is the second commonest cause of cancer-related deaths
- Most adenocarcinomas arise from adenomatous polyps, and risk of carcinoma is related to the number, size, and histology of adenomas
- Typical presenting features depend on the site of the tumor
- Anemia of unexplained origin, rectal bleeding, and altered bowel habit are the common presenting features
- The regional lymph nodes and the liver are the main sites for metastasis
- The definitive treatment for cure is resection
- Adjuvant chemotherapy or radiotherapy may be indicated, depending on the site and stage of the tumor
- Prognosis depends on the stage at the time of diagnosis
- Staging of colorectal cancer is based on either the tumor-node-metatases (TNM) staging system or Dukes' classification

The preferred staging system of colorectal carcinoma is the TNM classification, which has five stages (0–IV):

- Stage 0 – carcinoma in situ (Tis, N0, M0)
- Stage I (Dukes' stage A) – tumor invades the submucosa or muscularis propria (T1–2, N0, M0)
- Stage II (Dukes' stage B) – tumor invades the muscularis propria into the subserosa, pericolonic or perirectal tissue, or invades adjacent structures and/or perforates the visceral peritoneum (T3–4, N0, M0)
- Stage III (Dukes' stage C) – primary tumors at any level of invasion with involvement of local lymph nodes (any T, N1–2, M0)
- Stage IV (Dukes' stage D) – primary tumors at any level of invasion, local lymph node involvement, and distant metastases (any T, any N, M1)

CAUSES

Common causes

- Most carcinomas arise from adenomatous polyps, which are found in 30% of middle-aged and elderly people – note that <1% of polyps undergo malignant transformation
- The propensity to become malignant increases with increasing adenoma size
- Villous adenomas carry the greatest risk, followed by tubulovillous and tubular adenomas

Rare causes

Several inherited autosomal-dominant disorders confer a very high risk of colorectal carcinoma:

- Familial adenomatous polyposis confers an almost 100% chance of developing colorectal cancer by age 40
- Gardner's syndrome is familial adenomatous polyposis syndrome with associated osteomas, epidermoid cysts, and sesmoid tumors
- People with hereditary nonpolyposis syndrome (Lynch's syndrome I and II) carries a high risk of developing colorectal cancer

Contributory or predisposing factors

- Inflammatory bowel disease is a known predisposing factor for colorectal carcinoma
- Ulcerative colitis, especially when there is long-standing pancolitis, is more of a risk than Crohn's disease, conferring a 7–10% cumulative risk over 20 years
- Family history, when there is a first-degree relative affected
- Family history of colorectal carcinoma at age <50 is linked to higher risk yet
- Previous diagnosis of colorectal cancer
- Diet that is high in animal fat, low in fiber, or low in calcium
- Smoking may increase the risk
- Radiation exposure

EPIDEMIOLOGY

Incidence and prevalence

Over 150,000 new cases are diagnosed yearly in the US.

INCIDENCE

The incidence is 0.19/1000 population for those younger than 65 years of age and 3.37/1000 among those older than 65 years of age.

FREQUENCY

- The lifetime risk of developing colorectal carcinoma is 2.5–5% for the general population. The risk is two to three times higher if a first-degree relative is affected
- It is the second leading cause of cancer deaths in the US
- 60,000 patients die each year from colorectal cancer

Demographics

AGE

- Peak incidence is in the seventh decade
- Incidence increases with increasing age
- The incidence is 0.19/1000 population for those younger than 65 years of age and 3.37/1000 among those older than 65 years of age
- Younger patients tend to have a worse prognosis

GENDER

- Men and women are affected equally
- Rectal carcinoma is more common in men

RACE

African-Americans and American-Hispanics tend to present later, and are 50% more likely to have fatal disease.

GENETICS

- Familial adenomatous polyposis patients have an almost 100% risk of developing colorectal carcinoma by age 40
- Autosomal inheritance of the gene for Lynch's syndrome I and II (hereditary nonpolyposis coli) confers an increased risk
- Patients with affected first-degree relatives have a 2- to 3-fold increased risk
- Carcinogenic agents can cause mutational activation of oncogenes (K-ras gene), and loss of tumor suppressor genes (p53)

GEOGRAPHY

There is some evidence of an increased incidence in Western countries.

SOCIOECONOMIC STATUS

There is an increased risk in prosperous and urban socioeconomic groups.

DIFFERENTIAL DIAGNOSIS

Differential diagnoses include other diseases that cause per rectum bleeding, altered bowel habits, abdominal pain, and obstruction.

Inflammatory bowel disease

Inflammatory bowel disease includes both ulcerative colitis and Crohn's disease.

FEATURES

- Usually present in young to middle age
- Rectal bleeding
- Abdominal pain
- Frequent stools or diarrhea
- Obstructive symptoms may be caused by inflammatory strictures

Diverticular disease

Diverticular disease is a disorder of the digestive tract consisting of sac-like outpouchings of mucosa and submucosa through the muscular layer.

FEATURES

- Constipation is usually present with diverticular disease, as it is important in the pathogenesis of the disorder
- Abdominal pain (colicky) and altered bowel habit are common
- Diverticulitis is associated with fever secondary to inflammation, and it may cause abdominal pain with localized or generalized peritonitis
- Blood and mucus per rectum
- Abscess formation may complicate diverticulitis
- Postinfective strictures may be seen

Hemorrhoids

Hemorrhoids are masses of dilated vascular tissue occurring in and around the anus and rectum which are responsible for most anorectal complaints.

FEATURES

- Constipation is the commonest cause
- Bright red bleeding per rectum is the usual presenting feature
- Pruritus ani and mucus discharge may occur
- Pain occurs when hemorrhoids thrombose

Extrinsic tumors

Tumors arising from the pelvis may cause obstructive bowel symptoms.

FEATURES

Ovarian tumors or cysts, uterine myomas, or local invasion from a prostate carcinoma may cause obstructive bowel symptoms.

Upper gastrointestinal tract disease

Various upper gastrointestinal diseases can mimic the clinical features of colorectal carcinoma.

FEATURES

- Vague right upper quadrant pain associated with right-sided colonic tumors may be similar to pain associated with cholelithiasis or gastroduodenal disease
- Bleeding from the upper gastrointestinal tract can result in iron-deficiency anemia
- Melena is often associated with upper gastrointestinal bleeding

Irritable bowel syndrome
Irritable bowel syndrome is a diagnosis of exclusion.

FEATURES
- Intermittent diarrhea
- Colicky abdominal pain relieved by bowel motions
- Bloated abdomen
- Symptoms may be precipitated by stress

SIGNS & SYMPTOMS
Signs
General:
- There may be no signs
- Cachexia may be present in advanced disease

Right-sided colonic lesions:
- Pallor secondary to anemia
- Abdominal mass is the presenting symptom in 10% of cases

Left-sided colonic and rectal lesions:
- Palpable mass, blood, or mucus on rectal examination
- Abdominal tenderness may suggest obstruction or perforation

Metastatic disease:
- Enlarged liver, possibly with an irregular edge, is suggestive of hepatic metastases
- Ascites secondary to peritoneal deposits

Symptoms
Right-sided colonic lesions:
- Because stool is relatively liquid as it passes through the ileocecal valve into the right colon, obstructive symptoms or changes in bowel habit are rarely noted. Consequently, patients with right-sided lesions present with symptoms due to anemia, including weakness, dyspnea on exertion, palpitations, and lethargy
- Abdominal pain is usually nonspecific or dull

Left-sided colonic and rectal lesions:
- Altered bowel habit. Alternating constipation and diarrhea is indicative of pseudo-obstruction
- Bleeding per rectum or hematochezia
- Tenesmus
- Cramping abdominal pain

Metastatic disease:
- Abdominal pain may be present secondary to liver metastases, or direct extension into adjacent organs
- Anorexia
- Dyspnea secondary to pulmonary metastases is a rare presenting symptom

ASSOCIATED DISORDERS
Other gastrointestinal disorders that may be related to a low-fiber diet include:
- Hemorrhoids, which are commonly caused by constipation and prolonged straining
- Diverticular disease

KEY! DON'T MISS!

- Synchronous colorectal carcinoma may be present in 5% of patients. The entire bowel should be investigated with colonoscopy in patients who are diagnosed with colonic neoplasm
- Patients presenting with iron-deficiency anemia (with the possible exception of a premenopausal, multiparous women) should be investigated for colorectal carcinoma

CONSIDER CONSULT

- Referral is usually required for colonoscopy, which is the diagnostic test of choice
- Iron-deficiency anemia requires investigation of the gastrointestinal tract, once age and menstruation (where appropriate) have been considered

INVESTIGATION OF THE PATIENT

Direct questions to patient

Q **Have you noticed a change in your bowel habit?** Alternating constipation and diarrhea is a common symptom of left-sided colonic tumors

Q **Have you been feeling lethargic or short of breath on exertion?** Anemia may be the only presenting feature of right-sided colonic lesions

Q **Have you noticed blood in your stool?** Bleeding per rectum requires investigation

Q **Have you experienced any abdominal pain?** Pain may be caused by the primary lesion or metastases

Q **Do you have a feeling of incomplete evacuation after passing a motion?** Tenesmus may be associated with rectal cancer

Q **Have you ever been investigated for colorectal carcinoma?** Screening is indicated for patients with no predisposing factors from the age of 50 years. Specific guidelines exists for those younger than 50 but at high risk

Contributory or predisposing factors

Q **Do you have a history of inflammatory bowel disease?** Ulcerative colitis and Crohn's disease increase the risk of colorectal cancer, and patients with these disorders should be monitored for development of cancer

Q **Do you have a previous diagnosis of colorectal cancer?** The cumulative risk for metachronous cancers is as high as 30% after 40 years

Q **Describe your diet.** A diet high in animal fat, low in fiber, or low in calcium may contribute to risk

Family history

Q **Is there a family history of bowel cancer?** A patient with a first-degree relative with colorectal cancer has a two to three times greater risk than the general population. This risk is higher still if the diagnosis was made before the age of 50

Q **Is there a genetic disease in your family associated with colorectal cancer?** Familial polyposis coli, Gardner's syndrome, and hereditary nonpolyposis syndrome all carry a very high risk of colorectal cancer; patients should inform family members of the need for screening

Examination

The aim of the physical examination is to determine the extent of local disease and to reveal the presence of distant metastases:

- **Perform a general inspection.** Conjunctival pallor may be present in anemic patients. Cachexia is a late sign in colorectal carcinoma
- **Palpate the supraclavicular lymph nodes:** may be enlarged secondary to nodal metastasis
- **Perform an abdominal examination.** Inspection and percussion may reveal ascites (caused by peritoneal deposits). Palpate the abdomen for a mass and for an enlarged liver with an irregular edge

- **Perform a rectal examination.** Assess for blood or a palpable rectal tumor. If a mass is palpated, the location and extent of fixation should be determined, as should the size of the rectal lumen
- **Perform a vaginal and rectovaginal examination.** This may be useful in women to assess the size of the tumor and to palpate for retrorectal nodes

Summary of investigative tests

- Complete blood count should be performed in any patient presenting with rectal bleeding or symptoms consistent with anemia. It will reveal a hypochromic, microcytic anemia in most cases
- Iron studies will reveal an iron-deficiency anemia
- Serum calcium and liver function tests may be required preoperatively, to aid detection of distant metastases
- Fecal occult blood testing is used as a screening test, but it may also be used in the initial workup. It is useful only in directing further investigation if the initial presentation is anemia. Fecal occult blood testing is not sensitive or specific for colorectal cancer; if clinical suspicion of colorectal cancer is high despite negative fecal occult blood, colonoscopy should be performed
- Colonoscopy, usually performed by a specialist, is the gold standard investigation. The entire bowel can be visualized and biopsies may be taken
- Double-contrast barium enema is used only when colonoscopy is not available. It is the best radiographic examination but may still have to be followed by colonoscopy. It may be useful when colonoscopy cannot be performed or provides inadequate information, and it should preferably be followed by sigmoidoscopy
- Carcinoembryonic antigen (CEA) plasma level is useful to monitor the postoperative course of the disease. A preoperative level is essential, and can be useful as a prognostic factor. Elevated CEA after resection may indicate disease recurrence if the primary tumor was also associated with a raised level. CEA is not appropriate for screening purposes. Higher levels of CEA are linked to hepatic metastasis
- Computed tomography (CT) scan of the abdomen and pelvis with contrast may identify liver or intraperitoneal metastases
- Chest X-ray is normally performed after the diagnosis has been made, to help in staging. The presence or absence of pulmonary metastases must be determined prior to surgery

DIAGNOSTIC DECISION

- A diagnosis of colonic neoplasm is suspected on the basis of the history and examination findings and confirmed by biopsy
- Right-sided lesions of the colon are characterized by anemia and right abdominal discomfort with or without an abdominal mass
- Carcinoma of the left colon and rectum typically demonstrate obstructive bowel symptoms and per rectum bleeding
- Biopsy at colonoscopy is required for definitive diagnosis. If an obstructing lesion cannot undergo biopsy, brush cytology may be feasible

Guidelines

The following guidelines are available at the National Guidelines Clearinghouse:

- The American Society of Clinical Oncology. 2000 update of recommendations for the use of tumor markers in breast and colorectal cancer: clinical practice guidelines of the American Society of Clinical Oncology [1]
- The American College of Gastroenterology. Polyp guideline: diagnosis, treatment, and surveillance for patients with colorectal polyps [2]

CLINICAL PEARLS

- People with a familial history of colonic neoplasms, especially those with relatives developing it before 50 years, are considered to be at high risk and should be included in screening programs
- Fecal occult blood testing is used for screening purposes. Be aware that false-positive results are not uncommon, owing to the lack of adequate preparation for the test – a special diet is required before testing

THE TESTS

Body fluids

COMPLETE BLOOD COUNT

Description

Venous blood sample.

Advantages/Disadvantages

- Advantage: simple, inexpensive test
- Disadvantage: nonspecific

Normal

- Hemoglobin: male, 13.5–18.0g/dL (2.09–2.79mmol/L); female, 11.5–16.0g/dL (1.78–2.48mmol/L)
- Mean cell volume: 76–96mcm^3 (76–96fL)
- Mean cell hemoglobin: 27–32pg (0.42–0.49fmol)
- Mean cell hemoglobin concentration: 30–36g/dL (18–22mmol/L)

Abnormal

- Results below the normal reference range
- There is a possibility of a false-positive result

Cause of abnormal result

Chronic blood loss from an ulcerated tumor.

Drugs, disorders and other factors that may alter results

- Poor iron intake or decreased absorption, or the administration of oral iron supplements may alter the results
- Sideroblastic anemia and anemia of chronic disease may cause a similar picture, but iron studies will differentiate

IRON STUDIES

Description

Venous blood sample.

Advantages/Disadvantages

Advantage: simple, inexpensive test

Normal

- Serum iron: male, 81–175mcg/dL (14–31mcmol/L); female, 64–173mcg/dL (11–30mcmol/L)
- Total iron-binding capacity: 300–417mcg/dL (54–75mcmol/L)
- Serum ferritin: 12–200ng/L (12–200mcg/L)
- Transferrin: 139.6–279.3mcg/dL (25–50mcmol/L)
- Transferrin saturation: 10–55%

Abnormal

- Serum iron, ferritin, and transferrin below normal reference range
- Raised total iron-binding capacity
- Keep in mind the possibility of a false-positive result

Cause of abnormal result

Chronic blood loss depletes iron stores.

Drugs, disorders and other factors that may alter results

Poor iron intake or decreased absorption, or the administration of oral iron supplements may alter the results.

SERUM CALCIUM

Description

Venous blood sample.

Advantages/Disadvantages

Advantages:

- Simple test
- May be useful in detecting bony metastases

Disadvantage: nonspecific

Normal

- Total calcium: 8.8–10.0mg/dL (2.2–2.25mmol/L)
- Ionized calcium: 4.69–5.09mg/dL (1.17–1.27mmol/L)

Abnormal

- Results above normal reference range when corrected for albumin
- Keep in mind the possibility of a false-positive result

Cause of abnormal result

- Bony metastases
- Hypercalcemia of malignancy

LIVER FUNCTION TESTS

Description

Venous blood sample.

Advantages/Disadvantages

Advantage: simple, inexpensive test

Disadvantages:

- Nonspecific
- May be normal with liver metastases

Normal

- Aspartate aminotransferase: 5–40mU/mL (5–40 IU/L)
- Alanine aminotransferase: 5–40mU/mL (5–40 IU/L)
- Gamma-glutamyltransferase: 5–60mU/mL (5–60 IU/L)
- Alkaline phosphatase: 30–110mU/mL (30–110 IU/L)
- Total bilirubin: 0.3–1.4mg/dL (6–24mcmol/L)
- Albumin: 3.9–4.8g/dL (39–48g/L)

Abnormal
- Results outside normal reference range
- There is a possibility of a false-positive result

Cause of abnormal result
Liver metastases may cause deranged liver function.

Drugs, disorders and other factors that may alter results
- Many medications can affect liver function tests
- Alcohol abuse can cause abnormal liver function tests

CARCINOEMBRYONIC ANTIGEN PLASMA LEVEL
Description
- Venous blood test
- The CEA level is measured by radioimmunoassay and related techniques

Advantages/Disadvantages
Advantages:
- Level may be measured postoperatively to assess recurrence (as long as the level was raised preoperatively and returned to normal by 6 weeks after resection)
- Simple blood test, so ongoing testing is usually well tolerated
- Elevation of serum CEA levels correlates with a number of parameters. Higher CEA levels are associated with histologic grade 1 or 2 tumors, more advanced stages of the disease, and the presence of visceral metastases
- Useful as an adjunct to clinical and pathologic staging methods

Disadvantages:
- Not specific; level may be raised with other gastrointestinal tumors, with nongastrointestinal malignancy, and in some benign diseases
- Less than half of patients with localized disease are CEA-positive
- Not useful as a diagnostic or screening tool

Normal
2.5ng/mL is the upper limit of normal.

Abnormal
- Results outside normal reference range
- Serial assays should be performed
- Keep in mind the possibility of a false-positive result

Cause of abnormal result
- Tumor releases the glycoprotein into the bloodstream
- Levels higher than 20ng/mL are highly suggestive of malignancy
- Levels may rise more rapidly with metastatic disease than with local recurrence
- Prognosis is worse with a high preoperative level

Drugs, disorders and other factors that may alter results
CEA is not specific for colorectal carcinoma. It may be raised secondary to other tumors, nonmalignant disease, and even smoking.

Imaging

DOUBLE-CONTRAST BARIUM ENEMA

Description

A fluoroscopic test used to study the colon.

Advantages/Disadvantages

Advantages:

- No sedation required
- Widely available

Disadvantages:

- False-negative rate is as high as 40% in single-contrast studies
- Colonoscopy will often be required for tissue sampling, and synchronous tumors should be ruled out
- The entire colon may not be visualized if there is an obstructing lesion
- Smaller tumors will not produce characteristic filling defects, giving a false-negative result

Abnormal

- Right-sided lesions appear as a fixed filling defect, usually a 2–6cm long annular or 'apple core' lesion
- Left-sided lesions are represented by a constriction or intraluminal mass; the mucosal pattern will be destroyed

Cause of abnormal result

Filling defects are caused by intraluminal tumors affecting the passage of the barium.

Drugs, disorders and other factors that may alter results

- Stool or bowel spasm may resemble tumors, producing a false-positive result
- Inadequate bowel preparation may affect images

COMPUTED TOMOGRAPHY SCAN OF ABDOMEN AND PELVIS WITH CONTRAST

Description

Imaging study using computed tomography.

Advantages/Disadvantages

Advantages:

- Noninvasive test
- Allows detection of metastases, usually in the liver
- Direct extension of the tumor beyond the bowel wall can be detected
- May be helpful for staging cancer

Disadvantages:

- Expensive
- May require specialist interpretation of films

Abnormal

Evidence of primary colorectal carcinoma or metastases (either local or distant).

CHEST X-RAY

Advantages/Disadvantages

Advantages:

- Simple test
- Widely available
- Chest X-ray showing metastatic images is usually sufficient to diagnose pulmonary metastatic disease

Disadvantages:
- Exposure to radiation
- Nonspecific

Abnormal
One or more discrete lesions in the lung field(s).

Cause of abnormal result
Pulmonary metastases.

Drugs, disorders and other factors that may alter results
- Primary lung malignancy
- Metastases from other cancers have a similar appearance

Special tests
COLONOSCOPY
Description
Colonoscopy should be performed in every patient with suspected or proven colorectal carcinoma. Visualization of the entire colon is possible.

Advantages/Disadvantages
Advantages:
- Biopsy and polyp removal can be performed
- Allows visualization of the entire colon to the cecum, enabling evaluation of coexisting disease and synchronous cancers or polyps
- Detects lesions that are missed on barium enema

Disadvantages:
- Invasive procedure requiring sedation, so may be difficult or impossible in some patients (e.g. in severe obstructive lung disease)
- Lesions may be hidden around folds or flexures
- Results depend on good bowel preparation
- There is a small risk (1 in 1000) of serious complications, such as perforation or hemorrhage

Normal
Appearance of normal bowel.

Abnormal
Appearance consistent with colorectal cancer or neoplastic polyps.

Drugs, disorders and other factors that may alter results
- Inadequate bowel preparation reduces visibility
- Obstructing lesions may prevent visualization of the entire bowel
- Lesions may be more difficult to differentiate or biopsy in the case of a chronically inflamed bowel or when there are multiple polyps

Other tests
FECAL OCCULT BLOOD TEST
Description
A guaiac-based test may be used for screening – two slides should be prepared from three consecutive stool samples. Color change is noted with the addition of hydrogen peroxide when the test is positive.

Advantages/Disadvantages

Advantages:

- May be used as a screening method
- Noninvasive

Disadvantages:

- Low specificity and sensitivity – <10% of all positive results are caused by malignant neoplasms
- Negative results do not rule out cancer – up to 50% of patients with colorectal carcinoma may have a negative result because of intermittent bleeding
- False-positive results can occur as a result of inadequate preparation for the examination

Normal

Negative for fecal occult blood.

Abnormal

- Positive for fecal occult blood
- A positive result in a screening test is defined as positivity in one or more slide windows

Cause of abnormal result

Blood loss from an ulcerated colonic neoplasm.

Drugs, disorders and other factors that may alter results

- Red meats, nonsteroidal anti-inflammatory drugs (NSAIDs), antacids, steroids, iron supplements, and vitamin C may disrupt results and should be avoided for 48h before testing
- Other gastrointestinal diseases may be the cause of the bleeding, including polyps, diverticular disease, hemorrhoids, and inflammatory bowel disease

CONSIDER CONSULT

- Referral to a surgeon for resection is indicated
- Referral to a stoma therapy nurse will normally be made by the surgeon when required
- The need for referral to an oncologist is case-specific. Patients presenting with stage IV disease may be referred directly to an oncologist. Patients with localized disease may require referral, depending on the extent of invasion. The surgeon and primary care physician (PCP) should decide together whether an oncology referral is required for adjuvant therapy
- The referral for adjuvant therapy must be made as soon as possible after the surgery

IMMEDIATE ACTION

Patients presenting with bowel obstruction or perforation require immediate hospital treatment.

PATIENT AND CAREGIVER ISSUES

Impact on career, dependants, family, friends

- Diagnosis is difficult for the patient and their family. There is an added impact of family history incurring an increased risk for relatives to develop colorectal cancer
- Surgical resection may require a colostomy. Counseling and education are recommended before and after surgery
- If chemotherapy and radiotherapy are to be instituted, the patient will need much support from family and friends, due to the many side-effects with these treatments
- Palliative therapy should be discussed with the patient and the patient's family when necessary

Patient or caregiver request

Q **Should I enter a clinical trial?** Patients with advanced disease may be interested in trials. Each patient should be well informed before deciding whether it is the right option

Q **Should my family be screened?** Investigation is required for patients with high risk of developing colorectal carcinoma. Specific guidelines exist. All people should be screened after the age of 50

Q **Will I need a colostomy?** A colostomy may be required, depending on the site of the tumor, and this possibility needs to be discussed with the patient

Q **Was the cancer caused by my diet?** Low-fiber, high-fat diets have been associated with colorectal carcinoma

Health-seeking behavior

Q **Have you been taking anything for your symptoms?** Patients may have been using hemorrhoidal treatment for rectal bleeding or vitamins for lethargy. This can delay the diagnosis being reached, and diagnostic delay is an important prognostic factor.

MANAGEMENT ISSUES

Goals

- Early diagnosis to reduce mortality and morbidity
- Referral to a colorectal surgeon for resection
- Avoidance of colostomy if possible
- Diagnosis and treatment of metastatic disease
- Referral for chemotherapy and radiotherapy if required
- Adequate symptomatic relief from disease and treatment effects
- Palliative treatment where appropriate

Management in special circumstances

COEXISTING DISEASE

Total colectomy may be necessary in patients with familial adenomatous polyposis or ulcerative colitis.

SPECIAL PATIENT GROUPS
- Patients may be managed more conservatively if they have a coexisting terminal disease
- Resection of the tumor would most likely be performed to prevent obstruction and further blood loss, but adjuvant therapy may not be required

PATIENT SATISFACTION/LIFESTYLE PRIORITIES
- Preservation of bowel continuity is attempted where possible
- Patients with a favorable prognosis will be concerned with return to work and a normal lifestyle
- Patients with a poor prognosis will be concerned with pain control, quality of life, and end-of-life issues
- Side-effects of chemoradiotherapy may affect quality of life

SUMMARY OF THERAPEUTIC OPTIONS

Choices

- A multidisciplinary approach is required for the management of colorectal carcinoma
- Surgery, chemotherapy, and radiotherapy are the major treatment options for the management of colorectal carcinoma

Treatment of the primary neoplasm:
- The first-line curative treatment for colorectal carcinoma is surgery
- If a malignant polyp has been completely removed at polypectomy, no further surgery is required. If there is invasion of the stalk, or the polyp is a villous or villoglandular adenoma, partial colectomy should be considered
- Neoadjuvant radiochemotherapy is indicated for rectal carcinoma, to improve resection and survival
- Surgery is indicated in nearly all patients presenting with colorectal carcinoma, for either the intention of cure or palliation
- Wide surgical resection of the tumor and the involved bowel segment as well as the draining lymph nodes (hemicolectomy) is the preferred surgical option for cure of colonic tumors
- In surgical resection of rectal carcinoma the preferred option is to preserve sphincter function and avoid colostomy, provided the entire tumor can be removed; transanal local excision or low anterior resection are the choices. Abdominoperineal resection may be required if the tumor is situated low in the rectum
- Nonsurgical transanal treatments for rectal cancer include fulguration, radiation therapy, and electrocoagulation; these may be suitable for small and well-differentiated cancers, or if palliation is the goal of treatment
- Radiation and chemotherapy are used as adjuvant therapy for selected advanced carcinomas
- Surgery alone is adequate for patients with stage I disease
- Patients with stage III (Dukes' C) colon cancer should be considered for adjuvant therapy with 5-fluorouracil (5-FU) for 6 months. Adjuvant chemotherapy for stage II colon cancer is under evaluation, with promising results, especially for patients with T4 lesions. They must preferentially be entered into a clinical trial
- Radiation therapy has proven benefit in rectal cancer, either pre- or postoperatively. Combined chemotherapy and pelvic radiation therapy are standard as adjuvant and neoadjuvant treatment for stages II and III rectal carcinoma. Improvement in local disease control with radiation therapy has been suggested for T3 and T4 colonic tumors

Treatment of distant metastases:
- Patients with solitary hepatic metastasis without clinical or radiographic evidence of additional tumor involvement should be considered for partial liver resection, because such procedures are associated with 5-year survival rates of 25–30% when performed by an experienced surgeon
- Resection of isolated pulmonary metastasis may result in 5- and 10-year survival rates of 40% and 20%, respectively

- The role of additional systemic chemotherapy after potentially curative resection of liver metastases is uncertain
- In stage IV and recurrent colon cancer, chemotherapy has been used, with 5-FU-based treatment considered to be standard. Irinotecan (CPT-11) is now considered standard second-line therapy for patients with stage IV disease who do not respond to or progress on 5-FU. Irinotecan has also been used by specialists in first-line chemotherapy for stage IV disease

Palliative treatment:
- Surgery is usually performed in patients for whom curative resection is not possible, to prevent obstruction and ongoing blood loss. Palliative resection or diverting colostomy may be performed
- Observation, or treatment with palliative chemotherapy or radiotherapy, may be considered. Palliative radiotherapy may be used at the site of the primary tumor or for the treatment of metastases

Guidelines
- National Comprehensive Cancer Network Practice Guidelines for colorectal cancer [3]
- The American College of Gastroenterology. Polyp guideline: diagnosis, treatment, and surveillance for patients with colorectal polyps [2]
- Society for Surgery of the Alimentary Tract. Management of colonic polyps and adenomas [4]
- Society for Surgery of the Alimentary Tract. Surgical treatment of cancer of the colon or rectum [5]

Clinical pearls

The possibility of a colostomy is a major concern for patients. Preoperative counseling is important in aiding acceptance.

Never

- Never give oral barium contrast for imaging studies, because it may precipitate acute bowel obstruction
- Never assume that rectal bleeding has a benign cause and treat as such without further investigation, even if coexisting disease (e.g. hemorrhoids) is present

FOLLOW UP

Plan for review

- Referral to a colorectal surgeon is the first priority after biopsy confirmation of primary colorectal carcinoma
- Following surgical resection, referral to an oncologist may be required. This referral must not be delayed. Adjuvant therapy should be initiated as soon as possible after the surgery
- Patients who present with stage IV disease will require direct referral to an oncologist, and the decision regarding the need for surgical referral will be made by the oncologist
- The patient will require support and symptomatic treatment, as well as management of side-effects caused by therapies
- After initial therapy, review should be focused on ensuring that there is no recurrence or distant metastases and no development of a new primary carcinoma
- Successfully treated patients require physical examination, with fecal occult blood testing, complete blood count (CBC), and blood chemistries, every 3 months for 2 years, and every 6 months to 5 years
- If carcinoembryonic antigen (CEA) was elevated at diagnosis or within one week of colectomy, repeat CEA every 6 months for 2 years and then annually for 5 years
- Colonoscopy should be performed within one year of the surgery. If there are no symptoms or polyps, investigation is recommended once every 3 years
- Follow up after removal of an adenomatous polyp requires colonoscopy every 3–5 years

Information for patient or caregiver

- Prognosis or 5-year survival rate can be adequately determined only after surgery (when staging is possible), unless distant metastases are present
- Prognosis for younger patients is worse
- Treatment is multidisciplinary
- The patient should be involved in management decisions

DRUGS AND OTHER THERAPIES: DETAILS

Surgical therapy

- Surgery is the first-choice treatment for cure of primary colorectal carcinoma
- Surgery should be performed by experienced colorectal surgeons

COLECTOMY WITH EN BLOC REMOVAL OF REGIONAL LYMPH NODES

- Wide resection of the affected bowel and the draining lymph nodes is the procedure of choice
- Primary anastomosis is performed whenever possible
- Hartmann's procedure may be performed if the patient presents with obstruction or perforation

Efficacy

- Surgery is the definitive curative treatment for colorectal carcinoma
- 70% of primary tumors are resectable for cure at the time of diagnosis
- 45% of patients are effectively treated by primary resection

Risks/Benefits

Risks:

- Operative complications, including the risk of anesthetic
- Postoperative complications, including infection, dehiscence, bleeding, and anastomotic leak

Benefits:

- Surgery represents the only possibility for cure of invasive tumors
- Prevents obstruction and further bleeding
- Allows intraoperative examination for synchronous cancers or metastases

Evidence

- Surgery is the preferred treatment for colorectal cancer. Primary surgical resection is indicated in nearly all patients with newly diagnosed colorectal cancer, unless survival is unlikely or life expectancy is very short [5] *Level C*
- If curative surgery is not possible, palliative surgery should be performed to prevent obstruction and further bleeding [5] *Level C*

Acceptability to patient

- Surgery is generally well accepted, as it presents the most positive treatment option for cure and will relieve symptoms
- The possibility of colostomy is a major concern for patients

Follow up plan

- Surgical follow up will be required. If pathology reveals a stage I (or possibly II) primary tumor, follow up by the surgeon and PCP may be adequate
- Oncology referral will be necessary for patients with more advanced disease. Discussion with the surgeon and review of the pathology results will determine whether referral to an oncologist is required
- Regular lifelong surveillance is necessary after surgery

- Successfully treated patients require physical examination, including digital rectal examination with fecal occult blood testing, CBC, and blood chemistries, every 3 months for 2 years, and every 6 months to 5 years
- If CEA was elevated at diagnosis or within one week of colectomy, repeat CEA every 6 months for 2 years and then annually for 5 years
- Colonoscopy should be performed within one year of the surgery. If there are no symptoms or polyps, investigation is recommended once every 3 years

Patient and caregiver information
- Bowel preparation is required preoperatively
- A colostomy will be necessary in certain cases and the patient will need pre- and postoperative counseling and education

Radiation therapy

EXTERNAL BEAM RADIATION THERAPY
- There is little proven role for radiotherapy in the management of cancer of the colon, except perhaps for palliation
- Radiation therapy for treatment of locally advanced colonic disease has been suggested, but there is no definitive answer about the efficacy of this treatment
- Adjuvant pelvic radiotherapy is used in conjunction with chemotherapy for invasive rectal malignancy

Efficacy

Effective for the managment of rectal malignancy, but has little or no role in the managment of colonic neoplasm, except perhaps for palliation.

Risks/Benefits

Risks:
- May have significant side-effects, including lethargy, nausea, vomiting, diarrhea, skin damage, wound infections, or anastomotic breakdown
- May increase the risk of thromboembolism, hip fracture, and postoperative fistula formation
- Radiation proctitis

Benefits:
- Relieves pain
- May prevent local recurrence of disease and improve survival when combined with chemotherapy in rectal tumors

Evidence

There is evidence for radiotherapy in the treatment of rectal malignancy.

Acceptability to patient

Provided there is adequate treatment of side-effects, radiotherapy is usually acceptable.

Follow up plan
- Patients should be followed during treatment for support and for treatment of side-effects
- Warn patient about the risk of skin irritation
- Aggressively manage nausea, vomiting, and diarrhea, which can limit patient compliance
- Oncology follow up will be required

Patient and caregiver information
- Therapy is usually 5 days per week for several weeks
- Radiotherapy causes lethargy, and adequate rest is important

Chemotherapy

- Adjuvant chemotherapy is used for stage III colon cancer, but its role is less certain for stage II
- Chemotherapy can be administered systemically or directly into the hepatic artery if it is being used for hepatic metastases
- Chemotherapy is also used as a palliative therapy for advanced stages
- An oncologist should be involved in the treatment of patients requiring chemotherapy

5-FLUOROURACIL

- May be used in combination with leucovorin (the standard regimen) or levamisole
- Several adjuvant regimens produce a similar benefit for stage III colon cancer. These include 5-FU and leucovorin for 6 months, 5-FU and low-dose leucovorin plus levamisole for 6 months, and 5-FU and levamisole for one year

Efficacy

- Adjuvant 5-FU used in combination with leucovorin/levamisole may produce a reduction in the rates of relapse and mortality for stage III colorectal carcinoma
- May be used as palliative therapy to reduce pain and other symptoms
- Palliative chemotherapy reduces the risk of death by up to 35%

Risks/Benefits

Risks:

- Significant side-effects may occur, including nausea and vomiting, lethargy, diarrhea, leukopenia, mucositis, and hand-foot syndrome
- Must be given intravenously
- Life-threatening toxicity may occur in about 5% of patients

Benefits:

- Reduces symptoms
- May prevent recurrence of disease and prolong survival

Evidence

- A systematic review compared adjuvant systemic chemotherapy with no adjuvant chemotherapy in patients with Dukes' C colon cancer, and Dukes' B or C rectal cancer. There was a small but significant improvement in overall survival in patients receiving chemotherapy (5% for colon; 9% for rectal). The results were less clear with Dukes' B tumors [6] *Level M*
- Pooled analysis of three randomized controlled trials (RCTs) of adjuvant 5-FU and folinic acid found a significant increase in survival for patients with Dukes' C colon tumors at 3 years, but no survival benefit for patients with Dukes' B tumors [7] *Level M*
- Another systematic review compared one week of continuing portal vein infusion chemotherapy (5-FU) commenced within 5–7 days of surgery vs no additional treatment after surgery in patients with Dukes' A, B, and C colorectal tumors. A significant survival advantage was seen at 6 years in the chemotherapy group. The benefit was only seen for patients with colon cancer [8] *Level M*
- An RCT compared adjuvant levamisole with placebo in patients with colorectal carcinoma and no evidence of residual disease. There was no significant difference in recurrence or survival at 3 years in patients treated with levamisole [9] *Level P*
- A systematic review found that palliative chemotherapy was effective for prolonging time to disease progression in patients with advanced colorectal cancer. An absolute improvement in survival of 16% was seen at 6 and 12 months [10] *Level M*

Acceptability to patient

- Usually acceptable if side-effects can be controlled

- Patients should be involved in the treatment decision
- 5-FU and low-dose leucovorin for 6 months is often recommended because it is as effective as the other regimens, but the duration of therapy is shorter

Follow up plan

- Ongoing review by an oncologist is essential
- Support and symptomatic treatment during therapy is required
- CBC should be monitored, as myelosuppression manifesting as granulocytopenia and thrombocytopenia are major toxicities occurring 2–4 weeks post-treatment
- Aggressively manage nausea, vomiting, and diarrhea
- Diarrhea should be managed with adequate hydration and loperamide; octreotide has been used for severe diarrhea
- Nausea can usually be controlled with antiemetics

Patient and caregiver information

- Adjuvant chemotherapy is usually started within 5 weeks of surgery if the aim is for cure
- It should be emphasized whether the treatment is aimed to palliate or to prevent recurrence

Endoscopic therapy

Definitive treatment of adenomatous polyps may be performed at colonoscopy.

POLYPECTOMY

- Electrocautery is the usual technique for removal of polyps
- Pedunculated polyps may be removed using snare polypectomy – large sessile polyps require piecemeal snare resection
- Surgical removal of polyps is required only if they cannot be removed safely at endoscopy or there is invasive malignancy

Efficacy

- Colonoscopic removal of adenomatous polyps (with or without carcinoma in situ) is the definitive treatment
- Polypectomy at colonoscopy is adequate for pedunculated polyps with invasive carcinoma if there is complete excision with adequate margins, well-differentiated histology, and no vascular or lymphatic invasion
- Resection of adenomatous polyps prevents the development of colorectal carcinoma
- If complete or safe removal is not possible, primary surgical therapy should be instituted

Risks/Benefits

Risk: perforation or bleeding

Benefits:

- Day stay for procedure
- Avoids the need for more invasive abdominal surgery

Evidence

- Colonoscopic removal of adenomatous polyps (with or without carcinoma in situ) is definitive treatment [5] *Level C*
- Polypectomy at colonoscopy is adequate for peduculated polyps with invasive carcinoma if there are adequate margins and complete excision, well-differentiated histology, and no vascular or lymphatic invasion [2,5] *Level C*
- Resection of adenomatous polyps prevents colorectal cancer [2] *Level C*

Acceptability to patient

Usually acceptable.

Follow up plan

- Follow-up colonoscopy should be performed at 3–6 months to confirm that resection was complete
- Ongoing surveillance is necessary, due to the risk of metachronous adenomas and carcinomas

Patient and caregiver information

- Bowel preparation is required before colonoscopy
- Patients should not drive after the procedure

EFFICACY OF THERAPIES

- Surgery is the most effective treatment for colorectal carcinoma
- 45% of patients are effectively treated by primary resection
- Surgery is carried out with the intent of cure in over 80% of patients, but approximately half suffer recurrence
- Adjunctive chemotherapy for selected patients reduces the risk of local recurrence and prolongs survival
- Radiotherapy is effective for selected patients with rectal malignancy
- Palliative surgery is effective in reducing pain as well as symptoms secondary to obstruction and blood loss
- Patients with advanced colorectal carcinoma have improved survival and time to disease progression when treated with palliative chemotherapy
- The effect of chemotherapy on quality of life related to side-effects of treatment and symptoms secondary to disease is undetermined
- Removal of polyps at colonoscopy is effective, provided that there is no invasive carcinoma
- Surgical resection of liver and pulmonary metastases is effective in some circumstances

Evidence

- Adjuvant systemic chemotherapy has been shown to significantly improve overall survival compared with no adjuvant chemotherapy in patients with Dukes' C colon cancer, and Dukes' B or C rectal cancer. The results were less clear with Dukes' B tumors [6] *Level M*
- Pooled analysis of three randomized controlled trials (RCTs) of adjuvant 5-fluorouracil (5-FU) and folinic acid found a significant increase in survival for patients with Dukes' C colon tumors at 3 years, but no survival benefit for patients with Dukes' B tumors [7] *Level M*
- A significant survival advantage was seen at 6 years in patients treated with one week of continuing portal vein infusion chemotherapy (5-FU) commenced within 5–7 days of surgery vs no additional treatment after surgery, in patients with Dukes' A, B, and C colorectal tumors. The benefit was only seen for patients with colon cancer [8] *Level M*
- A systematic review found that palliative chemotherapy was effective for prolonging time to disease progression in patients with advanced colorectal cancer. An absolute improvement in survival of 16% was seen at 6 and 12 months [10] *Level M*

Review period

Lifelong follow up is required, using a multidisciplinary approach.

PROGNOSIS

- Around 50% of patients have curable disease at the time of diagnosis
- Prognosis is determined by histology, morphology, and stage of the tumor
- Prognosis for young patients is worse, especially those under 30 years of age
- A high plasma level of carcinoembryonic antigen (CEA) indicates a worse prognosis
- Staging is possible at surgery unless there is gross evidence of distant metastases, and is classified according to the tumor-node-metastases (TNM) staging system or the Dukes' classification
- 5-year survival: stage I cancer has a 5-year survival of >90%, stage II is 70–80%, stage III is 35–65%, and stage IV is 5%
- Obstruction and perforation result in a worse prognosis
- Surgical therapy has better results for colonic carcinoma than for rectal carcinoma

Clinical pearls

- Younger patients have a worse prognosis
- Elevated plasma CEA level at follow up may indicate hepatic metastasis, which requires further investigation
- A solitary liver or pulmonary metastasis should be evaluated with the aim of resection. If resection is possible, the prognosis is improved, and cure may be possible for some patients

Therapeutic failure

Second-line chemotherapy (irinotecan) may be instituted if a patient with known metastatic disease progresses while on first-line chemotherapy.

Recurrence

- Local recurrence, especially at the suture line, may be suitable for treatment with further resection
- Liver resection or thoracic surgery may be considered in patients who develop a solitary distant metastasis
- Patients with unresectable liver metastases may be considered for a trial of fluorodeoxyuridine by hepatic artery infusion plus systemic chemotherapy
- Resection of isolated pulmonary or ovarian masses may be appropriate
- Most recurrences occur within the first 2 years after surgery
- A rising plasma CEA level postoperatively is suggestive of tumor recurrence in those patients who had a raised CEA at diagnosis. These patients should be referred for further investigation and treatment

Terminal illness

- Palliative resection should be performed in most patients to prevent obstruction and ongoing blood loss
- Palliative chemotherapy has been shown to improve survival
- Radiotherapy has been used as a palliative treatment
- Pain control and symptomatic management should be optimized

COMPLICATIONS

- Perforation of the bowel
- Acute or subacute bowel obstruction
- In the rare case where a patient presents with obstruction or perforation, the prognosis is worse
- Metastasis, either local or distant. Direct extension of the tumor, regional lymph node involvement, and hematogenous extension, most commonly to the liver and lungs. Transperitoneal metastases cause abdominal carcinomatosis or local implants
- Deep vein thrombosis is a recognized complication of malignancy

CONSIDER CONSULT

- Some patients may be suitable for participation in a clinical trial
- Refer to a pain specialist for intractable pain
- Referral to a palliative care team may be required in advanced disease

PREVENTION

Colorectal carcinoma patients have an improved outcome when the carcinoma is diagnosed early. Removal of adenomas can prevent the development of adenocarcinoma.

RISK FACTORS

- Familial adenomatous polyposis: sigmoidoscopy is recommended every 1–2 years, beginning at age 12 years. Genetic counseling and testing is needed
- Lynch's syndrome: colonoscopy every 2 years, then yearly after age 40 years; begin screening at age 25 years or at 10 years younger than the youngest affected relative. Consider genetic counseling and testing
- Adenomatous polyps: polyps seen at colonoscopy should be removed as there is a chance of malignant transformation, especially with villous adenomas. Ongoing monitoring is required for life
- Inflammatory bowel disease: after 8 years of pancolitis or 12–15 years after a diagnosis of left-sided colitis, patients require regular colonoscopy (every 1–2 years) to allow early diagnosis of tumors and polyps
- Family history: in a patient with first-degree relatives who have colorectal cancer, begin screening at age 40 years with fecal occult blood testing annually and sigmoidoscopy every 3–5 years or colonoscopy every 10 years. In a patient who has two first-degree relatives with colorectal cancer or one first-degree relative who was diagnosed with colorectal cancer at 50 years of age or younger, begin screening at age 40 years or at 10 years younger than the youngest affected relative – screen by colonoscopy every 3–5 years. In a patient with any distant relative who has colorectal cancer or polyps, screening as for the general population is adequate
- Previous diagnosis of colorectal cancer: requires examination of the colon within one year of primary resection. If this is normal, 3- to 5-yearly examination is adequate. There is a chance of metachronous cancer development
- Diet: a diet high in animal fat and low in calcium and fiber is considered a possible risk factor
- Excessive alcohol use and smoking: have been associated with a higher risk of colorectal cancer

MODIFY RISK FACTORS

Lifestyle and wellness

TOBACCO

Smoking should be discouraged.

ALCOHOL AND DRUGS

Excessive alcohol use should be avoided.

DIET

- A diet that is low in animal fat and high in fiber, fruits, vegetables, and calcium may reduce the risk of bowel cancer
- Increased calcium intake or calcium supplements lead to a moderate reduction in the risk of polyp recurrence

PHYSICAL ACTIVITY

A sedentary lifestyle and increased body mass has been thought to be associated with an increased risk of colorectal carcinoma. Exercise should be encouraged.

FAMILY HISTORY

Patients with a strong family history of colorectal carcinoma should be investigated early to allow prompt detection of disease.

CHEMOPROPHYLAXIS

- There is some suggestion that use of nonsteroidal anti-inflammatory drugs (NSAIDs) and aspirin may reduce the risk of colorectal carcinoma
- Folic acid or selenium supplements may be beneficial

Cost/efficacy

- Efficacy is not proven, but NSAIDs do suppress cell proliferation by inhibiting prostaglandin synthesis
- These therapies cannot yet be recommended

SCREENING

- Colorectal carcinoma is one of the leading causes of death in the US
- Most colorectal carcinomas arise from adenomatous polyps
- Less extensive surgery is required for tumors that are diagnosed early and are less invasive
- 5-year survival rate for noninvasive disease is 80–90%
- Tests recommended for initial screening include colonoscopy or fecal occult blood testing and sigmoidoscopy
- Colonoscopy has a higher diagnostic yield but is more expensive, and carries a greater risk of major complications such as perforation of the colon
- People aged over 50 years who do not have risk factors should have a total colon examination (10-yearly colonoscopy or 5- to 10-yearly double-contrast barium enema) or yearly fecal occult blood testing and 5-yearly flexible sigmoidoscopy
- The American Cancer Society has published guidelines for screening and surveillance for early detection of colorectal polyps and cancer
- There are specific guidelines for high-risk patients

Guidelines

The following guidelines are available at the National Guidelines Clearinghouse:

- The American Cancer Society guidelines on screening and surveillance for early detection of adenomatous polyps and cancer – update 2001 [11]
- The American Gastroenterological Association. Colorectal cancer screening: Clinical guidelines and rationale [12]
- The United States Preventive Services Task Force. Screening for colorectal cancer [13]
- Institute for Clinical Systems Improvement. Colorectal cancer screening [14]

FECAL OCCULT BLOOD TESTING

- May be used as a screening method, as polyps are usually asymptomatic, but do cause occult fecal blood loss
- Yearly screening is recommended for this method
- A positive test requires complete colon examination within 2–3 months
- Colonoscopy is the best method to completely investigate the colon after a positive result. If no clinically significant neoplasms are detected at colonoscopy, no further screening is required for 5 years

- Double-contrast barium enema has a sensitivity of 75–80% for evaluation after a positive fecal occult blood test. It is used in the workup of a positive fecal occult blood test, but not as a primary screening method. When combined with sigmoidoscopy, 98% of lesions can be detected. The cost and risk of using both methods to follow a positive fecal occult blood test is undetermined

Cost/efficacy

- Fecal occult testing has been shown to reduce mortality from colorectal carcinoma
- Noninvasive (thus increasing compliance) and inexpensive method of screening
- Risks from this form of screening include complications from colonoscopy and the stress of false-positive results, as well as the discomfort resulting from the tests themselves
- Screening has been shown to reduce mortality by 16%; when adjusted for attendance this figure rises to 23%
- A possible reduction in colorectal carcinoma incidence may be achieved by early detection and removal of polyps
- The American Cancer Society recommends that fecal occult blood testing should be accompanied by sigmoidoscopy to further reduce mortality rates
- More information is required on cost and harmful effects of screening before widespread screening can be recommended

FLEXIBLE SIGMOIDOSCOPY

Sigmoidoscopy using the 60cm flexible sigmoidoscope every 3–5 years is an alternative screening method.

Cost/efficacy

- There is insufficient evidence to recommend the timing of sigmoidoscopy as a screening method
- Sensitivity and specificity are high
- The cost of sigmoidoscopy is higher than for fecal occult blood testing, but there are fewer false-positive results
- The proximal bowel is not visualized
- Sigmoidoscopy alone detects only about half of all colorectal carcinomas and polyps, but there is evidence that screening with sigmoidoscopy and fecal occult blood testing reduces mortality
- There are complications associated with sigmoidoscopy, and the test is uncomfortable, which may reduce compliance
- Polyps <1cm seen at endoscopy should be biopsied. If adenomatous polyps or carcinoma are detected, the patient should be offered colonoscopy to remove polyps, to biopsy other lesions, and to examine the rest of the colon. If large polyps are detected (>1cm), colonoscopy should be recommended. People with tubular adenomas <1cm should decide with their physician whether to undergo colonoscopy

ASSOCIATIONS

American Society of Clinical Oncology
225 Reineker Lane, Suite 650
Alexandria, VA 22314
Tel: (703) 299-0150
E-mail:asco@asco.org
www.asco.org

American Cancer Society
1599 Clifton Road, NE
Atlanta, GA 30322
Tel: (800) ACS-2345
www.cancer.org

National Cancer Institute
NCI Public Enquiries Office
Building 31, Room 10A03
31 Center Drive, MSC 2580
Bethesda, MD 20892
Tel: (301) 405-3848 or (800) 4-CANCER
www.nci.nih.gov

American Gastroenterological Association
7910 Woodmont Ave., Seventh Floor
Bethesda, MD 20814
Tel: (301) 654-2055
Fax: (301) 652-3890
E-mail: mgoslin@gastro.org
www.gastro.org

KEY REFERENCES

- Best L, Simmonds P, Baughan C, et al. Palliative chemotherapy for advanced or metastatic colorectal cancer (Cochrane Review). In: The Cochrane Library, 1, 2002. Oxford: Update Software
- National Comprehensive Cancer Network Practice Guidelines for colorectal cancer, Version 2000
- Scholefield J. Colorectal cancer. Reviewed in: Clinical Evidence. London: BMJ Publishing Group 2001;5:303–9
- Towler BP, Irwig L, Glasziou P, et al. Screening for colorectal cancer using the faecal occult blood test, Hemoccult (Cochrane Review). In: The Cochrane Library, 1, 2002. Oxford: Update Software

Evidence references and guidelines:

1 The American Society of Clinical Oncology. 2000 update of recommendations for the use of tumor markers in breast and colorectal cancer: clinical practice guidelines of the American Society of Clinical Oncology. J Clin Oncol 2001;19:1865–78

2 The American College of Gastroenterology. Polyp guideline: diagnosis, treatment, and surveillance for patients with colorectal polyps. Am J Gastroenterol 2000;95:3053–63

3 National Comprehensive Cancer Network. Guidelines for colorectal cancer, version 2000. Available from www.nccn.org

4 Management of colonic polyps and adenomas. Manchester, MA: Society for Surgery of the Alimentary Tract; 2000

5 Surgical treatment of cancer of the colon or rectum. Manchester, MA: Society for Surgery of the Alimentary Tract; 2000
6 Dube D, Heyen F, Jenicek M. Adjuvant chemotherapy in colorectal carcinoma. Results of a meta analysis. Dis Colon Rectum 1997;40:35–41. Reviewed in: Clinical Evidence 2001;6:344–50
7 International Multicenter Pooled Analysis of Colon Cancer Trials (IMPACT) Investigators. Efficacy of adjuvant fluorouracil and folinic acid in colon cancer. Lancet 1995;348:939–44. Reviewed in: Clinical Evidence 2001;6:344–50
8 Liver Infusion Meta-analysis Group. Portal vein chemotherapy for colorectal cancer: A meta-analysis of 4000 patients in 10 studies. J Natl Cancer Inst 1997;89:497–505. Reviewed in: Clinical Evidence 2001;6:344–50
9 QUASAR Collaborative Group. Comparison of fluorouracil with additional levamisole, higher dose folinic acid or both as adjuvant chemotherapy for colorectal cancer: a randomised trial. Lancet 2000;355:1588–96. Reviewed in: Clinical Evidence 2001;6:344–50
10 Best L, Simmonds P, Baughan C, et al. Palliative chemotherapy for advanced on metastatic colorectal cancer (Cochrane Review). In the Cochrane Library, 1, 2002. Oxford: Update Software
11 The American Cancer Society guidelines on screening and surveillance for early detection of adenomatous polyps and cancer – update 2001. In: American Cancer Society guidelines for the early detection of cancer. CA Cancer J Clin 2001;51:44–54
12 The American Gastroenterological Association. Colorectal cancer screening: Clinical guidelines and rationale. Gastroenterology 1997;112:594–642
13 The United States Preventive Services Task Force. Screening for colorectal cancer. In: Guide to Clinical Preventive Services. 2nd edn; Baltimore, MD: Williams and Wilkins; 1996
14 Colorectal cancer screening. Bloomington, MN: Institute for Clinical Systems Improvement (ICSI); 2001

FAQS

Question 1

When should a carcinoembryonic antigen (CEA) level be ordered?

ANSWER 1

The CEA should be ordered: (1) before resection (to serve as basis for follow up and to assess the prognosis); (2) after surgery (to serve as basis for follow up); and (3) at follow up (every 3 months in the first 2 years). Elevation in two consecutive tests may indicate the development of metastasis, especially to the liver. CEA should not be used for screening purposes.

Question 2

How soon should adjuvant chemotherapy be commenced?

ANSWER 2

Patients suitable for adjuvant chemotherapy should be referred to an oncologist as soon as possible after surgery. Early chemotherapy is linked to better prognosis. Most chemotherapy trials commenced therapy within 8 weeks of surgery.

Question 3

Should patients with stage II disease receive adjuvant therapy?

ANSWER 3

There are conflicting data from studies performed with patients with stage II disease. Recent randomized clinical trials tend to show a benefit for the treatment arm, but the results are not conclusive. Patients with stage II tumors should be evaluated on an individual basis. A clinical trial is appropriate for most patients.

Question 4

What is the appropriate treatment for patients who do not have regional lymph node involvement?

ANSWER 4

The decision to offer adjuvant treatment should be made by an experienced team. Depending on factors such as age, tumor extension, and clinical conditions, adjuvant therapy may be offered.

Question 5

Are there serious side-effects related to adjuvant chemotherapy?

ANSWER 5

5-Fluorouracil (5-FU) is the most common agent used, and in general it is well tolerated. The mortality associated with this treatment is very low and the benefits outweigh the possible harms by a large margin.

CONTRIBUTORS

Fred F Ferri, MD, FACP
Otavio A Clark, MD
Sandeep Garg, MD

ESOPHAGEAL TUMORS

SUMMARY INFORMATION

DESCRIPTION

- Benign or malignant tumors that arise from the esophagus
- The most common esophageal tumors are squamous cell carcinoma and adenocarcinoma
- Squamous cell carcinoma arises in the squamous epithelium
- Adenocarcinomas arise in dysplastic columnar epithelium, usually in the distal esophagus
- Both squamous cell carcinoma and adenocarcinoma carry a poor prognosis
- Other types of esophageal tumor include leiomyomas and other rare benign tumors, carcinoid tumor, hemangioma, small cell carcinoma, and adenoid cystic carcinoma

URGENT ACTION

- Aortoesophageal fistula can result in life-threatening hemorrhage and mandates immediate surgical or endoscopic intervention
- Evidence of life-threatening esophageal/pulmonary hemorrhage mandates immediate endoscopic or surgical intervention
- Hematemesis demands endoscopy to evaluate ulceration or fistula
- Life-threatening airway compromise mandates immediate surgical evaluation or intubation and ventilatory support
- Evidence of deep vein thrombosis requires anticoagulation
- Severe hypercalcemia requires treatment and hospitalization

KEY! DON'T MISS!

- Don't mistake the vague, nonspecific symptoms of esophageal cancer for dyspepsia or peptic ulcer disease
- Always consider the possibility of esophageal cancer in patients with dysphagia; the clinical index of suspicion is heightened by age, race, and other risk factors
- If clinical index of suspicion for esophageal pathology is high, proceed with double-contrast esophageal barium radiogram followed by endoscopy if indicated
- Life-threatening esophageal/pulmonary hemorrhage mandates immediate surgical or endoscopic intervention
- Deep vein thrombosis requires anticoagulation

ICD9 CODE
- 150.0 Cervical esophagus
- 150.1 Thoracic esophagus
- 150.2 Abdominal esophagus
- 150.3 Upper third of esophagus (proximal third of esophagus)
- 150.4 Middle third of esophagus
- 150.5 Lower third of esophagus (distal third of esophagus)
- 150.8 Other specified part
- 150.9 Esophagus, unspecified

SYNONYMS
- Esophageal adenocarcinoma
- Esophageal cancer
- Squamous cell carcinoma of the esophagus
- Adenocarcinoma of the esophagus

CARDINAL FEATURES
- Benign or malignant tumors that arise from the esophagus
- Squamous cell carcinoma usually arises in proximal two-thirds of the esophagus
- Adenocarcinoma usually arises in the distal one-third of the esophagus; the incidence of esophageal adenocarcinoma has risen 4–10% yearly since 1976
- Other types of esophageal tumor include leiomyomas and other rare benign tumors, carcinoid tumor, hemangioma, small cell carcinoma, and adenoid cystic carcinoma
- Tobacco and alcohol increase risk of squamous cell carcinoma
- Barrett's esophagus is the most important risk factor for adenocarcinoma; the rising incidence of adenocarcinoma is attributed to increased incidence of Barrett's metaplasia
- Clinically esophageal tumors, especially squamous cell carcinoma, are often silent with nonspecific complaints
- Overt symptoms are usually indicative of advanced disease
- Late presentation and early lymphatic spread contributes to the poor prognosis
- Approx. 50% have extensive locoregional disease at diagnosis and <60% of those with locoregional disease are candidates for curative resection
- Treatment for early esophageal cancers is esophagectomy and lymphadenectomy with 5-year survival being 5–20%
- For most patients, the primary goal of treatment is to prolong survival or palliation

CAUSES
Common causes
- No definitive cause of adenocarcinoma or squamous cell carcinoma has been identified
- Etiology is probably multifactorial, incorporating environmental and genetic factors

Contributory or predisposing factors
For squamous cell carcinoma:
- Diet: diets high in nitrosamines, fungi (e.g. pickled vegetables), hot tea, and tannins increase risk. Vitamin and mineral poor diets also increase risk (e.g. molybdenum, vitamin A, and zinc), as does betal nut chewing
- Alcohol: risk is increased by potency and quantity of alcohol consumed
- Tobacco: smoking or chewing tobacco increases risk that is related to quantity consumed; tobacco and alcohol act synergistically
- Drug use: smoking opiates may increase risk

- Achalasia: patients with achalasia are 16 times more likely to develop squamous cell carcinoma with an interval from time of diagnosis of achalasia to squamous cell carcinoma of approx. 20 years
- Celiac sprue
- Esophageal diverticula, esophagitis, and esophageal strictures, especially radiation- and lye-induced, usually 40–50 years postinsult
- Esophageal web with brittle fingernails, cheilosis, glossitis, iron-deficiency anemia, koilonychia, and splenomegaly (also known as Plummer-Vinson syndrome, Patterson-Kelly syndrome in the UK); approx. 10% of patients develop esophageal/hypopharyngeal cancer
- Head and neck malignancy with concurrent alcohol abuse and smoking
- Human papilloma virus and fungal infection of the esophagus
- Partial and total gastrectomy increases risk, usually 20 years postgastrectomy
- Radiation therapy
- Tylosis (autosomal dominant palmar/plantar kyperkeratosis): dramatically increases risk with 95% of those afflicted developing squamous cell carcinoma of the esophagus by 65 years

For adenocarcinoma:
- Alcohol: risk is increased by potency and quantity of alcohol consumed
- Tobacco: smoking may increase risk of adenocarcinoma in Barrett's esophagus
- Achalasia
- Barrett's esophagus is the strongest risk factor, increasing risk 40-fold
- Gastroesophageal reflux disease, esophagitis, and hiatal hernia
- Obesity
- Scleroderma
- Zollinger-Ellison syndrome

EPIDEMIOLOGY

Incidence and prevalence

- In the US, esophageal cancer accounts for 1.5% of all malignancies and 7% of gastrointestinal tumors
- The incidence of squamous cell carcinoma has declined in the US over the past 20 years
- The incidence of adenocarcinoma has increased dramatically, especially among Caucasians, now accounting for over 50% of esophageal cancers
- Worldwide, esophageal carcinomas are the ninth most common malignant cancer
- In endemic regions, squamous cell carcinoma predominates over adenocarcinoma

INCIDENCE

Squamous cell carcinoma:
- 0.003–0.004/1000 Caucasians
- 0.0168/1000 African-Americans

Adenocarcinoma:

- 0.051/1000 persons
- 8/1000 in Barrett's esophagus

FREQUENCY

- 12,300 new cases in the US in 2000
- 12,100 deaths in the US in 2000

Demographics

AGE

- Squamous cell carcinoma usually presents in the sixth or seventh decade
- Adenocarcinoma usually presents in the sixth decade

GENDER

- Squamous cell carcinoma is four times more common in men than in women
- Adenocarcinoma is five times more common in men than in women

RACE

- Squamous cell carcinoma: African-Americans are more often affected than Caucasians
- African-Americans have the highest incidence and death rates for squamous cell carcinoma, which is their seventh leading cause of cancer death
- Adenocarcinoma: 95% of those affected are Caucasian males

GENETICS

Adenocarcinoma p53, aneuploidy, and microsatellite instability found in esophageal cancer.

GEOGRAPHY

- Squamous cell carcinoma is endemic in part of China, central Asia, Iran, Puerto Rico, and Africa
- The incidence is relatively low in the US

SOCIOECONOMIC STATUS

Squamous cell carcinoma may be associated with low socioeconomic status.

DIAGNOSIS

DIFFERENTIAL DIAGNOSIS

Achalasia of the esophagus

Motility disorder of the esophagus that results in a functional esophageal obstruction.

FEATURES

- Dysphagia to both solids and liquids
- Chest pain
- Vomiting or regurgitation of undigested food and nonacidic material
- Respiratory symptoms (cough, especially at night, wheeze, breathlessness) may develop
- Barium studies show a dilated, fluid-filled esophagus

Diffuse esophageal spasm

Barium studies show numerous, simultaneous, unco-ordinated contractions.

FEATURES

- Chest pain
- Odynophagia and dysphagia

Gastroesophageal reflux disease

Gastroesophageal reflux disease (GERD) is a passive reflux of gastric contents into the esophagus that causes symptoms or histopathologic changes in the esophageal epithelium (or both).

FEATURES

- Dysphagia
- Heartburn
- Regurgitation
- Patient is likely to have a long history of symptoms before presentation
- Weight loss and odynophagia are rare
- May have persisting cough or hoarseness mimicking signs of esophageal tumor
- Diagnosis is obtained by barium swallow, endoscopy, and distal esophageal pH probe study

Scleroderma

Scleroderma affecting the esophagus produces clinical features similar to those of GERD.

FEATURES

Esophageal manifestations:

- Heartburn
- Dysphagia
- Regurgitation of gastric contents

Nonesophageal manifestations:

- Shiny, taut skin, with loss of hair and normal creases, beginning on the hands and then on the face; skin tightening may eventually limit movement
- Raynaud's phenomenon
- Arthralgia and arthritis
- Myopathy
- Involvement of gastrointestinal tract other than the esophagus is not uncommon
- Pulmonary, cardiac, renal, and other organ involvement may all occur

Leiomyoma and other benign tumors of the esophagus

Leiomyoma is the most common benign esophageal tumor. Other benign tumors include fibroma, fibrovascular polyps, granular cell tumors, inflammatory polyp (also known as pseudotumor, eosinophilic granulomas), lipomas, lymphangiomas, neurofibromas, and squamous cell papilloma.

FEATURES

- Similar to squamous cell carcinoma and adenocarcinoma causing esophageal constriction but with normal mucosa
- Similar to squamous cell carcinoma and adenocarcinoma presenting with anorexia, bleeding, dysphagia, heartburn, chest pain
- Usually presents as solitary lesion but can be multifocal
- Variable morphologic presentation, often seen as incidental lesion on barium study
- Treatment includes surveillance, endoscopic resection, injection therapy, laser ablation, surgical resection or thoracoscopic resection
- Malignant transformation is rare

Other rare tumors of the esophagus

Nonsquamous cell, nonadenocarcinoma malignant tumors may rarely involve the esophagus:

- Carcinoid tumor (a tumor originating from enterochromaffin-like cells)
- Hemangioma (benign)
- Adenoid cystic carcinoma
- Small cell carcinoma
- Kaposi's sarcoma, which has an increased incidence in AIDS
- Leiomyosarcoma
- Lymphoma, which most commonly occurs in patients who are immunosuppressed
- Malignant melanoma
- Mucoepidermoid carcinoma (also known as adenosquamous carcinoma)

FEATURES

- Clinical presentation is often similar to that seen with squamous cell carcinoma and adenocarcinoma
- Carcinoid tumors may present with a wide range of neuroendocrine symptoms (e.g. vasomotor disturbance, bronchospasm, diarrhea)

Gastric cancer

Gastric cardia cancer with proximal extension can present at or near gastroesophageal junction.

FEATURES

- Similar to squamous cell carcinoma and adenocarcinoma, early disease being often asymptomatic with symptoms appearing late in disease
- Similar to squamous cell carcinoma and adenocarcinoma symptoms, including anorexia, dysphagia, nausea, vomiting, and weight loss
- Similar to squamous cell carcinoma and adenocarcinoma as diagnosis is obtained through barium study and endoscopy
- Unlike squamous cell carcinoma and adenocarcinoma tumor, as usually confined to stomach with exception of cardia tumors that can extend proximally

Breast cancer, metastatic

Metastatic breast cancer is the most frequent metastatic malignancy to esophagus.

FEATURES

- Similar to squamous cell carcinoma and adenocarcinoma, causing dysphagia with compressive lesion on barium study

- Similar to squamous cell carcinoma and adenocarcinoma in using stents for palliation
- Significant lesions usually present years after initial breast cancer diagnosis, with a mean presentation 8 years after diagnosis
- Other tumors that can metastasize to esophagus include bladder, cervix, kidney, lung, pancreas, stomach, and thyroid, usually by direct extension or nodal spread

SIGNS & SYMPTOMS

Signs

Clinically, esophageal tumors are often silent, with nonspecific complaints; signs are usually indicative of advanced disease, and may include:

- Weight loss, which may be severe and is usually late and of short duration
- Cervical lymphadenopathy
- Signs of aspiration pneumonia

Symptoms

Symptoms typically occur late and are usually indicative of advanced disease; esophageal obstruction of approx. 60% is generally required for symptoms to occur. Symptoms may include:

- Anorexia
- Vomiting
- Cough, often from tracheal involvement or aspiration
- Back pain, indicative of mediastinal invasion
- Dysphagia, initially intermittent dysphagia for solids, progressing to constant dysphagia for solids and ultimately to dysphagia for liquids
- Gastroesophageal reflux, especially with adenocarcinoma
- Hematemesis or hemoptysis, which may be massive, as a result of invasion by the tumor of a vascular structure
- Hoarseness, which may occur if the recurrent laryngeal nerve is involved
- Chest pain
- Odynophagia

ASSOCIATED DISORDERS

- Squamous cell carcinoma: increased incidence of concurrent head, neck, and lung cancer from alcohol and tobacco abuse
- Squamous cell carcinoma: second primary tumors of the esophagus may develop in patients with cancer of the head, neck, palate, and tonsil
- Adenocarcinoma: Barrett's esophagus with malignant transformation
- GERD

KEY! DON'T MISS!

- Don't mistake the vague, nonspecific symptoms of esophageal cancer for dyspepsia or peptic ulcer disease
- Always consider the possibility of esophageal cancer in patients with dysphagia; the clinical index of suspicion is heightened by age, race, and other risk factors
- If clinical index of suspicion for esophageal pathology is high, proceed with double-contrast esophageal barium radiogram followed by endoscopy if indicated
- Life-threatening esophageal/pulmonary hemorrhage mandates immediate surgical or endoscopic intervention
- Deep vein thrombosis requires anticoagulation

CONSIDER CONSULT

- Refer to gastroenterologist for possible endoscopy with biopsy
- Major hemorrhage mandates emergency surgical or gastroenterologic referral

INVESTIGATION OF THE PATIENT

Direct questions to patient

- Q **When did your symptoms begin?** Early esophageal cancer is often asymptomatic with symptoms appearing late in the disease
- Q **How is your appetite?** Patients with esophageal cancer may have anorexia
- Q **Do you have 'heart burn'?** Gastroesophageal reflux has been associated with adenocarcinoma
- Q **Do you have a cough?** Tracheal involvement or esophagopulmonary fistula with aspiration may cause cough. Simple GERD may also produce cough
- Q **Do you have trouble swallowing solids or liquids?** Dysphagia is the cardinal squamous cell carcinoma/adenocarcinoma symptom from esophageal obstruction and dysfunction
- Q **Do you have pain with swallowing?** Odynophagia may indicate mediastinal invasion
- Q **Do you have abdominal, back or chest pain?** Pain is often vague and nonspecific but may be related to extent and location of tumor
- Q **Have you vomited?** Esophageal or gastric obstruction may lead to vomiting
- Q **Have you regurgitated food?** Esophageal obstruction or dysfunction can cause regurgitation
- Q **Has your voice changed or become hoarse?** Hoarseness may indicate recurrent laryngeal nerve involvement
- Q **Have you vomited blood or coffee ground-like material?** Hematemesis can occur with squamous cell carcinoma/adenocarcinoma
- Q **Have you noticed any black stools or blood from your rectum?** Severe hemorrhage is an uncommon manifestation of esophageal cancer
- Q **Have you lost weight?** Anorexia and dysphagia can cause weight loss
- Q **Do you have leg pain or have noticed one or both legs swelling?** Cancer can induce a hypercoaguable state that can cause deep vein thrombosis

Contributory or predisposing factors

- Q **Does the patient smoke?** Smoking tobacco increases the risk for squamous cell carcinoma and adenocarcinoma
- Q **Does the patient abuse alcohol?** Alcohol abuse is a risk factor for squamous cell carcinoma and adenocarcinoma
- Q **What is the patient's diet?** Diets rich in nitrosamines, tannins, betal nuts, fungi, and hot tea can increase risk for squamous cell carcinoma as can diets low in zinc, molybdenum, and zinc
- Q **What is the patient's medical history?** Several medical conditions increase the risk of squamous cell carcinoma, including: achalasia, celiac sprue, esophageal diverticula, esophageal fungal infection, esophageal stricture/web, esophagitis, gastrectomy, head and neck malignancy, and human papillomavirus infection. Radiation therapy also increases the risk of squamous cell carcinoma. Conditions that increase the risk of adenocarcinoma include: achalasia, GERD, esophagitis, obesity, scleroderma, and Zollinger-Ellison syndrome
- Q **Does the patient have a history of tylosis (autosomal dominant with palmar/plantar hyperkeratosis)?** Risk of squamous cell carcinoma increased 95% by tylosis
- Q **Does the patient have a history of Barrett's esophagus?** Barrett's esophagus is the most influential risk factor for adenocarcinoma, increasing risk 40-fold
- Q **Has the patient recently emigrated?** The worldwide incidence of esophageal cancer varies widely from nation to nation, with China having one of the highest rates
- Q **What is the patient's socioeconomic status?** Squamous cell carcinoma may be associated with low socioeconomic status
- Q **What is the patient's race?** Squamous cell carcinoma is more common in African-Americans, and adenocarcinoma is common in Caucasians

Examination

- **Is there lymphadenopathy?** Esophageal cancer often spreads to local lymph nodes
- **Is the patient pale?** Esophageal bleeding my cause anemia
- **Is the patient's voice hoarse?** Recurrent laryngeal nerve involvement may cause hoarseness
- **Is there evidence of weight loss?** Patients may be cachetic
- **Is there lower extremity edema?** Venous thrombosis is a recognized complication of neoplastic disease classically presenting as an edematous lower extremity

Summary of investigative tests

Initial studies to document disease include:

- Biphasic barium esophagram: the usual initial test of choice to demonstrate esophageal lesion
- Flexible upper endoscopy with biopsy of the lesion is needed to establish a definitive diagnosis. The biopsy alone is diagnostic in 70% of the patients and the brushing in 90%. The combination of both is diagnostic in 95% of the cases

Staging the tumor can be done using the following:

- Computed tomography (CT) scan of the chest and abdomen to evaluate presence of locally advanced or metastatic disease and to determine resectability. CT is less accurate than endoscopic ultrasonography for staging the tumor depth and lymph node spread
- Endoscopic ultrasonography is used for staging and biopsy. Gives a better estimate of the degree of invasion and extension to lymph nodes than CT
- Laparoscopy may be indicated for staging if tumor located at gastroesophageal junction
- Bronchoscopy, laparoscopy, thoracoscopy, and thoracotomy can play a role in complication management and staging and are normally ordered, performed, and interpreted by a specialist
- If complete upper endoscopy is not possible then double-contrast barium radiogram of upper gastrointestinal tract should be performed

The National Comprehensive Cancer Network Practice (NCCN) Practice Guidelines for Esophageal Cancer 2000 [1] state that those with a new diagnosis of esophageal cancer should have:

- Complete history and physical examination
- Complete upper endoscopy
- Complete blood count, serum electrolytes, and coagulation panel
- CT scan of the chest and abdomen

DIAGNOSTIC DECISION

- Early clinical presentation is often vague and does not suggest neoplastic disease; early diagnosis is therefore difficult, and most patients present with advanced disease
- Always consider the possibility of malignancy in patients with esophageal complaints, clinical index of suspicion heightened by age, race, and other risk factors
- If clinical index of suspicion for esophageal pathology is high then the patient should undergo double-contrast barium esophagram
- Once a esophageal lesion is identified, a flexible upper endoscopy with biopsy is needed to establish a definitive diagnosis

Diagnostic workup also aims to stage the tumor affecting the treatment and prognosis. The tumor-node-metastases (TNM) classification is commonly used.

In the TNM classification, disease is first classified according to the characteristics of the tumor itself:

- Primary tumor (T)
- TX: primary tumor cannot be assessed
- T0: no evidence of primary tumor
- Tis: carcinoma in situ
- T1: tumor invades lamina propria or submucosa

- T2: tumor invades muscularis propria
- T3: tumor invades adventitia
- T4: tumor invades adjacent structures

Disease is next classified according to lymph node involvement:
- Regional lymph nodes (N)
- NX: regional lymph nodes cannot be assessed
- N0: no regional lymph node metastasis
- N1: regional lymph node metastasis

Disease is next classified according to the presence and extent of metastases:
- Distant metastasis (M)
- MX: presence of distant metastasis cannot be assessed
- M0: no distant metastasis
- M1: distant metastasis

Tumors of the lower thoracic esophagus:
- M1a: metastasis in celiac lymph nodes
- M1b: other distant metastasis

Tumors of the midthoracic esophagus:
- M1a: not applicable
- M1b: nonregional lymph nodes and/or other distant metastasis

Tumors of the upper thoracic esophagus:
- M1a: metastasis in cervical nodes
- M1b: other distant metastasis

TNM staging:
- Stage 0: Tis, N0, M0
- Stage I: T1, N0, M0
- Stage IIA: T2, N0, M0
- Stage IIA: T3, N0, M0
- Stage IIB: T1, N1, M0
- Stage IIB: T2, N1, M0
- Stage III: T3, N1, M0
- Stage III: T4 any N, M0
- Stage IV: any T, any N, M1
- Stage IVA: any T, any N, M1a
- Stage IVB: any T, any N, M1b

Guidelines

The American College of Gastroenterology treatment guideline: esophageal cancer [2].

THE TESTS

Biopsy

FLEXIBLE UPPER ENDOSCOPY WITH BIOPSY

Description

- Esophageal tissue obtained endoscopically with biopsy or snare polypectomy
- Patients suspected of having an esophageal lesion should undergo endoscopy with biopsy and brush cytology
- Squamous cell carcinoma can appear as small bumps/polypoid masses with denuded epithelium or ragged ulcerated lesions

- Adenocarcinoma can appear as flat ulcerated lesions to fungating/polypoid mass
- Adenocarcinoma and squamous cell carcinoma are grossly similar and biopsy with histologic review is necessary to differentiate
- Adenocarcinoma and Barrett's esophagus are often diagnosed concurrently

Advantages/Disadvantages

Advantages:

- Invasive diagnostic procedure of choice
- Provides tissue for definitive diagnosis of gastric malignancy
- Can be used to stage esophageal malignancy
- High sensitivity and specificity especially using both biopsy and brush cytology
- Well tolerated by patients

Disadvantages:

- Insufficient tissue obtained in 33% of endoscopic biopsies secondary to inadequate forceps tissue penetration
- Random biopsy surveillance endoscopy for high-grade dysplasia or Barrett's esophagus is subject to sampling error
- Sedation frequently needed for procedure
- Complications include bleeding and esophageal/gastric perforation

Normal

- No gastric lesion identified
- No abnormal histology

Abnormal

- Gastric lesion identified
- Abnormal histology identified

Cause of abnormal result

Esophageal or gastric tumor.

Imaging

DOUBLE-CONTRAST BARIUM ESOPHAGEAL RADIOGRAM

Description

- Barium contrast study used to highlight mucosal detail and identify esophageal lesion
- Procedure of choice for initial investigation of dysphagia
- Low specificity

Advantages/Disadvantages

Advantages:

- Initial diagnostic procedure of choice to identify gastric lesion
- Can identify esophageal fistula, obstruction, or stenosis
- Good sensitivity and specificity for advanced lesions

Disadvantages:

- Can only determine if esophageal lesion is present, biopsy needing for definitive diagnosis
- Cannot determine resectability
- Complications include barium aspiration
- Poor sensitivity and specificity for early lesions
- Fails to identify 73% of early esophageal lesions

Normal

No esophageal lesion identified.

Abnormal
Esophageal lesion identified.

Cause of abnormal result
- Esophageal tumor
- Esophageal web
- Esophageal diverticulum
- Esophageal fistula

ENDOSCOPY WITH ULTRASOUND IMAGING
Description
- Endoscopic ultrasound is used to highlight mucosal detail and identify esophageal lesions
- Useful adjunct to endoscopy for imaging lesion
- Endoscopic ultrasonography has emerged as a leading staging modality for determining tumor invasion and lymph node status

Advantages/Disadvantages
Advantages:
- Can identify esophageal fistula, obstruction, or stenosis for biopsy
- Can determine tumor invasion and lymphadenopathy
- Identifies early tumors with good sensitivity and specificity

Disadvantages:
- Specialist test
- Sedation frequently needed for procedure
- Complications include bleeding and esophageal/gastric perforation

Normal
No esophageal lesion identified.

Abnormal
Esophageal lesion identified.

Cause of abnormal result
Esophageal tumor.

COMPUTED TOMOGRAPHY SCAN OF THE CHEST AND ABDOMEN
Description
Used for staging and formulating treatment plan.

Advantages/Disadvantages
Advantages:
- Painless
- A very low-risk procedure
- Relatively inexpensive

Disadvantage: less accurate than endoscopic ultrasonography for staging the tumor depth and lymph node spread

Abnormal
Presence of invasion into nearby tissues and of enlarged local lymph nodes.

Cause of abnormal result
Possible metastases or localized spread.

TREATMENT

CONSIDER CONSULT

Multidisciplinary team approach enhances patient satisfaction and may improve survival:

- Refer to oncologist for initial planning and chemotherapy
- Refer to radiation oncologist for radiation therapy
- Refer to dietitian for nutritional support
- Referral to a clinical trial may be appropriate

IMMEDIATE ACTION

- Evidence of life-threatening esophageal/pulmonary hemorrhage mandates immediate endoscopic or surgical intervention
- Evidence of deep vein thrombosis requires anticoagulation

PATIENT AND CAREGIVER ISSUES

Forensic and legal issues

- Most patients will be able to consent for treatment
- If patient cannot give consent, determine who has authority to consent, especially in life-threatening esophageal/pulmonary hemorrhage and other emergencies

Impact on career, dependants, family, friends

- Overall prognosis is poor and the patients, their families, and friends will have to deal with end-of-life issues
- Psychologic impact of cancer diagnosis is profound with patients, families, and friends experiencing a variety of emotions including anger, anxiety, denial, depression, and grief
- Potential significant impact on career given physical and psychologic demands of diagnosis/treatment and poor overall prognosis

Patient or caregiver request

- Green tea: there is no available evidence that green tea can prevent esophageal cancer
- Garlic: there is no available evidence that garlic can prevent esophageal cancer

MANAGEMENT ISSUES

Goals

- To achieve complete curative resection if possible
- To prolong survival and improve quality of life in nonresectable patients
- To palliate symptoms in end-stage patients
- To achieve adequate pain control
- To ensure adequate nutrition
- To evaluate social support

Management in special circumstances

COEXISTING DISEASE

Patients with comorbidities tend to have worse prognosis.

PATIENT SATISFACTION/LIFESTYLE PRIORITIES

- Patients will have questions regarding treatment and prognosis
- Patients will be especially concerned with pain control and quality of life
- Patients with advanced disease will need assistance with end-of-life issues
- Side-effects of chemoradiotherapy may lead to poor quality of life
- Severe disability may occur with terminal disease

SUMMARY OF THERAPEUTIC OPTIONS

Choices

- Treatment for esophageal tumors requires specialist input
- Treatment modalities can be used for curing the disease or palliation

Curative treatments:

- Surgery including esophagectomy and periesophageal lymphadenectomy for early-stage disease can be curative if complete resection is achieved
- Chemoradiotherapy is sometimes given before surgery in attempt to improve the resectability, but is an experimental treatment. It is also an alternative to esophagectomy for locoregional disease
- Radiation therapy and chemotherapy (5-fluouracil (5-FU)/cisplatin) are often given after surgery

Palliative treatments:

- Palliation uses external beam radiation therapy, but has been superseded by chemoradiotherapy
- Photodynamic therapy is an experimental treatment that destroys tumor tissue without damaging normal tissue
- Endoscopic therapy may be used for palliation including esophageal stenting

Guidelines

- National Comprehensive Cancer Network. NCCN Practice Guidelines for Esophageal Cancer 2000 [1]
- The American College of Gastroenterology treatment guideline: esophageal cancer [2]

FOLLOW UP

- Follow up primarily to evaluate treatment efficacy and manage complications
- Specific areas of investigation include evaluation of recurrence or spread and complications related to surgery and chemoradiotherapy

Plan for review

- Following treatment, evaluate symptom relief and disease recurrence or spread
- Repeat endoscopy several months postresection to determine efficacy
- Evaluate patient for signs and symptoms of postoperative complications
- Evaluate patient for signs and symptoms of chemotherapeutic toxicity
- Evaluate patient for signs and symptoms of radiation toxicity
- Abdominal or chest computed tomography may be indicated to evaluate efficacy and to rule out metastasis

Information for patient or caregiver

- Patients need to know that esophageal cancer has significant morbidity and mortality
- Patients should understand that the only hope for cure is curative resection
- Many patients will have to decide on end-of-life issues and be informed of their treatment choices
- Appropriate hospice, skilled nursing facility, or home health care referral may need to be made depending on the patient's medical condition, personal preference, and social/financial support

DRUGS AND OTHER THERAPIES: DETAILS

Surgical therapy

- Complete tumor resection with microscopically negative resection margins and lymphadenectomy (R0 resection) is curative
- Goal of surgical intervention is curative resection and resumption of swallowing
- Palliative surgery should be avoided for advanced or unresectable disease
- Patients with positive resection margins should be offered radiotherapy and chemotherapy

ESOPHAGECTOMY AND PERIESOPHAGEAL LYMPHADENECTOMY

- Half the patients will not be surgical candidates at diagnosis due to unresectable disease or poor operative risk
- Standard surgical approach includes near total resection of the esophagus with regional lymphadenectomy and cervical or intrathoracic anastomosis using a variety of approaches including, but not limited to, left thoracoabdominal esophagectomy, transhiatal esophagectomy, and Ivor Lewis esophagogastrectomy
- The stomach is a common anastomotic conduit although the bowel may also be used
- Resection margin of at least 5cm should be attempted
- Extended lymphadenectomy does not improve survival but may improve local control
- Treatment of choice for resectable tumors following neoadjuvant chemoradiation

Efficacy

- Complete tumor resection with microscopically negative resection margins and lymphadenectomy offers only hope for cure
- Morbidity and mortality are surgeon- and patient-dependent, with postoperative mortality in specialized centers approx. 5%
- Overall 5-year survival after surgery is 5–20%

Risks/Benefits

Risks:

- Operative mortality: <5%
- Postoperative mortality: 10–15%
- Perioperative morbidity: 29–75%
- Complications include anastomotic fistula leak, bleeding, abdominal/chest infection, pulmonary disease, subphrenic abscess, and wound infection
- Advancing age and comorbidity increase the risk of perioperative morbidity and mortality

Benefit: overall 5-year survival after surgery is 5–20%

Evidence

- Patients with early disease (stages 0, I, and IIA) are usually cured with surgery alone [2] *Level C*
- Surgery is recommended for stage I–III resectable disease [1] *Level C*

Acceptability to patient

Esophagectomy may be associated with significant morbidity that can be unacceptable to some patients.

Follow up plan

- No further treatment is required following successful R0 resection with no evidence of metastatic disease
- Ensure adequate postoperative pain control
- Observe for bleeding, fistula formation, wound infection, and other postoperative complications

According to the National Comprehensive Cancer Network (NCCN), follow up should include:

- History and physical examination
- Complete blood count (CBC) and serum electrolytes 4-monthly for one year then 6-monthly for 2 years, then annually
- Chest X-ray every 6–12 months

Patient and caregiver information

Patients and caregivers need to be able to recognize major postoperative complications such as bleeding and wound infection.

Radiation therapy

Radiation therapy is used extensively for palliation and as an adjunct to curative resection.

EXTERNAL BEAM RADIATION THERAPY

- External beam radiation therapy as single agent therapy is rarely used (being superseded by chemoradiotherapy)
- External beam radiation therapy primarily used for advanced disease and palliation
- Squamous cell carcinoma is more radiosensitive than adenocarcinoma

Efficacy

- 5-year survival for locoregional disease treated with external beam radiotherapy alone is 5%; median survival of 12 months
- Preoperative radiotherapy does not improve survival
- Radiotherapy is used for palliation when chemotherapy cannot be tolerated
- Patients with positive resection margins should be offered radiotherapy and chemotherapy
- Unresectable disease (T4) or those refusing surgery should be treated with 50–60Gy radiotherapy and chemotherapy

For squamous cell carcinoma:

- Favorable response with females, proximal tumors, and tumors under 5cm; recurrence rate 62–84%
- Impact on survival is variable and depends on stage, tumor response, and concurrent surgery/chemotherapy
- Preoperative radiotherapy not recommended in those eligible for curative resection secondary to increased morbidity and mortality

For adenocarcinoma:

Radiotherapy is primarily for palliation as adenocarcinoma is not radiosensitive.

Risks/Benefits

Risks:

- Early complications include esophagitis and stricture
- Late complications occur within 2–60 months and include Brown-Sèquard's syndrome, constrictive pericarditis, gastric ulcers, pericardial effusion, pneumonitis, pulmonary fibrosis, and transverse myelitis

Benefits:

- Can reduce tumor size and pain
- Useful for palliation of esophageal malignancy

Evidence

There is no consistent evidence that preoperative radiotherapy is effective for the treatment of esophageal carcinoma.

- There is no clear evidence that preoperative radiotherapy alone improves survival in patients with potentially resectable esophageal tumors. Results indicate that any survival benefit noted was modest (absolute improvement of 3–4%) [3] *Level M*
- A randomized controlled trial (RCT) compared preoperative radiotherapy with no preoperative treatment in patients with squamous cell carcinoma of the esophagus. No survival benefit was noted in the treatment group, and there was a nonsignificant increase in mortality associated with radiotherapy [4] *Level P*
- A RCT compared preoperative radiation therapy, chemotherapy, and combination radiochemotherapy with surgery alone in patients with squamous cell esophageal carcinoma. Radiotherapy-treated patients had an improved 3-year survival compared with chemotherapy, and surgery alone [5] *Level P*

There is no evidence that postoperative adjuvant radiotherapy improves survival.

- A RCT compared postoperative radiation therapy with no adjuvant therapy in patients following curative resection of squamous cell carcinoma of the esophagus. There was no significant difference noted in survival. Quality of life was adversely affected in the radiation-treated group [6] *Level P*
- Postoperative radiotherapy was compared with surgery alone in a RCT. Intrathoracic recurrence was reduced in the radiotherapy group, but overall median survival was decreased [7] *Level P*

Acceptability to patient

- Treat nausea, vomiting, and diarrhea which can limit patient compliance
- Profound fatigue is common during radiation therapy, instruct patient to get adequate rest
- Warn patient about potential skin irritation over radiated site

Follow up plan

According to the NCCN, follow up should include:

- History and physical examination
- CBC and serum electrolytes 4-monthly for one year, then 6-monthly for 2 years, then annually
- Chest X-ray every 6–12 months
- Evaluate patient for tumor burden reduction

Patient and caregiver information

- Advise patient to receive adequate rest to limit profound fatigue
- Warn patient that radiation therapy may cause nausea, vomiting, and diarrhea but emphasize that these side-effects can be managed

CHEMORADIOTHERAPY

- Chemoradiotherapy combines both radiotherapy and chemotherapy and improves survival and reduces relapse
- It is an alternative to esophagectomy for locoregional disease
- Multiple RCTs have demonstrated that concomitant chemotherapy with radiotherapy is superior to radiotherapy in unresectable disease and can reduce recurrence
- Neoadjuvant chemoradiotherapy used preoperatively is an emerging treatment modality that may enhance surgical therapy
- It increases the rate of curative resection by improving resectability and treating micrometastases

Efficacy

Neoadjuvant chemoradiotherapy:

Neoadjuvant chemoradiotherapy is an emerging treatment modality that may enhance surgical therapy; however, there is a lack of consistent evidence regarding impact on overall survival.

Chemoradiotherapy:

- 5-year survival for locoregional disease treated with primary chemoradiotherapy is 29%, median survival is 20 months
- Multiple RCTs have demonstrated that concomitant chemotherapy with radiotherapy is superior to radiotherapy alone, and can reduce recurrence
- In one RCT, median survival of 5-flurouracil/mitomycin with radiotherapy was 14.8 vs 9.2 months for radiotherapy alone
- No survival advantage following multiple courses of chemoradiotherapy
- Patients with positive resection margins should be offered chemoradiotherapy
- Unresectable disease (T4) or those refusing surgery should be treated with 50–60Gy radiotherapy and chemotherapy

Risks/Benefits

Risks:

- Complications of chemotherapy component includes myelosuppression, nausea, nephrotoxicity, neuropathy, ototoxicity, and vomiting
- Nephrotoxicity and ototoxicity are cumulative, ototoxicity is irreversible
- Complications from radiation exposure/damage to surrounding organs

Benefits:

- Can reduce tumor size and pain
- Can permit surgical resection of the tumor if used as a neoadjuvant therapy
- Can improve survival

Evidence

There is limited evidence on the efficacy of neoadjuvant chemoradiotherapy.

- A RCT compared surgery alone with combined surgery and preoperative chemoradiation (flurouracil and cisplatin) therapy. A significant survival advantage was noted for combined therapy at 3 years follow up [8] *Level P*
- Neoadjuvant chemoradiotherapy (5-flurouracil and cisplatin) was not shown to improve survival in another RCT when compared with surgery alone [9] *Level P*

Chemoradiotherapy may improve survival when used for selected patients as the primary mode of therapy.

- A systematic review has found combined chemoradiotherapy to be superior to radiotherapy alone for the primary treatment of esophageal carcinoma (when a nonoperative approach is selected). Significant toxicity is associated with this form of treatment [10] *Level M*
- A RCT compared chemoradiation therapy with radiotherapy alone for patients with esophageal carcinoma (T1–3, N0–1, M0). At 5-year follow up, the overall survival rates were 26% in the combined group, and 0% in the radiotherapy group. The combination group had a higher incidence of severe acute toxic effects [11] *Level P*

Acceptability to patient

- Treat nausea, vomiting, and diarrhea, which can limit patient compliance
- Profound fatigue is common during radiation therapy; instruct patient to get adequate rest
- Warn patient about potential skin irritation over radiated site

Follow up plan

Following chemoradiotherapy, surgery may be possible and further endoscopic evaluation is appropriate.

According to the NCCN, follow up should include:

- History and physical examination
- CBC and serum electrolytes 4-monthly for one year, then 6-monthly for 2 years, then annually
- Chest X-ray every 6–12 months
- Evaluate patient for tumor burden reduction
- Endoscopy is recommended 4–6 months postchemoradiotherapy

Patient and caregiver information

- Advise patient to receive adequate rest to limit profound fatigue
- Warn patient that radiation therapy may cause nausea, vomiting, and diarrhea; however, emphasize that these side-effects can be managed

Chemotherapy

- Most chemotherapeutic regimens include 5-FU/cisplatin combined with another agent
- Patients with positive resection margins should be offered radiotherapy with or without chemotherapy

- Most chemotherapeutic regimens are limited to clinical trials; consider entry into clinical trial, especially for palliative chemotherapy
- Chemotherapy has not demonstrated significant efficacy, with little if any impact on survival as responses are only partial
- Chemoradiotherapy is the emerging treatment of choice

CISPLATIN

- Most common chemotherapeutic regimen with 5-FU showing a 20–50% response rate
- Cisplatin is emerging as the chemotherapeutic agent of choice
- Chemoradiotherapy can improve survival and reduce relapse and is an alternative to esophagectomy for locoregional disease
- Resectable disease (stages I–III or T1–T3) should be treated with esophagectomy or chemoradiotherapy using 50–60Gy radiotherapy with 5-FU combined with cisplatin or mitomycin
- Unresectable disease (T4) or those refusing surgery should be treated with 50–60Gy radiotherapy with 5-FU combined with cisplatin or mitomycin
- Palliative chemotherapy outside a clinical trial may consist of cisplatin with paclitaxel or 5-FU

Efficacy

- Cisplatin as a single agent is efficacious with a response rate of approx. 20%
- Cisplatin with 5-FU is a common chemotherapeutic regimen, with 20–50% response rates

Risks/Benefits

Risks:

- Should not be used in patients with hearing impairment
- Should not be used in myelosuppressed patients
- High side-effect profile includes myelosuppression, nausea, nephrotoxicity, neuropathy, ototoxicity, and vomiting
- Nephrotoxicity and ototoxicity are cumulative, ototoxicity is irreversible
- Adequate hydration may temporize nephrotoxicity
- Perform frequent neurologic examinations during treatment and evaluate for signs and symptoms of neuropathy
- Side-effects include arrhythmias, glucose intolerance, ischemic vascular events, pancreatitis, seizures and vision change, fatigue, nausea and vomiting, hair loss, bone marrow suppression, anorexia, astomatitis, sexual dysfunction

Benefits:

- Acts synergistically with surgery, radiotherapy, and other chemotherapeutic agents
- May permit surgical resection of tumor if used as a neoadjuvant therapy

Evidence

The combination of chemotherapy and surgery has not been shown to improve survival.

- A systematic review found no current strong evidence to support preoperative chemotherapy alone in the management of surgically resectable thoracic esophageal carcinomas [12] *Level M*
- Chemotherapy with surgery was not found to improve survival when compared with surgery alone in a RCT of patients with squamous cell carcinoma of the esophagus. Cisplatinum, bleomycin, and vinblastine were used [13] *Level P*
- Preoperative chemotherapy using cisplatin and 5-FU for patients with squamous cell carcinoma of the esophagus was compared with surgery alone in a RCT. Patients treated with chemotherapy had an increased likelihood of complete resection; however, there was no survival benefit noted [14] *Level P*

- A RCT compared surgery alone, and in combination with chemotherapy (cisplatin and vindesine) in patients with squamous cell carcinoma of the esophagus. There was no significant difference in survival between the two groups [15] *Level P*

Acceptability to patient
- Side-effect profile dependent on agents used
- Compliance may be limited by nausea, vomiting, ototoxicity, and neuropathy
- Neuropathy is usually reversible

Follow up plan
Following chemotherapy, surgical resection may be possible and endoscopic evaluation is appropriate.

According to the NCCN, follow up should include:
- History and physical examination
- CBC and serum electrolytes 4-monthly for one year, then 6-monthly for 2 years, then annually
- Chest X-ray every 6–12 months
- Evaluate patient for tumor burden reduction
- Endoscopy is recommended 4–6 months postchemoradiotherapy
- Audiogram should be performed every 2–3 cycles

Patient and caregiver information
Warn patient about side-effects; however, emphasize that these problems can be managed.

5-FLUOROURACIL
- Most common chemotherapeutic regimen is 5-FU with cisplatin, with a 20–50% response rate
- Chemoradiotherapy can improve survival and reduce relapse and is an alternative to esophagectomy for locoregional resectable disease (stages I–III or T1–T3) which should be treated with esophagectomy or chemoradiotherapy using 50–60Gy radiotherapy with 5-FU combined with cisplatin or mitomycin
- Unresectable disease (T4) or those refusing surgery should be treated with 50–60Gy radiotherapy with 5-FU combined with cisplatin or mitomycin
- Palliative chemotherapy outside a clinical trial may consist of 5-FU with paclitaxel or cisplatin

Efficacy
For squamous cell carcinoma:
- Goal of preoperative chemotherapy is to enhance resectability
- Preoperative chemotherapy produces 45–75% response and may offer a survival advantage; however, use is limited to clinical trials
- Preoperative chemoradiotherapy produces up to 24% response, but impact on survival is minimal and not consistent

For adenocarcinoma:
- Neoadjuvant chemoradiotherapy with 5-FU and mitomycin produced a 63% response
- When compared with surgery alone, neoadjuvant chemoradiotherapy with 5-FU and cisplatin improved 3-year survival and reduced metastasis

Risks/Benefits
Risks:
- Specialist advice must be followed
- Bone marrow suppression
- Impaired hepatic or renal function

- High-dose pelvic irradiation
- Previous use of alkylating aents
- Discontinue as soon as signs of toxicity appear (diarrhea, watery stools, frequent bowel movements, gastrointestinal ulceration and bleeding, hemorrhage, leukopenia, stomatitis or esophagopharyngitis, thrombocytopenia, vomiting)

Benefit: acts synergistically with surgery, radiotherapy, and other chemotherapeutic agents

Side-effects and adverse reactions:

- Alopecia, dermatitis, photosensitivity, hyperpigmentation
- Biliary sclerosis, cholestatic jaundice
- Gastrointestinal ulceration, nausea, diarrhea
- Myelosuppression, sepsis
- Myocardial ischemia, neurologic toxicity
- Severe vomiting and diarrhea can be complicated by dehydration and hypotension
- Therapy may have to be suspended or interrupted secondary to diarrhea or mucositis
- 5-FU can increase dermatologic toxicity of radiotherapy
- Catheter-related complications include hemorrhage, infection, thrombosis and catheter migration into receiving artery

Evidence

The combination of chemotherapy and surgery has not been shown to improve survival.

- A systematic review has found no current strong evidence to support preoperative chemotherapy alone in the management of surgically resectable thoracic esophageal carcinomas [12] *Level M*
- Preoperative chemotherapy using cisplatin and 5-FU for patients with squamous cell carcinoma of the esophagus was compared to surgery alone in a RCT. Patients treated with chemotherapy had an increased likelihood of complete resection; however, there was no survival benefit noted [14] *Level P*

Acceptability to patient

- Side-effect profile dependent on agents used
- Compliance may be limited by nausea, vomiting, diarrhea, gastrointestinal ulceration, and neurologic toxicity manifesting as ataxia and somnolence
- Warn patient about possibility of alopecia and skin rash

Follow up plan

According to the NCCN, follow up should include:

- History and physical examination
- CBC and serum electrolytes 4-monthly for one year, then 6-monthly for 2 years, then annually
- Chest X-ray every 6–12 months
- Evaluate patient for tumor burden reduction
- Endoscopy is recommended 4–6 months postchemoradiotherapy
- Audiogram should be performed every 2–3 cycles
- Pay particular attention to CBC as myelosuppression manifesting as granulocytopenia and thrombocytopenia are a major toxicities occurring 2–4 weeks post-treatment initiation

Patient and caregiver information

Warn patient about side-effects but emphasize that these problems can be managed.

Other therapies

PALLIATIVE THERAPY

Endoscopic balloon dilation or bougienage:

- Relieves dysphagia in 90%, although repeated dilatations every 4 weeks is often necessary
- Dilation can be combined with other palliative therapies
- Complications include bacteremia, bleeding, bronchospasm, chest pain and perforation (1 in 500 dilations)
- Prior radiation therapy increases perforation risk

Esophageal stenting:

- Can reduce dysphagia in 90–95%
- Complications include perforation and stent migration/occlusion
- Complication rate is 10%
- Self-expanding metal stents may have fewer complications than plastic stents
- Significant esophageal pain can result from stent-induced ulceration or radial tension and requires adequate analgesia

Endoscopic laser therapy:

- Restores esophageal patency in 90–95% and relieves dysphagia in 75–85%
- Complications include bleeding, edema, and perforation
- Complication rate approx. 8.7%, virtually no mortality associated with laser ablation
- Perforation rate of 2.1%

Bipolar electrocoagulation:

- Restores esophageal patency in 90%
- Complications include fever, fistula, perforation, and stricture

Photodynamic therapy (PDT):

- PDT laser ablation after administration of a photosensitizer is an emerging palliative modality for high-grade dysplasia, squamous cell carcinoma, and adenocarcinoma
- Experimental treatment that aims to destroy tumor leaving surrounding normal tissue undamaged
- Complications include fever, fistula, perforation, photosensitivity, stricture, and sunburn
- Barrett's esophagus post-PDT still requires surveillance endoscopy due to persistent risk of adenocarcinoma and high-grade dysplasia

Injection therapy, direct injection of absolute alcohol, or other cytotoxic agent into tumor:

- Usually combined with other palliative modality
- Results unpredictable and usually transient requiring monthly treatment
- Several cytotoxic agents are under investigation

Acceptability to patient

Palliative therapy is usually well accepted by most patients, especially when dysphagia is relieved.

Follow up plan

- Evaluate for evidence of recurrent dysphagia or obstruction
- Ensure adequate postoperative pain control
- Observe for bleeding, fistula formation, wound infection, and other postoperative complication

Patient and caregiver information

Patients and caregivers need to be able to recognize major postoperative complications including bleeding, further obstruction, and ulceration.

OUTCOMES

EFFICACY OF THERAPIES

- Medical, surgical, and endoscopic outcomes similar for advanced esophageal cancer
- Surgery is more effective at relieving obstruction than radiotherapy with overall 5-year patient survival being between 5% and 20%
- Single-agent chemotherapy can reduce tumor size in 15–25%
- Cisplatin-based multiagent chemotherapy can reduce tumor size in 30–60%
- Chemoradiotherapy with or without surgery may be of benefit
- Adjuvant chemoradiotherapy may provide a survival benefit
- Chemoradiotherapy offers a survival advantage when compared with radiotherapy alone
- Neoadjuvant chemoradiotherapy is an emerging treatment modality that may enhance surgical therapy; however, there is a lack of consistent evidence regarding impact on overall survival
- Photodynamic therapy (PDT) is experimental and still under evaluation

Evidence

- There is no clear evidence that preoperative radiotherapy alone improves survival in patients with potentially resectable esophageal tumors. Results indicate that any survival benefit noted is modest (absolute improvement of 3–4%) [3] *Level M*
- Surgery plus neoadjuvant chemoradiation therapy has been shown to confer a significant survival advantage at 3 years follow-up in a randomized controlled trial (RCT), compared with surgery alone [8] *Level P*
- Neoadjuvant chemoradiotherapy was not shown to improve survival in another RCT when compared with surgery alone [9] *Level P*
- A systematic review has found combined chemoradiotherapy to be superior to radiotherapy alone for the primary treatment of esophageal carcinoma (when a nonoperative approach is selected). Significant toxicity is associated with this form of treatment [10] *Level M*
- A systematic review has found no current strong evidence to support preoperative chemotherapy alone in the management of surgically resectable thoracic esophageal carcinomas [12] *Level M*

PROGNOSIS

- Prognosis depends on stage as determined by The American Joint Commission on Cancer tumor-node-metastases (TNM) classification system
- 5-year survival variable (4.1–60.4%), depending on stage
- Median survival post-R0 resection: 18 months
- 5-year survival postresection: 10–35%
- Most present with advanced disease, approx. 50% have extensive locoregional disease at diagnosis, <60% of those with locoregional disease are candidates for curative resection
- Postresection 60–70% of specimens have lymph node involvement
- Squamous cell carcinoma and adenocarcinoma have similar prognosis for stage
- Several prognostic markers are under investigation and include DF3 monoclonal antibodies, cyclin D1, and tumor growth factor-alpha
- Tumors of the lower esophagus have a worse prognosis than middle or upper-third esophageal cancers

Survival according to stage:

- T1: 5-year survival 46.1%
- T2: 5-year survival 29.5%
- T3: 5-year survival 21.7%
- T4: 5-year survival 7.0%

- Stage I: 5-year survival 60.4%
- Stage II: 5-year survival 31.3%
- Stage III: 5-year survival 19.9%
- Stave IV: 5-year survival 4.1%

For squamous cell carcinoma:
- Early disease: 5-year survival approx. 90%, 8–12% are diagnosed early
- Most present at stage III
- Regional lymph node metastasis: 5-year survival 39.9% with surgery, 16.8% without
- Distant lymph nodes metastasis: 5-year survival 5.2%
- 42–67% have lymph node metastasis
- Organ metastasis: 5-year survival 3.0%
- 25–30% have bone, liver, or lung metastasis
- Pulmonary fistula: survival 1.4–4 months
- Spread can be lymphatic, hematogenous or direct extension; cancer tends to spread to liver, lung, pleura, and local/supraclavicular lymph nodes

For adenocarcinoma:
- Poor prognosis, most present at stage III or IV
- Early lymph node metastasis with extension to diaphragm, liver, and stomach

Therapeutic failure
- Consider entry into clinical trial
- Pain control and quality of life should be a priority
- Consider installing a feeding tube by gastrostomy or endoscopy

Recurrence
- Patients who experience recurrence postresection and who have not previously received chemotherapy or radiotherapy should be offered surgery or chemoradiotherapy [1]
- Patients who experience resectable recurrence postchemoradiotherapy should be offered surgery. If the patient has another relapse post-resection the cancer should be deemed incurable and palliation should be offered [1]
- Laser ablation and PDT can be used for unresectable disease [1]
- Entry into clinical trial should be strongly considered
- Pain control and quality of life should be a priority
- Consider installing a feeding tube by gastrostomy or endoscopy

Deterioration
- Entry into clinical trial should be strongly considered
- Pain control and quality of life should be a priority
- Consider installing a feeding tube by gastrostomy or endoscopy

Terminal illness
- Pain control and quality of life should be a priority
- Assist patient and family in dealing with end-of-life issues
- Have patient evaluated for hospice or home health care
- Dysphagia should be aggressively managed either endoscopically or surgically (e.g. gastrostomy/jejunostomy)
- Tracheoesophageal fistula may necessitate surgical intervention
- Malnutrition risk high and best managed by team approach utilizing nutritionist, surgeon, internist, and endoscopist

COMPLICATIONS

- Aortoesophageal fistula can result in massive hematemesis
- Esophagopulmonary fistula can result in aspiration and pneumonia
- Ulceration can result in hematemesis and gastrointestinal bleed
- Stricture managed with endoprosthesis or dilation
- Hypercalcemia, from bony metastasis or parathormone-related peptide, can complicate squamous cell carcinoma
- Weight loss can be severe and often necessitates nutritional support
- Esophageal obstruction can be relieved by laser treatment, PDT, radiotherapy, stenting, or multimodal therapy
- Recalcitrant esophageal obstruction managed by an endoscopically, radiographically or surgically placed feeding tube, percutaneous endoscopic gastrostomy tube (PEG) is preferred
- Pain may be severe and should be managed aggressively
- Deep vein thrombosis is a recognized complication of malignancy

CONSIDER CONSULT

- Consider referral to an academic-university center for clinical trial entry
- Consider referral to hospice for treatment failure, clinical deterioration, or terminal disease
- Consider referral to a psychiatrist/psychologist for emotional support and insight
- Consider referral to a pain specialist for intractable pain

PREVENTION

There are no known interventions that can prevent esophageal cancer.

RISK FACTORS

- Low socioeconomic status may increase risk of squamous cell carcinoma
- Coexisting medical history: many medical conditions increase the risk of squamous cell carcinoma, including tylosis, esophageal strictures, and esophageal webs. Barrett's esophagus is the strongest risk factor for adenocarcinoma although its ablation does not reduce esophageal tumor risk
- Surgical history: gastrectomy increases risk of squamous cell carcinoma

MODIFY RISK FACTORS

Lifestyle and wellness

TOBACCO

- Smoking increases risk of squamous cell carcinoma/adenocarcinoma
- Smoking cessation should be encouraged

ALCOHOL AND DRUGS

- Excessive alcohol is associated with increased risk of squamous cell carcinoma and of adenocarcinoma and should be discouraged
- Opiate smoking increases the risk of squamous cell carcinoma and should be discouraged

DIET

- Diets high in nitrosamines, fungi, betal nuts, hot tea, and tannin increase risk of squamous cell carcinoma
- A diet rich in vitamins (especially vitamin A) and minerals (especially zinc and molybdenum) may be protective against esophageal carcomina
- Raw vegetables may decrease risk of squamous cell carcinoma/adenocarcinoma

SCREENING

- In the US, population screening for esophageal cancer is not recommended
- Biannual endoscopy performed in most screening programs
- Given high incidence of squamous cell carcinoma with tylosis, surveillance endoscopy is recommended
- Surveillance endoscopy is recommended for esophageal metaplasia and Barrett's esophagus
- Patients with achalasia or history of caustic injury over 20 years ago may benefit from annual screening endoscopy
- In endemic areas like Linxian, China, screening has reduced squamous cell carcinoma mortality

ESOPHAGEAL ENDOSCOPY

Endoscopic examination of the esophagus to evaluate presence of malignant and premalignant lesions.

Cost/efficacy

Esophageal tumors discovered as a consequence of surveillance endoscopy for Barrett's are usually stage I or II.

PREVENT RECURRENCE

Recurrence can be prevented/delayed by:

- Choosing appropriate surgical candidates
- Multimodal therapy
- Assuring macroscopic-/microscopic-free resection margins

Reassess coexisting disease

PATIENT SATISFACTION/LIFESTYLE PRIORITIES

- Most patients with recurrence will be concerned with quality-of-life and end-of-life issues
- Pain control and patient comfort should be a priority

ASSOCIATIONS

American Association for Cancer Research
Public Ledger Building, Suite 826
150 South Independence Mall West
Philadelphia, PA 19106–3483
Tel: (215) 440-9300
Fax: (215) 440-9313
www.aacr.org

American Cancer Society
1599 Clifton Road NE
Atlanta, GA 30329
Tel: (800) 227-2345 (800-ACS-2345)
www.cancer.org

American Society for Clinical Oncology
1900 Duke Street, Suite 200
Alexandria, VA 22314
Tel: (703) 299-0150
Fax: (703) 299-1044
E-mail: asco@asco.org
www.asco.org

Cancer Hope Network
Two North Road
Chester, NJ 07930
Tel: (877 467-3638 (877-HOPENET)
E-mail: info@cancerhopenetwork.org
www.cancerhopenetwork.org

Cancer Links USA
9737 NW 41st Street, Suite 183
Miami, FL 33178
E-mail: lynx@cancerlinks.com
www.cancerlinksusa.com

Cleveland Clinic – Department of Gastroenterology
9500 Euclid Avenue
Cleveland, OH 44195
Tel: (800) 223-2273, ext. 4-6536
www.clevelandclinic.org/gastro

National Cancer Institute
Public Inquires Office
Building 31, Room 10A03
31 Center Drive, MSC 2580
Bethesda, MD 20892–2580
Tel: (800) 422-6237 (800-4-CANCER)
E-mail: cancermail@cips.nci.nih.gov
www.cancer.gov

National Coalition for Cancer Survivorship
1010 Wayne Avenue, Suite 505
Silver Springs, MD 20910–5600
Tel: (800) 622-7337
E-mail: info@cansearch.org
www.cansearch.org

National Comprehensive Cancer Network
50 Huntington Pike, Suite 200
Rockledge, PA 19046
Tel: (215) 728-3877 or (888) 909-6226 (888-909-NCCN)
E-mail: information@nccn.org
www.nccn.org

National Hospice and Palliative Care Organization
1700 Diagonal Road, Suite 300
Alexandria, VA 22314
Tel: (800) 658-8898
E-mail: helpline@nhpco.org
www.nhpco.org

The Cancer Group Institute
17620 NE 9th Avenue
North Miami Beach, FL 53162
Tel: (305) 493-1980
E-mail: info@cancergroup.com
www.cancergroup.com

KEY REFERENCES

- DeVita VT, Hellman S, Rosenberg SA. Cancer: principles & practices of oncology. 5th edn. New York: Lippincott-Raven, 1997, p980–1021
- Coia LR, Mkinsky BD, John MJ, et al. Patterns of care study decision tree and management guidelines for esophageal cancer. American College of Radiology. Radiat Med 1998;16:321–7
- De Palma GD, di Matteo E, Romano G, et al. Plastic prosthesis versus expandable metal stents for palliation of inoperable esophageal thoracic carcinoma: a controlled prospective study. Gastrointest Endosc 1996;43;478–82
- Forastiere AA, Orringer MB, Perez-Tamayo C, et al. Preoperative chemoradiation followed by transhiatal esophagectomy for carcinoma of the esophagus: final report. J Clin Oncol 1993;11:1118–23
- Gaspar LE, Nag S, Herskovic A, et al. American Brachytherapy Society (ABS) consensus guidelines for brachytherapy of esophageal cancer. Clinical Research Committee, American Brachytherapy Society, Philadelphia, PA. Int J Radiat Oncol Biol Phys 1997;38:127–32
- Gignous M, Roussell A, Paillot B, et al. The value of preoperative radiotherapy in esophageal cancer: results of a study of the EORTC. World J Surg 1987;11:426–32
- Ginsberg R, Roth J, Fergusson M. Esophageal cancer surgical practice guidelines. Esophageal Cancer Practice Guidelines Committee. Oncology 1997;11:1059–62
- Hatlevol R, Hagen S, Hansen HS, et al. Bleomycin/cis-platin as neoadjuvant chemotherapy before radical radiotherapy in localized, inoperable carcinoma of the esophagus: a prospective randomized multicentre study. The second Scandinavian trial in esophageal cancer. Radiother Oncol 1992;24:114–6
- Herskovic A, Martz K, Al-Sarraf M, et al. Combined chemotherapy and radiotherapy compared with radiotherapy alone in patients with cancer of the esophagus. N Engl J Med 1992;326:1593–8
- Jensen DM, Machicado G, Randall G, et al. Comparison of low-power YAG laser and BICAP tumor probe for palliation of esophageal cancer strictures. Gastroenterol 1988;94;1263–70

Evidence references and guidelines

1 National Comprehensive Cancer Network. NCCN Practice Guidelines for Esophageal Cancer, 2000
2 Lightdale, CM. The American College of Gastroenterology treatment guideline: esophageal cancer. Am J Gastroenterol 1999;94:20–9
3 Arnott SJ, Duncan W, Gignoux M, et al. (Oeosphageal Cancer Collective Group). Preoperative radiotherapy for esophageal carcinoma (Cochrane Review). In: The Cochrane Library, 4, 2001. Oxford: Update Software
4 Launois B, Delarue D, Campion JP, et al. Preoperative radiotherapy for carcinoma of the esophagus. Surg Gynecol Obstet 1981;153:690–2. Medline
5 Nygaard K, Hagen S, Hansen HS, et al. Pre-operative radiotherapy prolongs survival in operable esophageal carcinoma: a randomized, mutlicenter study of preoperative radiotherapy and chemotherapy. The second Scandinavian trial in esophageal cancer. World J Surg 1992:16;1104–10. Medline
6 Zieren HU, Muller JM, Jacobi CA, et al. Adjuvant postoperative radiation therapy after curative resection of squamous cell carcinoma of the thoracic esophagus: a prospective randomized study. World J Surg 1995;19:444–9. Medline
7 Fok M, Sham JS, Choy D, et al. Postoperative radiotherapy for carcinoma of the esophagus: a prospective, randomized controlled study. Surgery 1993;113:138–47. Medline
8 Walsh TN, Noonan N, Hollywood D, et al. A comparison of multimodal therapy and surgery for esophageal adenocarcinoma. N Engl J Med 1996;335:462–7. Medline
9 Le Prise E, Etienne PL, Meunier B, et al. A randomized study of chemotherapy, radiation therapy, and surgery versus surgery for localized squamous cell carcinoma of the esophagus. Cancer 1994;73:1779–84. Medline
10 Wong R, Malthaner R. Combined chemotherapy and radiotherapy (without surgery) compared with radiotherapy alone in localized carcinoma of the esophagus (Cochrane Review). In: The Cochrane Library, 4, 2001. Oxford: Update Software
11 Cooper JS, Guo MD, Herskovic A, et al. Chemoradiotherapy of locally advanced esophageal cancer: long term follow-up of a prospective randomized trial (RTOG 85–01). Radiation Therapy Oncology Group. JAMA 1999;281:1623–7. Medline
12 Malthaner R, Fenlon D. Preoperative chemotherapy for resectable thoracic esophageal cancer (Cochrane Review) In: The Cochrane Library, 4, 2001. Oxford: Update Software
13 Maipang T, Vasinanukorn P, Petpichetchian C, et al. Induction chemotherapy in the treatment of patients with carcinoma of the esophagus. J Surg Oncol 1994;56:191–7. Medline
14 Law S, Fok M, Chow S, et al. Preoperative chemotherapy versus surgical therapy alone for squamous cell carcinoma of the esophagus: a prospective randomized trial. J Thorac Cardiovasc Surg 1997;114:210–17. Medline
15 Ando N, Iizuka T, Kakegawa T, et al. A randomized trial of surgery with and without chemotherapy for localized squamous carcinoma of the thoracic esophagus: the Japan Clinical Oncology Group Study. J Thorac Cardiovasc Surg 1997;114:205–9. Medline

CONTRIBUTORS

Russell C Jones, MD, MPH
Otavio A Clark, MD
Naixi N Chen, MD

GASTRIC MALIGNANCY

SUMMARY INFORMATION

DESCRIPTION

- Gastric adenocarcinoma is the 11th most common cancer in the US and the 14th leading cause of cancer death; it is the second most common cancer and cause of cancer death worldwide
- Gastric adenocarcinomas represent 90% of all gastric malignancies and are divided into intestinal and diffuse forms; the prognosis of each is different
- Often clinically silent and diagnosed endoscopically at an advanced stage
- The overall 5-year survival rate in the US ranges from 5 to 15%
- Prognostic factors relate to tumor extent and include nodal involvement and extension beyond the gastric wall. Ploidy may be an independent prognostic factor
- Gastrectomy with regional lymphadenectomy is the treatment of choice. Postoperative adjuvant chemoradiation using 5-fluorouracil and leucovorin is now the standard of care for resected patients able to tolerate such treatment

URGENT ACTION

- Evidence of life-threatening gastric hemorrhage mandates immediate endoscopic or surgical intervention
- Evidence of deep vein thrombosis requires anticoagulation

KEY! DON'T MISS!

- Do not mistake the vague nonspecific symptoms of gastric adenocarcinoma for those of dyspepsia or peptic ulcer disease
- Always consider the possibility of malignancy in patients with gastrointestinal complaints; clinical index of suspicion is heightened by age, race, family history, and other risk factors

ICD9 CODE

- 151 Malignant neoplasm of stomach
- 151.0 Malignant neoplasm of stomach, cardia
- 151.1 Malignant neoplasm of stomach, pylorus
- 151.2 Malignant neoplasm of stomach, antrum (pyloric)
- 151.3 Malignant neoplasm of stomach, fundus
- 151.4 Malignant neoplasm of stomach, body
- 151.4 Malignant neoplasm of stomach, corpus
- 151.5 Malignant neoplasm of stomach, lesser curvature
- 151.6 Malignant neoplasm of stomach, greater curvature
- 151.8 Malignant neoplasm of stomach, contiguous site
- 151.8 Malignant neoplasm of stomach, wall, anterior
- 151.8 Malignant neoplasm of stomach, wall, posterior
- 151.9 Malignant neoplasm of stomach, wall

SYNONYMS

- Gastric cancer
- Stomach cancer
- Cancer of the stomach
- Gastric adenocarcinoma
- Gastric carcinoma

CARDINAL FEATURES

- Remains 11th most common cancer and 14th leading cause of cancer death in US
- Worldwide it is the second most common cancer and the second most common cause of cancer death
- Mortality rate and incidence have decreased markedly over the past 60 years. Although the incidence of gastric cancer has decreased dramatically over the past century, the decline has been limited to cancers below the gastric cardia. The number of newly diagnosed patients with proximal gastric and gastroesophageal junction adenocarcinomas has increased markedly since the mid-1980s
- About 95% of gastric cancers are adenocarcinomas; the rest are leiomyosarcomas, lymphomas, carcinoids, squamous cancers, or other rarer types
- Gastric adenocarcinomas are divided into intestinal and diffuse forms, each with its own prognostic factors
- Intestinal-type gastric cancers are usually well differentiated and have more distal location, occur in younger patients, are more frequently endemic, and are associated with inflammatory changes and with *Helicobacter pylori* infection
- Diffuse-type gastric cancer is associated with hereditary factors and a proximal location and does not appear to occur in the setting of intestinal metaplasia or dysplasia. Diffuse-type generally occurs in patients <50 years of age and is more common in women. Diffuse-type gastric cancer is usually less differentiated and thickens the stomach wall (linitis plastica, 'leather bottle' stomach) rather than forming a discrete tumor mass. It carries a poorer prognosis than intestinal-type gastric cancer
- Often clinically silent with nonspecific complaints, and often diagnosed at late stage
- Double-contrast gastric radiograph followed by endoscopic biopsy is the typical diagnostic protocol
- Endoscopy with biopsy is the primary diagnostic modality
- Poor prognosis overall, with 5-year survival rate of 5–15%
- Prognosis is dependent on the degree of invasion, extension, and spread

- Treatment is primarily surgical, and gastrectomy with lymphadenectomy offers the only hope of cure
- Postoperative chemoradiation using 5-fluorouracil and leucovorin is now the standard of care for resected patients able to tolerate such treatment

CAUSES

Common causes

- No definitive cause has been identified
- Etiology is probably multifactorial, including environmental and genetic factors

Contributory or predisposing factors

- Diet: dietary factors that may be associated with an increased risk for stomach cancer include high salt consumption, high nitrate consumption, low dietary vitamin A and C, poor food preparation (smoked, salt cured), lack of refrigeration, and water from wells (which may contain high concentrations of nitrates or *H. pylori*). Antioxidants, which can prevent the conversion of nitrates to nitrosamine, appear to be protective
- Gastric polyps: patients with familial adenomatous polyposis (FAP) have a higher incidence of gastric cancer. Patients with adenomatous polyps or FAP should have endoscopic surveillance
- Chronic atrophic gastritis, pernicious anemia, achlorhydria: chronic gastritis increases the risk of gastric cancer, and the increased risk usually manifests itself 10–15 years after the diagnosis. In Ménétrier's disease (hypertrophic gastritis), an increase in the incidence of gastric cancer is also observed. Pernicious anemia increases relative risk for gastric cancer by 3–18 times, and endoscopic monitoring is suggested
- *H. pylori* infection increases the risk of gastric cancer between 3-fold and 6-fold, but its precise role the etiology of gastric cancer remains unknown. A higher incidence of *H. pylori* infection is found in patients with intestinal rather than diffuse-type gastric cancer
- Previous partial gastric resection increases the risk of gastric stump cancer. The increased risk is observed only after a latency period of at least 15 years, involves patients operated on for gastric ulcer but not for duodenal ulcer, and is slightly higher in women than in men
- High-grade dysplasia is considered to be a marker for future gastric cancer
- Intestinal metaplasia (the replacement of gastric glandular epithelium with intestinal mucosa) is associated with intestinal-type gastric cancer
- Heredity and race: African, Asian, and Hispanic Americans have a higher risk of gastric cancer than Caucasians
- Gastric cancer is more common in men older than 50 years of age and in people with blood type A. Gastric cancer is consistently seen more commonly among those of lower socioeconomic class across the world. Possible occupational relationships include coal mining and rubber or asbestos workers. Risk is increased in cigarette smokers and people with radiation exposure

EPIDEMIOLOGY

Incidence and prevalence

- Incidence of distal intestinal-type gastric cancer has declined steadily in the US over the past 60 years for unknown reasons
- Incidence of proximal gastric and gastroesophageal junction adenocarcinomas has increased dramatically over past 10–15 years in Western nations for unknown reasons

FREQUENCY

In the US:

- 21,900 new cases during 1999
- Annual mortality rate: 2.3/100,000 females, 5.2/100,000 males
- 13,500 deaths during 1999
- The incidence of early gastric cancers is less than 5% in most of the US
- Lifetime risk is 1 in 60
- Lifetime probability is 1–2%

Demographics

AGE

- Incidence increases from fourth decade on, peaking in the seventh decade in men and slightly later in women
- Mean age at diagnosis in the US is 63 years

GENDER

In the US, stomach cancer occurs at a higher incidence in men than in women (ratio of approximately 2:1).

RACE

More frequent in African-American men than in Caucasian men (1.5:1).

GENETICS

- Familial clusters of gastric cancer exist. The best example is the Bonaparte family: Napoleon, his father, and his grandfather all died of gastric carcinoma
- Blood type A confers an increased risk of gastric cancer
- Gastric cancer occurs with increased frequency in family members diagnosed with hereditary nonpolyposis colorectal cancer and Li-Fraumeni syndrome
- Several genetic anomalies, including DNA mismatch repair, mutated p53, and E-cadherin genes, have been observed in association with gastric adenocarcinoma

GEOGRAPHY

Incidence is related to geography:

- Epidemic in Japan, China, eastern Europe, Middle East, Russia, and South America
- Japan has highest incidence of 1:1000. The incidence is intermediate in Japanese immigrants to the US; first-generation Japanese Americans have an incidence comparable with that of other Americans
- Low incidence in Australia, Israel, New Zealand, North America, and western Europe
- Intestinal-type gastric cancer is more prevalent in endemic regions

SOCIOECONOMIC STATUS

- Low socioeconomic status related to distal gastric cancer
- Medium to high socioeconomic status related to proximal gastric cancer

DIAGNOSIS

DIFFERENTIAL DIAGNOSIS

Several benign and malignant gastric lesions share a similar constellation of symptoms and radiographic appearance. Diagnosis ultimately depends on endoscopy with biopsy.

Peptic ulcer disease

Peptic ulcer disease is a benign ulcerative disease of the stomach and duodenum.

FEATURES

- Common: lifetime prevalence 12% for men, 10% for women
- Peptic ulcer disease is strongly associated with *H. pylori* infection
- Epigastric pain that radiates to the back is common
- Water brash may be noted
- Differentiation from gastric adenocarcinoma is difficult owing to similar clinical, radiographic, and macroscopic appearance
- Bleeding is a common complication
- Diagnosis depends on double-contrast barium study followed by endoscopy with biopsy

Gastric polyps

Polypoid lesions of the stomach, usually benign.

FEATURES

- Common, 25% incidence: gastric polyps rarely undergo malignant transformation (3% after 7 years), but many contain independent carcinoma
- Histologically classified as hyperplastic, inflammatory, fundic gland, and adenomatous
- Adenomatous polyps have high malignant potential
- Range morphologically from small bumps to polypoid mass that can mimic gastric cancer
- Occur throughout the stomach
- Gastric polyps are associated with atrophic gastritis, gastroenterostomy anastomoses, *H. pylori* infection, hypochlorhydria, intestinal metaplasia, and polyposis syndromes
- Benign polyps rarely produce symptoms; 85% are hyperplastic
- Visualized radiographically or endoscopically; often an incidental finding

Primary gastric lymphoma

Lymphoma involving the stomach.

FEATURES

- Differentiation from gastric adenocarcinoma is difficult owing to similar clinical, radiographic, and macroscopic presentation
- Primary gastric lymphoma may be associated with *H. pylori* infection
- Anorexia, early satiety, and epigastric pain are common
- Fatigue is often present
- Biopsy is required for diagnosis, and deep biopsy is recommended given submucosal location
- Histologically, most are nonHodgkin's B cell lymphomas
- Better prognosis than for gastric adenocarcinoma

Gastric (nonlymphoid) sarcoma

Rare group of stromal tumors representing 1–3% of stomach cancers.

FEATURES

- Leiomyosarcoma is the most common type
- Normally found in anterior or posterior fundal wall

- Can ulcerate and bleed, often slow-growing
- Epigastric pain is common
- Biopsy required for diagnosis
- Usually does not involve lymph nodes

Metastases to stomach

Rare: accounts for less than 1% of gastric tumors. Tumors that metastasize to the stomach include primaries of the breast, colon, liver, lung, ovary, parotid gland, and testis, and malignant melanomas.

Rare malignant tumors

Extremely rare, representing less than 1% of gastric cancers. Rare malignant tumors include adenosquamous, choriocarcinoma, gastrinoma, glomus tumor, Kaposi's sarcoma, leiomyoblastoma, myenteric schwannoma, parietal cell carcinoma, small cell carcinoma, and squamous cell carcinoma.

Carcinoid tumor

Tumors originating from enterochromaffin-like cells.

FEATURES

- Most commonly found in appendix and small bowel but can occur throughout the gastrointestinal tract
- Gastric carcinoids are rare, accounting for 0.3% of gastric tumors, usually involving the fundus
- Carcinoid tumor may display a benign or malignant course
- Associated with chronic atrophic gastritis, pernicious anemia, multiple endocrine neoplasia type 1 (MEN-1) syndrome, and Zollinger-Ellison syndrome
- 80% of gastric carcinoids are asymptomatic
- Carcinoid syndrome most commonly characterized by flushing and diarrhea; however, a wide range of symptoms may manifest involving multiple organ systems
- Diagnosed endoscopically with deep biopsy given submucosal location
- Prognosis better than gastric cancer: 5-year survival rate often greater than 50%

Ménétrier's disease

Benign lesion of stomach characterized by tortuous giant gastric folds.

FEATURES

- Rare, unknown etiology, usually diagnosed after 50 years of age
- Histologically characterized by marked foveolar hyperplasia, gland atrophy, and increased mucosal thickness
- Symptoms include anemia, anorexia, diarrhea, edema, epigastric pain, nausea, vomiting, and weight loss
- Course often complicated by protein-losing gastropathy resulting in hypoalbuminemia
- Ménétrier's disease may be associated with increased risk of gastric cancer
- Diagnosed endoscopically with deep biopsy to rule out malignancy

Rare benign tumors

Extremely rare, accounting for less than 1% of gastric tumors. Rare benign tumors of the stomach include juvenile polyps, pancreatic rest, Peutz-Jeghers polyps, and xanthelasma.

SIGNS & SYMPTOMS

Signs

- Abdominal mass (30%) is usually indicative of extensive disease
- Ascites

- Hepatomegaly, or hepatic mass
- Skin pallor secondary to iron-deficiency anemia
- Jaundice is a late sign
- Left axillary lymphadenopathy (Irish's node)
- Ovarian mass (Krukenberg's tumor)
- Periumbilical lymphadenopathy (Sister Joseph's nodules)
- A large peritoneal implant in the pelvis felt as mass palpable on rectal or vaginal examination (Blumer's shelf)
- Supraclavicular lymphadenopathy (Virchow's node)
- Weight loss and cachexia are indicative of serious disease, and patients often present late with such nonspecific signs

Symptoms

- Symptoms, if present, are often vague and nonspecific
- In early disease, approximately 80% of patients are asymptomatic
- Significant symptoms suggest advanced disease and may reflect a pattern of local extension or metastases
- Most patients have symptoms for less than one year
- Abdominal or epigastric discomfort or pain (60%) can range from mild to severe and unrelenting
- Anorexia, weight loss (50%) point to a significantly shorter survival
- Hematemesis, melena (10–15%)
- Nausea, vomiting (40%)
- Dysphagia is indicative of cardia or gastroesophageal junction tumor
- Early satiety may indicate diffusely infiltrative carcinoma
- Fatigue
- Postprandial fullness
- Persistent vomiting is indicative of pyloric obstruction or antral tumor

ASSOCIATED DISORDERS

Several paraneoplastic disorders are associated with gastric malignancy and include:

- Acanthosis nigricans
- Polymyositis, dermatomyositis
- Circinate erythemas, pemphigoid
- Dementia, cerebellar ataxia
- Migratory thrombophlebitis (Trousseau syndrome)
- Ectopic Cushing's syndrome or carcinoid syndrome (rare)
- Seborrheic keratosis (Leser-Trélat sign)
- Microangiopathic hemolytic anemia

KEY! DON'T MISS!

- Do not mistake the vague nonspecific symptoms of gastric adenocarcinoma for those of dyspepsia or peptic ulcer disease
- Always consider the possibility of malignancy in patients with gastrointestinal complaints; clinical index of suspicion is heightened by age, race, family history, and other risk factors

CONSIDER CONSULT

- Refer undiagnosed patients for possible upper endoscopy with biopsy
- Major hemorrhage mandates emergency surgical or gastroenterologic referral

INVESTIGATION OF THE PATIENT

Direct questions to patient

Q **When did your symptoms begin?** Early gastric cancer is often asymptomatic, with symptoms appearing late in the disease

- Q **How is your appetite?** Patients with gastric cancer may have anorexia
- Q **Does your stomach 'fill up' easily?** Early satiety is an uncommon complaint but, when present, may indicate diffusely infiltrative tumor
- Q **Do you have trouble swallowing solids or liquids?** Dysphagia may be indicative of tumor in the cardia or gastroesophageal junction
- Q **Have you noticed any dark urine or pale stools?** Jaundice from biliary obstruction is usually a late manifestation of gastric cancer, indicating extensive disease
- Q **Do you have abdominal pain?** Abdominal pain is often vague and nonspecific but may be related to the extent and location of tumor
- Q **Have you vomited?** Persistent vomiting may be indicative of an antral tumor obstructing the pylorus
- Q **Have you vomited blood or 'coffee-ground' material?** Hematemesis occurs in 10–15% of patients with gastric cancer
- Q **Have you noticed any black stools or blood from your rectum?** Severe hemorrhage is an uncommon manifestation of gastric cancer
- Q **Have you noticed any weight loss?** Weight loss occurs late in the disease
- Q **Do you have leg pain, or have you noticed one or both legs swelling?** Cancer can induce a hypercoagulable state that can cause deep vein thrombosis

Contributory or predisposing factors

- Q **Do you smoke?** Tobacco abuse is a risk factor for proximal gastric cancer
- Q **What is your occupation?** Rubber and coal workers may have an increased risk of developing gastric cancer
- Q **Have you emigrated?** The worldwide incidence of gastric cancer varies widely from nation to nation, with Japan, for example, having one of the highest rates
- Q **What is your diet?** Diets rich in nitrates can increase the risk of gastric cancer, as can diets that are low in protein and vitamins A, C, and E. High-fat diets are associated with proximal gastric cancer
- Q **Describe your home or social situation.** Distal gastric cancer is related to low socioeconomic status, inadequate refrigeration, and ingestion of water from wells. Proximal gastric cancer is related to medium or high socioeconomic status
- Q **Do you have a history of chronic atrophic gastritis, pernicious anemia, intestinal metaplasia, or *H. pylori* infection?** All of these conditions increase the risk of gastric malignancy. The relationship between gastric ulcer disease and gastric cancer remains controversial. There is no association between duodenal ulcer and gastric cancer
- Q **Do you have a history of partial gastrectomy for benign gastric ulcer disease?** A history of partial gastrectomy increases the risk of gastric cancer; increased risk observed 15 years postgastrectomy
- Q **Do you have a history of Ménétrier's disease?** Ménétrier's disease increases risk of gastric cancer by 10–15%
- Q **Do you have a history of gastroesophageal reflux disease (GERD)?** GERD may be associated with proximal gastric cancer

Family history

- Q **Do you have a family history of gastric cancer?** Familial clusters of gastric cancer have been described.

Examination

- **Is the patient jaundiced?** Biliary obstruction may occur depending on the location and extent of gastric malignancy; look for yellow skin and icteric sclera
- **Are there excoriations?** Pruritus secondary to jaundice can result in intense scratching with superficial trauma
- **Is there conjunctival pallor?** Iron-deficiency anemia may result from chronic gastrointestinal blood loss

- **Is the patient obese?** Obesity may be linked to proximal gastric cancer
- **Is there a palpable abdominal mass?** An abdominal mass may be palpated depending on the location and extent of the tumor
- **Is there any evidence of ascites?** Malignant ascites may be present with advanced disease
- **Is there lymphadenopathy?** Gastric cancer often spreads to superficial lymph nodes, especially the left axillary (Irish's node), supraclavicular (Virchow's node), and periumbilical nodes (Sister Joseph's nodules)
- **Is there a palpable liver?** Hepatomegaly may result from obstruction or liver metastasis
- **Is there bitemporal wasting or evidence of weight loss?** Patients may be cachectic
- **Is there lower-extremity edema?** Venous thrombosis is a recognized complication of neoplastic disease classically presenting as an edematous lower extremity

Summary of investigative tests

Initial studies to document disease include the following:

- Double-contrast barium gastric radiograph or flexible upper endoscopy is the usual initial test to demonstrate gastric lesion; an endoscopy would be performed by a specialist
- Once a gastric lesion is identified, biopsy is needed to establish definitive diagnosis; a biopsy would be performed by a specialist

Once a gastric malignancy is confirmed, the following tests are used to further evaluate and stage the cancer:

- Complete blood count with differential and liver function tests are needed
- Computed tomography (CT) scan of the abdomen, pelvis, and chest is useful for assessing the presence of locally advanced or systemic metastatic disease and to determine resectability
- Laparoscopy: up to 50% of patients have more extensive disease at laparotomy than was predicted by preoperative CT. Laparoscopy can identify patients with regionally advanced or disseminated disease who are not candidates for immediate potentially curative surgical intervention and is normally performed by a specialist. Laparoscopy, whenever feasible, should eliminate the need for patients undergoing laparotomy without resection
- Endoscopic ultrasonography can accurately determine depth of gastric invasion and lymph node status; it is normally performed by a specialist in radiology
- CT, endoscopic ultrasonography, and laparoscopy are considered complementary tests
- Serologic markers have not demonstrated adequate sensitivity or specificity to encourage use

DIAGNOSTIC DECISION

- Early diagnosis is difficult; most patients present with advanced disease, and clinical presentation of gastric adenocarcinoma is often vague and nonspecific and may not suggest neoplastic disease
- Always consider the possibility of malignancy in patients with gastrointestinal complaints; clinical index of suspicion is heightened by age, race, and other risk factors
- Upper endoscopy is always indicated in patients 45 years of age or older who present with new-onset dyspepsia
- A lower age threshold for endoscopy may be appropriate for those with alarm symptoms (anemia, dysphagia, vomiting, and weight loss), those with empiric therapy failure, and those from high-risk groups
- If clinical index of suspicion for gastric pathology is high, the first diagnostic test is usually double-contrast barium upper gastrointestinal series or endoscopy
- Laboratory testing cannot establish or exclude a diagnosis of gastric cancer
- Definitive diagnosis requires biopsy

THE TESTS

Body fluids

COMPLETE BLOOD COUNT WITH DIFFERENTIAL

Description

Venous blood sample.

Advantages/Disadvantages

- Advantage: simple, inexpensive, and readily available test
- Disadvantage: nonspecific

Normal

- Hemoglobin: males, 13.6–17.7g/dL (8.4–11.0mmol/L); females, 12.0–15.0g/dL (7.4–9.3mmol/L)
- Mean cell volume: 76–100mcm^3 (76–100fL)
- Mean cell hemoglobin: 27–33pg
- Mean cell hemoglobin concentration: 33–37g/dL (330–370g/L)
- Hematocrit: males: 39–49%; females 33–43%
- Platelets: 130–400x10^3 cells/mm^3 (130–400x10^9 cells/L)
- White cell count: 3200–9800 cells/mm^3 (3.2–9.8x10^9 cells/L)
- Basophils: 10–1000 cells/mm^3 (<0.01–1.0x10^9 cells/L)
- Eosinophils: 40–400 cells/mm^3 (0.04–0.4 x10^9 cells/L)
- Lymphocytes: 1500–4000 cells/mm^3 (1.5–4.0x10^9 cells/L)
- Monocytes: 200–800 cells/mm^3 (0.2–0.8x10^9 cells/L)
- Neutrophils: 3500–7500 cells/mm^3 (3.5–7.5x10^9 cells/L)

Abnormal

- Results outside normal reference range
- Keep in mind the possibility of a falsely abnormal result

Cause of abnormal result

Anemia due to chronic blood loss or malignancy.

LIVER FUNCTION TESTS

Description

Venous blood sample.

Advantages/Disadvantages

- Advantage: simple, inexpensive, and readily available test
- Disadvantage: nonspecific, may not be abnormal even in the presence of liver metastases

Normal

- Aspartate aminotransferase (AST): 5–40mU/mL (5–40 IU/L)
- Alanine aminotransferase (ALT): 5–40mU/mL (5–40 IU/L)
- Gamma-glutamyl transferase: 5–60mU/mL (5–60 IU/L)
- Alkaline phosphatase: 30–110mU/mL (30–110 IU/L)
- Total bilirubin: 0.3–1.4mg/dL (6–24mcmol/L)
- Albumin: 3.9–4.8g/dL (39–48g/L)

Abnormal

- Results outside normal reference range
- Keep in mind the possibility of a falsely abnormal result

Cause of abnormal result

Elevated alkaline phosphatase, gamma-glutamyl transpeptidase, hepatic aminotransferases, and bilirubin are indicative of biliary, pancreatic, or hepatic involvement but are not diagnostic.

Drugs, disorders and other factors that may alter results

There are many medications and conditions that cause abnormal liver function.

Biopsy

FLEXIBLE UPPER ENDOSCOPY WITH BIOPSY

Description

Gastric tissue obtained endoscopically with biopsy or snare polypectomy. Needle aspiration is occasionally used.

Advantages/Disadvantages

Advantages:

- Invasive diagnostic procedure of choice
- Provides tissue for definitive diagnosis of gastric malignancy
- Helpful in the staging process of gastric malignancy
- Diagnostic yield increased if between six and 10 biopsy specimens are taken from edge and base of ulcer – 95% accurate
- Usually well tolerated by patients

Disadvantages:

- Superficial biopsy of gastric lesion may yield false-negative results
- Supravital stains are occasionally used to identify suspicious lesions
- Sedation frequently needed
- Complications include bleeding and esophageal or gastric perforation

Normal

- No gastric lesion identified
- No abnormal histology

Abnormal

- Gastric lesion identified
- Abnormal histology identified
- Keep in mind the possibility of a falsely abnormal result

Cause of abnormal result

Gastric malignancy.

Drugs, disorders and other factors that may alter results

Ménétrier's disease may make gastric mucosa visualization and biopsy technically difficult.

Imaging

DOUBLE-CONTRAST BARIUM GASTRIC RADIOGRAPH

Description

Barium study of stomach to highlight mucosal detail.

Advantages/Disadvantages

Advantages:

- Relatively accurate: can identify 75% of 5- to 10-mm lesions
- Sensitivity high for detecting gastric lesions: >90%

Disadvantages:

- Can only determine whether gastric lesion is present; biopsy is needed for definitive diagnosis
- Cannot determine resectability
- Specificity very low

Normal

No mucosal or gastric lesion identified.

Abnormal

- Mucosal or gastric lesion identified
- Keep in mind the possibility of a falsely abnormal result

Cause of abnormal result

Gastric malignancy, which is highlighted on the X-ray films.

Drugs, disorders and other factors that may alter results

- Gastric distention may be impaired by diffusely infiltrating tumors
- Ménétrier's disease may make gastric mucosa visualization and biopsy technically difficult
- Gastric lymphoma may cause a very similar appearance to an adenocarcinoma
- Benign and malignant gastric ulcers may be difficult to differentiate. Given the challenges inherent in clinically differentiating benign peptic ulcer disease from gastric cancer, many physicians perform endoscopic biopsy and brush cytology on all gastric lesions to rule out malignancy

COMPUTED TOMOGRAPHY SCAN

Description

CT scanning of the abdomen, pelvis, and chest is used for staging, to determine resectability, and to rule out metastasis.

Advantages/Disadvantages

Advantages:

- Initial noninvasive imaging procedure of choice for staging once diagnosis is established
- Can accurately identify metastasis, upwards of 90%

Disadvantages:

- Can only identify lesion and cannot determine whether lesion is benign or malignant
- Cannot accurately stage many gastric cancers (approximately 50% of gastric cancers are understaged, and approximately 15% are overstaged)
- Given accuracy problems, should not be used as sole staging modality if curative resection is intended

Abnormal

- Evidence of local or metastatic tumor invasion
- Keep in mind the possibility of a falsely abnormal result

Cause of abnormal result

Invasive or metastatic gastric malignancy.

TREATMENT

CONSIDER CONSULT

Multidisciplinary team approach enhances patient satisfaction and may improve survival:

- Any patient with confirmed diagnosis of gastric carcinoma should be referred to an oncologist
- Refer to experienced gastric surgeon for possible resection
- Refer to radiation oncologist for radiation therapy
- Refer to oncologist for chemotherapy
- Refer to dietitian for nutritional support
- Referral to a clinical trial may be appropriate

IMMEDIATE ACTION

- Evidence of life-threatening gastric hemorrhage mandates immediate endoscopic or surgical intervention
- Evidence of deep vein thrombosis requires anticoagulation

PATIENT AND CAREGIVER ISSUES

Forensic and legal issues

- Most patients will be able to give consent for treatment
- If patient cannot give consent, determine who has authority to consent
- With the exception of life-threatening gastric hemorrhage, deep vein thrombosis, or other life-threatening emergency, the treatment of gastric cancer can be delayed until consent is obtained
- Obtain and keep on the file advance directives of the patient with gastric carcinoma

Impact on career, dependants, family, friends

- Given the overall poor prognosis, many patients and their families and friends will have to deal with end-of-life issues
- Psychological impact of cancer diagnosis is profound, with patients, family, and friends experiencing a variety of emotions, including (but not limited to) anger, anxiety, bereavement, denial, depression, and grief
- Potential significant impact on career, given physical and psychological demands of diagnosis and treatment and the poor overall prognosis

Patient or caregiver request

- **Can green tea prevent stomach cancer?** There is no evidence that green tea can prevent stomach cancer
- **Is there a link between H_2-blockers and stomach cancer?** There is no clear association between histamine-2 receptor antagonists and gastric cancer

MANAGEMENT ISSUES

Goals

- Initiate evaluation for surgical and chemoradiotherapy
- Achieve complete curative resection if possible
- Prevent spread of disease
- Enhance survival and quality of life
- Achieve adequate pain control
- Ensure adequate nutrition
- Evaluate social support
- Determine code status
- Determine attitudes toward hospice
- Prepare patient for end of life

Management in special circumstances

COEXISTING DISEASE

Patients with comorbidities tend to have worse prognosis.

PATIENT SATISFACTION/LIFESTYLE PRIORITIES

- Patients will have questions regarding treatment and prognosis
- Patients will be especially concerned with pain control and quality of life
- Patients with advanced disease will need assistance with end-of-life issues
- Side-effects of chemoradiotherapy may have a negative impact on quality of life
- Severe disability is possible with terminal disease

SUMMARY OF THERAPEUTIC OPTIONS

Choices

Surgery:

- Surgery is an option for less than one-third of patients but is the only possibility of cure
- Curative resection (total gastrectomy) should be offered to all patients unless there are distant metastases or the patient is not a surgical candidate
- Subtotal gastrectomy with adequate disease-free margin and regional lymph node dissection is the treatment of choice and is generally considered the only potentially curative approach for patients with gastric cancer

Postoperative chemoradiotherapy:

- Postoperative (adjuvant) chemoradiotherapy should be considered for all patients at high risk for recurrence after curative resection, especially those with T3 or T4 tumors or with positive lymph nodes
- Following curative gastrectomy (subtotal or total) with positive resection margins, chemoradiotherapy may be prescribed or patient entered into trials
- Neoadjuvant chemotherapy is still considered an experimental therapy. Studies indicate a possible increase in resection rates, but there is a high incidence of locoregional relapse

For unresectable disease and palliation:

- For unresectable or locally advanced disease, combined external beam radiation therapy plus chemotherapy or intraoperative irradiation produces long-term survival in 10–20% of patients in most trials; external beam radiation therapy is also used for pain palliation
- Patients with unresectable disease should be offered supportive care, chemoradiotherapy, surgical debulking, and entry into a clinical trial
- Debulking is used for palliation and may enhance the response to chemoradiotherapy
- For nonsurgical candidates, consider palliation with endoscopic stenting, electrocautery/laser ablation, and gastrostomy/jejunostomy tube
- Patients submitted to gastrostomy/jejunostomy may have a better quality of life
- For palliation, multiple drug chemotherapy regimens have response rates of 30–50%; some regimens improve the survival
- Immunotherapy, intraperitoneal adjuvant therapy, and superselective intra-arterial chemotherapy are under investigation
- Endoscopic mucosal resection may be an emerging treatment for superficial gastric cancer
- Consider entry into clinical trial

FOLLOW UP

- Follow up is primarily to evaluate efficacy of treatment and manage complications
- Specific areas of investigation include evaluation of recurrence or spread and complications related to surgery or chemoradiotherapy

Plan for review

- After treatment, evaluate symptom relief and disease recurrence or spread
- Repeat endoscopy several months after resection to determine efficacy
- Evaluate patient for signs and symptoms of postoperative complications and of chemotherapeutic or radiation toxicity
- Abdominal/pelvic/chest CT scanning may be indicated to evaluate efficacy and rule out metastasis

Information for patient or caregiver

- Patients need to know that gastric cancer has significant morbidity and mortality rates
- Patients should understand that the only hope for cure is curative resection
- Many patients will have to decide on end-of-life issues and be educated regarding options
- Appropriate hospice, skilled nursing facility, or home health care referral may need to be made depending on the patient's medical condition, personal preference, and social/financial support

DRUGS AND OTHER THERAPIES: DETAILS

Surgical therapy

GASTRECTOMY, TOTAL

- Resection of entire stomach with local lymphadenectomy
- Treatment of choice for proximal tumors
- Recommended in stage I–III resectable disease
- Some surgeons advocate total gastrectomy 'de principe' for diffuse distal gastric cancer
- Vascular invasion/encasement, metastatic disease, peritoneal disease, and extensive local disease usually preclude resection

Considerable controversy among different methods to perform the resection exists. Some advocate a broader resection of lymph nodes based on results from some Japanese trials, whereas others do not agree with this view and perform a narrower resection.

Efficacy

Complete tumor resection with microscopically negative resection margins and lymphadenectomy offers only hope for cure.

Risks/Benefits

Risks: complications include abdominal/chest infection, anastomotic leak, bleeding, fistula, nutritional defects, and wound infection

Benefits:

- Palliative gastrectomy improves survival
- There is no evidence that total gastrectomy has a higher perioperative mortality rate than subtotal gastrectomy
- Curative resection has 7–10% perioperative mortality rate (morbidity and mortality rates are surgeon- and patient-dependent)

Acceptability to patient

Gastrectomy may be associated with a significant morbidity rate that can be unacceptable to some patients.

Follow up plan

- Follow up should be as clinically indicated and should include history and physical examination, complete blood count (CBC), serum electrolytes every 3 months for 2 years (then every 6 months for 3 years), and chest X-ray every 6–12 months. Other studies, including (but not limited to) endoscopy and CT, may be indicated

- Educate patient regarding nutritional deficiencies, and refer to a nutritionist
- Vitamin B12 supplementation is necessary
- Ensure adequate postoperative pain control
- Observe for bleeding, fistula formation, wound infection, and other postoperative complications
- Following curative gastrectomy without evidence of metastatic disease or positive resection margins, observation without further treatment is warranted; entry into a clinical trial may also be offered

Patient and caregiver information

- Patients and caregivers need to be aware of the nutritional difficulties after gastrectomy that patients can experience
- Patients and caregivers need to be able to recognize major postoperative complications, such as bleeding and wound infection

GASTRECTOMY, SUBTOTAL

- Resection of distal two-thirds to four-fifths of the stomach
- Treatment of choice for distal tumors
- Recommended in stage I–III resectable disease
- Given the improved quality of life and nutritional status following subtotal vs total gastrectomy, many surgeons recommend subtotal gastrectomy when appropriate
- Vascular invasion/encasement, metastatic disease, peritoneal disease, and extensive local disease usually preclude resection

Efficacy

For distal tumors, survival is similar for total and subtotal gastrectomy.

Risks/Benefits

Risks:

- Complications include abdominal/chest infection, anastomotic leak, bleeding, fistula, nutritional defects, and wound infection
- Subtotal gastrectomy may have a lower postoperative morbidity rate than total gastrectomy and a shorter length of stay (morbidity and mortality rates are surgeon- and patient-dependent)

Benefits:

- Treatment of choice for distal tumors
- Offers improved postoperative quality of life and nutritional status

Acceptability to patient

Subtotal gastrectomy may be associated with a significant morbidity rate that can be unacceptable to some patients; however, morbidity rate tends to be less than that associated with total gastrectomy.

Follow up plan

- Follow up should be as clinically indicated and should include history and physical examination, CBC, serum electrolytes every 3 months for 2 years (then every 6 months for 3 years), and chest X-ray every 6–12 months. Other studies, including (but not limited to) endoscopy and CT, may be indicated
- Vitamin B12 supplementation is necessary
- Educate patient regarding nutritional deficiencies, and refer to a nutritionist
- Ensure adequate postoperative pain control
- Observe for bleeding, fistula formation, wound infection, and other postoperative complications

Patient and caregiver information

- Patients and caregivers need to be aware of the nutritional difficulties that postgastrectomy patients can experience; however, these tend to be less those that associated with total gastrectomy
- Patients and caregivers need to be able to recognize major postoperative complications, such as bleeding and wound infection

LYMPHADENECTOMY

Resection of local lymph nodes.

Efficacy

There is no survival advantage from extended/regional lymph node resection (D-2, D-3 resection) vs local lymph node resection (D-1 resection).

Risks/Benefits

Risk: there is an increased perioperative mortality rate from extended/regional lymph node resection (D-2, D-3 resection) vs local lymph node resection (D-1 resection)

Acceptability to patient

Patients submitted to gastrectomy experience problems with deglutition, but this is the only possibly curative approach. Of more concern can be the symptoms from the adjuvant therapy with chemoradiation. This approach improves survival and diminishes recurrence rates but is associated with potentially severe toxicity. A careful balance between possible benefits and toxicity must be performed.

Follow up plan

There are no systematic studies that address the impact of a follow-up plan in gastric carcinomas. Recurrence occurs mostly during the first 2 years, and most attention should be given to this period. Endoscopic examinations during this period may be useful.

Patient and caregiver information

- Specialized nutritional care can be required for patients submitted to gastrectomy and also for those submitted to gastrostomy/jejunostomy
- Adverse events of the adjuvant chemoradiation are common. Specialized oncology care will be required

Radiation therapy

- Primarily used for palliation
- Gastric adenocarcinomas are radioresistant
- Radiation therapy has minimal impact on survival when used for palliation
- Restage inoperable patients after chemoradiotherapy and observe to see if there is a complete response
- Salvage therapy may be indicated for inoperable patients after chemoradiotherapy if residual or M1 disease is present

EXTERNAL BEAM RADIATION THERAPY

- Primarily used for palliation and advanced disease
- Adjuvant and intraoperative radiotherapy are being investigated

Efficacy

- No significant impact on survival if used alone
- Postoperative combined chemoradiotherapy has shown a definite survival advantage in patients at high risk for recurrence after curative resection

- Combined external beam radiation therapy and adjuvant chemotherapy may improve survival after noncurative resection
- May offer small survival benefit in unresectable disease when combined with 5-fluorouracil (5-FU)

Risks/Benefits

- Risk: complications primarily from radiation exposure/damage to surrounding organs (e.g. bowel, spinal cord)
- Benefit: can reduce tumor size and pain

Acceptability to patient

Aggressively manage nausea, vomiting, and diarrhea, which can limit patient compliance.

Follow up plan

- Follow-up should be as clinically indicated and should include history and physical examination, CBC, serum electrolytes every 3 months for 2 years (then every 6 months for 3 years), and chest X-ray every 6–12 months. Other studies, including (but not limited to) endoscopy and CT, may be indicated
- Evaluate patient for symptomatic improvement
- Evaluate patient for tumor burden reduction

Patient and caregiver information

- Advise patient to receive adequate rest to limit profound fatigue
- Warn patient that radiation therapy may cause nausea, vomiting, and diarrhea; however, emphasize that these side-effects can be managed

Chemotherapy

ADJUVANT CHEMOTHERAPY

5-FU and doxorubicin are usually combined with cisplatin, methotrexate, or mitomycin-C.

Efficacy

- May improve survival after noncurative resection
- Postoperative adjuvant chemoradiation therapy can result in improvement in both disease-free and overall survival
- For palliation, chemotherapy induces response but has little impact on survival
- May prolong relapse interval
- Multiagent chemotherapy provides 30–50% partial response in advanced disease, but the overall impact on survival is controversial
- There may be a survival advantage with superselective intra-arterial chemotherapy when used for palliation

Risks/Benefits

Risks:

(In general):

- Must be administered under specialist supervision
- Use caution with renal and hepatic impairment
- Should not be used in myelosuppressed patients
- Risk of myelosuppression

(5-Fluorouracil)

- High-dose pelvic irradiation
- Previous use of alkylating agents
- Discontinue as soon as signs of toxicity appear (diarrhea, watery stools, frequent bowel movements, gastrointestinal ulceration and bleeding, hemorrhage, leukopenia, stomatitis or esophagopharyngitis, thrombocytopenia, vomiting)

(Cisplatin)
- Should not be used in patients with hearing impairment
- Peripheral blood counts should be monitored weekly

(Methotrexate)
- Use caution with peptic ulceration and ulcerative colitis
- Use caution with the elderly

(Mitomycin)
Risk: acute shortness of breath and severe bronchospasm

Benefit (In general): Several meta-analyses of isolated adjuvant chemotherapy RCTs found weak evidence of survival benefit; however, there is no consistent evidence that adjuvant chemotherapy improves survival

Side-effects and adverse reactions
(5-Fluorouracil)
- Cardiovascular system: angina, myocardial ischemia
- Central nervous system: headache, nystagmus, acute cerebellar syndrome
- Gastrointestinal: stomatitis, esophagopharyngitis, diarrhea, emesis, nausea, vomiting
- Hematological: bone marrow suppression, leukopenia, thrombocytopenia, agranulosis, pancytopenia, anemia
- Ophthalmic: photophobia
- Skin: alopecia, dermatitis, photosensitivity

(Methotrexate)
- Central nervous system: fatigue
- Eyes, ears, nose, and throat: ototoxicity
- Gastrointestinal: nausea, vomiting, anorexia
- Genitourinary: sexual dysfunction
- Hematologic: bone marrow suppression
- Metabolic: renal toxicity
- Skin: alopecia

(Mitomycin)
- Cardiovascular system: pulmonary toxicity, cardiac toxicity
- Central nervous system: fever, anorexia
- Gastrointestinal: nausea, and vomiting
- Hematologic: thrombocytopenia and/or leukopenia, hemolytic uremic syndrome (HUS)
- Metabolic: renal toxicity
- Skin: cellulitis, extravasation, delayed erythema

Interactions (other drugs)
(5-Fluorouracil)
- Leucovorin calcium
- Cimetidine
- Filgrastim
- Metronidazole

(Methotrexate)
Pyridoxine plus hexmethylmelamine (may affect response duration).

Contraindications
(5-Fluorouracil)
- Hypersensitivity to fluorouracil
- Severe hematologic toxicity
- Serious infections
- Gastrointestinal hemorrhage
- Depressed bone marrow
- Poor nutritional state

(Mitomycin)

- **Demonstrated a hypersensitive or idiosyncratic reaction to it in the past**
- **Thrombocytopenia, coagulation disorder, or an increase in bleeding tendency due to other causes**
- **Safe use of mitomycin in pregnant women has not been established.**

Acceptability to patient

- Side-effect profile dependent on agents used
- Compliance may be limited by nausea, vomiting, diarrhea, gastrointestinal ulceration, and neurologic toxicity
- Warn patient about possibility of alopecia and skin rash

Follow up plan

- Follow up should be as clinically indicated and should include history and physical examination, CBC, serum electrolytes every 3 months for 2 years (then every 6 months for 3 years), and chest X-ray every 6–12 months. Other studies, including (but not limited to) endoscopy and CT, may be indicated
- Follow CBC because myelosuppression is a major toxicity
- Aggressively manage nausea, vomiting, and diarrhea
- Monitor fluid status in patients with profound diarrhea/vomiting
- Restage inoperable patients after chemoradiotherapy, and observe to see if there is a complete response

Patient and caregiver information

Warn patient about side-effects; however, emphasize that these problems can be managed.

Other therapies

PALLIATIVE THERAPY

- Debulking is for palliation and may enhance the response to chemoradiotherapy
- For nonsurgical candidates, consider endoscopic stenting, electrocautery/laser ablation, and gastrostomy/jejunostomy tube to relieve obstruction

Efficacy

- Debulking procedures may improve quality of life by enhancing the response to chemoradiotherapy
- Palliative debulking can relieve obstruction in 50% of patients
- Palliative gastrectomy improves survival

Risks/Benefits

Risk: palliative resection has 15–20% perioperative mortality rate

Acceptability to patient

Generally acceptable measures because gastric obstruction is relieved, leading to greater patient comfort.

Follow up plan

- Patients should be followed for symptomatic improvement
- Palliative care patients do not require extensive follow up with investigations

Patient and caregiver information

Patients should be aware that palliative treatment, including surgical debulking procedures, is not curative.

OUTCOMES

EFFICACY OF THERAPIES

- Surgery: survival is dependent on complete tumor resection
- Palliative gastrectomy: palliative gastrectomy improves survival
- Subtotal gastrectomy: for distal tumors, survival is similar for total and subtotal gastrectomy
- Postoperative morbidity rate: subtotal gastrectomy may have a lower postoperative morbidity rate and a shorter length of stay than total gastrectomy
- Lymphadenectomy, survival: there is no survival advantage from extended/regional lymph node resection (D-2, D-3 resection) vs local lymph node resection (D-1 resection)
- Lymphadenectomy, mortality rate: there is an increased perioperative mortality rate from extended/regional lymph node resection (D-2, D-3 resection) vs local lymph node resection (D-1 resection)
- Adjuvant chemoradiotherapy: a national intergroup trial showed that postoperative adjuvant chemoradiation therapy resulted in a significant improvement in both disease-free and overall survival. The median overall survival in the surgery-only group was 27 months compared with 36 months in the chemoradiotherapy group
- Adjuvant chemotherapy and palliation: there may be a survival advantage with superselective intra-arterial chemotherapy when used for palliation

PROGNOSIS

- Cure rates of 80% or higher are achieved only with early lesions (nodes negative, confined to mucosa or submucosa), which are uncommon in the US
- Overall prognosis is poor, with 5-year survival rate of 5–15%
- Without treatment the mean survival is less than 6 months
- Prognosis depends on the stage as determined by The American Joint Commission on Cancer tumor-node-metastases (TNM) classification system
- Prognosis is good for early gastric cancer (confined to mucosa or submucosa), with high cure rates following surgical resection
- Intramucosal gastric cancer has the best 5-year survival rate (over 90%)
- Following complete resection, the 5-year survival rate is approximately 10% for proximal cancers and 20% for distal cancers
- Over 50% have lymph node or adjacent organ involvement at diagnosis
- Aneuploidy, lymph node involvement, vascular invasion, and weight loss confer a poor prognosis
- CD44, erbB-2, and p-53 expression may be associated with a poor prognosis
- Signet ring features and estrogen receptor status may confer poor prognosis
- There is a wide disparity in outcomes between Western and Japanese studies

TNM staging system for gastric carcinoma:

- Stage 0 cancer is limited to the mucosa
- Stage IA is when the tumor invades the submucosa or lamina propria
- Stage IB is when the tumor invades through the muscularis propria
- Stage II is when the cancer has invaded the stomach wall without lymph node involvement, or the tumor is invading the mucosa but is confined to the wall, and lymph nodes are involved
- Stage IIIA cancers have positive nodes and invasion of the muscularis propria or the entire wall
- Stage IIIB tumors have no nodal involvement but adherence to adjacent structures
- Stage IV indicates distant metastases, or positive nodes and adherence to adjacent structures

Clinical pearls

In Japan there are reports of successful programs of screening for gastric cancer, but some studies indicate that this rate of success can be due to differences in the anatomopathologic criteria used to differentiate severe dysplasia from carcinoma in situ.

Therapeutic failure

- Consider entry into a clinical trial
- Pain control and quality of life should be a priority

Recurrence

- Recurrence occurs in 80% within 5 years of resection
- Most recurrences are local; however, over 50% relapse at multiple local sites
- Postoperative chemoradiotherapy can reduce recurrence
- Entry into clinical trial should be strongly considered
- Pain control and quality of life should be a priority

Deterioration

- Entry into a clinical trial should be strongly considered
- Pain control and quality of life should be a priority

Terminal illness

- Pain control and quality of life should be a priority
- Assist patient and family in dealing with end-of-life issues
- Have patient evaluated for hospice or home health care

COMPLICATIONS

- Common metastatic sites include liver, lung, bone, and peritoneum
- Tumor may cause biliary or pancreatic duct obstruction; refer to a gastroenterologist or surgeon for appropriate management
- Gastrointestinal obstruction can be relieved by laser treatment, photodynamic therapy, radiotherapy, stenting, or multimodal therapy
- Transverse colon fistula and bowel obstruction may occur secondary to local spread
- Pain may be severe and should be managed aggressively
- Gastrointestinal bleeding may occur; it may require urgent referral for surgical or endoscopic intervention if life-threatening, or it may present as anemia requiring transfusion
- Deep vein thrombosis is a recognized complication of malignancy
- Nutritional deficits are especially common after total gastrectomy and may require a percutaneous endoscopic gastronomy

CONSIDER CONSULT

- Consider referral to an academic-university center for clinical trial entry for patients with incurable disease
- Consider referral to hospice for treatment failure, clinical deterioration, or terminal disease
- Consider referral to psychiatrist or psychologist for emotional support and insight
- Refer to pain specialist for intractable pain

PREVENTION

There are no known interventions that can prevent gastric adenocarcinoma.

RISK FACTORS

- Tobacco: smoking increases relative risk
- Alcohol: excessive alcohol consumption is associated with increased risk
- Diet: diets high in nitrates and fat increase risk, as do diets low in protein and vitamins A, C, and E
- Environment: unknown environmental exposure may increase risk, especially early in life
- Family history: familial clusters of gastric cancer are described
- Coexisting medical history: gastric atrophy, gastritis, and *H. pylori* infection increase risk
- Surgical history: partial gastrectomy increases risk
- Occupational: coal and rubber workers have increased risk
- Socioeconomic status: poor refrigeration and use of water from wells that harbor high concentrations of nitrates and *H. pylori* are associated with increased risk

MODIFY RISK FACTORS

There are no studies documenting that risk factor modification can reduce the incidence of gastric cancer.

Lifestyle and wellness

TOBACCO

Smoking cessation should be encouraged.

ALCOHOL AND DRUGS

Excessive alcohol use should be discouraged.

DIET

- Reduce intake of nitrate-rich foods (e.g. dried, salted, or smoked foods)
- Adopt a high-fiber diet rich in raw fruits and vegetables
- Adopt a diet high in vitamins A, C, and E
- Adopt a low-fat diet

ENVIRONMENT

Ensure adequate refrigeration and safe drinking water.

FAMILY HISTORY

- Familial clusters reported
- Associated with blood type A

DRUG HISTORY

No established association between gastric cancer and H_2 receptor antagonists.

SCREENING

- Japanese mortality rates have declined secondary to mass screening with double-contrast barium radiograph or endoscopy
- Mass screening is most successful in epidemic areas
- In the US, mass screening for gastric cancer is not recommended
- Endoscopic surveillance is recommended for patients with Barrett's esophagus, gastric adenomas, familial adenomatous polyposis, and high-grade gastric dysplasia

PREVENT RECURRENCE

Recurrence can be prevented/delayed by choosing appropriate surgical candidates, choosing multimodal therapy, and ensuring macroscopic/microscopic free resection margins.

Reassess coexisting disease

PATIENT SATISFACTION/LIFESTYLE PRIORITIES

- Most patients with recurrence will be concerned with quality-of-life and end-of-life issues
- Pain control and patient comfort should be a priority

RESOURCES

ASSOCIATIONS

American Cancer Society
1599 Clifton Road NE
Atlanta, GA 30329
Tel: (800) 227-2345 (800-ACS-2345)
www.cancer.org

National Cancer Institute
Public Inquires Office
Building 31, Room 10A03
31 Center Drive, MSC 2580
Bethesda, MD 20892–2580
Tel: (800) 422-6237 (800-4-CANCER)
www.cancer.gov

National Comprehensive Cancer Network
50 Huntington Pike, Suite 200
Rockledge, PA 19046
Tel: (215) 728-3877, (888) 909-6226 (888-909-NCCN)
www.nccn.org

National Hospice and Palliative Care Organization
1700 Diagonal Road, Suite 300
Alexandria, VA 22314
Tel: (800) 658-8898
www.nhpco.org

KEY REFERENCES

- Allum WH, Hallissey MT, Kelly KA. Adjuvant chemotherapy in operable gastric cancer. 5-year follow-up of the first British Stomach Cancer Group trial. Lancet 1989;1:571–4
- American Gastroenterological Association medical position statement: evaluation of dyspepsia. Gastroenterology 1998;114:579–81
- Boddie AW Jr, McMurtrey MJ, Giacco GG, et al. Palliative total gastrectomy and oesophagogastrectomy: an evaluation. Cancer 1983;51:1195–2000
- Bonenkamp JJ, Hermans J, Sasako M, et al. Extended lymph-node dissection for gastric cancer. N Engl J Med 1999;340:908–14
- Bonenkamp JJ, Songun I, Hermans J, et al. Randomised comparison of morbidity after D1 and D2 dissection for gastric cancer in 996 Dutch patients. Lancet 1995;345:745–8
- Bozzette F, Marubini E, Bonfanti G, et al. for the Italian Gastrointestinal Study Group. Total versus subtotal gastrectomy: surgical morbidity and mortality rates in a multicenter Italian randomized trial. The Italian Gastrointestinal Tumor study Group. Ann Surg 1997;226:613–20
- Bozzette F, Marubini E, Bonfanti G, et al. for the Italian Gastrointestinal Study Group. Subtotal versus total gastrectomy for gastric cancer: five-year survival rates in a multicenter randomized Italian trial. Ann Surg 1999;230:170–8
- Cotran RS, et al. Robbins Pathological Basis of Disease, 5th edn. Philadelphia: WB Saunders, 1994, p779–83
- Cuschieri A, Fayers P, Fielding J, et al. Postoperative morbidity and mortality after D1 and D2 resections for gastric cancer: preliminary results of the MRC randomised controlled surgical trial. Lancet 1996;347:995–9
- Cuschieri A, Weedon S, Fielding J, et al. Patient survival after D1 and D2 resections for gastric cancer; long-term results of the MRC randomised surgical trial. Br J Cancer 1999;79:1522–30
- Dent DM, Madden MV, Price SK. Randomised comparison of R1 and R2 gastrectomy for gastric carcinoma. Br J Surg 1988;75:110–12
- DeVita VT, Hellman S, Rosenberg SA. Cancer: principles & practices of oncology. 5th edn. New York: Lippincott-Raven, 1997, p1021–1054

- Earle CC, Maroun JA. Adjuvant chemotherapy after curative resection for gastric cancer in non-Asian patients: revisiting a meta-analysis of randomised trials. Eur J Cancer 1999;35:1059–1064
- Feldman M, et al. Sleisenger & Fordtran's Gastrointestinal and Liver Disease. 6th edn. New York: WB Saunders, 1998, p733–57
- Gouzi JL, Huguier M, Fagniez PL, et al. Gastrectomie totale contre gastrectomie partielle pour adeno-cancer de l'antre. Ann Chir 1989;43:356–60
- Gouzi JL, Huguier M, Fagniez PL, et al. Total versus subtotal gastrectomy for adenocarcinoma of the gastric antrum. A French prospective controlled study. Ann Surg 1989;209:162–6
- Haugstvedt T. Benefits of resection in palliative surgery. Dig Surgery 1994;11:121–5
- Hermans J, Bonenkamp JJ, Ban MC, et al. Adjuvant therapy after curative resection for gastric cancer: a meta-analysis of randomised trials. J Clin Oncol 1993;11:1441–7
- Jaki RJ, Miholic J, Koller R, et al. Prognostic factors in adenocarcinoma of the cardia. Am J Surg 1995;169:316–19
- Mari E, Floriani I, Tinazzi A, et al. Efficacy of adjuvant chemotherapy after curative resection for gastric cancer: a meta-analysis of published randomised trials. A study of the GISCAD (Gruppo Italiano per lo Studio dei Carcinomi dell'Apparato Digerente). Ann Oncol 200;11:837–43
- McCulloch P. Should general surgeons treat gastric carcinoma? an audit of practice end results. Br J Surg 1994;81:417–20
- Maruyama K, Okabayashi K, Kinoshita T. Progress in gastric cancer surgery in Japan and its limits of radicality. World J Surg 1987;11:418–25
- Robertson CS, Chung SCS, Woods SDS, et al. A prospective randomised trial comparing R1 subtotal gastrectomy with R3 total gastrectomy for antral cancer. Ann Surg 1994;220:176–82
- Yu W, Whang I, Suh I, et al. Prospective randomized trial of early post-operative intraperitoneal chemotherapy as an adjuvant to resectable gastric cancer. Ann Surg 1998;228:347–54
- Shchepotin IB, Chorny V. Hanfelt J, et al. Palliative superselective intra-arterial chemotherapy for advanced nonresectable gastric cancer. J Gastrointest Surg 1999;3:426–31

FAQS

Question 1

What staging examination should be requested?

ANSWER 1

An abdominal CT scan, endoscopy, chest X-ray, and, if available, an endoscopic ultrasonograph.

Question 2

Does the carcinoembryonic antigen (CEA) have a value as a prognostic or diagnostic marker in gastric cancer?

ANSWER 2

No. The CEA can be elevated in gastric cancer, but it is not a maker for gastric cancer and must not be used as one. Some in-course studies are evaluating its value in follow up, but no conclusion can be drawn up to now.

Question 3

Do the new STI571 work for gastric cancer?

ANSWER 3

Only for a specific subset of gastric cancers (the gastrointestinal stromal tumors), and it is still considered experimental.

CONTRIBUTORS

Martin L Kabongo, MD, PhD
Otavio A Clark, MD
Sandeep Garg, MD

HEMOPHILIA

SUMMARY INFORMATION

DESCRIPTION

- Hereditary bleeding disorders with an X-linked recessive inheritance pattern
- Two main types – A (classic hemophilia) and B (Christmas disease) are clinically indistinguishable
- Caused by low levels of factor VIII (hemophilia A) or factor IX (hemophilia B)
- Almost all affected patients are male but it can occur in females
- Disease severity is determined by amount of coagulant factor present

URGENT ACTION

For acute bleeds where coagulation disorder is suspected but not confirmed:

- Urgent admission for transfusion of blood products
- Patients with active life-threatening bleeding who are suspected of having a congenital bleeding disorder can be supported with fresh frozen plasma, 15mL/kg, while diagnostic studies are being done (rarely needed nowadays)
- The risk of viral transmission of hepatitis B or C or HIV must be considered

For acute bleeds in known hemophiliacs:

- Significant bleeds require urgent admission for transfusion
- Factor VIII or IX concentrate infusion is urgently needed
- Quantity required depends on site and nature of the bleed. Usually raising clotting factor levels to 30% is sufficient to control hemorrhage
- Major surgery or life-threatening bleeds require the level to be raised to 100%, and then maintained at 30–50% for 2 weeks to prevent secondary hemorrhage
- Desmopressin acetate 0.3mcg/kg may be used in mild hemophilia A
- Aminocaproic acid (EACA) 4g orally every 4h can be given as an adjunct treatment for persistent bleeding unresponsive to factor VIII concentrate or desmopressin in hemophilia A, but consider inhibitor and use of high-dose factor VIII or factor VIIa

For acute hemarthroses:

- Prompt treatment is essential
- Patients can be taught to give replacement therapy at home
- Refer for urgent orthopedic assessment as aspiration may be considered (if a response to treatment is not noted)

Intracranial bleeding is the most common emergent cause of death:

- Life-threatening bleeding in the hemophilic patient is caused by bleeding into vital structures (CNS, upper airway) or by exsanguination (external, gastrointestinal, or iliopsoas hemorrhage)
- Prompt treatment with clotting factor concentrate for these life-threatening hemorrhages is imperative

BACKGROUND

ICD9 CODE

- 286.0 Hemophilia A
- 286.1 Hemophilia B

SYNONYMS

Hemophilia A:

- Classic hemophilia
- Factor VIII-deficient hemophilia

Hemophilia B:

- Christmas disease
- Factor IX-deficient hemophilia
- Acquired hemophilia
- Heckathorn's disease is a poorly understood variant of hemophilia A that is inherited as an X-linked recessive trait

CARDINAL FEATURES

- Congenital disorder of coagulation factors VIIIc (hemophilia A) or IX (hemophilia B)
- Mainly males are affected but females may also be affected
- Factor VIII or IX levels are low (<20U/dL or 20%)
- Most patients have a reduction in the amount of clotting factor protein; however, 5–10% of hemophilia A and 40–50% of hemophilia B patients make a dysfunctional protein
- The platelet plug forms, but formation of the fibrin clot that follows it is delayed and is not robust
- 70% are of a sex-linked recessive nature
- The remaining 25–30% have no family history and are believed to result from a spontaneous genetic abnormality
- Mild cases may not present until major challenge, e.g. major surgery, trauma, childbirth
- Moderate cases may present with bleeding after dental hemorrhage or tonsillectomy
- Severe cases usually present at birth or when first walking
- Antenatal diagnosis is available using DNA analysis
- Repeated bleeding into a joint causes joint destruction – a major cause of morbidity in hemophilia and virtually diagnostic of coagulation factor defects
- Intracranial bleeding is the major cause of death for all age groups of hemophiliacs
- Currently around 70% of diagnosed hemophiliacs are HIV-positive

CAUSES

Common causes

The cause of hemophilia is genetic.

Hemophilia A:

- Low or absent factor VIII anticoagulant (VIIIc) activity
- Factor VIII normally circulates in the plasma bound to a larger molecule, the von Willebrand factor (VWF), as part of the factor VIII complex
- The functional attribute of this complex is VIIIc
- Factor VIIIc is aberrant or deficient in patients with hemophilia A
- The severity in hemophilia A may be directly related to the level of factor VIII coagulant (factor VIIIc) activity
- In severe cases of hemophilia A, factor VIIIc level is <1% and spontaneous joint and muscle bleeds occur
- In moderate cases of hemophilia A, factor VIIIc levels are 1–5% and these patients bleed after minor trauma

- In mild cases of hemophilia A, factor VIIIc levels are >5% and bleeds usually only occur after major surgery. Presentation may be delayed until early adulthood
- VWF apparently is qualitatively normal and is present in normal or increased amounts
- Evidence suggests that reinforcement of platelet plugs with fibrin is defective. Patients with hemophilia do not bleed more rapidly but have a slowing of the rate of clot formation. The clot may be friable, and rebleeding occurs during the physiologic lysis of clots or with minimal trauma, typically delayed after trauma

Hemophilia B (Christmas disease):
- Low levels of factor IX anticoagulant activity
- Congenital
- X-linked recessive inheritance

Rare causes

Acquired hemophilia A:
- Acquired factor VIII autoantibodies are seen in 0.2–1 per million population annually and can arise spontaneously in association with various autoimmune and chronic inflammatory diseases, such as systemic lupus erythematosus, rheumatoid arthritis, and ulcerative colitis
- Antibodies to factor VIII can develop in the puerperium, usually appearing at term or within several months after parturition in association with a first pregnancy. The antibody may disappear spontaneously in postpartum patients after 12–18 months
- Acquired hemophilia may also be seen in association with hematologic malignancies and solid tumors; certain medications such as penicillin, sulfa antibiotics, chlorpromazine, and phenytoin; and dermatologic conditions such as psoriasis and pemphigus vulgaris
- Most often, acquired factor VIII antibodies are idiopathic, particularly in older patients without apparent underlying disease
- The immunologic mechanism that underlies inhibitor induction is unclear. Underlying genetic susceptibility factors have been suggested
- No evidence exists that exogenous factor VIII acts as an antigen in nonhemophilic patients
- Acquired factor VIII inhibitors may explain some reports of hemophilia in women and may also underlie apparent occult hemophilia presenting later in life
- The bleeding manifestations resulting from antibodies to factor VIII are often similar to those seen in hemophilia A, but prognosis is worse

Hemophilia B Leyden:
- Rare variant form
- The clinical manifestations tend to diminish with advancing age in association with a rise in the factor IX level from as low as 1U/dL in childhood to levels of 20U/dL or more in adult life
- The basis for this variant is that mutations responsible for hemophilia B Leyden occur in the factor IX gene promoter region; this region contains an androgen response element that, with age, stimulates factor IX gene transcription and protein synthesis

Contributory or predisposing factors

- Positive family history in 70%
- Can predict risk to offspring using simple Mendelian genetics for an X-linked recessive disorder

EPIDEMIOLOGY

Incidence and prevalence

PREVALENCE
- Hemophilia A: 0.1/1000 males
- Hemophilia B: 0.02/1000 males
- Hemophilia A is the second most common of the inherited coagulation disorders

FREQUENCY
Hemophilia A and B and von Willebrand's disease together account for >90% of all inherited bleeding disorders.

Demographics

AGE
- Both are congenital conditions
- Severe disease generally noted at birth or in first year
- Mild disease may not be diagnosed until young adulthood
- Mean age of onset of symptoms is 1.5 years for severe disease (often noted in first year), 3 years for moderate disease, and 5 years or later for mild disease

GENDER
- Most patients are male
- Females are usually asymptomatic carriers of hemophilia A unless their factor level is <40%
- Factor IX levels below 10% have been documented in a few women, including some with chromosomal abnormalities. Unlike hemophilia A, the spontaneous mutation rate is low, and most patients with hemophilia B have positive family histories

GENETICS
- X-linked autosomal recessive
- Women can be carriers and may have lower than normal levels of factor VIII on testing
- The genes for both factor VIII and factor IX are carried near the terminus of the long arm of the X chromosome and are therefore X-linked traits
- Approximately 45–50% of patients with severe hemophilia A have the same mutation, in which there is an internal inversion within the factor VIII gene that results in no protein being produced
- This mutation can be detected in the blood of patients or carriers and in the amniotic fluid by molecular techniques
- Because of the multiple genetic causes of either factor VIII or factor IX deficiency, however, most patients are classified based upon the amount of factor VIII or factor IX clotting activity
- The defective gene is located on the X chromosome
- In males who lack a normal allele, the defect is manifested by clinical hemophilia. The affected male will not transmit the disorder to his sons, because his Y chromosome is normal. However, all of his daughters will be carriers of the trait because they inherit his X chromosome. Most of these women will be unaffected clinically because of the presence of a normal allele from the mother. The female carrier will transmit the disorder to half of her sons
- The mutation rate for the responsible gene may be unusually high: no evidence or history of abnormal bleeding is found in other members of the families of at least one-third of all hemophiliacs. In other instances, neonatal deaths or the passage of the trait through a succession of female carriers may explain the negative family history. For practical purposes, therefore, a negative family history is of little value in excluding the possibility of hemophilia A
- About 40% of severe hemophilia A results from a major inversion of a section of the tip of the long arm of the X chromosome, one break point of which is situated within intron 22 of the factor VIII gene. These results indicate that a substantial number of families with severe hemophilia A can undergo accurate gene tracking and carrier analysis. In affected females, X-chromosome inactivation may occur at an unusually early stage of embryogenesis, resulting in low levels of factor VIII
- Homozygous hemophilia A is now well authenticated in several women and resembles the disorder seen in affected males in all respects
- In several other instances of female hemophilia A, the disorder appears to have developed as the result of a newly mutated gene

- A chromosomal abnormality in the female rarely may be responsible, such as 46XX/45X mosaicism, 46XY karyotype, inactive X isochromosome, or deleted X chromosome (Turner's syndrome)
- Unusual degrees of X-chromosome inactivation (hyperlyonization) may produce severe factor VIII deficiency in some carriers of hemophilia A
- Hemophilia B is inherited as an X-linked recessive trait, but the locus on the X chromosome of the gene controlling factor IX production is remote from that involved with factor VIII biosynthesis

GEOGRAPHY

Hemophilia A has been recognized in all areas of the world where adequate information is available.

DIFFERENTIAL DIAGNOSIS

Most of the following disorders are seldom associated with a prolonged partial thromboplastin time (PTT) and a normal prothrombin time (PT), a combination that strongly suggests an inherited disorder or an inhibitor.

Von Willebrand's disease

- Von Willebrand's disease (VWD) is a congenital deficiency of von Willebrand's factor (VWF)
- There are several subtypes
- 80% are type 1, caused by a quantitative decrease in VWF
- Type 2A and 2B are results of qualitative protein abnormalities
- Type 3 is a rare autosomal recessive disorder with near-complete quantitative VWF deficiency
- Severe VWD in males may be indistinguishable from mild hemophilia A associated with a prolonged bleeding time, even if the latter abnormality is an inconsistent finding
- Confirmatory tests for VWD are needed to make this distinction
- Patients with the uncommon type 2N VWD may also be clinically indistinguishable from patients with hemophilia A
- An X-linked family history of bleeding supports a diagnosis of hemophilia A in these patients, and an autosomal recessive family history of bleeding supports a diagnosis of type 2N VWD

FEATURES

- Mucosal bleeding (gingival, epistaxis) and gastrointestinal bleeding
- Menorrhagia
- Easy bruising
- Postpartum bleeding
- Bleeding after surgery or dental extraction
- Decreased factor VIII activity
- Prolonged bleeding time
- Decreased VWF antigen
- PTT prolonged

Other coagulation factor deficiencies

With the exception of von Willebrand's disease, the inherited coagulation disorders associated with bleeding produce similar signs and symptoms, regardless of the particular factor that is lacking. The other inherited coagulation disorders affect at most 1 in 10,000–15,000 people. Diagnosis of these factor deficiencies can be established by laboratory testing for the various factors.

Factor XI deficiency (hemophilia C):

- Autosomal deficiency associated with mild to moderate bleeding symptoms
- Frequently encountered in Ashkenazi Jews but has been found in many other ethnic groups
- In Israel, 1/1000 to 3/1000 are homozygous for this deficiency. Sephardic Jews are rarely affected
- While the condition is referred to as hemophilia C, the bleeding tendency is not as great as in factor VIII or factor IX deficiency

Deficiencies of the contact factors (nonbleeding disorders):

- Deficiencies of the contact factors prolong the PTT but are not causes of clinical bleeding. Clinical history, therefore, can exclude this diagnosis in the presence of a prolonged PTT
- These factors include factor XII, prekallikrein, and high molecular weight kininogen. Because these contact factors function at the step of initiation of the intrinsic clotting system, the PTT is markedly prolonged when these factors are absent

- It is important that these individuals be well informed about the meaning of their clotting factor deficiency, as they do not need treatment even if major surgery is undertaken
- On rare occasions, factor XII deficiency is associated with VWD and has been termed von Willebrand San Diego. Thus, if a patient with reduced factor XII is identified who has bleeding symptoms, it is advisable to carry out von Willebrand screening

Factor VII deficiency:

- Rare bleeding disorder that is usually detected only in the homozygous state
- Spontaneous intracranial hemorrhage and frequent mucocutaneous bleeding. Markedly prolonged PT but a normal PTT
- Plasma half-life of factor VII is 2–4h, so therapy with fresh frozen plasma (FFP) is difficult and often complicated by fluid overload

Factor X deficiency:

- Rare autosomal disorder that results in mucocutaneous and post-traumatic bleeding
- Reduced factor X level is associated with a prolongation of both the PT and the PTT
- Systemic amyloidosis may be associated with factor X deficiency due to the adsorption of factor X on the amyloid
- Transfusion therapy is often not successful because of rapid clearance

Prothrombin (factor II) deficiency:

- This deficiency is caused either by a markedly reduced prothrombin level (hypoprothrombinemia) or by a functionally abnormal prothrombin (dysprothrombinemia)
- Laboratory testing in homozygous patients demonstrates a prolonged PT and PTT
- Treatment can be achieved using either prothrombin complex concentrates or FFP. In prothrombin deficiency, FFP is useful, because the half-life of prothrombin is 3.5 days

Fibrinogen deficiency:

- Congenital afibrinogenemia is a rare autosomal recessive disorder in which there is an absence of fibrinogen
- Patients do not bleed as frequently as hemophilia patients and rarely have hemarthroses
- Affected patients may present in the neonatal period with gastrointestinal hemorrhage or hematomas following vaginal delivery
- Laboratory testing demonstrates a marked prolongation of the PTT, PT, and thrombin time

Factor V deficiency:

- The deficiency of factor V, also known as labile factor, is an autosomal recessive, mild to moderate bleeding disorder that has also been termed parahemophilia
- Hemarthroses occur rarely; mucocutaneous bleeding and hematomas are the most common symptoms
- Severe menorrhagia is a frequent symptom in women
- Laboratory evaluation demonstrates a prolonged PTT and PT
- The only currently available therapeutic product that contains factor V is FFP

Combined deficiency of factor V and factor VIII:
Combined deficiency of factor V and factor VIII has been demonstrated to be secondary to the absence of an intracellular transport protein, ERGIC-53, which is responsible for transporting factor V and factor VIII from the endoplasmic reticulum to the Golgi compartments.

Factor XIII deficiency (fibrin-stabilizing factor or transglutaminase deficiency):

- Since factor XIII is responsible for the cross-linking of fibrin or the stabilization of fibrin clot, symptoms of delayed hemorrhage are secondary to poor maintenance of hemostasis

- Patients will have trauma on one day and then develop a bruise or hematoma on the following day
- In patients with significant bleeding symptoms, prophylaxis can be achieved with infusion of cryoprecipitate every 3–4 weeks

Antiplasmin or plasminogen activator inhibitor (PAI) deficiency:

- Deficiency of either of these two antifibrinolytic proteins results in increased plasmin generation and the premature lysis of fibrin clots
- Patients have mucocutaneous bleeding but rarely have joint hemorrhages
- Treatment is with fresh frozen plasma

FEATURES

Deficiency of factors V and VIII:

- Inherited as an autosomal recessive trait
- Combined deficiency of factors V and VIII manifests clinically with mild mucosal and cutaneous bleeding. Severe post-traumatic and postsurgical bleeding is common. Hemarthrosis is rare. Laboratory findings in homozygous patients include a prolonged PTT and prothrombin time, and levels of factor VIIIc and Vc that average 15U/dL. Levels of factor VIIIAg (VIIIcag) and VAg are low

Abnormalities of protease inhibitors:

- Alpha-2 antiplasmin deficiency
- Severe bleeding, including hemarthrosis, may be associated with deficiency of alpha-2 antiplasmin. This disorder appears to be inherited as an autosomal recessive trait, in which heterozygotes have detectable deficiencies of this antiprotease but only mild bleeding
- When assayed qualitatively by fluorometric or photochromogenic techniques, alpha-2 antiplasmin levels usually are below 10U/dL. Bleeding episodes can be treated with tranexamic acid/EACA (aminocaproic acid)

Plasminogen activator inhibitor-1 deficiency:

Deficiency of this inhibitor to tissue plasminogen activator is also associated with a bleeding disorder. The basis of the bleeding is similar to that described for alpha-2 antiplasmin deficiency: excessive plasmin activity, caused in this case by excessive activation of plasminogen.

Vitamin K deficiency

- Causes hemorrhagic disease of the newborn
- Can occur early (first week of life) or in weeks 1–8
- May occur in breast-fed infants only
- Infants of mothers taking anticonvulsants are at increased risk
- Prevented by giving all newborn infants vitamin K

FEATURES

- Bruising
- Hematemesis
- Melena
- Prolonged bleeding of cord stump or after circumcision
- Intracranial hemorrhage

Thrombocytopenia

- Thrombocytopenia is an acquired disorder
- Most common form is immune mediated: immune-mediated thrombocytopenic purpura (ITP)
- Usually develops when platelet count falls below $20x10^9/L$

- Hemorrhage likely if platelet count <10x10^9/L
- Multiple causes
- Petechiae are characteristic
- Deep dissecting hematomas are rare
- Superficial ecchymoses are usually small and multiple
- Hemarthrosis is rare
- Delayed bleeding is rare
- Bleeding from superficial cuts and scratches is minimal
- 80–90% of inherited forms occur only in male patients

FEATURES
- Purpura in acutely unwell children
- Increased bone marrow megakaryocytes in ITP
- Mainly affects children aged 2–10 years
- Purpura and superficial bruising
- Epistaxis and other mucosal bleeding
- Intracranial bleeding is rare
- Acute and self-limiting in 90%
- Treatment is controversial
- Corticosteroids and immunoglobulins are sometimes used
- Can become chronic
- Sudden onset in children, insidious in adolescents and adults
- Adults and adolescents more likely to have protracted course

Disseminated intravascular coagulation
- A chronic form may present with low platelets, reduced/normal fibrinogen and only mild bleeding
- Treatment relies on correcting the underlying cause while providing intensive care
- FFP is used to replace clotting factors
- Therapy with heparin and antithrombin III remains controversial

FEATURES
- Purpura in acutely unwell children
- Other signs of sepsis and life-threatening illness

Nonaccidental injury
- Multiple bruising in small children may be due to bleeding diathesis, but nonaccidental injury is common
- Look for other marks, old injuries, bruising at unusual sites, failure to thrive, history of abuse of other siblings
- Look for evidence of neglect – poor nutrition, lack of hygiene, infestation, developmental delay, disturbed behavior
- Look for expression of frozen watchfulness by the child

FEATURES
- Late presentation
- Denial by parent of pain from an obviously painful injury
- Disclosure by child
- Disclosure by other, e.g. sibling
- Inconsistent story re injury – either story changes or story does not fit injury
- Presence of coagulation disorder does not exclude nonaccidental injury: children with chronic disease are more likely to be abused than normal children

Acute bone marrow failure

- Bone marrow failure – e.g. in aplastic anemia, marrow replacement by tumor or myelofibrosis – will result in acute deficiency of platelets and therefore bruising characteristic of thrombocytopenia
- Anemia also will result in poor wound healing and secondary infection leading to secondary bleeding

FEATURES

- Pancytopenia on blood count
- Marrow failure confirmed on bone marrow sampling

Platelet dysfunction – inherited intrinsic

- Group of mild bleeding disorders
- Caused by disorder of the amplification of platelet activation
- Two main types: thrombasthenia and Bernard-Soulier's syndrome

FEATURES

Thrombasthenia:

- Rare hereditary platelet defect affecting platelet surface membrane glycoproteins
- Autosomal recessive with consanguinity in affected families
- Severe mucosal bleeding requiring platelet transfusions
- Platelets lack membrane glycoprotein GP IIb-IIIa
- Fail to bind fibrinogen during platelet activation so fail to aggregate
- Laboratory findings show failure of platelet aggregation with agents including ADP, absence of clot retraction, and single platelets on a peripheral blood smear

Bernard-Soulier's syndrome:

- Rare autosomal recessive disorder affecting surface membrane glycoproteins
- Severe mucosal bleeding requiring platelet transfusions
- Large platelets are present that do not agglutinate with ristocetin
- Aggregate normally with agent ADP
- Surface membrane glycoprotein GP Ib-IX is absent
- Platelets do not adhere normally to subendothelium despite normal VWF levels

Platelet dysfunction – acquired

- These disorders are relatively common due to aspirin use
- Other medications affect platelet function
- Clinical disorders can cause platelet dysfunction, e.g. myeloproliferative and myelodysplastic disorders

FEATURES

- Platelet dysfunction appears to be due to activation of fibrinolysis on the platelet surface leading to loss of GP Ib binding site for VWF
- Aspirin may markedly prolong the bleeding time if there is an underlying platelet disorder or severe coagulation defect
- Platelets can dysfunction during a cardiopulmonary bypass operation using a pump oxygenator
- Patients should be given platelet transfusions regardless of platelet numbers if postoperative bleeding is excessive

Liver disease

Liver disease leads to a complicated bleeding disorder.

FEATURES

- The liver is involved in the clotting process through three functions: synthesis of clotting factors, absorption of vitamin K, and platelet function
- Vitamin K is required for the synthesis of factors II, VII, IX, and X
- Therefore the hematologic effect of liver disease is complicated
- Investigations will reveal a raised PT, bleeding time, and PTT
- Treatment includes parenteral vitamin K, platelet and FFP transfusions

SIGNS & SYMPTOMS

Signs

- Mild cases may be asymptomatic in childhood and present only in response to major trauma or surgery
- Mild to moderate cases may present with prolonged oozing after dental extraction
- Mild cases may not be diagnosed until young adulthood
- Even severe cases usually cause few problems in the first year of life
- When the child starts to ambulate, abnormal bleeding may be noted
- Sites of bleeding frequently include joints and muscles
- Nonaccidental injury is often suspected
- Large superficial ecchymoses may be seen
- Hot, swollen, painful joints resulting from hemarthroses
- Joint deformities from hemarthroses
- Hematuria may be present
- Postpartum hemorrhage
- Menorrhagia
- Hemorrhage after tooth extraction
- Bleeding into serous cavities and internal fascial spaces often occurs
- Retroperitoneal hemorrhage or bleeding into the psoas sheath may mimic appendicitis, and hemorrhage into the bowel wall may be confused with intestinal obstruction
- Hemoptysis rarely is associated
- Spontaneous hemorrhage may be cyclic in nature
- Petechiae are rare but have been noted in severely affected patients during an exacerbation of bleeding
- Mucocutaneous bleeding can occur, but is more common in platelet disorders
- Pulmonary and pleural bleeding are uncommon, although mediastinal and pleural shadows have been noted radiographically and presumably originate from fresh or old hematomas
- Intraocular hemorrhage is uncommon, but bleeding into the orbit and conjunctiva occurs often
- Spontaneous rupture of the spleen has been reported
- Wound healing is often slow, probably because of continued or intermittent hemorrhage or complicating infection

Neonatal signs:

- Many infants with inherited coagulation disorders do not bleed significantly in the neonatal period
- Occasionally, neonates with hemophilia may sustain intracranial hemorrhage
- About 30% of affected male infants with hemophilia bleed with circumcision
- Small cephalohematomas and petechiae are common in the newborn as a result of the trauma of delivery
- Large cephalohematomas that progressively increase in size may result from hemophilia, but are more common in association with acquired bleeding disorders such as hemorrhagic disease of the newborn
- Hemorrhage from the umbilical cord or stump is unusual
- The onset of bleeding from the umbilical cord may be delayed

Infants:

- Infants usually are asymptomatic because they are insulated from trauma
- Hematomas are seen first when children become active, and hemarthroses seldom develop until they begin to walk
- The earliest joint bleeds appear most commonly in the ankle, because of the lack of stability of this joint as the toddler assumes an upright posture
- In the older child and adolescent, hemarthroses of the knees and elbows are the most debilitating
- While the child's early joint bleeds are recognized only following major swelling and fluid accumulation in the joint space, older children are frequently able to recognize bleeding earlier than the physician

Symptoms

- Patient may comment on easy bruising and prolonged bleeding time
- Wound healing is often slow, probably because of continued or intermittent hemorrhage or complicating infection
- Joint pains and stiffness from hemarthroses
- Onset of bleeding after trauma often is delayed. Bleeding after a tooth extraction may stop completely, then recur in a matter of hours or even after 1–3 days and persist despite use of styptics, vasoconstrictors, and packing. The temporary hemostatic adequacy of the platelet plug despite defective blood coagulation may explain this phenomenon

CONSIDER CONSULT

- Refer all patients for specialist management
- Management should be supervised by a hemophilia comprehensive care center providing medical, nursing, and psychosocial support for patients and their families
- These centers are also supported by specialist laboratories, able to undertake specific assays to monitor therapy, and physiotherapists to preserve muscle strength and avoid harm from immobilization

INVESTIGATION OF THE PATIENT

Direct questions to patient

All of these questions are looking for evidence that the patient bleeds more easily or for longer than other people. People with normal hemostasis may believe they bleed excessively. Bleeding after trauma in a person with hemophilia differs from normal in amount, duration, and magnitude. The need for transfusions, the number administered, and the patient's statement concerning the duration of bleeding more are the most reliable indicators of bleeding severity.

Q **Have you ever needed a transfusion of blood or blood products?**

Q **Have you ever had major surgery?** The patient is likely to forget procedures or injuries that were uncomplicated. A history of surgical procedures or significant injury without abnormal bleeding is good evidence against the presence of hemophilia

Q **Does excessive bleeding occur after tooth extraction or small cuts? Does bruising occur spontaneously? Are there lumps with bruises for which there is minimal trauma?**

Q **Do you heal well?** Delayed or slow healing of superficial injuries may suggest a hereditary bleeding disorder

Q **In postpubertal females: are your periods heavy?** As some common bleeding disorders such as VWD have a fairly high prevalence and are genetic, mothers and family members may have the same mild bleeding disorder and may not realize that the child's menstrual history is abnormal

Q **Do you have any problems taking aspirin?** Medication, such as aspirin and other nonsteroidal anti-inflammatory agents, may inhibit platelet function and increase bleeding symptoms in patients with a low platelet count or abnormal hemostasis

- Q **Have you ever had bleeding problems following tooth extraction?** The removal of molar teeth is a major challenge to hemostasis, as is a tonsillectomy. Few hemophiliacs, even mildly affected, can withstand these procedures without excessive bleeding
- Q **Do you bleed excessively from small cuts and nicks?** Patients with coagulation disorders seldom bleed abnormally from small superficial cuts such as razor nicks
- Q **Do you experience delayed bleeding after trauma or tooth extraction?** Bleeding after trauma often is delayed. Bleeding after a tooth extraction may stop completely, then recur in a matter of hours and persist despite use of styptics, vasoconstrictors, and packing. The temporary hemostatic adequacy of the platelet plug despite defective blood coagulation may explain this phenomenon
- Q **For how long have you had these problems?** An inherited bleeding disorder is suggested by the onset of bleeding symptoms in infancy and childhood
- Q **Does spontaneous bruising or muscle bleeding occur?** Large superficial ecchymoses may be seen and the most characteristic lesion is the large spreading hematoma. These may arise spontaneously or after trivial trauma, and often spread to involve an entire limb by dissecting within muscles and deep fascial spaces, often with minimal discoloration of the overlying skin
- Q **Have you ever been transfused or treated with blood products?** This is a good guide to history of excessive bleeding

In children:

- Q **Does your child bruise easily?** This can be very difficult to evaluate as many patients with normal coagulation believe that they bruise easily
- Q **Did your child have bruising at birth?** Bleeding during the first month of life may be the first evidence of an inherited disorder of hemostasis. Small cephalohematomas and petechiae are common in the newborn but large cephalohematomas that progressively increase in size may result from hemophilia
- Q **Did your child have bleeding after birth?** Bleeding from the umbilical stump occurs in hemophilia. The onset of bleeding from the umbilical cord may be delayed
- Q **Have you ever felt your child had more bruises than other children?**
- Q **Does your child have nosebleeds?** Epistaxis and mucous membrane bleeding may be seen but is more characteristic of platelet disorders
- Q **Does your child ever limp or complain of painful joints?** Hematomas may first be seen only when the child becomes active. Hemarthrosis commonly does not develop until a child is 3 or 4 years of age
- Q **Has your child ever bled after dental extractions or surgery?** A history of uncomplicated previous surgery or dental extraction suggest bleeding tendency is acquired rather than inherited

In adults:

- Q **Have you ever had surgery? Did you bleed or bruise more than you expected?** A history of uncomplicated previous surgery or dental extraction suggest bleeding tendency is acquired rather than inherited
- Q **Have you any painful joints?**
- Q **Do you have heavy periods?** Menorrhagia tends to be more a feature of VWD but may occur in hemophilia
- Q **Did you ever have heavy bleeding after any surgical procedure?** The absence of bleeding after an episode of major surgery virtually excludes hemophilia
- Q **Are you taking any medication?** Many commonly used drugs, notably aspirin, impair platelet function and produce abnormal findings in laboratory tests. The same drugs may provoke bleeding when administered to patients with hemophilia A

Family history

- Q **Have you ever heard of any member of your family having bleeding or bruising problems?** Hemophilia is an X-linked recessive disorder, the clinical condition expressed only in males with bleeding, bruising, hemarthrosis. The presence of typical bleeding manifestations in male siblings and maternal uncles is virtually diagnostic of X-linked recessive inheritance

Q **Do you know of any ancestors who died in childhood? If so, do you know what they died of?** Prior to availability of clotting factors, moderate or severe hemophilia was usually fatal by late childhood. 30–40% of patients with hemophilia A have a negative family history. The family history usually is negative in the autosomal recessive traits and consanguinity

Examination

- **Is there evidence of bruising or bleeding?**
- **Where has the bleeding been?** Mucous membrane bleeding and skin hemorrhage is characteristic of platelet disorders and VWD. Bleeding into muscles or joints is characteristic of severe clotting factor deficiencies. Scarring and delayed healing is more suggestive of connective tissue disorders such as Marfan's syndrome or factor XIII deficiency
- **Is there evidence of joint deformity?**
- **In children, does the history of how the bruising was acquired match the injury, and is the story consistent? Was there delay in presentation?** Always consider child abuse, and always remember that children with clotting disorders may also be abused. Indeed, children with chronic health problems are slightly more likely to be abused than children in good health. Severe bruising would obviously be painful, and failing to present to a physician might be a cause for concern of child abuse
- **Are there any petechiae, ecchymoses, hematomas, hemarthroses, or mucous membrane bleeding?** Patients with defects in platelet-blood vessel wall interaction (VWD or platelet function defects) usually have mucous membrane bleeding (epistaxis, menorrhagia, hematuria, gastrointestinal bleeding); petechiae on the skin and mucous membranes; and small, ecchymotic lesions of the skin sometimes associated with hematomas

Summary of investigative tests

- Partial thromboplastin time (PTT)
- Prothrombin time (PT)
- Thrombin time
- Platelet count
- Factor VIIIc level
- Factor IX level
- A PTT-mixing study to exclude an inhibitor
- Factor VIII antigen
- Von Willebrand factor levels
- Bleeding time
- Skeletal survey would normally be ordered by a specialist and is not usually performed in children >3 years old. In young children with unexplained or inadequately explained bruising, consider X-rays and full skeletal survey to try to exclude nonaccidental injury
- Hemophilia A carrier detection compares the ratio of factor VIII to von Willebrand factor protein and is predictive in 70–80% of cases. Rarely done nowadays; usually performed by a specialist
- Molecular diagnosis is preferred for carrier testing. Usually performed by a specialist

DIAGNOSTIC DECISION

- The diagnosis of hemophilia A is seldom difficult in the severely affected patient
- Hemarthrosis with significant orthopedic disability is rare in patients with coagulation disorders other than hemophilia A and hemophilia B
- Hemophilia A is diagnosed by factor VIII level <50%
- Hemophilia B is diagnosed by factor IX level <60%
- In patients with the mild forms of the disorder, however, failure to recognize the existence of the disease or to make the correct diagnosis is more likely
- A normal PTT value cannot exclude the possibility of hemophilia. In the mildly affected patient, specific factor assays must be performed to confirm or exclude the diagnosis of hemophilia

CLINICAL PEARLS

Normal PTT does not rule out the diagnosis of mild hemophilia, as the detection threshold for PTT in most labs is between 25–40% of normal factor level.

THE TESTS

Body fluids

PARTIAL THROMBOPLASTIN TIME

Description

- The PT and PTT are the basic laboratory diagnostic tools used in the evaluation of coagulation disorders and can be used to organize the approach to their diagnosis
- The PTT as performed in the clinical laboratory is actually an 'activated' PTT (or APTT)
- This test measures the initiation of clotting at the level of factor XII through sequential steps to the final clot end point. It does not measure factor VII, factor XIII, or anticoagulants
- The PTT is usually prolonged in patients with hemophilia A. Abnormal results are usually obtained if the factor VIIIc level is less than 25% of normal

Advantages/Disadvantages

Disadvantage: some PTT reagents are insensitive to mild factor VIII deficiency

Normal

Check with lab: performed against control. Because of different reagents and laboratory instruments the normal range for the PTT varies between one hospital laboratory and another.

Abnormal

- Increased
- The laboratory screening test that is affected by a reduced level of factor VIII or factor IX is the PTT. In severe hemophilia, this is usually 2–3 times the upper limit of normal
- Two groups of inherited disorders manifest an isolated elevation in the PTT. The first group is the contact factors, e.g. XII (Hageman factors), prekallikrein (Fletcher factor), and high-molecular-weight kininogen. They cause a benign disorder in which the PTT is elevated but the patient has no bleeding diathesis. These deficiencies exist as isolated laboratory abnormalities, and thus they should not be invoked as a cause of the patient's bleeding problem. They may be specifically assayed when precise diagnosis is necessary

Cause of abnormal result

Among the inherited disorders characterized by raised PTT and normal PT (hemophilia A, hemophilia B, and deficiencies of factors XI, XII, prekallikrein, and high-molecular-weight kininogen), deficiency of the latter three factors can be readily excluded because their deficiency is not associated with excessive clinical bleeding. Factor XI deficiency in males may mimic mild hemophilia, and hemophilia B is clinically identical to hemophilia A.

Drugs, disorders and other factors that may alter results

- Heparin therapy
- Liver disease
- Vitamin K deficiency
- Disseminated intravascular coagulation
- Warfarin therapy
- Nephrotic syndrome

PROTHROMBIN TIME

Description

The PT measures the extrinsic clotting system following the activation of clotting by tissue factor (thromboplastin) in the presence of calcium. It is not prolonged with deficiencies of factors VIII, IX, XI, or XII. An elevated PT reflects an extrinsic pathway abnormality via factor VII deficiency. As factor VII has the shortest half-life (3–5h) of the coagulation factors, it is the first to manifest a deficiency when its active form is underproduced.

Advantages/Disadvantages

Advantage: blood test – easy and quick

Normal

- In most laboratories the normal PT ranges between 10 and 13s. The PT has been standardized using the International Normalized Ratio (INR) so that values can be compared from one laboratory or instrument to another
- PT is normal in hemophilia
- Normal range varies between laboratories – result is set against control

Abnormal

Outside normal range.

Cause of abnormal result

Normal in hemophilia. Increased by:

- Liver disease
- Warfarin
- Heparin
- Disseminated intravascular coagulation (DIC)
- Vitamin K deficiency
- Afibrinogenemia

Drugs, disorders and other factors that may alter results

Increased by:

- Salicylate ingestion
- Chloral hydrate
- Estrogens
- Antacids
- Phenylbutazone
- Quinidine
- Antibiotics
- Allopurinol
- Anabolic steroids

THROMBIN TIME

Description

Blood test. The thrombin time measures the final step of the clotting cascade in which fibrinogen is converted to fibrin.

Advantages/Disadvantages

Advantage: easy, simple, quick.

Normal
10–16s.

Abnormal
Increased.

Cause of abnormal result
Prolongation of the thrombin time occurs with reduced fibrinogen levels (hypofibrinogenemia or afibrinogenemia), with dysfunctional fibrinogen (dysfibrinogenemia), or by substances that interfere with fibrin polymerization such as heparin or fibrin split products. This test is normal in hemophiliac patients.

Drugs, disorders and other factors that may alter results
Thrombolytic and heparin therapy.

PLATELETS
Description
- Blood test
- The platelet count is essential in the evaluation of patients with a positive bleeding history
- Thrombocytopenia is the most common acquired cause of a bleeding diathesis in children

Normal
130–400x10^9/L. Patients with a platelet count above 50x10^9/L rarely have significant clinical bleeding. Hemophiliacs have a normal platelet count.

Abnormal
Outside normal range.

Cause of abnormal result
- Usually normal in hemophilia
- May be elevated. Thrombocytosis may reflect a response to acute or chronic hemorrhage, but in many hemophiliacs it has been found in the absence of significant bleeding
- Decreased in thrombocytopenia, due to increased destruction (immune, trauma, drugs, hypersplenism, transfusion reactions) or decreased production (marrow failure, hereditary abnormalities)

MIXING STUDIES
Description
Laboratory test with blood sample and stored plasma to quantify inhibitor level, also called Bethesda assay. If there is prolongation of the PT or PTT, a mixing study is usually performed. Normal plasma is added to the patient's plasma, and the PTT or PT is repeated. In patients with hemophilia A, inhibitors of factor VIII may develop after exposure to replacement therapy.

Normal
- Correction of the PT or PTT by 1:1 mixing with normal plasma suggests the deficiencies of a clotting factor, as a 50% level of individual clotting proteins is sufficient to produce a normal PT or PTT
- Unless the patient has an inhibitor to factor VIII, the mixing of normal plasma with patient plasma results in correction of the PTT

Abnormal
- Positive
- To quantitate the amount of inhibitor present, the standardized clinical assay of these clotting inhibitors is termed the Bethesda assay

- One Bethesda Unit is defined as the amount that will inhibit 50% of the clotting factor in normal plasma

Cause of abnormal result

- If the clotting time is not corrected or only partially corrected, an inhibitor is usually present
- If the mixing study does not correct or becomes more prolonged and the patient has clinical bleeding, an inhibitor against factor VIII, IX, or XI may be present
- If the patient has no bleeding symptoms and both the PTT and the mixing study are prolonged, a lupus-like anticoagulant is often present

Drugs, disorders and other factors that may alter results

Inhibitors are sometimes found in:

- Systemic lupus erythematosus (SLE) and autoimmune diseases
- Pregnancy

FACTOR VIIIC ASSAY

Description

- Blood test
- Each of the clotting factors can be measured in the clinical laboratory using individual factor-deficient plasmas
- Both factor XI deficiency and hemophilia B must be distinguished from hemophilia A in the laboratory. The best way of evaluating patients with an isolated prolonged PTT is by performing specific assays of these three factors in the order of their statistical frequency, that is, VIIIc, IX, and XI
- Factor VIII testing measures the ability of the patient's plasma to correct the prolonged PTT of plasma deficient in factor VIII. This ability is compared with that of normal plasma and is given as a percentage of normal. The test measures the procoagulant activity of factor VIII but does not discriminate between abnormal activity resulting from an abnormal factor VIII or low levels of normal factor VIII. The two forms of this deficiency are hemophilia A and VWD

Advantages/Disadvantages

Advantages:

- Hemophilia A – diagnostic test is low factor VIII
- Assay of factor VIIIc is a simple technique. The one-stage techniques are used most widely because they are simple to perform. Two-stage assays detect approximately 20% more factor VIIIc than do one-stage methods
- Assays for both factor VIIIc and VWF may be carried out with reasonable accuracy on material obtained by fetoscopy, that is, mixtures of blood and amniotic fluid or unmixed fetal blood
- Bedside measurement of factor VIIIc activity may be accomplished using a whole blood factor VIIIc assay, achieving more rapid results

Disadvantages:

- The factor VIIIc assay has a large potential for error, even in expert hands. Therefore, when borderline values are obtained, the assay should always be repeated
- Samples that are frozen and subsequently thawed might lose 15–20% of their activity; therefore these assays are best performed on fresh plasma
- Cord blood testing a neonate can be accurate for factor VIII; however, it will not be accurate for factor IX, as liver function in neonates is not as high as in adults

Normal

For most clotting factors the normal range is between 50 and 150U/dL (50–150%). Factor VIII normal is 50–170%.

Abnormal
Less than 50%. In general, severe deficiency of factor VIII is less than 1% of normal plasma (<1U/dL or <1%), moderate deficiency between 1 and 5% of normal, and mild deficiencies greater than 5% and below the normal range.

Cause of abnormal result
Hemophilia A.

FACTOR IX ASSAY
Description
- Blood test
- Each of the clotting factors can be measured in the clinical laboratory using individual factor-deficient plasmas
- Both factor XI deficiency and hemophilia B must be distinguished from hemophilia A in the laboratory. The best way of evaluating patients with an isolated prolonged PTT is by performing specific assays of these three factors in the order of their statistical frequency, that is, VIIIc, IX, and XI

Normal
For most clotting factors the normal range is between 50 and 150U/dL (50–150%). Factor IX normal is 60–136%.

Abnormal
Less than 60%. In general, severe deficiency of factor IX is less than 1% of normal plasma (<1U/dL or <1%), moderate deficiency between 1 and 5% of normal, and mild deficiencies greater than 5% and below the normal range.

Cause of abnormal result
Hemophilia B.

FACTOR VIII INHIBITORS
Description
- Blood test
- In patients with hemophilia A or hemophilia B, inhibitors of factor IX may develop after exposure to replacement therapy
- To quantitate the amount of inhibitor present, the standardized clinical assay of these clotting inhibitors is termed the Bethesda assay
- One Bethesda Unit is defined as the amount that will inhibit 50% of the clotting factor in normal plasma
- In 14–25% of patients who receive infusions of factor VIII or factor IX, a factor-specific antibody may develop
- These antibodies are directed against the active clotting site and are termed inhibitors
- The majority of antibodies to factor VIII are IgG immunoglobulins that appear to be specific for the coagulant subunit of the factor VIII molecule (VIIIc). IgA or IgM inhibitors are rare, as are antibodies that inhibit both VIIIc and VWF
- Antibodies to factor VIII are disproportionately often of the IgG4 subclass and do not fix complement
- Antibodies inactivate factor VIII
- The inactivation of factor VIII is usually irreversible
- Factor IX antibodies are usually not clinically active

Normal
Negative.

Abnormal
Positive.

Cause of abnormal result
- Presence of antibodies to factor VIII or IX, a common complication of therapy with clotting factors
- In acquired hemophilia this test will also be positive

VON WILLEBRAND FACTOR LEVELS
Description
Definitive diagnosis for VWD requires measuring:
- Total plasma VWF antigen
- VWF function
- Plasma factor VIII level
- Agarose gel electrolysis of VWF multimers

VWF function is determined by the ability of plasma to support the agglutination of normal platelets by ristocetin.

Advantages/Disadvantages
Advantages:
- Diagnostic of VWD
- The test levels will determine the severity of the disease

Disadvantages:
- Specialized tests – require laboratory and specialist interpretation
- Expensive

Abnormal
- In patients with the common type 1 form of VWD, results are concordant, i.e. VWF antigen, VWF function and plasma factors VIII levels are equally depressed
- The degree of depression varies around 15–60% of normal
- The test levels will determine the severity of the disease
- In patients with type 2 VWD, there is abnormal synthesis of VWF molecules, resulting in deficiency
- Diagnosis is confirmed by reduced large VWF multimers on agarose gel electrophoresis

Cause of abnormal result
- Von Willebrand's disease
- Healthy blood group O individuals also have reduced levels of VWF antigen: 40–60% of normal

Tests of function
BLEEDING TIME
Description
- The bleeding time assesses the function of platelets and their interaction with the vascular wall
- Disposable standardized devices have been developed that control the length and depth of the skin incision
- A blood pressure cuff is applied to the upper arm and inflated to 40mmHg for children and adults
- In term newborns and young children a modified device has been developed and used with a lower cuff pressure
- Following the incision with the bleeding time device, blood is blotted from the margin of the incision at 30-s intervals until bleeding ceases. While each laboratory must establish its own normal range, bleeding usually stops within 4–8min

Advantages/Disadvantages

Advantages:

- The bleeding time test may be valuable when carefully performed
- An abnormal bleeding time result in a patient with a personal or family history of excessive mucocutaneous bleeding would justify further hemostatic testing for platelet dysfunction, such as platelet aggregation studies or specific tests for VWD

Disadvantages:

- The bleeding time is a difficult laboratory test to standardize, and there is much interlaboratory and interindividual variation
- Normally performed by specialist in laboratory setting

Normal

Bleeding time (template) 3–9min.

Cause of abnormal result

- Bleeding time is prolonged in 15–20% of patients with hemophilia A. Although platelet counts less than 100,000/mm^3 are associated with prolonged bleeding times, disproportionate prolongations of the bleeding times may suggest a qualitative platelet defect or VWD
- This test is only inconsistently abnormal in most disorders attributed to abnormalities of the vessels
- The bleeding time usually is prolonged in some patients with inherited afibrinogenemia, probably as the result of platelet dysfunction
- The bleeding time decreases slightly with advancing age in both men and women

Drugs, disorders and other factors that may alter results

Recent aspirin use will increase bleeding time, leading to confusion with VWD.

CONSIDER CONSULT

All hemophiliacs should already be under the umbrella of specialist services, under regular review, and with open access. Review is needed urgently for:

- Acute bleeds
- Suspected intracranial bleeds
- Known hemophiliacs developing complications
- New onset of resistance to coagulation factors needing assessment for inhibitors
- New hemarthrosis or major bleed
- Psychosocial and family issues related to disease
- Any suspicion of self-harm or nonaccidental injury
- Pregnancy in hemophiliacs
- Acquisition of bloodborne disease

IMMEDIATE ACTION

- Urgent transfusion with factor concentrates and blood may be necessary
- Urgent orthopedic, surgical, or neurosurgical referral may be necessary for acute bleeds, dependent on site

PATIENT AND CAREGIVER ISSUES

Forensic and legal issues

- Where life-threatening hemorrhage occurs in a child and the parents conscientiously object, e.g. as Jehovah's Witnesses, emergency life-saving treatment can generally be given
- Permission of court to continue therapy may be necessary
- No adult person of sound mind may be given transfusion against their will

Impact on career, dependants, family, friends

- Severe hemophilia is a crippling disease that will have profound impact on family, the patient, and careers
- Mild hemophilia may seem to have little aspect but, conversely, it may be a huge shock to the patient and family if sudden surgical complications arise
- The impact of genetic disease on the family in terms of guilt and blame related to carrier status should not be underestimated
- Adolescents frequently rebel when restrictions on contact sports are placed upon them. Sometimes it is necessary for all to compromise so that life may be lived, but there can be long-term consequences of any injury

Patient or caregiver request

- Parents at first may believe this is a terminal condition based on historical knowledge, and need to be reassured that with adequate treatment it is possible for their child to lead a very normal life
- Most hemophiliacs and their families are able to manage their illness well, but it is important that even mild hemophiliacs are aware of the considerable risk posed by head injury and subsequent silent intracranial bleeding

Health-seeking behavior

Ask if the patient uses aspirin or other nonsteroidal anti-inflammatory drugs (NSAIDs). Advise not to do so.

MANAGEMENT ISSUES

Goals

- Prevention of spontaneous bleeding
- Prevention of excessive bleeding during any surgical intervention
- Prevention of acquired bloodborne diseases, particularly hepatitis and HIV
- Genetic counseling

Management in special circumstances

COEXISTING DISEASE

- Nearly 70% of hemophiliacs are currently HIV-seropositive
- This affects life expectancy but does not affect treatment of the hemophilia

COEXISTING MEDICATION

Avoid NSAIDs.

SPECIAL PATIENT GROUPS

Pregnancy:

- The vast majority of females are asymptomatic carriers, although an occasional carrier will bleed at times of surgery. They require no specific treatment during pregnancy or delivery
- Prenatal diagnosis previously required sampling fetal blood for coagulant activity. Newer prenatal detection schemes detect an identifiable restriction fragment length polymorphism or a gene deletion or rearrangement in a sample of chorionic villus or from fluid obtained at amniocentesis

Female hemophiliacs:

- Hemophilia has been well documented in human females. The most common form is that seen in a minority of heterozygous carriers, in whom X-chromosome inactivation may occur at an unusually early stage of embryogenesis, resulting in low levels of factor VIII
- A second cause is homozygous female hemophilia that was once thought to be lethal and to inhibit the development of the embryo
- Unusual degrees of X-chromosome inactivation (hyperlyonization) may produce severe factor VIII deficiency in some carriers of hemophilia A

PATIENT SATISFACTION/LIFESTYLE PRIORITIES

- Avoidance of contact sports is advisable
- Patient education regarding their disease: promotion of exercises such as swimming
- Avoidance of aspirin and other NSAIDs
- Hepatitis vaccination

SUMMARY OF THERAPEUTIC OPTIONS

Choices

There are three general forms of treatment for hemophilia, namely pharmacologic (antifibrinolytics and DDAVP), plasma-derived clotting factors, and recombinant clotting factors.

Hemophilia A and B treatments:

- Outpatient home infusion therapy
- Inpatient for infusions following significant bleeding episodes
- Factor VIII concentrate
- Factor IX concentrate
- Recombinant factor VIII and IX
- Recombinant factor VIIa
- Cryoprecipitate
- Desmopressin acetate (DDAVP) (mild hemophilia A only)
- Aminocaproic acid
- Tranexamic acid
- Danazol
- Cyclophosphamide with prednisone is a treatment for acquired hemophilia only
- Plasmapheresis
- Gene therapy
- Surgical or radionucleotide synovectomy may be necessary in selected patients
- Joint replacement, in selected patients
- The primary care practitioner (PCP) should be aware of the orthopedic treatment of hemophilia and refer appropriately

Important points for treatment:

- Avoid aspirin or aspirin-containing drugs
- Treat early. Symptoms often precede obvious bleeding
- An uncomplicated, soft-tissue bleed or an early hemarthrosis requires a single infusion to 20–30% activity
- More extensive hemarthrosis requires infusions twice daily for 72h or more to 25–50% activity
- Life-threatening bleeding into the central nervous system (CNS) requires maintaining levels greater than 50% activity for 2 weeks
- Major surgery requires greater than 50% activity preoperatively, continued for 1–2 weeks postoperatively
- Orthopedic care and physical therapy to prevent contractures and maintain joint mobility
- Vaccinate against hepatitis B at time of diagnosis
- Maintain good dental care
- Annual evaluation in a comprehensive hemophilia center
- Consideration for prophylaxis three times weekly in severe factor VIII deficiency
- Gene therapy is a development under investigation

Clinical pearls

If a patient with hemophilia who responds suboptimally to treatment (or a patient who is not known to have hemophilia, including females, usually older ones) suddenly develops symptoms and signs of bleeding diathesis, then suspect an inhibitor against coagulation factor(s) (usually factor VIII inhibitor).

Never

Never take aspirin or aspirin-containing drugs.

FOLLOW UP

Plan for review

- Regular evaluations every 6–12 months include a musculoskeletal evaluation, an inhibitor screen, liver tests, and tests for antibodies to hepatitis viruses and human immunodeficiency virus (HIV)
- More frequent reviews may be necessary depending on patient's age and clinical state

Information for patient or caregiver

- Avoid aspirin or aspirin-containing drugs
- Treat early. Symptoms often precede obvious bleeding
- Maintain good dental care
- Vaccinate against hepatitis B at time of diagnosis
- Teach patient and family about signs and symptoms to watch for
- Genetic counseling
- Home care with self-administered replacement therapy is often used
- Printed patient information available from: National Hemophilia Foundation, 110 Green Street, Room 406, New York, NY, 10012, Tel: (212) 219–8180

DRUGS AND OTHER THERAPIES: DETAILS

Drugs

FACTOR VIII

- Bleeding in severe hemophilia is treated by prompt adequate infusion of factor concentrate
- Mild hemophilia can usually be managed without factor concentrates
- 5–20% develop antibodies to factor VIIIc
- Recombinant or monoclonal factor VIII is treatment of choice for hemophilia A patients who are HIV-negative and who have had minimal prior concentrate exposure
- In patients with hemophilia A, the hemostatic level of factor VIIIc is approximately 25–30U/dL
- For patients with major trauma or those undergoing surgery, higher plasma levels of these coagulation proteins should be achieved (i.e. 100% for factors VIII or IX)

Dose

- Usually raising the level to 30% is sufficient to control hemorrhage
- Major surgery or life-threatening bleeds require correction to 100% and then maintenance at 30–50% for two subsequent weeks to avoid secondary hemorrhage
- Initial loading dose of factor VIII should always be administered
- Sufficient factor VIII must be given often enough to ensure that the blood level does not fall below 30U/dL for any length of time
- Maintenance doses usually are given every 8–12h
- Regimens of continuous infusion of factor VIII are being used with increasing frequency
- The administration of 2U/kg/h of factor VIII produces a mean factor VIIIc level in the plasma of approximately 50U/dL and appears to be more cost-effective than twice-daily intravenous bolus treatments in patients with mild hemophilia A
- Most authors recommend treatment for 10–14 days after major surgical procedures
- Therapeutic doses may be administered by a syringe
- The response to therapy can be monitored by clinical improvement, a decreasing partial thromboplastin time (PTT), and optimally, serial factor VIIIc activity levels
- The lack of a response to factor VIII administration should raise the question of circulating antibodies
- Peak factor levels should be monitored to document attainment of the expected response; dosage adjustment can then be made, if needed

Efficacy

- One unit of factor VIII (the amount in 1mL of plasma) per kg of body weight will raise the plasma level of the recipient by 2%
- Preparations of factor VIII are capable of correcting all coagulation abnormalities in the blood of hemophiliacs; they are equally effective in vitro and in vivo, and their administration can prevent and arrest hemorrhage in patients with hemophilia A
- Factor VIII of animal origin has been purified as much as 1000-fold from porcine plasma
- Such preparations are of proven clinical effectiveness, and are particularly valuable in the treatment of hemophiliacs with high-titer factor VIII inhibitors
- This product is antigenic, a drawback that limits its use to a single therapeutic course

Risks/Benefits

Risks:

- Persistent hepatitis B surface antigen occurs in the blood of 5% of hemophiliacs, whereas the anti-B surface antigen is found in 80%
- This problem has been overshadowed by the association of acquired immunodeficiency syndrome (AIDS) with hemophilia. The association is related to blood product use, and although the total number is low, the incidence is high: 3.6/1000 hemophilia A patients
- Activated prothrombin concentrate has a high risk of thrombosis; its use should be restricted to hematologists familiar with its administration

Side-effects and adverse reactions

- Central nervous system: mild chills
- Gastrointestinal: nausea
- Skin: stinging at infusion site

Interactions (other drugs)

No drug interactions known.

Contraindications

Hypersensitivity to the product.

Acceptability to patient
Very acceptable.

Follow up plan
As for underlying disease.

Patient and caregiver information
May self-infuse.

FACTOR IX

- Purified factor IX concentrates are recommended for the treatment of major or minor hemorrhage because of the thrombotic potential of prothrombin complex concentrates
- At least two purified factor IX products are available that are not thrombogenic
- Recombinant factor IX appears to be equivalent to plasma-derived, purified factor IX products and is now available for clinical use

Dose

- Because of the low initial in vivo recovery and the rapid initial disappearance of factor IX from the circulation, loading doses are recommended, even for the treatment of minor bleeding
- For patients with major trauma or those undergoing surgery, higher plasma levels of these coagulation proteins should be achieved (that is, 100%)
- One unit/kg will raise levels 1%, or use the following formula to calculate a replacement dose: [desired level (%) – actual level (%)] * kg BW
- Replacement products can be given on the basis of body weight or plasma volume

Efficacy

- One unit/kg will raise levels 1%
- Purified factor IX is now used. The plasma prothrombin complex (factors II, VII, IX, and X) still is useful, but it has a higher risk of viral transmission and venous or arterial thrombosis. The maintenance dosage schedule is increased to every 18–24h because of the longer half-life of factor IX

Risks/Benefits
Risk: hemophilia B – some factor IX concentrates contain trace amounts of activated vitamin K-dependent factors, therefore are thrombogenic and carry a risk for thromboembolism

Side-effects and adverse reactions

- Central nervous system: chills, headache, fever
- Gastrointestinal: nausea, vomiting
- Skin: stinging at injection site
- Allergic reactions

Interactions (other drugs)
No drug interactions known.

Contraindications
Hypersensitivity to product.

Acceptability to patient
Usually very acceptable.

Follow up plan
As appropriate to general condition.

RECOMBINANT FACTOR VIII AND IX

- In 1985 the genes for both factor VIII and factor IX were cloned
- This has resulted in the development of recombinant factor VIII and factor IX for treating patients with hemophilia and avoids the infection risk of plasma-derived transfusion-transmitted diseases
- There are factor VIII and factor IX concentrates prepared from human plasma using a monoclonal antibody method plus either heat or detergent treatment of the concentrate
- These monoclonal-prepared concentrates have the lowest risk for hepatitis B and essentially no risk for HIV infection
- Recombinant factor IX became available in mid-1997, and has no risk of viral infection
- Recombinant factor IX is the treatment of choice for hemophilia B patients who are HIV-negative and who have had minimal prior concentrate exposure
- More expensive than purified concentrates

Dose

- Recombinant factor VIII and IX is also now available for clinical use
- Dosages are calculated as for nonrecombinant factors

Efficacy

Highly effective.

Risks/Benefits

Risks:

- Although in vitro studies suggest that the nonhigh-purity factor VIII products have immunosuppressive properties, the clinical importance of these studies is uncertain
- The significant cost difference between products enters into this controversy
- A report that parvovirus B19 DNA is present in recombinant factor VIII products (a likely result of the addition of human albumin as a stabilizer) has also contributed to this discussion

Benefit: prevents transmission of bloodborne viruses

Side-effects and adverse reactions

- Central nervous system: anaphylactic shock, fever
- Gastrointestinal: nausea, retching, vomiting
- Respiratory: dyspnea
- Skin: urticarial rashes

Interactions (other drugs)

No known drug interactions.

Contraindications

None known.

Acceptability to patient

Highly acceptable.

Follow up plan

As appropriate to general condition.

RECOMBINANT FACTOR VIIA

- Recombinant factor VIIa is a promising agent for treating inhibitor patients, but it is not yet routinely available
- Recombinant factor VIIa is being studied primarily for treatment of bleeding episodes in patients with hemophilia with inhibitors

Dose

- This should be administered by a hematologist
- The typical dosage in the literature is 90–120mcg/kg body weight every 2–4h

Efficacy

Recombinant activated factor VIIa has been found helpful in these circumstances but it is also very expensive.

Risks/Benefits

Risk: monitor if signs or symptoms of activation of the coagulation system or thrombosis develop

Side-effects and adverse reactions

- Central nervous sytem: fever
- Cardiovascular system: hypertension, hemorrhage
- Musculoskeletal: hemarthrosis

Interactions (other drugs)

No known drug interactions.

Contraindications

Hypersensitivity to product.

Acceptability to patient

Experimental treatment, unknown.

Follow up plan

As appropriate to general condition.

CRYOPRECIPITATE

- Cryoprecipitate is the cold precipitable protein fraction derived from fresh frozen plasma (FFP) thawed at 1–6°C
- Cold insoluble material obtained from plasma contains high concentrations of factor VIII, fibrinogen, and factor XIII; it was once the mainstay of hemophilia A therapy
- It may be used when noninfectious factor VIII concentrates are not available
- Cryoprecipitate, which for many years was discarded during clarification of plasma, is prepared by slowly thawing rapidly frozen plasma at 2–4°C and then harvesting the precipitate by centrifugation

Dose

- Titrated against effect
- Cryoprecipitate prepared from 200mL of fresh plasma (1 unit) contains 50–120 units of factor VIII, approximately 250mg of fibrinogen, and therapeutically useful amounts of factor XIII and von Willebrand's factor (VWF) that is rich in the high-molecular-weight multimers
- Cryoprecipitation provides 7- to 20-fold purification of factor VIII with respect to plasma
- With the widespread availability of factor VIII concentrates to treat hemophilia A and von Willebrand's disease (VWD), cryoprecipitate is now used mainly to treat hypofibrinogenemia

Efficacy

- Although effective in minor bleeding, plasma or cryoprecipitate is not currently used in the treatment of patients with hemophilia A. Factor VIII concentrates are now widely available and are the most useful therapeutic materials
- However, it is important for clinicians to be aware of its use in life-threatening bleeds where factor concentrates are not available

Acceptability to patient

Not currently recommended except when factor concentrates are unavailable.

DESMOPRESSIN

- Infusions of desmopressin cause endogenous release of factor VIII and are therefore useful in hemophilia A
- Only useful in hemophilia A and type 1 VWD (first-line therapy in type 1 VWD)
- It allows minor surgery and dental extractions to be carried out without blood products
- Only small amounts of factor VIII are produced by DDAVP in severely affected hemophiliacs, and the use of this drug in patients with factor VIII levels below 5U/dL is not recommended, even for minor bleeding manifestations
- DDAVP also induces the release of endothelial cell-derived plasminogen activators and has produced exaggerated fibrinolytic phenomena in several cases. For this reason, it is often given with aminocaproic acid (EACA) or other fibrinolytic enzyme inhibitors

Dose

- It is given intravenously in a 0.3mcg/kg dose or as a nasal spray (150mcg/nostril = 300mcg total). Benefits are primarily noted in patients with mild disease and last for 4–6h
- Side-effects are more prominent if the total dose exceeds 24mcg
- Both parenteral and intranasal administration produce significant increases in factor VIIIc and VWF
- Repeated doses of DDAVP at approximately daily intervals may produce useful increments of factor VIII in many patients
- At least 24h should elapse before repeat administration of the drug (as VWF stores are exhausted and rebuilt)
- Patients should be tested for their response to DDAVP by documenting factor VIII levels 30–60min after treatment, before surgery. This ensures that the drug will be effective in appropriate responders

Efficacy

- With mild factor VIII hemophilia A, the patient's endogenously produced factor VIII can be released by the administration of DDAVP
- In moderate or severe factor VIII-deficient patients, the stored levels of factor VIII in the body are inadequate, and the DDAVP is ineffective
- Repeated doses of DDAVP at approximately daily intervals may produce useful rises in factor VIII levels
- Most centers administer a trial of DDAVP to determine the level of factor VIII achieved following its infusion
- DDAVP is not effective in the treatment of factor IX-deficient hemophilia B

Risks/Benefits

Risks:

- Use caution in cystic fibrosis, children, and the elderly
- DDAVP is a pressor agent and an antidiuretic. Neither effect has proved to be a problem in its therapeutic use, but clinicians should use caution when treating patients with hypertension or congestive heart failure. Repeated doses of DDAVP may produce progressively diminishing amounts of VWF (tachyphylaxis), presumably because of exhaustion of stored VWF and its precursors

Benefits:

- It is particularly useful because the biohazards of blood products are avoided
- May assist in achieving bladder control overnight

Side-effects and adverse reactions

- Cardiovascular system: hypertension
- Central nervous system: headache, flushing, drowsiness
- Eyes, ears, nose, and throat: rhinitis, epistaxis
- Gastrointestinal: abdominal pain, nausea, heartburn

Interactions (other drugs)

■ Carbamazepine ■ Chlorpropamide ■ Cisplatin ■ Clofibrate ■ Cyclophosphamide ■ Demeclocycline ■ Epinephrine ■ Ethanol ■ Fludrocortisone ■ Heparin ■ Indomethacin ■ Lithium ■ Vincristine

Contraindications

■ Cardiac insufficiency and other conditions treated with diuretics ■ Desmopressin should not be prescribed to patients over the age of 65 for primary nocturnal enuresis ■ Type IIB von Willebrand's disease

Acceptability to patient

Usually very acceptable.

Follow up plan

As for underlying disease. Patients should be tested for their response to DDAVP by documenting factor VIII levels 30–60min after treatment, before surgery. This ensures that the drug will be effective in appropriate responders.

AMINOCAPROIC ACID

- Useful in hemophilia A and in VWD only
- Aminocaproic acid (epsilon-aminocaproic acid, EACA) can be used for minor dental work following a single factor VIII infusion
- Aminocaproic acid greatly enhances the risk of thromboembolism and should be used with caution with factor IX concentrates
- Inhibitors of fibrinolysis such as EACA or tranexamic acid may diminish bleeding in patients with inherited coagulation disorders, particularly that which arises in the mouth, tongue, frenulum, tonsils, and pharynx and that associated with operative dental procedures
- Acts to protect labile hemostatic plugs from fibrinolytic degradation
- This is an off-label indication

Dose

- EACA has been administered together with DDAVP in an attempt to minimize fibrinolysis
- For maximal effectiveness, antifibrinolytic drugs should be given before oral surgical procedures
- EACA should be administered in oral doses (pills or syrup) of 6g every 6h to adults and 100mg/kg every 6h to children, for 3–4 days after tooth extraction. The drug can be given intravenously (1g/h) for patients who cannot swallow

Efficacy

- Antifibrinolytic therapy, such as the administration of EACA, may be helpful in patients with factor VIII inhibitors, especially in dental procedures
- This therapy should be used cautiously in muscle bleeds because it appears to be less effective
- This therapy should not be used in conjunction with the prothrombin complex concentrates or activated prothrombin complex concentrates
- Some clinicians have used EACA as an adjunct to single-dose or various other replacement regimens

- Hematuria or abnormal renal function is a contraindication to the use of this drug because of the hazard of intrarenal or ureteral obstruction by blood clots
- EACA also should not be given to patients with disseminated intravascular coagulation or active hepatitis or patients receiving prothrombin complex concentrates
- These drugs may be teratogenic and should be used with caution in pregnant women

Risks/Benefits

Risks:

- Use caution in renal, hepatic, and cardiac disease
- Use caution in thrombosis

Side-effects and adverse reactions

- Cardiovascular system: bradycardia, dysrhythmias, hypotension
- Central nervous system: dizziness, headache, seizures, cerebral ischemia, hallucinations
- Eyes, ears, nose, and throat: conjunctival suffusion, nasal congestion, tinnitus
- Gastrointestinal: diarrhea, nausea, abdominal cramps, vomiting
- Genitourinary: renal failure, dysuria, ejaculatory failure, frequency, menstrual irregularities, myoglobinuria, oliguria
- Hematologic: thrombosis
- Musculoskeletal: malaise, fatigue, myopathy, rhabdomyolysis
- Skin: rash

Interactions (other drugs)

No known drug interactions.

Contraindications

- Upper respiratory tract bleeding
- Disseminated intravscular coagulation

Acceptability to patient

Usually very acceptable and well tolerated.

Follow up plan

As for underlying condition.

TRANEXAMIC ACID

- Useful in hemophilia A and VWD only
- Antifibrinolytic useful to achieve hemostasis and reduce the required dose of factor VIII
- Tranexamic acid (cyclokapron) can be used for minor dental work following a single factor VIII infusion
- Tranexamic acid greatly enhances the risk of thromboembolism and should be used with caution with factor IX concentrates
- Inhibitors of fibrinolysis such as tranexamic acid may diminish bleeding in patients with inherited coagulation disorders, particularly that which arises in the mouth, tongue, frenulum, tonsils, and pharynx and that associated with operative dental procedures
- Acts to protect labile hemostatic plugs from fibrinolytic degradation

Dose

Adult oral dose: 1–1.5g four times daily.

Efficacy

Antifibrinolytic therapy, such as the administration of tranexamic acid, may be helpful in patients with factor VIII inhibitors, especially in dental procedures.

Risks/Benefits

Risks:

- Use caution in pregnancy
- Use caution in renal impairment and thromboembolic disease (however, long-term studies in Sweden have not confirmed an increased rate of thrombosis compared with women not on treatment)

Benefits:

- Antifibrinolytic used as an adjunct to factor VIII transfusions for hemostasis
- Useful as prophylaxis to bleeding in minor surgical procedures for hemophilia A patients

Side-effects and adverse reactions

- Cardiovascular system: thromboembolism (rare)
- Central nervous system: headache
- Eyes, ears, nose, and throat: disturbances in color vision (discontinue)
- Gastrointestinal: nausea, vomiting, diarrhea

Interactions (other drugs)

None recorded.

Contraindications

- Acquired defective color vision
- Subarachnoid hemorrhage
- Active intravascular clotting

Acceptability to patient

Usually very acceptable and well tolerated.

Follow up plan

As for underlying condition.

DANAZOL

- An early study using the anabolic steroid, danazol, suggests its administration can increase plasma factor VIIIc concentrations
- However, subsequent trials with danazol do not demonstrate similar results
- Currently, danazol is not considered routine therapy for hemophilia

Dose

Not recommended in this disorder.

Efficacy

Not of proven benefit.

Risks/Benefits

Risks:

- Use caution in cardiac, renal, and hepatic disease
- Use caution in epilepsy and migraine
- Use caution in diabetes mellitus

Side-effects and adverse reactions
- Central nervous system: dizziness, nervousness, mood changes, anxiety, headache
- Gastrointestinal: nausea, vomiting, weight gain, hepatitis, cholestatic jaundice
- Genitourinary: menstrual disturbances, vaginal dryness and irritation, change in breast size
- Hematologic: thrombocytopenia, leukopenia, thrombotic events
- Metabolic: insulin resistance, lipoprotein alteration
- Musculoskeletal: joint pain, swelling
- Skin: acne, oily skin, hirsutism

Interactions (other drugs)
■ **Carbamazepine** ■ **Cyclosporine, tacrolimus** ■ **Statins** ■ **Oral anticoagulants**

Contraindications
■ **Porphyria** ■ **Pregnancy** ■ **Severe renal, cardiac, or hepatic disease** ■ **Undiagnosed abnormal genital bleeding**

Acceptability to patient
Currently, danazol is not considered routine therapy for hemophilia.

STEROIDS AND CYTOTOXIC THERAPY
- In patients with low-titer inhibitors who do not have any clinical bleeding and for whom no surgical procedures are foreseen, the most reasonable approach may be to monitor the abnormal laboratory finding. Resorting to early immunosuppressive therapy has led to variable results
- Steroids and cytotoxic therapy are usually ineffective when inhibitors arise in patients with congenital hemophilia A
- Standard immunosuppression should probably be reserved for patients with autoantibodies because this therapy is rarely beneficial in the alloimmune setting

Dose
- Prednisone in doses of 1–1.5mg/kg/day
- Cyclophosphamide 2–3mg/kg/day
- These may be administered alone or together

Efficacy
- Not usually effective or recommended in hemophilia A
- Sometimes effective in acquired hemophilia

Risks/Benefits
Risk: the risks of bone marrow supression and hepatotoxicity must be weighed against the limited evidence for real therapeutic benefit in established renal involvement in Henoch-Schoenlein purpura

Side-effects and adverse reactions
- Cardiovascular system: cardiotoxicity (at high doses)
- Central nervous system: dizziness, headache
- Gastrointestinal: nausea, vomiting, diarrhea
- Genitourinary: amenorrhea, azoospermia, ovarian fibrosis, sterility, hematuria, hemorrhagic cystitis, neoplasms
- Hematologic: leukopenia, myelosuppression, pancytopenia, thrombocytopenia
- Metabolic: bone marrow supression
- Respiratory: fibrosis
- Skin: alopecia, dermatitis

Interactions (other drugs)
■ Allopurinol (increased cyclophosphamide toxicity) ■ Clozapine (may cause agranulocytosis) ■ Digoxin (decreased digoxin absorption from tablet form) ■ Pentostatin (increased toxicity with high-dose cyclophosphamide) ■ Phenytoin (reduced absorption of phenytoin) ■ Warfarin (inhibits hypoprothrombinemic response to warfarin) ■ Succinylcholine (prolonged neuromuscular blockade) ■ Suxamethonium (enhanced effect of suxamethonium)

Contraindications
■ Serious infections, including chickenpox and herpes zoster ■ Myelosuppression

Acceptability to patient
Not recommended.

Other therapies

PLASMAPHERESIS
Plasma exchange may be useful in patients with high levels of factor VIII inhibitors.

Efficacy
Patients with inhibitors to factor VIII may require intensive plasmapheresis, large doses of concentrate, infusion of prothrombin complex concentrates (bypassing products), or porcine factor VIII.

GENE THERAPY
Gene therapy for the inherited bleeding disorders is under active investigation. Viral and nonviral constructs containing genes for factor VIII or factor IX have been used, as well as modified retrovirus or adenovirus vectors.

Efficacy
Experimental.

Risks/Benefits
Not known.

LIFESTYLE

- Avoidance of contact sports
- Encouragement of low-impact exercise such as swimming
- Attempt to lead as normal a life as possible
- Restrict activities in proportion to the degree of factor deficiency, but maintaining a trim physical condition is important
- The prevention of trauma is important to the care of the child with hemophilia, but bleeds may occur in the absence of trauma
- Early psychosocial intervention helps the family achieve a balance between overprotection and permissiveness
- Aspirin and other nonsteroidal anti-inflammatory drugs that affect platelet function should be avoided by patients with hemophilia
- Although recombinant products may avoid exposure to transfusion-transmitted diseases, immunization against hepatitis B virus in the neonatal period in case plasma-derived products are used with future bleeds
- Patients should be periodically screened for hepatitis and abnormalities in liver function

RISKS/BENEFITS
Risk: particularly for adolescents, there are psychological problems associated with the restriction in activities

PATIENT AND CAREGIVER INFORMATION

- There is increased risk of psychological problems – affects children and adolescents with chronic conditions
- Children's intelligence and temperament appear to contribute to their ability to adapt to the extra stresses of the illness
- Parents' self-esteem, mental health, social support network, and beliefs about health care all have an impact on the success of children's adaptation as does the cohesiveness, flexibility, and effectiveness of shared communication within the family
- It may be appropriate for some children and adolescents to be referred for mental health services
- The prevention of psychosocial complications of childhood chronic illness is met best by a family- and community-centered approach
- The involvement of school, friends, the extended family, and the pediatrician is all important in this. No family should become an island due to their child's ill health

EFFICACY OF THERAPIES

- The principal treatment is intravenous administration of the required factor in the form of blood products derived from normal people or animals or recombinant coagulation proteins
- Some authors advocate prophylactic factor therapy in patients with severe disease
- Desmopressin acetate (DDAVP) and epsilon-aminocaproic acid (EACA) have a role in mild hemophilia A
- Cryoprecipitate may be used in an emergency
- Danazol has been suggested but is of no proven benefit
- Plasmapheresis may be helpful in acquired hemophilia where there are high circulating antibody levels
- Gene therapy is currently under investigation

Hemophilia A treatment of minor bleeding:

- DDAVP is effective in the treatment of minor bleeding manifestations in hemophiliacs with baseline factor VIIIc levels greater than 5U/dL
- EACA (6g orally every 6h) or tranexamic acid (25mg/kg orally every 6–8h) has been administered together with DDAVP in an attempt to minimize fibrinolysis. For maximal effectiveness, antifibrinolytic drugs should be given before oral surgical procedures
- Although effective in minor bleeding, cryoprecipitate is not currently used in the treatment of patients with hemophilia A. Factor VIII concentrates are now widely available and are the most useful therapeutic materials

Hemophilia A treatment of major bleeding:

- Treatment must always be with factor VIII
- Recombinant factor VIII and IX offer the advantage of no risk of viral transmission. Although HIV and hepatitis screening is now carried out on purified factor products there is evidence that parvovirus transmission may occur

Hemophilia B treatment of major or minor bleeding:

- In patients with hemophilia B, purified factor IX concentrates are recommended for the treatment of major or minor hemorrhage because of the thrombotic potential of prothrombin complex concentrates
- In the treatment of major bleeding, the in vivo levels of the deficient factor should be maintained above the hemostatic level
- In bleeding of a critical nature, such as intracranial hemorrhage, or for the prevention of excessive bleeding during neurosurgery, factor levels should be maintained at 100% of normal
- Small cuts and scratches, removal of stitches or drains, superficial ecchymoses, and small hematomas may require no replacement therapy

Long-term management approach:

- Involves care of the child and family
- Planning for emergency situations is essential
- Psychological support is often necessary
- Complications should be managed as they arise
- Severe joint destruction may be managed orthopedically

Approach:

- The therapy of hemophilia involves a team effort of physicians, specialized nurses, physical therapists, social workers, the patient, and the patient's family
- The therapeutic responsibility of the emergency physician consists of: preparation for and identification of the problem, initial evaluation, and admission of new bleeders; replacement therapy for bleeding episodes; and the anticipation of potential life threats and the admission of known bleeders for observation in selected circumstances

- At one time the treatment of hemophilia-associated bleeding was a relatively common emergency medicine activity
- Since 1975, hemophilia home therapy has increasingly been instituted
- A co-operative effort should be made between the emergency department and the hematology service to generate a file of known hemophiliacs in the area who are followed at the hospital
- The file should include the primary physician, diagnosis, factor VIII activity level, blood type, presence of antihemophilia factor antibodies, and time of last hospitalization. A protocol should be developed for ordering and administering factor VIII

Home treatment programs:

- In general, replacement therapy of hemarthrosis is more effective, and subsequent joint damage is minimized if treatment is begun immediately after the onset of symptoms
- The availability of factor VIII concentrates that are stable in home refrigerators led to the development of various early home care programs
- Parents and patients are trained to administer the material at the first sign of bleeding
- Such programs have resulted in improved preservation of joint function
- Although the amount of factor VIII used may increase during the initial phase of home treatment, subsequent requirements are approximately the same as with traditional hospital-based care; the total cost, when ancillary hospital charges are included, is less
- Absenteeism from school and work is significantly diminished
- The patient is able to develop a more active and mobile lifestyle
- Some claim that the self-reliance engendered by home care may improve family interactions and minimize some of the serious psychosocial consequences of hemophilia
- Effective home care requires a high level of intelligence, motivation, and co-operation on the part of the patient and his or her family, and time-consuming special efforts by the physician and other health care providers
- Problems with home care are uncommon, and this practice is now firmly incorporated into the programs of most hemophilia treatment centers
- Because of the delayed bleeding pattern in hemophiliacs, it may be especially hazardous to transfer them over long distances. Therefore the importance of advance knowledge and preparation is re-emphasized
- Outpatients are usually managed under the auspices of the hematologic consultant. Early notification and appropriate follow up arrangements should be made with these specialists
- Epistaxis often stops spontaneously, and usually only conservative treatment is required. Intranasal tamponade has proved helpful in managing this complication
- Hematuria may be virtually intractable, and some patients do not respond even to vigorous replacement therapy
- Narcotics should be used for pain relief only when absolutely necessary because of the possibility of addiction

Treatment of complications:
(Antibodies to coagulation factors)

- Many hemophiliacs develop antibodies (inhibitors) to factor VIII
- The 7–20% of patients who develop inhibitors usually have a severe deficiency, necessitating multiple factor VIII transfusions. The treatment may be complex, and hospitalization is necessary
- This complication is less common in patients with hemophilia B and other inherited coagulation disorders
- Many patients who develop an inhibitor lose this inhibitor with continued regular infusions
- Others develop a higher titer with subsequent infusions and may need to go through desensitization programs
- If desensitization fails, these patients are treated with either activated prothrombin complex concentrates or factor VIIa

(Hemarthroses)

- All patients with hemarthroses should receive adequate replacement therapy, so permanent disability resulting from repeated bleeding into the joints is minimized
- Daily or alternate-day prophylactic therapy with factor concentrates may prevent or significantly delay progression of hemophilic arthropathy

(Intracranial bleeding)

Patients should immediately receive sufficient concentrate to raise the plasma level of deficient factor to 100U/dL.

(Hematomas, psoas and retroperitoneal hematomas)

- Urgent factor replacement to 100% is required as for major bleeds above
- Release operations and fasciotomy may be necessary

(Thrombocytopenia)

- Mild to moderate thrombocytopenia is common in hemophiliacs who receive large amounts of factor VIII concentrates
- Because of the desire to avoid steroid therapy or splenectomy in this immunocompromised population, immune thrombocytopenia in these patients has been treated with intravenous immunoglobulin G (IgG) or anti-Rh(D)

Review period

Regular evaluations every 6–12 months include a musculoskeletal evaluation, an inhibitor screen, liver tests, and tests for antibodies to hepatitis viruses and human immunodeficiency virus (HIV).

PROGNOSIS

- Survival is of normal life expectancy in HIV-negative patients with mild disease
- Repeated hemarthroses result in eventual deformity and crippling
- Survival is normal for those with mild disease, and mortality is increased 2- to 6-fold in those with moderate to severe disease, primarily due to complications of infection
- Median life expectancy with this condition peaked in late 1970s at 68 years, and is now declining due to the AIDS epidemic
- Up to 70% are HIV-seropositive, especially those with severe disease, and 4% with severe disease develop AIDS. Younger patients whose treatment began since the mid-late 1980s are largely HIV-negative and are not expected to be exposed by modern replacement products. The proportion of HIV-positive hemophiliacs is therefore declining
- A recent retrospective analysis of hemophilia mortality between 1900 and 1990 indicates that although survival in this population improved after widespread use of factor concentrates between 1971 and 1980 (median life expectancy of 68 years), median life expectancy in the next decade (1981–90) declined to 49 years. This increase in relative mortality in hemophilia patients was attributed primarily to AIDS. It is likely that in the absence of viral infection, the life expectancy of patients with hemophilia would be similar to that of the general male population
- A major cause of death in all hemophiliacs of all severities is intracranial hemorrhage

Clinical pearls

Prognosis of nonhemophilic patients with inhibitors is worse than hemophilic patients with inhibitors (the death rate may approach 20%).

COMPLICATIONS

Antibodies to coagulation factors:

- The 7–20% of patients who develop inhibitors usually have a severe deficiency, necessitating multiple factor VIII transfusions. The treatment may be complex, and hospitalization is necessary

- This complication is less common in patients with hemophilia B and other inherited coagulation disorders
- Such antibodies may seriously complicate the treatment of these patients
- This condition may have serious consequences, and fatal events are seen in 10–20% of clinically symptomatic patients
- Antibodies to factor VIII arising during pregnancy may cross the placenta
- Infusion of the deficient clotting factor may initiate an immune response in patients with either factor VIII or factor IX deficiency
- The antibody to factor VIII or factor IX is usually an antibody that blocks the clotting activity and is therefore defined as an inhibitor
- Inhibitors are suspected clinically when patients who have responded well to replacement therapy suddenly become less responsive or are identified during routine follow up testing
- Many patients who develop an inhibitor lose this inhibitor with continued regular infusions
- Others develop a higher titer with subsequent infusions and may need to go through desensitization programs, in which high doses of factor VIII or factor IX are infused in an attempt to saturate the antibody and to permit the body to develop tolerance
- If desensitization fails, these patients are treated with either activated prothrombin complex concentrates or factor VIIa
- The use of these products bypasses the inhibitor in many instances but increases the risk for thrombosis
- Inhibitor patients require referral to a hospital that cares for many such patients and has a comprehensive hemophilia program

Hemarthroses:

- Hemarthrosis is common, painful, and debilitating
- Bleeding originates from the synovial vessels and develops spontaneously or as the result of imperceptible or trivial trauma
- Some hemophiliacs report a characteristic warm, tingling sensation before the onset of hemarthrosis; this is called the aura
- The earliest definite symptom is pain, which may be excruciating. Physical examination reveals muscle spasm and limited motion. The joint may be warm, distended, and discolored, but external evidence of bleeding may be minimal or absent in chronically damaged joints because of thickening of the articular capsule
- The knee is most commonly affected and is the joint most often permanently crippled. Other joints that may be involved are the ankles, elbows, hips, wrists, shoulders, and small joints of the hands and feet, the vertebral articulations, and the temporomandibular joints
- Hemorrhage occurs into the joint cavity or into the diaphysis or epiphysis of the bone. In the acute stage, the synovial space is distended with blood
- The joint may regain normal function after the first episodes of hemarthrosis. More often, however, the joint remains swollen, tender, and painful for months or years, often in the absence of bleeding
- Acute hemarthroses almost invariably recur
- The terminal stage of hemarthrosis is called chronic hemophilic arthropathy. It is less common now because of widespread use of prophylactic replacement therapy
- All patients with hemarthroses should receive adequate replacement therapy, so permanent disability resulting from repeated bleeding into the joints is minimized
- Pain is usually relieved promptly and is a reliable index of the therapeutic response
- Supportive therapy includes immobilization and the administration of analgesics. The value of packing the joint in ice is uncertain
- Early but careful physiotherapy aimed at restoring the full range of motion of the joint should be instituted as soon as the acute stage of hemarthrosis has resolved. More energetic physiotherapeutic techniques should be carried out only in conjunction with an adequate course of replacement therapy

- Orthopedic devices have proved useful in reducing the frequency of recurrent hemarthrosis, particularly in the knee and ankles
- Chronic degenerative joint disease in hemophiliacs is difficult to treat effectively. Nonsteroidal anti-inflammatory agents may be helpful. In particular, salsalate or choline magnesium trisalicylate may be useful in patients with bleeding disorders because these drugs have anti-inflammatory activity, but do not impair platelet function
- Daily or alternate-day prophylactic therapy with factor concentrates may prevent or significantly delay progression of hemophilic arthropathy
- Many reconstructive surgical procedures greatly improve the function of chronically damaged joints
- Synovectomy is effective in reducing the frequency of hemarthrosis that cannot be controlled by replacement therapy

Hemophilic cysts:
- Serious complication in patients with severe hemophilia A or B
- Gradually expanding blood-filled loculations that apparently originate from hemorrhages into confined subperiosteal, tendinous, or fascial spaces
- Further influx of fluid, together with recurrent bleeding, explaining the progressive increase in the size of the cyst and its ability to erode contiguous structures
- Cysts most commonly develop in the thigh, and may destroy bone as well as the soft tissues as they increase in size
- These lesions are more readily prevented than treated. Hemophilic pseudocysts may require radical surgical procedures, such as extensive resections or amputations
- The modern use of home prophylaxis has made pseudotumors an unusual complication of hemophilia at this time

Intracranial bleeding:
- Intracranial hemorrhage is a common cause of death in hemophiliacs. Approximately 50% of cases are associated with head injury
- Etiology is not apparent in 38% of cases (spontaneous cases)
- Bleeding may be subdural, epidural, or intracerebral
- Subarachnoid bleeding occurs least commonly, but it carries the best prognosis
- Hemorrhage also may develop in the spinal cord or spinal meninges
- Significant head injury must be treated early and intensively
- Patients should immediately receive sufficient concentrate to raise the plasma level of deficient factor to 100U/dL
- Samples for essential coagulation studies should be drawn before administration of replacement therapy, but treatment should not be delayed while waiting for results of these studies
- Radiologic procedures, such as computed tomography (CT) scanning, can be done while the therapeutic material is administered
- In cases involving major cranial trauma the administration of factor VIII or factor IX concentrates should continue on a schedule in doses sufficient to keep the nadir levels of the deficient factor above 30U/dL. Treatment should be maintained for 10–14 days
- Because of these risks, patients with hemophilia should always have ready access to factor concentrates, even those with mild disease

Hematomas:
- Large ecchymoses and subcutaneous and intramuscular hematomas are common and characteristically spread within fascial spaces and dissect deeper structures
- Subcutaneous bleeding may extend over as much as one-half of the body
- At the site of origin, the tissue is hard, indurated, raised, and purplish black. From this center, the hemorrhage extends in all directions, with each successive concentric extension less deeply colored

- The point of origin of the hemorrhage may be absorbed entirely while the margin is still progressing
- Intramuscular and subcutaneous hematomas may produce leukocytosis, fever, and severe pain in the absence of significant discoloration of the overlying skin
- Hematomas may produce serious consequences from the compression of vital structures. Bleeding into the tongue, throat, or neck may develop spontaneously and is especially dangerous because it may compromise the airway
- Gangrene may result from pressure on arteries, and ischemic contractures are common sequelae of hemorrhage into the calves or forearms, as in Volkmann's contracture
- Peripheral nerve lesions of varying severity are common complications of hemorrhage into joints or muscles, as in femoral nerve compression caused by hematomas of the iliacus

Psoas and retroperitoneal hematomas:

- Bleeding into or around the iliopsoas muscle produces pain of progressively increasing severity and tenderness; when it occurs on the right side, it may closely simulate acute appendicitis
- Femoral nerve involvement may be partial or complete, with the development of pain on the anterior surface of the thigh. The psoas sign is positive, and the hip is held in partial flexion
- Paresthesias, partial or complete anesthesia, and ultimately weakness or paralysis of the thigh extensors with eventual muscular atrophy may ensue
- Retroperitoneal hemorrhage and intraperitoneal hemorrhage also are common
- A deep hematoma may be mistaken for a suppurative condition and surgical drainage may be attempted
- Intra-abdominal bleeding raises serious diagnostic and therapeutic problems. Intraperitoneal hemorrhage and bleeding into and around other viscera may simulate perforating peptic ulcer, bowel obstruction, or virtually any acute intra-abdominal condition. CT scanning and sonography may be particularly helpful in differentiating between intra-abdominal conditions that require surgical intervention and retroperitoneal and psoas hemorrhages

Gastrointestinal and genitourinary bleeding:

- Hemorrhage from the mouth, gums, lips, frenulum, and tongue is common and often serious
- The eruption and shedding of deciduous teeth usually occurs without abnormal bleeding, but it may be accompanied by hemorrhage that lasts for days or weeks
- Epistaxis occurs in many patients and may be of exsanguinating proportions
- Hematemesis, melena, or both are not uncommon. The source of the blood is usually the upper gastrointestinal tract. In most patients it originates from a structural lesion, most commonly a peptic ulcer or gastritis
- Hemorrhage may be accompanied by abdominal pain, distention, increased peristalsis, fever, and leukocytosis
- Intramural bleeding into the intestinal wall may result in intussusception or obstruction
- Hematuria, although more common than gastrointestinal bleeding, is less often the result of a demonstrable pathologic condition in the genitourinary tract. The bleeding may persist for days or weeks. When clots form, ureteral colic may develop

Traumatic bleeding:

- After larger injuries, hemorrhage out of proportion to the extent of the injury is characteristic and may persist as a slow continuous oozing for days, weeks, or months, or it may be massive and life-threatening
- Delayed bleeding is common. This phenomenon apparently occurs because the processes of primary hemostasis are temporarily effective. Delayed bleeding is a significant hazard after minor surgical procedures, particularly those performed on an outpatient basis, such as tooth extractions and tonsillectomy
- Subcutaneous, intracutaneous, and small intramuscular injections seldom produce hematomas if firm finger pressure is maintained for at least 5min. Large intramuscular injections should be avoided

Psychosocial complications:
- Serious psychological and sociological problems often arise in families affected with the inherited coagulation disorders
- Increased risk-taking may occur as a neurotic response to the disease
- At times of emotional stress, spontaneous bleeding has been observed
- Parental guilt feelings are common, and the emotional interaction between carrier mothers and affected males often is abnormal
- Suicide and suicidal gestures are not uncommon, and drug addiction often is a serious problem. Management of these problems is an important part of the overall care of the hemophilic patient

Acquired immune deficiency syndrome:
- AIDS was first recognized in 1978, and HIV was found to be transmitted in blood products soon thereafter. A high degree of viral contamination was found in concentrated preparations of factor VIII and IX. Such therapeutic materials are prepared by pooling the plasma of multiple donors. This practice produced rapid and widespread dissemination of HIV in the hemophilic population
- Serologic evidence of HIV is most common in severe hemophiliacs, as distinguished from mildly affected patients
- In the 1980s, more than 90% of patients requiring extensive replacement therapy developed positive results of screening tests for HIV antibody and ultimately full-blown AIDS
- Many of these patients have died of the disease
- The advent of sterile concentrates, together with rigid donor testing instituted in 1985, as well as the availability of recombinant products, have greatly diminished the risk of blood product administration
- Many seropositive patients remain who do not yet have the diagnosis of AIDS, but who constitute a pool of patients at high risk
- Cases of AIDS in association with hemophilia B are less common, probably because of the rarity of the disorder

Thrombocytopenia:
- Mild to moderate thrombocytopenia is common in hemophiliacs who receive large amounts of factor VIII concentrates
- Most of these patients have positive tests for HIV, and their clinical findings are consistent with AIDS-related complex. The clinical features resemble the idiopathic thrombocytopenic purpura (ITP) syndrome
- Because of the desire to avoid steroid therapy or splenectomy in this immunocompromised population, immune thrombocytopenia in these patients has been treated with intravenous IgG or anti-Rh(D)

Hepatitis:
- 75% of hemophiliacs have abnormalities of liver function that may persist for years, even though clinical evidence of hepatic dysfunction is minimal
- Liver biopsies have confirmed the presence of chronic active hepatitis mostly due to persistent infection with hepatitis viruses, most being non-A, non-B (hepatitis C)
- Postnecrotic cirrhosis may occur in some cases
- Serologic tests for hepatitis B are positive in as many as 90% of older patients
- There is evidence that other viruses may be responsible in some patients
- Modern sterilization methods appear to render factor concentrates virus-free, especially the lipid-enveloped viruses
- Patients who are seronegative for the hepatitis B virus should receive immunization for this virus. Standard solvent-detergent inactivated products may still transmit nonlipid-enveloped viruses such as parvovirus and hepatitis A

- The availability of a hepatitis A vaccine should lead to decreased transmission of this latter virus. An unresolved issue is the transmission potential of the agent causing Creutzfeldt-Jakob disease
- Concern about transmission of human viruses has led many clinicians and patients to use recombinant factor products exclusively
- Parvovirus and hepatitis A are nonenveloped viruses that may escape solvent-detergent treatment and heat treatment. Thus, plasma-derived products may continue to transmit these infectious agents. The potential for Creutzfeldt-Jakob disease to be transmitted through blood remains controversial but unsubstantiated

Other complications of bleeding:

- Pulmonary and pleural bleeding are uncommon, but mediastinal and pleural shadows have been noted radiographically and presumably originate from fresh or old hematomas
- Intraocular hemorrhage is uncommon, but bleeding into the orbit and conjunctiva occurs often
- Spontaneous rupture of the spleen has been reported
- Wound healing is often slow, probably because of continued or intermittent hemorrhage or complicating infection
- Bleeding into a small joint may produce a clinical and radiologic picture suggestive of sarcoma; when larger joints are involved, findings simulate tuberculosis, arthritis, or Perthes disease
- Bleeding elsewhere may suggest local causes such as kidney tumor, pulmonary disease, or peptic ulcer

CONSIDER CONSULT

All hemophilia patients should receive regular follow up from a hematologist or a hemophilia clinic.

- Significant bleeding episodes require inpatient treatment
- Orthopedic referral may be indicated for patients with severe joint deformity and crippling – joint replacement may be considered
- Referral of all patients who develop factor VIII antibodies, even if hemophilia is mild, is essential

PREVENTION

The only prevention possible of the disease is through genetic counseling, offering prenatal testing for carrier females who may choose to terminate affected male pregnancies – carrier females have a 50% chance that a male fetus will be affected and a 50% chance that a female fetus will be a carrier.

Prevention of major complications involves:

- Drug therapy
- Physical therapy
- Immunization
- Lifestyle adjustment
- Prophylaxis for surgical and dental procedures
- Family and caregiver education
- Attention to general health
- Availability of emergency treatment

Prophylactic therapy against bleeding:

- Prophylactic therapy may have a role for the occasional patient with severe, frequently recurring spontaneous bleeding manifestations that appear to be otherwise unmanageable
- The administration of 1500–3000U of factor VIII three to four times a week significantly reduces the incidence of hemarthrosis
- Trials with smaller or less frequent administration of factor VIII have yielded less dramatic results
- The expense of these regimens probably is not a valid argument against their use
- Additionally, these regimens may reduce the necessity for synovectomy or joint replacement
- Consideration is being given to instituting primary prophylaxis at an early age (1–2 years) to prevent recurrent joint bleeding with subsequent development of chronic joint disease
- The goal of such therapy is to maintain the trough factor VIII or IX level above 1%, which usually can be accomplished by giving 25–40U/kg factor VIII three times per week, or 25–40U/kg factor IX twice weekly

Dental care:

- Special attention should be given to preventive dental care to minimize the complications, expense, and hazards of operative dental procedures
- The extraction of even a single tooth requires replacement therapy
- Multiple extractions create a major bleeding hazard
- Acrylic splints, orthodontic rubber bands, and other specialized dental techniques reduce the chance of serious postoperative bleeding
- The suturing of bleeding tooth sockets after extractions, particularly of the third molar, should be avoided because it may lead to extension of bleeding into the neck
- Most authorities recommend that dental procedures in patients with inherited coagulation disorders be carried out under cover of replacement therapy and EACA
- Probably the safest practice is to regard tooth extractions, particularly of molar or multiple contiguous teeth, as a major bleeding hazard, although only 1–3 days of replacement therapy + EACA are usually needed

SCREENING

- There is currently no screening program indicated for individuals in unaffected families
- Formal blood testing may be appropriate where there is a strong family history

BLOOD TESTING

However, in mild disease there may be no symptoms until early adulthood, so this would justify screening individuals from affected families so that their coagulant factor levels could be monitored before clinical problems occur

Cost/efficacy

Inexpensive as blood tests are simple and straightforward and few patients are involved.

PREVENT RECURRENCE

Prevent recurrence of symptomatic disease by monitoring factor VIII levels.

ASSOCIATIONS

National Hemophilia Foundation
110 Green Street, Room 406
New York, NY 10002
Tel: (212) 219-8180
www.hemophilia.org

KEY REFERENCES

- Psychosocial Risks of Chronic Health Conditions in Childhood And Adolescence Policy Statement. Psychosocial Risks of Chronic Health Conditions in Childhood And Adolescence (RE9338). American Academy of Pediatrics. Psychological risks of chronic conditions. Recommendations for pediatric care. Pediatrics 1993;92:6;876–8 Committee on Children With Disabilities and Committee on Psychosocial Aspects of Child and Family Health. Available online: http://www.aap.org/policy/05127.html
- Ashenhurst JB, Langehennig PL, Seeler RA. Early treatment of bleeding episodes with 10 U/kg of factor VIII. Blood 1977;50:181–2
- Levine PH. Efficacy of self-therapy in hemophilia: A study of 72 patients with hemophilia A and B. N Engl J Med 1974;291:1381–5
- Levine PH, Britten AFH. Supervised patient management of hemophilia. Ann Intern Med 1973;78:195
- Bona RD, Weinstein RA, Weisman SJ, et al. The use of continuous infusion of factor concentrates in the treatment of hemophilia. Am J Hematol 1989;32:8–13
- Rodgers GM, Ford MH. Lack of response to commercial factor VIII concentrate in hemophilia A. Am J Hematol 1991;37:288
- Kim HC, McMillan CW, White GC, et al. Purified factor IX using monoclonal immunoaffinity technique: clinical trials in hemophilia B and comparison to prothrombin complex concentrates. Blood 1992;79:568–75
- White GC, Beebe A, Nielsen B. Recombinant factor IX. Thromb Haemost 1997;78:261–5
- Helske T, Ikkala E, Myllyla G, et al. Joint involvement in patients with severe haemophilia A in 1957–59 and 1978–79. Br J Haematol 1982;51:643–7
- Strawczynski H, Stachewitsch A, Morgenstern G, Shaw ME. Delivery of care to hemophilic children: home care versus hospitalization. Pediatrics 1973;51:986–991
- Lazerson J. Hemophilia home transfusion program: effect on school attendance. J Pediatr 1972;81:330–2
- Agle D. Psychological factors in hemophilia: the concept of self-care. Ann NY Acad Sci 1975;240:221–5
- Lusher JM. Approach to the bleeding patient. In: Hematology of infancy and childhood, 5th edn. Nathan DG, Orkin SH, eds. Philadelphia: WB Saunders, 1998, p1574–84
- Montgomery RR, Scott JP. Hemostasis: diseases of the fluid phase. In: Hematology of infancy and childhood, 4th edn. Nathan DG, Orkin SH, eds. Philadelphia: WB Saunders, 1993, p1605–50
- Hirschman RJ, Itscoitz SB, Shulman NR. Prophylactic treatment of factor VIII deficiency. Blood 1970;35:189–94
- Montgomery RR, Behrman JP. Section 7 – Hemorrhagic and thrombotic diseases. In: Nelson textbook of pediatrics, 16th edn. Philadelphia: WB Saunders, 2000
- Jones PK, Ratnoff OD. The changing prognosis of classic hemophilia (factor VII 'deficiency'). Ann Int Med 1991;114(8):641–8
- Schwartz RS, Abildgaard CF, Aledort LM, et al. Human recombinant DNA-derived antihemophilic factor (Factor VIII) in the treatment of hemophilia A. N Engl J Med 1990;323:1800–5
- Lee GR. Wintrobe's clinical hematology, 10th edn. Philadelphia: Lippincott Williams & Wilkins, 1999
- Ball L. In: Haematological disorders in illustrated textbook of paediatrics. Lissauer T, Clayden G. eds. Philadelphia: Mosby, 1998, chapter 19
- Kurachi K, Yao S-N, Furukawa M, et al. Deficiencies in factors IX and VIII: what is now known. Hosp Pract 1992;27:41
- Pfaff JA, Geninatt M. Hemophilia. Emerg Med Clin North Am 1993;11:337
- Brettler DB, Levine PH. Factor concentrates for treatment of hemophilia: which one to choose? Blood 1989;73:2067
- Pierce GF, Lusher JM, Brownstein AP, et al. The use of purified clotting factor concentrates in hemophilia: influence of vial safety, cost, and supply on therapy. JAMA 1989;261:3434
- National Hemophilia Foundation Medical and Scientific Advisory Council: Recommendations concerning AIDS and therapy of hemophilia. New York: National Hemophilia Foundation, 1984
- Kohler M, Hellstern P, Miyashita C, et al. Comparative study of intranasal, subcutaneous and intravenous administration of desamino-D-arginine vasopressin (DDAVP). Thromb Haemost 1986;55:108–11

- Ashenhurst JB, Langehennig PL, Seeler RA. Early treatment of bleeding episodes with 10 U/kg of factor VIII. Blood 1977;50:181–2
- Bona RD, Weinstein RA, Weisman SJ, et al. The use of continuous infusion of factor concentrates in the treatment of hemophilia. Am J Hematol 1989;32:8–13
- Hathaway WE, Christian MJ, Clarke SL, Hasiba U. Comparison of continuous and intermittent factor VIII concentrate therapy in hemophilia A. Am J Hematol 1984;17:85–8
- Rodgers GM, Ford MH. Lack of response to commercial factor VIII concentrate in hemophilia A. Am J Hematol 1991;37:288
- Kim HC, McMillan CW, White GC, et al. Purified factor IX using monoclonal immunoaffinity technique: clinical trials in hemophilia B and comparison to prothrombin complex concentrates. Blood 1992;79:568–75
- White GC, Beebe A, Nielsen B. Recombinant factor IX. Thromb Haemost 1997;78:261–5
- Lozier JN, Brinkhous K. Gene therapy and the hemophilias. JAMA 1994;271:47–51
- Andes WA, Wulff K, Smith WB. Head trauma in hemophilia. Arch Intern Med 1984;144:1981–3
- Seeler RA, Imana RB. Intracranial hemorrhage in patients with hemophilia. J Neurosurg 1973;39:181–5
- Curran JW, Lawrence DN, Jaffe H, et al. Acquired immunodeficiency syndrome (AIDS) associated with transfusions. N Engl J Med 1984;310:69–75
- Jones PK, Ratnoff OD. The changing prognosis of classic hemophilia (factor VIII 'deficiency'). Ann Intern Med 1991;114:641–8
- Triemstra M, Rosendaal FR, Smit C, et al. Mortality in patients with hemophilia: Changes in a Dutch population from 1986 to 1992 and 1973 to 1986. Ann Intern Med 1995;123:823–7

FAQS

Question 1

In a patient with negative family history and no previous bleeding, is hemophilia still in the differential diagnosis?

ANSWER 1

Yes. In about 30% of cases, no family history is elicited (new mutations). It is not infrequent that mild to moderate cases of hemophilia are diagnosed during a recent surgery such as dental extraction.

Question 2

What are the most important screening tests in the detection of bleeding disorders?

ANSWER 2

Carefully elicited history remains the most important diagnostic test to rule out bleeding diathesis. If the history is negative, the positive results of tests such as bleeding time, prothombin time/partial thromboplastin time are most likely false-positive (and therefore should not be done).

Question 3

In a patient with hemophilia and gastrointestinal bleeding should gastrointestinal workup be done?

ANSWER 3

Yes. Bleeding should not be assumed to be due to hemophilia, but most likely due to some underlying gastrointestinal structural abnormalities.

Question 4

What is the difference between the 'ristocetin-induced platelet agglutination' and 'ristocetin-cofactor assay'?

ANSWER 4

The ristocetin-induced platelet agglutination (RIPA) tests whether the patient's von Willebrand factor (VWF) is capable of binding to the Gplb/IX receptor on his/her own platelets. Ristocetin is added to the patient's blood sample; if platelet clumps form, the patient's platelets and VWF interact appropriately. The ristocetin-cofactor assay is used to detect VWF activity and tests VWF function in the patient's plasma. A fixed platelet preparation is used to replace the patient's own platelets and tested with various concentration of ristocetin. The latter test is probably the most sensitive test for the diagnosis of von Willebrand's disease (any type) while RIPA is the most useful for the diagnosis if type 2B VWD.

CONTRIBUTORS

Randolph L Pearson, MD
Benjamin Djulbegovic, MD, PhD
Dinesh S Rao, MD

HEPATOCELLULAR CARCINOMA

SUMMARY INFORMATION

DESCRIPTION

- Relatively rare in the US and other Western countries, but one of the most common types of cancer in areas where chronic hepatitis or liver diseases are prevalent
- Men are more likely to develop this disease, as are patients with cirrhosis or a chronic liver disease such as hepatitis B or C
- Usually asymptotic until later stages, and prognosis is generally very poor
- Treatment may include surgical resection (very rarely, due to level of progression), chemotherapy, and/or radiation therapy
- Hepatitis B vaccine reportedly helps prevent the disease

KEY! DON'T MISS!

- Hepatic abscess as cause of a hepatic mass requires prompt treatment
- Patients with hepatitis B and C have a very high risk of developing hepatocarcinoma. Proper follow up can be effective in detecting small lesions
- Patients with hepatitis B and C who do not drink alcohol have less chance of developing hepatocarcinoma than those who drink

ICD9 CODE
155.0 Hepatocellular carcinoma.

SYNONYMS
Hepatoma.

CARDINAL FEATURES
- Among the 10 most common cancers worldwide; more common in regions where chronic hepatitis B or C is prevalent
- Associated with cirrhosis, chronic hepatitis B or C infection, chronic liver disease, and mycotoxin exposure
- Usually asymptomatic until late stages of the disease; symptoms usually include abdominal pain and an abdominal mass, and may also include fever, anorexia, stomach fullness, edema, and jaundice
- Prognosis is generally very poor, with fewer than 5% of symptomatic patients surviving for more than 2 years
- Treatments include total surgical resection if possible, systemic chemotherapy, hepatic arterial chemotherapy, hepatic arterial chemoembolization, radiation therapy, percutaneous ethanol injection, radiofrequency ablation, and liver transplantation
- Screening at-risk patients (cirrhotic disease, chronic hepatitis B or C infection, or other liver injury) with alpha-fetoprotein tests and ultrasound may detect disease in early stages
- Preventive measures include hepatitis B vaccination, elimination of aflatoxin exposure, and decreased alcohol intake

CAUSES
Common causes
- Idiopathic neoplasia
- Hepatitis B or C virus chronic carrier state
- Liver cirrhosis

Rare causes
Environmental exposures, including alcohol, aflatoxin B1, vinyl chloride, Thorotrast, or estrogen.

Serious causes
- Cirrhosis: risk of cancer in a cirrhotic liver is 3% per year; 60–90% of hepatocellular carcinoma occurs in cirrhotic livers
- Hepatitis C: annual incidence in hepatitis C virus carriers is 1.5–4%

Contributory or predisposing factors
- Chronic hepatitis B and C
- Concomitant infection by B and C viruses increases the risk
- Chronic liver disease
- Cirrhosis
- Hepatotoxins: alcohol
- Mycotoxins: aflatoxin B1 exposure
- High-dose anabolic steroids
- Vinyl chloride exposure
- Thorotrast (a contrast medium) exposure
- Estrogen (possibly)
- Systemic liver diseases: alpha-1-antitrypsin deficiency, hemochromatosis, tyrosinemia, porphyria cutanea tarda, galactosemia, citrullinemia, and Wilson's disease
- Tobacco use

EPIDEMIOLOGY
Incidence and prevalence
INCIDENCE
- 14,500–19,000 cases/year in the US
- 350,000 to 1 million cases/year worldwide
- Increasing incidence in the US: 1.4/100,000 in the period 1976–1980 to 2.4/100,000 in the period 1991–1995

PREVALENCE
- 0.02–0.04/1000 in North and South America, north and central Europe, and Australia
- 0.2/1000 in Mediterranean countries
- 1.5–5/1000 in Korea, Taiwan, Mozambique, and southeast China

FREQUENCY
- Cirrhotic patients are 40 times more likely to develop hepatocellular carcinoma; 70–90% of cases are associated with cirrhosis
- 36% of cases in the US are seropositive for hepatitis B virus; hepatitis C virus is also associated with hepatocellular carcinoma, especially in the Far East

Demographics
AGE
- Incidence increases with age and peaks between 30 and 50 years
- In the Western world, usually occurs between 50 and 70 years of age
- In areas where hepatitis B virus is prevalent, usually occurs between 20 and 40 years of age

GENDER
- Males are eight times more likely to develop hepatocellular carcinoma than females in areas where disease is highly prevalent
- In the US, males are four times more likely to develop disease than females

RACE
Incidence rates among African-Americans are four times higher than among Caucasians.

GEOGRAPHY
More common in regions with a high prevalence of hepatitis B, including sub-Saharan Africa, southeast Asia and China, Japan, Korea, Taiwan, and Mozambique.

DIFFERENTIAL DIAGNOSIS

The liver is a common site for metastatic disease; therefore it is especially important to determine if current disease is metastatic or primary in nature.

Metastatic liver tumors

Secondary cancer that has metastasized from another primary cancer site such as colon, stomach, breast, lung, or pancreas.

FEATURES

- Enlarged or tender liver
- Signs and symptoms associated with the primary cancer
- If there is no knowledge of a previous tumor, the diagnosis is usually made only by biopsy

Cholangiocarcinoma

Rare cancer of the bile ducts of the liver.

FEATURES

Hematogenous metastases in 50% of cases.

Benign liver tumors

Including adenomas, focal nodular hyperplasia, and hemangiomas.

FEATURES

- Adenomas are most common in women between 30 and 40 years of age and are frequently associated with use of birth control pills
- Focal nodular hyperplasia is also more common in women but is not associated with use of birth control pills

Focal fatty infiltration

Infiltration of hepatic tissue with fat.

FEATURES

- Can occur as the result of alcohol use
- Considered benign

Hepatic abscess

- Infectious mass within liver
- Can include bacterial (Gram-negative enterics), fungal (*Candida* spp.) and parasitic (amebic) etiologies
- Consider diagnosis in immunosuppressed patients or those who have history of travel
- Use of multiple imaging modalities can clarify the matter

FEATURES

With bacterial and fungal etiologies, fevers and other signs of infection may be present.

Hepatic cyst

Imaging can usually help differentiate cyst from hepatocellular carcinoma.

FEATURES

History of polycystic kidney disease: occurs in 50–70%.

Focal nodular hyperplasia

Pathologically defined lesion that occurs as nodules in the liver regenerate after acute liver injury. Can be differentiated from hepatocellular carcinoma by history and imaging studies.

FEATURES

History of acute liver injury.

SIGNS & SYMPTOMS

Signs

- Signs of associated cirrhosis are common, including weight loss, ascites, malnutrition, and liver failure
- Jaundice
- Clubbing, palmar erythema
- Peripheral edema due to decreased plasma albumin levels
- Tender, enlarged liver
- Hepatic bruit
- Enlarged spleen
- Anemia

Symptoms

- 33% of patients are asymptomatic
- Abdominal pain, especially in epigastrium or right upper quadrant
- Abdominal mass
- Weight loss
- Malaise
- Anorexia
- Cachexia
- Jaundice, pale stools, dark urine
- Fever

ASSOCIATED DISORDERS

Paraneoplastic disorders may result:

- Erythrocytosis
- Thrombocytosis
- Hypoglycemia
- Hypercholesterolemia
- Hypercalcemia
- Dysfibrinogenemia
- Cryoyfibrinogenemia
- Porphyria cutanea tarda
- Hypertrophic osteoarthropathy

KEY! DON'T MISS!

- Hepatic abscess as cause of a hepatic mass requires prompt treatment
- Patients with hepatitis B and C have a very high risk of developing hepatocarcinoma. Proper follow up can be effective in detecting small lesions
- Patients with hepatitis B and C who do not drink alcohol have less chance of developing hepatocarcinoma than those who drink

CONSIDER CONSULT

- Refer for alpha-fetoprotein levels and liver function tests based on physical examination and suspicion of diagnosis
- Refer for imaging studies based on laboratory test and liver biopsy results
- Refer for liver biopsy based on laboratory and imaging study results

INVESTIGATION OF THE PATIENT

Direct questions to patient

- Q **What symptoms do you have?** Abdominal pain and an abdominal mass are usually the first indications for this disease. Most patients are asymptomatic until late stages of disease
- Q **Do you have chronic liver disease, such as hepatitis B or C infection or cirrhosis?** Chronic liver disease is one of the most common causes for hepatocellular carcinoma

Contributory or predisposing factors

- Q **Do you have hepatitis B or C virus infection?** People who have hepatitis B or C infection have an increased risk for developing hepatocellular carcinoma
- Q **Do you drink excessive amounts of alcohol?** Does the patient have signs and symptoms of cirrhotic disease? Alcohol-induced cirrhosis is one of the most important contributory factors of hepatocellular carcinoma among patients in the Western world
- Q **Have you ever been exposed to any environmental toxins? Do you have a history of working with dyes? Have you ever undergone radiographic examination with Thorotrast?** Other environmental toxins that are considered hepatocarcinogenic are aflatoxin B1, nitrosamines, carbon tetrachloride, and polyvinyl chloride

Family history

- Q **Do you have a family history of liver disease of any type?** Hereditary disorder-induced cirrhosis, including hemochromatosis, alpha-1-antitrypsin deficiency, type I glycogen storage disease, hypercitrullinemia, porphyria, tyrosinemia, and Wilson's disease, are contributory factors for cirrhotic disease and therefore put affected people at increased risk for hepatocellular carcinoma.

Examination

- **What is patient's overall physical condition? Does he/she complain of weight loss, abdominal pain, weakness, fatigue, or fever?** Loss of hepatic function can lead to these constitutional symptoms. However, presence of acute-onset fever and chills should raise possibility of hepatic abscess
- **Does patient complain of abdominal pain in right upper quadrant? Does palpation detect an abdominal mass?** Mass may indicate presence of a hepatic lesion
- **Does patient have signs of obvious jaundice or edema in the extremities?** The liver conjugates and excretes bilirubin, and jaundice can be a consequence of liver failure. A failure of the liver's synthetic function in producing albumin leads to a decrease in plasma oncotic pressure and edema

Summary of investigative tests

- Routine tests of liver function include serum bilirubin, prothrombin time, serum albumin, alkaline phosphatase, and serum alanine (ALT) and aspartate (AST) aminotransferases
- Other laboratory tests include alpha-fetoprotein and tumor markers (des-gamma-carboxy prothrombin, plasma urokinase-like plasminogen activator, alpha-L-fucosidase, and transcobalamin I), which may indicate underlying chronic liver disease
- Tests and imaging studies usually ordered by a specialist, including abdominal ultrasound, computed tomography (CT), and magnetic resonance imaging (MRI), can be used to define size and severity of tumoral invasion and associated lesions. Other variations of these tests using interventional radiography can be used to detect smaller lesions
- CT scans with standard iodinated contrast media are less accurate than abdominal ultrasounds in the evaluation of hepatocellular carcinoma tumors <2cm in diameter
- Optimal imaging technique (80–90% detection rate) is dynamic bolus injection with power injectors and rapid table incrementation during contrast infusion
- CT arteriography (CTA) – bolus infusion of the contrast media into the celiac or hepatic artery during CT procedure – has a 94% detection rate and is particularly effective in detecting tumors <1cm in diameter

- CT angioportography (CTAP) – a contrast media is injected into the superior mesenteric artery before the liver CT is performed – has a 85–90% detection rate for hepatocellular carcinoma tumors >2cm
- CT with ethiodized oil emulsion (CTEOE) – ethiodized oil emulsion is injected into the hepatic artery and a CT scan is performed 7–14 days later – has a 90% detection rate for small tumors
- MRI scans are more accurate than CT scans but are more expensive
- Liver biopsy (percutaneous or fine-needle aspiration) studies support diagnosis if cancerous cells are present

DIAGNOSTIC DECISION

The following diagnostic parameters are generally recommended:

- When symptomatic, hepatocellular carcinoma is usually unresectable, the best approach is to screen 'at-risk' patients (e.g. cirrhotics) by alpha-fetoprotein screening of the serum, ultrasound, and MRI
- Presence of a hepatic mass on CT or MRI consistent with hepatocellular carcinoma and alpha-fetoprotein >500 are strongly suggestive of hepatocellular carcinoma but are not enough to firm the diagnosis
- Presence of cirrhosis or hepatitis further supports diagnosis of hepatocellular carcinoma
- Use of fine-needle aspiration for cytologic evaluation is necessary when the above do not provide a conclusive diagnosis
- Definitive diagnosis requires biopsy and pathologic diagnosis

CLINICAL PEARLS

A high alpha-fetoprotein level can also be indicative of gonadal tumors that are potentially curable, even when metastatic.

THE TESTS

Body fluids

ALPHA-FETOPROTEIN LEVEL

Description

Blood sample.

Advantages/Disadvantages

Advantages:

- Valuable diagnostic test: elevated levels occur in 70% of patients with hepatocellular carcinoma
- Useful for monitoring progress of treatment; gradually decreasing levels are indicative of good response

Disadvantage: relatively expensive

Normal

<15ng/mL in men and nonpregnant women.

Abnormal

>15ng/mL.

Cause of abnormal result

Alpha-fetoprotein is an intracellular protein found in several tissues of the gastrointestinal tract, including hepatocellular cells. Conditions that compromise hepatocellular integrity (e.g. cirrhosis, hepatitis) or increase growth and turnover of cells (cancers) will lead to elevated alpha-fetoprotein levels.

Drugs, disorders and other factors that may alter results
- Hemolysis caused by rough or inappropriate blood sample handling
- Pregnancy
- Other tumors, such as some gonadal tumors, can cause an elevation on the levels of alpha-fetoprotein

ALKALINE PHOSPHATASE
Description
Blood sample.

Advantages/Disadvantages
Advantages:
- Quick, easy, widely available
- Useful for monitoring disease progression
- Good indicator of cholestasis

Normal
- 98–251U/L for men 19 years of age or older
- 81–213U/L for women 24–45 years of age
- 84–309U/L for women 45 years of age or older

Abnormal
Elevated values.

Cause of abnormal result
Sharply elevated alkaline phosphatase levels are indicative of complete biliary obstruction resulting from malignancy or fibrotic infiltrations.

Drugs, disorders and other factors that may alter results
- Hemolysis due to inappropriate handling techniques or delayed analysis
- Vitamin D intake
- Albumin infusion
- Drugs that influence liver function, including barbiturates, chlorpropamide, oral contraceptives, halothane, isoniazid, methyldopa, phenothiazines, phenytoin, rifampin
- Bone disease (Paget's, osteomalacia, bony metastasis)
- Renal failure

SERUM ALBUMIN
Description
Venous blood sample.

Advantages/Disadvantages
Advantages:
- Quick, inexpensive, widely available
- Measures protein synthetic activity of liver
- Level correlates well with severity of liver disease
- Useful for monitoring disease progression

Normal
4–6g/dL (40–60g/L).

Abnormal
- <4g/dL
- >6g/dL
- Keep in mind the possibility of a false-positive result

Cause of abnormal result

Loss of functioning liver tissue resulting in decreased albumin synthesis.

Drugs, disorders and other factors that may alter results

- Genetic abnormalities leading to absence of albumin or abnormal molecular forms
- Nephrotic syndrome
- Protein-losing enteropathy
- Malabsorption
- Malnutrition
- Iatrogenic from intravenous infusions

SERUM BILIRUBIN

Description

Venous blood sample.

Advantages/Disadvantages

Advantages:

- Serves as a general assessment of hepatic cellular uptake and synthetic and secretary functions
- Quick, inexpensive, widely available

Normal

- Total: 0.2–1.0mg/dL (2.0–10mg/L)
- Conjugated: 0–0.2mg/dL (0–2.0mg/L)

Abnormal

- Any value above upper limit of normal range
- Keep in mind the possibility of a false-positive result

Cause of abnormal result

- Hepatocytes function to remove, conjugate, and excrete bilirubin. Compromise of this function leads to increased levels of bilirubin in the blood
- Blockage of the common bile duct (mass leading to obstruction)

Drugs, disorders and other factors that may alter results

- Hemolysis
- Viral infection (hepatitis, Epstein-Barr virus)
- Autoimmune diseases
- Primary biliary cirrhosis
- Gallstone disease
- Pancreatic carcinoma
- Lymphoma (enlarged nodes in the porta hepatis)
- Drugs such as paracetamol, barbiturates, methyldopa
- Rare syndromes such as Gilbert's, Crigler-Najjar, Wilson's

PROTHROMBIN TIME

Description

- Measure of activity of extrinsic and common coagulation pathways
- Samples consist of venous blood collected via routine venipuncture into vessel containing a noncalcium-containing anticoagulant

Advantages/Disadvantages

Advantages:

- Can evaluate competency of extrinsic and common coagulation pathways, in which factors synthesized in the liver are involved
- Quick, inexpensive, widely available
- Useful for planning management

Normal

10–14s.

Abnormal

- Any value outside control range
- Keep in mind the possibility of a false-positive result

Cause of abnormal result

- Liver synthesizes these coagulation factors. Their deficiency indicates a deficiency in synthetic capacity of the liver, which can be caused by hepatocellular carcinoma
- Loss of the liver's functional reserve

Drugs, disorders and other factors that may alter results

- Congenital disorders, factor VIII and factor IX deficiency
- Disseminated intravascular coagulation
- Malabsorption leading to vitamin K deficiency
- Anticoagulants

SERUM ALANINE AMINOTRANSFERASE AND ASPARTATE AMINOTRANSFERASE

Description

Venous blood sample.

Advantages/Disadvantages

Advantages:

- Identifies and evaluates hepatic injury
- Inexpensive
- Simple test with rapid result
- Good indicator of disease progression

Disadvantage: nonspecific

Normal

ALT and AST: 0–35U/L.

Abnormal

- Any values above the upper limit of normal
- Keep in mind the possibility of a false-positive result

Cause of abnormal result

These two enzymes are present in high levels in hepatocytes. When there is damage to the liver, they are released into the bloodstream.

Drugs, disorders and other factors that may alter results
- Skeletal muscle damage or myocardial infarction. These enzymes are also present in other cell types and are released upon cellular damage
- Viral infections, hepatitis, Epstein-Barr virus, infectious mononucleosis
- Cirrhotic liver disease
- Drugs, e.g. lipid-lowering medications

Biopsy

PERCUTANEOUS OR FINE-NEEDLE ASPIRATION LIVER BIOPSY

Description

Core tissue sample from liver.

Advantages/Disadvantages

Advantage: gives a definitive tissue diagnosis

Disadvantages:
- Need to perform imaging studies first
- Invasive procedure requiring a skilled practitioner
- Risk of bleeding, infection, and perforation
- Biopsy is contraindicated in patients with platelet count of <100,000/mcL, prothrombin time of longer than 15s, or empyema of the biliary tract, liver, lungs, peritoneum, or vascular tumors

Abnormal
- Abnormal cells consistent with hepatocellular carcinoma seen on aspirate
- Beware of false-negative results

Cause of abnormal result

Hepatocellular carcinoma cells are abnormal with a high mitotic index and are often binucleate.

Drugs, disorders and other factors that may alter results
- Improper handling and evaluation
- Inaccurate sampling where the lesion has been missed

Imaging

ABDOMINAL ULTRASOUND

Description

Patient must have fasted for 8–12h before the test, which usually takes 15–30min.

Advantages/Disadvantages

Advantages:
- Noninvasive
- Can show organ size, shape, and position
- Can detect suspicious regions in liver not detected by radionuclide tests and whether regions are abscesses, cysts, or tumors

Disadvantages:
- Ultrasonography of the liver or abdomen may not detect hepatocellular carcinoma tumors in early stage; therefore consider ultrasonography of the liver and spleen
- Cannot distinguish hepatocellular carcinoma tumors from other tumors; therefore pathologic evaluation is required for a definitive diagnosis of hepatocellular carcinoma
- Operator-dependent test. Most experienced physicians will achieve a more accurate result
- Ribs, gas, or residual barium in stomach or colon can make scan difficult to interpret
- Dehydration can obscure boundaries between organs and tissues

Normal
No organomegaly, free fluid, masses.

Abnormal
- Liver mass/lesion
- Enlarged liver or spleen
- Free fluid, ascites
- Shrunken or cirrhotic liver

Cause of abnormal result
Hepatocellular carcinoma.

Drugs, disorders and other factors that may alter results
- Metastatic deposits rather than primary liver tumor. Secondary liver deposits are by far the most common cause of a liver mass
- Cysts, hydatid, amebic, congenital liver cysts, and polycystic liver disease
- Abscesses
- Syphilitic gumma
- Hemangioma

COMPUTED TOMOGRAPHY SCAN
Description
Patient must be in a fasted state only if an oral contrasting agent is used.

Advantages/Disadvantages
Advantage: CT scans are the preferred imaging study for obese patients and patients with livers located high under the rib cage

Disadvantages:
- Although CT scans are generally noninvasive, contrasting agents may be used and are administered orally or intravenously
- Intravenous contrast agents may cause transient discomfort, and some patients may be allergic to them
- Intravenous contrast agents should not be used in patients with severe hepatic or renal disease or those who are allergic to iodine
- Patients are exposed to radiation
- CT scans and ultrasonography are equally effective in detecting hepatocellular carcinoma, but CT scans are more expensive
- CT scanning may miss small lesions depending on the resolution of the scan

Normal
- No evidence of liver mass
- Beware of false-negative results

Abnormal
- Single or multiple solid lesions
- Parenchymal disease
- Cirrhosis
- Fat deposition

Cause of abnormal result
Hepatocellular carcinoma.

Drugs, disorders and other factors that may alter results
CT scanning cannot differentiate between primary hepatocellular carcinoma and metastatic lesions. Secondary lesions are the most common cause of a liver mass and usually arise from a primary in the stomach, lung, colon, breast, or uterus.

MAGNETIC RESONANCE IMAGING
Description
Dual-contrast MRI is the preferred test and uses chondroitin sulfate iron colloid as the negative contrast and gadopentetate dimeglumine as the positive contrast.

Advantages/Disadvantages
Advantages:
- Can detect tumor spread
- Can distinguish small hepatocellular carcinoma tumors from small hemangiomas

Disadvantage: more expensive than CT scans

Normal
- No evidence of liver mass
- Beware of false-negative results

Abnormal
- Single or multiple solid lesions
- Parenchymal disease
- Cirrhosis
- Fat deposition

Cause of abnormal result
Hepatocellular carcinoma.

Drugs, disorders and other factors that may alter results
MRI scanning cannot differentiate between primary hepatocellular carcinoma and metastatic lesions. Secondary lesions are the most common cause of a liver mass and usually arise from a primary in the stomach, lung, colon, breast, or uterus.

Special tests

TUMOR MARKERS

Description

- Examples include des-gamma-carboxy prothrombin and alpha-L-fucosidase
- Blood sample

Advantages/Disadvantages

Advantages:

- Both are easy and quick to measure
- Alpha-L-fucosidase is inexpensive

Disadvantages:

- Des-gamma-carboxy prothrombin is expensive
- Both are less sensitive in African-Americans
- Tumor markers are not specific enough to be used for diagnosis. Their main value is for monitoring disease progression

Normal

- Values within the normal limits
- Beware of false-negative results

Abnormal

Values above the upper limits of normal.

Cause of abnormal result

In des-gamma-carboxy prothrombin:

- Benign hepatic parenchymal disease
- Hepatic metastases
- Hepatic abscesses

Drugs, disorders and other factors that may alter results

Other diseases and malignancies can lead to abnormal results.

TREATMENT

CONSIDER CONSULT

Refer patient for treatment when diagnosis is suspected or made. Treatment is contingent on tumor size, liver function, and extrahepatic disease status.

IMMEDIATE ACTION

Immediate action is usually unnecessary for hepatocellular carcinoma itself, but hepatic abscess requires prompt institution of antibiotic treatment.

PATIENT AND CAREGIVER ISSUES

Forensic and legal issues

Because the prognosis is very poor, practical end-of-life measures such as filing a will and nominating a next-of-kin should be addressed.

Impact on career, dependants, family, friends

Patients with liver tumors usually have an aggressive disease with high mortality rate. The patient should be made aware of the prognosis.

Patient or caregiver request

- **What options do I have?** There are many therapies that have been tried in treating liver cancer. These include chemotherapy, radiotherapy, and liver transplantation. Unfortunately, none of these therapies has been shown to improve survival. Surgical resection of small tumors is possible but only improves survival in 50% of cases
- **How long do I have to live?** Three-year survival for hepatocellular carcinoma is 13%. Because the disease may have been asymptomatic, patient presentation may not occur until he/she is terminally ill. Death is usually within 6 months of diagnosis

MANAGEMENT ISSUES

Goals

- To provide treatment that is potentially life-saving
- To reduce level of pain
- If treatment is successful, to prevent recurrence

Management in special circumstances

COEXISTING DISEASE

- Coexisting cirrhosis can make treatment even more difficult. Underlying coagulation disturbances and low albumin production are associated with a poorer prognosis
- Cirrhosis may make the treatment of complications such as gastrointestinal bleeding, edema, and others very difficult to manage

SPECIAL PATIENT GROUPS

Some younger patients with a fibrolamellar subtype usually have a better prognosis. A few can achieve a long-term survival or even cure if resection is performed.

PATIENT SATISFACTION/LIFESTYLE PRIORITIES

- Pain management
- Symptom control of nausea, shortness of breath, and edema

SUMMARY OF THERAPEUTIC OPTIONS

Choices

- Treatment is dependent on disease status, including size of tumor(s), liver function, and any other coexisting medical conditions

- Most patients present after the disease is symptomatic and advanced, making most treatment options unsuccessful. There is no standard treatment for patients with advanced primary liver cancer, and to consider referring for clinical trials is a reasonable option
- Treatment for hepatocellular carcinoma is usually managed by a specialist in a hospital setting
- Resection is the primary treatment option if tumor is localized in one hepatic lobe and cirrhotic disease is not observed. Recurrence rates after surgical resection are high. In patients without cirrhosis (comprising 50% of all hepatocellular carcinoma patients in the US), surgical mortality rate is 5%
- Liver transplantation is usually limited to select patients (localized disease, no extrahepatic disease states), requires lifelong immunosuppression therapy, and has a high recurrence rate. Patients who are candidates for liver transplantation should cease smoking, drinking, and taking drugs if they wish to join the transplantation list
- Chemotherapy is considered to be palliative in nature and can be used adjunctively with surgical resection or liver transplantation. However, response rate is very low (<20%). Additionally, toxicity associated with chemotherapy and effect on patient's quality of life should be considered. Single-agent chemotherapy has been studied but resulted in low response rates and high rates of disease progression. Combination chemotherapy regimens are offered only in clinical trials
- Intra-arterial chemotherapy with floxuridine, doxorubicin, and cisplatin as single agents or part of a combination regimen are under investigation
- Biologic and hormonal therapies are expensive and painful. They are being evaluated in clinical studies (www.cancer.gov/clinical_trials)
- Chemoembolization with contrast agents and chemotherapeutic agents may decrease size of tumor to a level where surgical resection is possible
- Percutaneous ethanol injection has been used to treat hepatocellular carcinoma tumors <5cm in diameter, but patients are required to have adequate coagulation and platelet count. Risk of tumor dissemination is high. This treatment needs to be studied further
- Radiation therapy requires total doses of irradiation in excess of 30Gy, which can result in radiation hepatitis and death. Therefore combining radiation therapy and a new 3-D administration program and combining radiation therapy with antiferritin antibody treatment have been studied
- Participation in clinical studies is encouraged
- Undergoing no treatment is an option but is associated with a 100% mortality rate

Clinical pearls

Some young patients with a fibrolamellar subtype can achieve a long-term survival.

Never

Never forget that a patient with an elevation in alpha-fetoprotein levels can have a gonadal, potentially curable tumor.

FOLLOW UP

- Hepatocellular carcinoma progresses rapidly after it is diagnosed in the late stages
- Survival time is usually <2 years and can be as quick as 1–4 months if no treatment is provided
- If a treatment plan is instigated, follow up will include joint care of the patient with a specialist (oncologist, surgeon, hematologist, or gastroenterologist)
- If palliation only is required, follow up should be at regular intervals to check for symptom control, side-effects from medication, and pain management. The patient may indicate how much medical intervention he/she prefers

Plan for review

Laboratory tests, including alpha-fetoprotein levels, liver function tests, and tumor markers, are useful in evaluating patients for response to treatment.

DRUGS AND OTHER THERAPIES: DETAILS

Surgical therapy

SURGICAL RESECTION

- Resection is only possible in a small percentage of patients
- Surgical resection is limited to patients who do not have extrahepatic disease, cirrhosis, chronic hepatitis, and who have good residual liver function
- Resectability is defined by the anatomic location of the tumor and is most effective when tumor is limited to one lobe of the liver

Efficacy

5-year survival rates of 10–30% have been reported for patients who have undergone surgical resection of localized tumors.

Risks/Benefits

Risks:

- High mortality rate
- High recurrence rate

Benefit: only chance for curative intervention

Acceptability to patient

High recurrence rates may make this option less acceptable to patients.

Follow up plan

- Follow up laboratory tests for alpha-fetoprotein levels, liver function, and tumor markers are useful tools for following progress of the disease
- Follow up of the resection should be performed by a surgeon

LIVER TRANSPLANTATION

- Liver transplantation is limited to patients with localized tumor and no extrahepatic disease
- Patients with fibrolamellar type can have a great benefit from transplantation

Efficacy

20–30% survival rates in patients with small localized cancers.

Risks/Benefits

Risks:

- Requires extensive surgical procedure
- Requires specialized care with lifelong immunosuppression drugs
- High recurrence rate

Acceptability to patient

- High recurrence rates may make this option less acceptable to patients
- Younger patients with fibrolamellar type cancer are more likely to accept the risks due to the chance of improved long-term survival

Follow up plan

- Monitor for immunosuppression
- Monitor liver function for signs of rejection
- Monitor for signs of infection
- Follow up of the transplantation should be performed by a specialist transplantation team

Radiation therapy

RADIATION THERAPY

New radiation regimens are being investigated, including combining radiation therapy with a 3-D administration technique and radiation therapy combined with antiferritin antibody treatment.

Efficacy

- Unproven efficacy
- Used palliatively for unresectable tumors

Risks/Benefits

Risks:

- Associated with radiation hepatitis
- High recurrence rates
- Death

Acceptability to patient

- Patients can be alarmed by risk of radiation hepatitis
- Noninvasive and can be used in the palliative setting
- This treatment modality is still experimental and should be used only in the context of a clinical trial

Follow up plan

- Follow up laboratory tests for alpha-fetoprotein levels, liver function, and tumor markers are useful tools for following progress of the disease
- Follow up of the radiotherapy should be performed by a specialist

Chemotherapy

CHEMOTHERAPY

Chemotherapy, including single-agent chemotherapy, combination chemotherapies, regional chemotherapy, intra-arterial regional chemotherapy, or combination chemotherapy and radiation therapy, is offered in clinical trials.

Efficacy

Response rates ranging from 10–30% have been reported. Substantial controversy about benefits of chemotherapy in liver cancer exist.

Acceptability to patient

- Most chemotherapy regimens are associated with some degree of toxicity. Toxic effects will affect patient's quality of life
- High recurrence rates may make this option less acceptable to patients
- Chemotherapy should be offered only in the context of a clinical trial

Follow up plan

- Follow up laboratory tests for alpha-fetoprotein levels, liver function, and tumor markers are useful tools for following progress of the disease
- Follow up of the chemotherapy should be performed by a specialist

Other therapies

PERCUTANEOUS ETHANOL INJECTION (ALCOHOL INJECTION)

- Alcohol injection has been used to treat small hepatocellular carcinoma tumors, usually less than 5cm in diameter
- Patients must have adequate coagulation profile and platelet count

Efficacy

Has been evaluated in nonrandomized clinical trials, but no definitive conclusion exists. Remissions have been reported, but the effect on clinical outcomes is unknown.

Risks/Benefits

Risks:

- High recurrence rates
- Peritoneal hemorrhage
- Liver failure or infarction
- Peritoneal seeding of tumor

Acceptability to patient

High recurrence rates and the unknown benefits may make this option less acceptable to patients.

Follow up plan

- Follow up laboratory tests for alpha-fetoprotein levels, liver function, and tumor markers are useful tools for following progress of the disease
- Follow up of this therapy should be performed by a specialist

EFFICACY OF THERAPIES

- Hepatocellular carcinoma is almost always fatal within 2 years of diagnosis, and average survival is 6 months
- There is no standard treatment for patients with advanced primary liver disease
- Surgical resection is the treatment of choice in patients whose tumor is localized and who have good residual liver function
- Long-term survival can be achieved in fibrolamellar subtypes

PROGNOSIS

- Prognosis is very poor
- Fewer than 5% of patients diagnosed with unresectable hepatocellular carcinoma survive for 2 years
- Average survival is 6 months
- Surgical intervention can improve survival in a select group of patients
- Other therapies have not been proven to improve prognosis

Clinical pearls

Younger patients with fibrolamellar type can achieve long-term survival, even when the tumor is not completely resected.

Recurrence

Recurrence rates are high regardless of treatment.

Deterioration

Patients who are diagnosed with advanced hepatocellular carcinoma rapidly deteriorate, and the majority die within 2 years of diagnosis.

Terminal illness

- Surgical resection is the preferred treatment but is rarely possible
- There is no standard therapy for patients with metastatic disease. These patients should be entered into clinical trials

COMPLICATIONS

- Metastasis
- Biliary obstruction
- Heart failure
- Renal failure
- Intraperitoneal bleeding
- Treatment with surgical resection is associated with a high degree of postoperative complications, such as bleeding, infection, and tumor seeding
- Treatment with chemotherapy and radiotherapy have many toxic side-effects
- Liver transplantation necessitates lifelong immunosuppression, which predisposes to overwhelming infection

CONSIDER CONSULT

- All patients with treatment failure should be referred to a medical oncologist for evaluation (clinical trials vs palliative treatment)

RISK FACTORS

- Cirrhotic disease: patients with cirrhosis are at increased risk for developing hepatocellular carcinoma
- Chronic hepatitis B or C infection: the most significant risk factors for hepatocellular carcinoma
- Aflatoxin exposure: patients who eat foods contaminated with aflatoxins are at increased risk for developing hepatocellular carcinoma

MODIFY RISK FACTORS

Lifestyle and wellness

TOBACCO

- Tobacco use is associated with an increased risk of hepatocellular carcinoma
- It is also a major risk factor for lung, stomach, and colon cancers as well as being a risk factor for coronary artery disease (a major contributor to mortality and morbidity)
- All patients who smoke should be advised to give up

ALCOHOL AND DRUGS

- Alcohol-induced cirrhotic liver disease coexists in 50% of patients with hepatocellular carcinoma
- Alcohol abuse not only increases the risk of hepatocellular carcinoma but also damages the brain and heart, leading to multiorgan failure
- Alcoholics need to be encouraged to give up alcohol and join support groups
- Social drinkers need to be advised of the recommended daily limits
- Intravenous drug users are at increased risk of exposure to hepatitis B and C, both of which are associated with developing hepatocellular carcinoma. Addicts should be encouraged to join a drug rehabilitation program and advised to use clean needles if they do take drugs

DIET

Food contaminated with aflatoxin should be avoided.

SEXUAL BEHAVIOR

Do not have unprotected sex with a partner who is positive for hepatitis.

ENVIRONMENT
Environmental toxins associated with hepatocellular carcinoma should be avoided, including vinyl chloride, dye production, and Thorotrast (a contrast medium).

FAMILY HISTORY
If there is a family history of systemic liver disease, screening programs should be participated in.

IMMUNIZATION
Participation in hepatitis vaccination programs.

SCREENING

ALPHA-FETOPROTEIN LEVEL

- At-risk patients and those with cirrhosis, chronic hepatitis B or C, or other chronic liver disease should have this test regularly
- Elevated serum alpha-fetoprotein levels are indicative of hepatocellular carcinoma but are not specific

Cost/efficacy

- Inexpensive
- About 70% of patients with hepatocellular carcinoma have elevated alpha-fetoprotein levels

ABDOMINAL ULTRASOUND
At-risk patients and those with cirrhosis, chronic hepatitis B or C, or other chronic liver disease should have abdominal ultrasounds regularly.

Cost/efficacy

- Inexpensive, quick, noninvasive
- An effective tool for detecting hepatocellular carcinoma tumors

PREVENT RECURRENCE

High recurrence rate with current treatments and is almost always fatal.

RESOURCES

ASSOCIATIONS

American Cancer Society
1599 Clifton Road, NE
Atlanta, GA 30329
Tel: (800) 227-2345
www.cancer.org

American Liver Foundation
75 Maiden Lane, Suite 603
New York, NY 10038
Tel: (800) GOLIVER (800-465-4837)
www.liverfoundation.org

National Cancer Institute Cancer Information Service
Tel: (800) 4-CANCER (800-422-9237)
http://cis.nci.nih.gov/

KEY REFERENCES

- Neoplasms, liver cancer. In: Diseases, 2nd edn. Eckman M, Priff N, eds. Springhouse: Springhouse Corporation, 1997, p334–6
- Watkins KT, Curley SA. Liver and bile ducts. In: Clinical oncology. 2nd edn. Abeloff, ed. New York: Churchill Livingstone, 2000, p1681–721
- Feldman M. Hepatic tumors. In: Sleisenger & Fordtran's gastrointestinal liver Disease. 6th edn. Sleisenger MH, Fordtran JS, Weisiger RA, Bilhartz CE, eds. Philadelphia: WB Saunders, 1998, p1365–74
- Iwatsuki S, Starzl TE, Sheahan DG, et al. Hepatic resection versus transplantation for hepatocellular carcinoma. Ann Surgery 1991;214:221–9
- Pichlmayr R, Weimann A, Oldhafer KJ, et al. Appraisal of transplantation for malignant tumors of the liver with special reference to early stage hepatocellular carcinoma. Eur J Surg Oncol 1998;24:60–7
- CancerNet: Adult primary liver cancer (p 1–12). In http://www.cancer.gov/

FAQS

Question 1

Should patients with high levels of alpha-fetoprotein always be considered to have a hepatocellular carcinoma?

ANSWER 1

No. The level of alpha-fetoprotein can also be high in other diseases, particularly gonadal tumors. Special attention should be given to detecting gonadal tumors as they are potentially curable.

Question 2

Should a patient with established hepatocellular carcinoma and alcoholic cirrhosis be asked to stop drinking alcohol, even if the disease is metastatic?

ANSWER 2

Yes. Liver function could improve, thereby decreasing some of the symptoms of disease.

Question 3

How often should a patient with hepatitis B or C be followed up?

ANSWER 3

There is no general consensus, but at least 6-monthly/yearly unless complications arise.

Question 4

Is there any way to distinguish between a metastatic carcinoma to the liver and a primary hepatocellular carcinoma?

ANSWER 4

Only a biopsy can distinguish between the two. Usually imaging techniques can help but are not always able to give a definitive diagnosis. Even a high level of alpha-fetoprotein is not enough to firm the diagnosis.

CONTRIBUTORS

Kenneth L Evans, MD
Otavio A Clark, MD
Dinesh S Rao, MD

HODGKIN'S DISEASE

SUMMARY INFORMATION

DESCRIPTION

- Malignant tumor of the lymphatic system that can occur at all ages
- Presents with painless lymphadenopathy, fever, and weight loss
- Characterized histologically by the presence of multinucleated giant cells (Reed-Sternberg cells) and associated abnormal and smaller mononuclear cells originating from B lymphocytes in germinal centers of lymphoid tissue
- Several types and accurate classification of the type, together with accurate staging of the disease, will determine the most favorable treatment options and prognosis
- Eminently treatable and overall prognosis for cure is very good, especially in children

URGENT ACTION

- Lymphadenopathy that persists for more than 2–3 weeks requires investigation
- Symptoms of night sweats, fever, weight loss, and pruritus that accompany the lymphadenopathy require urgent investigation

KEY! DON'T MISS!

- Alcohol intake associated with pain is a characteristic of this disease
- Don't omit to carry out a careful neurologic examination in all cases of possible Hodgkin's disease to exclude spinal cord compression
- If the Hodgkin's diagnosis is confirmed, fertility tests and gonadal tissue harvesting may be offered to patients, especially younger ones. The treatment for this disease usually leads to infertility

ICD9 CODE

- 201.9 Hodgkin's disease, unspecified
- 201.4 Hodgkin's disease, lymphocyte predominance
- 201.5 Hodgkin's disease, nodular sclerosis
- 201.6 Hodgkin's disease, mixed cellularity
- 201.7 Hodgkin's disease, lymphocyte depletion

SYNONYMS

Hodgkin's lymphoma.

CARDINAL FEATURES

- Palpable lymphadenopathy, often painless, nontender and no alteration on the skin
- The neck region is most commonly involved
- Symptoms are not always present, but weight loss and fevers are the most important symptoms
- Pruritus may be an important diagnostic factor as it is a poor prognostic predictor
- Hodgkin's disease is diagnosed by histologic examination of biopsied tissue from one or more peripheral lymph nodes
- Characteristic histologic finding is the Reed-Sternberg cell

CAUSES

Common causes

- Probably caused by a combination of environmental and genetic factors along with a susceptible immune system
- Exact triggers and factors are not known

Contributory or predisposing factors

- Epstein-Barr virus has been found in the Reed-Sternberg cells of about 50% of patients with Hodgkin's disease and appears to have a crucial role in the development of Hodgkin's disease
- Patients who had developed mononucleosis, a disease caused by Epstein-Barr virus, have a 2- to 3-fold risk of developing Hodgkin's disease
- The virus may protect the Reed-Sternberg cell from apoptosis and from the immune response of killer T cells
- The presence of the virus has a higher incidence in patients with the mixed cellularity subtype of Hodgkin's disease and a lower incidence in the nodular sclerosis subtype

EPIDEMIOLOGY

Incidence and prevalence

INCIDENCE

- 0.04/1000
- About 7200 new cases a year are diagnosed in the US
- 3200 deaths per year in the US

Demographics

AGE

- Can occur at all ages
- Bimodal distribution of the most common age ranges of occurrence: 15–30 years and over 50 years

GENDER

- Male:female ratio in general is 1.4:1
- Male:female ratio in children is 4:1

RACE
More common in Caucasians.

GENETICS
There is a concordance for Hodgkin's disease in identical twins, suggesting that there may be an underlying genetic susceptibility to the disease.

GEOGRAPHY
More common in people living in temperate climates.

SOCIOECONOMIC STATUS
More common in higher socioeconomic groups.

DIFFERENTIAL DIAGNOSIS

- The main differential diagnoses are those disorders that present with lymphadenopathy
- It is necessary to have a lymph node biopsy examination for the correct diagnosis of Hodgkin's disease

Mononucleosis

Infectious mononucleosis causes lymphadenopathy.

FEATURES

- Especially common in adolescents and young adults
- Lymphadenopathy, usually cervical, affecting posterior triangle in particular
- Pharyngitis and tonsillitis
- May be associated with hepatic involvement
- Splenomegaly
- Fever, fatigue, and malaise
- Rash
- Positive heterophil antibody (monospot)
- Atypical lymphocytes with relative lymphocytosis on peripheral blood film

AIDS and acute retroviral syndrome

AIDS is associated with lymphadenopathy.

FEATURES

- Can present with fever, weight loss, and anorexia
- Pharyngitis
- Lymphadenopathy
- Maculopapular rash
- Opportunistic infections often present
- Serology for HIV tests positive

NonHodgkin's lymphoma

NonHodgkin's lymphoma is a lymphoproliferative disease without the Reed-Sternberg cell.

FEATURES

- Difficult to distinguish from nonHodgkin's lymphoma except histologically
- NonHodgkin's lymphoma usually presents in late middle-age
- About one-third of nonHodgkin's lymphoma originates extranodally
- Fever, night sweats, weight loss, and pruritus are less common than in Hodgkin's disease
- The differentiation is possible only after lymph node biopsy and examination by a pathologist

Tuberculosis

Tuberculosis is an infection caused by *Mycobacterium tuberculosis*.

FEATURES

- Fever, night sweats, weight loss
- Cough, hemoptysis
- Pleuritic chest pains
- Primary pulmonary tuberculosis may be asymptomatic or present with systemic symptoms rather than respiratory symptoms

Leukemias

A total blood cell examination can help in distinguishing lymphomas from leukemias.

FEATURES

Acute lymphoblastic:

- Primarily a disease of children
- Lymphadenopathy, hepatosplenomegaly
- Pallor, malaise, purpura
- Weight loss, fever

Acute myelogenous:

- Affects adults
- Anemia, bleeding, purpura
- Hepatosplenomegaly and lymphadenopathy can occur
- Fever, malaise, weakness

Chronic lymphocytic:

- Affects the middle-aged and elderly
- Lymphadenopathy and splenomegaly are common
- Hepatomegaly may occur
- Fatigue, weakness
- Often asymptomatic, especially in the early stages

Chronic myelogenous:

- Splenomegaly and hepatomegaly may occur
- Lymphadenopathy is rare
- Weakness and malaise
- Abdominal pain from splenic enlargement

Sarcoid and other chronic granulomatous diseases

Sarcoidosis can lead to lymphadenopathy.

FEATURES

- Bilateral hilar lymphadenopathy
- Noncaseating epithelioid cell granulomas on histology
- Night sweats
- Often asymptomatic
- Raised serum angiotensin-converting enzyme levels in the blood

Myeloma

Myeloma is a plasma cell neoplasm producing diffuse bone marrow infiltration and focal osteolytic deposits.

FEATURES

- Fatigue and weakness
- Bone pain, swellings of bones, especially ribs and vertebrae
- Weight loss

Toxoplasmosis

Toxoplasmosis is a protozoan infection with *Toxoplasma gondii.*

FEATURES

- Common cold symptoms
- Nodes usually confined to one side
- Mild lymphocytosis
- Asymptomatic or mildly tender posterior triangle adenopathy
- Hepatosplenomegaly

Cytomegalovirus infection

Primary infection with cytomegalovirus in a young adult can produce an infectious mononucleosis syndrome with fever, lymphadenopathy, and relative lymphocytosis.

FEATURES

- Pronounced splenomegaly
- Sore throat and lymphadenopathy, both variable
- Hepatic enzymes are frequently elevated
- Typhoid-like symptoms

Skin infections

Skin infections can result in local or generalized lymphadenopathy.

FEATURES

- Rash or other lesion usually apparent
- Systemic symptoms unlikely unless severe infection occurs

Tularemia

Tularemia is a systemic infection caused by *Francisella tularensis.*

FEATURES

- Fever, chills
- Fatigue and malaise
- Skin papules that ulcerate are not always present
- Pharyngitis; may be severe
- Regional lymphadenopthy is common

SIGNS & SYMPTOMS

Signs

- Lymphadenopathy, which can be regional, generalized, or local. The most common site is the neck region. Easily palpable, smooth, and may have a rubbery feel
- Hodgkin's disease usually spreads by contiguity from one lymph node chain to those adjacent
- Splenomegaly and hepatomegaly may be present and are associated with disease below the diaphragm
- Peripheral weakness and numbness with attenuated reflexes if spinal cord compression is present
- Plethora and distended neck and facial veins if there is superior venous cava syndrome
- Ear, nose, and throat examination is usually normal
- Presence of bulky disease worsens the prognosis

Symptoms

- Fever of 38°C, especially if in a cyclical pattern of days or weeks of fever alternating with afebrile periods (Pal-Epstein fever)
- Weight loss of more than 10% of body weight over the last 6 months for which there is no other explanation
- Night sweats that can be severe and drenching, requiring one or more changes of bedclothes per night
- Pruritus, generalized, and severe
- Malaise
- Persistent nonproductive cough if there is mediastinal enlargement
- Pain associated with alcohol ingestion in specific sites or regions
- Headache and facial fullness if there is superior vena cava obstruction
- Weakness and numbness, especially of the lower limbs, if there is spinal cord compression

- Fever, night sweats, and weight loss are classified as B symptoms and have prognostic importance: presence of B symptoms worsens the prognosis
- Fever and weight loss are more significant prognostic indicators than night sweats
- Recurrent, generalized, and otherwise unexplained pruritus may be the equivalent of a B symptom, especially when the severity of the pruritus rises and falls parallel to disease activity

KEY! DON'T MISS!

- Alcohol intake associated with pain is a characteristic of this disease
- Don't omit to carry out a careful neurologic examination in all cases of possible Hodgkin's disease to exclude spinal cord compression
- If the Hodgkin's diagnosis is confirmed, fertility tests and gonadal tissue harvesting may be offered to patients, especially younger ones. The treatment for this disease usually leads to infertility

CONSIDER CONSULT

- Refer unexplained lymphadenopathy that persists more than 2–4 weeks
- Refer more readily if there are any B symptoms, and immediately with signs and symptoms of spinal cord compression
- As soon as diagnosis is made, refer with the diagnosis workup as complete as possible. This includes excisional biopsy results, computed tomography (CT) scans of thorax and abdomen, lactate dehydrogenase (LDH), and liver function tests
- Refer all patients with persistent enlargement of lymph nodes for biopsy

INVESTIGATION OF THE PATIENT

Direct questions to patient

- Q **Do you have any night sweats?** These can be drenching, requiring changing of the patient's nightwear and bedclothes
- Q **Have you lost any weight?** Weight loss, otherwise unexplained, of 10% of body weight over 6 months is especially significant
- Q **Do you have any fever?** Recurrent fevers of >38°C, especially over several days or weeks alternating with afebrile periods, are significant
- Q **Have you developed any problems when you drink alcoholic drinks?** Such drinks can cause nonspecific pain at sites of eosinophil infiltration of tumor, or there may be indifference to or nonspecific intolerance of alcohol
- Q **Do you have persistent or recurrent itching of the skin?** Pruritus is often associated with Hodgkin's disease
- Q **How do you feel within yourself?** There may be nonspecific fatigue or malaise

Contributory or predisposing factors

- Q **What is the patient's HIV status?** Hodgkin's disease may arise more commonly in patients with AIDS, although there is a stronger likelihood of HIV-positive patients developing nonHodgkin's lymphoma.

Examination

- **Palpate the lymph nodes:** the cervical and supraclavicular nodes are most commonly enlarged in Hodgkin's disease
- **Examine the abdomen:** look for hepatic and splenic enlargement
- **Auscultate the chest:** auscultation will usually be normal unless there is segmental collapse or other diagnoses (e.g. tuberculosis, lung cancer)
- **Examine the throat and tonsils (Waldeyer's ring):** pathology of these sites may account for the cervical lymphadenopathy
- **Examine the nervous system:** careful examination may reveal signs of spinal cord compression before any corresponding symptoms occur
- **Examine the venous system:** to exclude superior vena cava compression

Summary of investigative tests

- Complete blood count (CBC) is necessary to exclude leukemias, mononucleosis, and other causes of lymphadenopathy. The degrees of any anemia, leukocytosis, and lymphopenia carry prognostic indications in Hodgkin's disease
- Erythrocyte sedimentation rate (ESR) is raised in Hodgkin's disease and very many other conditions. An ESR of >70mm in the first hour carries an unfavorable prognosis in Hodgkin's disease
- Liver function and serum protein tests (including serum albumin and (LDH)). The level of any rise in LDH and fall in albumin levels in Hodgkin's disease has prognostic significance
- Lymph node biopsy is essential. Excisional node biopsy is better than fine-needle or core-needle biopsy – it allows the diagnosis of lymphomas based on the morphology of the lymph node, which is not offered by needle biopsy. Biopsy of peripheral or mediastinal or intra-abdominal nodes may be needed, and is normally performed by specialists
- Chest X-ray is needed to assess any intrathoracic lymphadenopathy and mediastinal expansion
- CT scans of the thorax and abdomen are useful in staging Hodgkin's disease
- Lymphangiography is usually performed by specialists. It may be useful if there is subdiaphragmatic presentation of Hodgkin's disease with equivocal abdominal CT findings, or there is subdiaphragmatic presentation of Hodgkin's disease with the intention to treat with radiotherapy alone
- Gallium scans can be useful if CT scanning produces equivocal results. Specialists perform these scans in some centers if mediastinal or hilar nodes are involved and as a baseline in patients with bulky disease for better determination of response during and after therapy
- Laparotomy may be needed to stage Hodgkin's disease, but usually only if contemplating supradiaphragmatic radiotherapy and only in patients who do not have lymphocyte-predominant Hodgkin's disease. Staging laparotomy is not recommended routinely and it should not be done in patients who require combination chemotherapy
- Bone marrow biopsy is indicated for staging purposes and is normally carried out by a specialist
- Fertility tests and gonadal tissue harvesting may be requested by the patient as the treatment usually leads to unfertility. This is necessary if the patient wishes to maintain the option of future parenthood, as they are likely to receive high-dose radiotherapy and/or chemotherapy that may render them permanently infertile. Men need to produce a fresh semen sample. Women need oophoropexy at laparotomy if also being performed, or as a separate laparoscopic procedure
- Heterophil antibody test may be performed, which is rapid and inexpensive but may not always be accurate
- HIV tests are necessary in patients with suspected Hodgkin's disease

DIAGNOSTIC DECISION

Diagnosis is from histologic examination of biopsied tissue. Excisional nodal biopsy is required; fine-needle aspiration is inadequate. The biopsied tissue should provide proof of the diagnosis and of the subtype of Hodgkin's disease. A positive biopsy should be followed by attempts to accurately stage the disease.

The natural history, treatment options, and prognosis of Hodgkin's disease depend on:

- The histologic subtype of the disease – this is based on the number of lymphocytes and Reed-Sternberg cells, and of fibrous tissue
- The stage of the disease as defined by the Ann Arbor classification, later modified by the Cotswold convention. Staging depends on the presence of symptoms, the extent of the disease, and its spread

The histologic subtypes of Hodgkin's disease are listed below. In about 5% of patients with Hodgkin's disease, there are no clear classifiable features.

Nodular sclerosis:

- More common in younger patients and in developing countries
- The most common subtype, representing about 60% of cases
- The mediastinal lymph nodes are often first affected

Mixed cellularity:

- Occurs mainly in middle-aged patients
- Is the most common among HIV-infected patients
- The second most common subtype in non-HIV patients, representing about 25% of cases

Lymphocyte depleted:

- Occurs mainly in the elderly
- Represents about 5% of cases, but represents up to 20% of the cases among HIV-infected patients
- Indicates extensive disease and a poorer prognosis
- Has a propensity to involve retroperitoneal lymph nodes and extralymphatic sites
- Most difficult to distinguish from nonHodgkin's lymphoma

Lymphocyte predominant:

- Patients with this subtype are usually young men, often with no symptoms
- Represents about 5% of cases
- Slow-growing and with the best prognosis
- The lymphocytic and histiocytic cells found in this subtype differ from the Reed-Sternberg cells found in the other subtypes
- The disease transforms to nonHodgkin's lymphoma in about 3% of patients with this subtype

One subtype of Hodgkin's disease, nodular lymphocyte-predominant Hodgkin's lymphoma, is considered to be a clinicopathologic entity of B cell origin different from classic Hodgkin's disease. These patients have better prognosis and the REAL Classification of Lymphoid Neoplasms proposed separating nodular lymphocyte-predominant Hodgkin's disease on the basis of immunophenotypic differences.

Staging of Hodgkin's disease:

- Stage I: involvement of a single lymph node region (I), or localized involvement of a single extralymphatic organ or site (IE)
- Stage II: involvement of two or more lymph node regions on the same side of the diaphragm (II), or localized involvement of a single associated extralymphatic organ or site and its regional lymph node(s) with or without involvement of other lymph node regions on the same side of the diaphragm (IIE). The number of lymph node regions may be indicated by a subscript, e.g. II_3
- Stage III: involvement of lymph node regions on the both sides of the diaphragm (III), which may also be accompanied by localized involvement of an associated extralymphatic site or organ (IIIE), by involvement of the spleen (IIIS), or both (IIIE-S)
- Stage IV: disseminated (multifocal) involvement of one or more extralymphatic organs with or without associated lymph node involvement, or isolated extralymphatic organ involvement with distant (nonregional) nodal involvement
- Suffix A: no systemic symptoms
- Suffix B: presence of unexplained fever, night sweats, or weight loss (>10% body weight over preceding 6 months)
- Suffix X: indicates bulky disease – either mediastinal mass occupying over one-third of the mediastinal diameter, or >10cm maximum dimension of a nodal mass on a chest X-ray
- Suffix E: indicates extranodal disease, and the following letters the organ involved: H = liver, L = lung, M = bone marrow, S = spleen, P = pleura, O = bone, D = skin

THE TESTS

Body fluids

COMPLETE BLOOD COUNT WITH DIFFERENTIAL

Description

Venous blood sample.

Advantages/Disadvantages

Advantages:

- Inexpensive
- Readily available

Normal

- Hemoglobin concentration above 12g/dL (7.4mmol/L)
- Total leukocyte count less than 11,000/mcL
- Relative lymphocyte percentage 15–40%
- Absolute lymphocyte count 800–2200/mcL

Abnormal

- The CBC and differential may be entirely normal
- Keep in mind the possibility of false-positive results: atypical lymphocytes seen in a variety of systemic viral illnesses; reactive lymphocytes can be confused with lymphoblasts
- Anemia may occur (Hb less than 10.5g/dL (6.5mmol/L))
- Leukocyte count may be high (up to 15,000/mcL)
- Lymphopenia may occur (lymphocyte count less than 800/mcL)

Cause of abnormal result

- Bone marrow infiltration may be present if there is pancytopenia
- Mild abnormalities of the CBC are nonspecific
- Infectious mononucleosis
- Multiple other causes including cytomegalovirus, human herpesvirus 6, rubella, hepatitis, and toxoplasmosis

ERYTHROCYTE SEDIMENTATION RATE

Description

Venous blood sample.

Advantages/Disadvantages

Advantage: inexpensive

Normal

- Values vary with age
- Less than 20mm in the first hour for adults

Abnormal

Up to 30mm in the first hour.

Drugs, disorders and other factors that may alter results

The ESR is raised in a variety of disorders:

- Infections
- Collagen vascular diseases
- Inflammatory states
- Hyperthyroidism
- Hypothyroidism
- Many neoplasms, especially of the urinary tract

LIVER FUNCTION TESTS AND SERUM PROTEINS

Description

Venous blood sample.

Advantages/Disadvantages

Advantage: inexpensive

Normal

- Alanine aminotransferase (ALT): 0–35U/L
- Serum albumin: 4–6g/dL
- Aspartate aminotransferase (AST): 0–35U/L
- LDH: 50–150U/L

Abnormal

Keep in mind the possibility of a false-positive result for any of these tests.

Cause of abnormal result

Abnormal liver function.

Drugs, disorders and other factors that may alter results

Elevated ALT or AST:

- Alcohol
- Liver disease, e.g. hepatitis, cirrhosis
- Hepatic congestion
- Infectious mononucleosis
- Myocardial infarction
- Myocarditis
- Severe muscle trauma
- Dermatomyositis
- Polymyositis
- Muscular dystrophy
- Drugs, e.g. antibiotics, antihypertensives, heparin, nonsteroidal anti-inflammatory drugs (NSAIDs), amiodarone, chlorpromazine, phenytoin
- Malignancy
- Renal and pulmonary infarction
- Convulsions
- Eclampsia

Elevated LDH:

- Biliary obstruction, cirrhosis, and other liver disease
- Bone disorders, e.g. Paget's disease, rickets, osteomalacia, neoplasms, and metastases
- Hyperthyroidism and hyperparathyroidism
- Ulcerative colitis
- Infectious mononucleosis
- Cytomegalovirus infection
- Sepsis
- Pulmonary infarction
- Congestive heart failure
- Leukemia
- Multiple myeloma
- Pregnancy
- Puberty
- Drugs, e.g. estrogens, albumin, antibiotics

Low serum albumin:
- Liver disease
- Nephrotic syndrome
- Poor nutritional status
- Rapid intravenous hydration
- Inflammatory bowel disease
- Malignancy, e.g. lymphomas
- Chronic inflammatory diseases, e.g. glomerulonephritis
- Pregnancy
- Drugs, e.g. oral contraceptives
- Prolonged immobilization

Biopsy

LYMPH NODE BIOPSY

Description
- Biopsy of suspect tissue, usually from palpable peripheral lymph nodes, but biopsy from mediastinal or intra-abdominal nodes may be required
- Fine-needle aspiration alone is insufficient, as it does not offer diagnosis relayed on the morphology of the lymph node and may delay diagnosis
- Excisional nodal biopsy is recommended as it offers diagnosis relayed on the morphology of the lymph node
- Staining with hematoxylin and eosin can be complemented by immunohistochemistry and flow cytometry
- An experienced pathologist must perform the examination of the specimen. Accurate histologic examination is crucial in making the diagnosis and for staging of the disease

Advantages/Disadvantages

Disadvantages:
- Requires anesthesia
- Risks of infection, hemorrhage, and pain

Abnormal
- Presence of Reed-Sternberg cells
- Relative abundance or paucity of lymphocytes and of fibrous tissue is also important
- Keep in mind the possibility of false-positive results

Cause of abnormal result

Malignant transformation of B cells or their precursors within the lymph nodes, and failure of the helper T cells in destroying the mutated and abnormal B cells.

Drugs, disorders and other factors that may alter results
- NonHodgkin's lymphoma can mimic Hodgkin's disease
- Infections and inflammatory disorders can distort the normal histology of the lymph nodes, causing histologic confusion

Imaging

CHEST X-RAY

Advantages/Disadvantages

Advantages:
- Inexpensive
- Readily available

Disadvantages:
- Interpretation is subjective
- Not accurate enough to evaluate intra-thorax involvement

Abnormal
- There may be hilar enlargement or mediastinal widening
- If the maximum width of any mass on the chest X-ray is more than one-third of the maximum intrathoracic diameter, there is by definition bulky disease, which is an unfavorable prognostic factor
- Another measurement of bulk is of any mass greater than 10cm in maximum diameter. Such bulky masses rarely occur outside the mediastinum

Cause of abnormal result
Hodgkin's disease infiltrating and enlarging mediastinal or hilar lymph nodes.

Drugs, disorders and other factors that may alter results
Any other causes of hilar or mediastinal enlargement may alter the results, e.g. primary lung malignancies, nonHodgkin's lymphoma, TB, sarcoidosis, secondary cancers.

CT SCAN OF THORAX AND/OR ABDOMEN AND PELVIS
Description
Computerized axial tomograms of the abdomen and pelvis; a mandatory procedure for staging.

Advantages/Disadvantages
Advantages:
- Inexpensive and readily available
- Visualization of the extent of any splenic or hepatic enlargement
- Ability to assess stage and spread of the Hodgkin's disease

Disadvantages:
- Interpretation is subjective
- Radiation exposure is not negligible, especially to the ovaries and (to a lesser extent, as they are easier to shield) the testes
- Children and any confused or agitated patient may require sedation

Abnormal
- Evidence of involvement of mesenteric, hepatic, portal, splenic hilar, and retroperitoneal lymph nodes
- Splenic or hepatic enlargement

Cause of abnormal result
Hodgkin's disease affecting subdiaphragmatic sites.

Drugs, disorders and other factors that may alter results
Any other causes of intra-abdominal lymph node enlargement may alter the results, e.g. nonHodgkin's lymphoma, TB, sarcoidosis, secondary cancers.

Special tests
LAPAROTOMY
Description
Inspection of the abdominopelvic contents under direct vision at operation. At the same procedure, the surgeon may undertake:
- Splenectomy
- Random sampling of retroperitoneal nodes
- Liver biopsy
- Oophoropexy if indicated – can be indicated in young patients when fertility is an issue and the plan for irradiation compromises the pelvic area

- Laparotomy is not required for staging Hodgkin's disease in most cases. It has been replaced by CT or magnetic resonance imaging (MRI) examinations for this purpose. Laparotomy has been reserved for those patients with early disease who will be treated with radiation alone
- Laparoscopy is not suitable for staging

Advantages/Disadvantages

Advantages:

- Allows direct inspection of the intra-abdominal and pelvic organs and an opportunity to assess the extent of any spread of the Hodgkin's disease to the lymph nodes, liver, or spleen
- Allows biopsies to be taken from as many sites as needed
- Allows oophoropexy if required and requested

Disadvantages:

- Requires a general anesthetic with the risks of infection, pain, and hemorrhage, and of perioperative death
- It is generally not indicated in patients who have a large mediastinal mass, who will generally receive combined radiotherapy and chemotherapy, patients with clinical stage I disease, and patients who are at low risk of abdominal disease (e.g. females with supradiaphragmatic disease)

Abnormal

- The quality of clinical information gained from laparotomy will depend on the surgeon and pathologist – there will be subjective assessments of normality and degree of abnormality
- There is, therefore, always the possibility of false-positive and of false-negative results

Cause of abnormal result

Spread or extension of Hodgkin's disease.

Drugs, disorders and other factors that may alter results

Any other causes of lymph node, hepatic, or splenic enlargement may alter the results, e.g. primary lung malignancies, nonHodgkin's lymphoma, TB, sarcoidosis, secondary cancers.

Other tests

HETEROPHIL ANTIBODY TEST

Description

Venous blood sample.

Advantages/Disadvantages

Advantage: Rapid, inexpensive, can be performed in the office

Disadvantages:

- Not always accurate – some false-positive results
- Antibodies may not be detectable until 2–3 weeks into illness
- Antibodies not usually detectable in young children
- Antibodies last for months or even lifelong, so does not improve acute infection
- Antibody titer does not correlate with severity of illness
- Normal result may be misleading in immunocompromised patients

Normal

No heterophil antibodies present.

Abnormal

- Keep in mind the possibility of a false-negative or a false-positive result
- Heterophil antibodies present

Cause of abnormal result
Infectious mononucleosis.

Drugs, disorders and other factors that may alter results
Immunocompromised patients may not produce antibodies even when suffering from disease.

HIV TESTS
Description
- Venous blood sample
- HIV status is necessary in patients with suspected Hodgkin's disease as AIDS or AIDS syndromes can produce similar signs and symptoms
- If a patient has both diagnoses, their prognosis for each is worse

Abnormal
Positive HIV tests (HIV antibody, type 1 and HIV type 1 antigen).

Cause of abnormal result
Infection with HIV.

CONSIDER CONSULT

- All patients who have been diagnosed with Hodgkin's disease should be referred for careful staging and treatment planning
- Referral should result in decisions being taken by a multidisciplinary team of cancer specialists

IMMEDIATE ACTION

Refer for immediate specialist care if there is any suspicion of spinal cord compression.

PATIENT AND CAREGIVER ISSUES

Forensic and legal issues

- If storage of sperm or ovarian tissues is offered, the conditions of their ownership, storage, and when and if such material can be utilized and by whom must be agreed
- Arrangements for the use or destruction of such material after the patient's death must also be made

Impact on career, dependants, family, friends

- The diagnosis will cause grave concern to the patient and his or her caregiver
- The overall favorable prognosis should be clarified and emphasized

Health-seeking behavior

- Patients who have painless lymphadenopathy may not seek medical help for some weeks or months
- Adolescents and young adults are notoriously slow to seek medical attention

MANAGEMENT ISSUES

Goals

- To cure Hodgkin's disease
- To prevent recurrences
- To prevent the occurrence of second malignancies after treatment
- To provide the most effective, least incapacitating therapy with fewest side-effects and best long-term safety
- To reduce symptoms and alleviate them at all times, especially if no further active cure is possible

Management in special circumstances

COEXISTING DISEASE

- HIV and AIDS are often associated with malaise, weight loss, and lymphadenopathy
- TB, mononucleosis, and sarcoid can also create diagnostic problems, especially if Hodgkin's disease develops in patients known to have any of these diseases

SPECIAL PATIENT GROUPS

Pregnant women:

- Hodgkin's disease affects primarily young adults, so concomitant pregnancy and Hodgkin's disease are not uncommon
- Treatment choices must be individualized – the wishes of the mother, the severity of the Hodgkin's disease, and the length of the remaining pregnancy must be considered
- Most oncologists would recommend therapeutic abortion in the first trimester
- Chemotherapy treatment in the first trimester is associated with congenital abnormalities in up to 30% of infants
- In the first trimester, radiotherapy above the diaphragm or with uterine shielding is associated with remarkably few congenital abnormalities, but there is no consensus that it should be administrated

- In later pregnancy, aim for induction of delivery at 32–36 weeks
- If there are many symptoms and the treatment cannot be postponed, vinblastine is the chemotherapeutic agent of choice with or without glucocorticoid steroids
- The long-term effects on progeny after chemotherapy in utero are unknown, although present evidence is so far reassuring

Children:

- Refer all children with suspected Hodgkin's disease to centers with a multidisciplinary team of cancer specialists experienced in managing childhood cancers
- Cure rates of >90% are possible in childhood Hodgkin's disease
- Treatment options are broadly similar to those for adults. There will be risks to growth and skeletal maturation, to fertility, to damage of the heart and lungs, and of secondary malignancies
- These secondary malignancies include nonHodgkin's lymphoma, hematopoietic malignancies (e.g. acute myelogenous leukemia) that are associated with chemotherapy, and solid tumors (e.g. sarcomas and breast cancer) associated with radiotherapy
- Children who have had a splenectomy or received high-dose radiation to the spleen should receive immunization with polyvalent pneumococcal vaccine, Hib conjugate vaccine, and meningococcal vaccines as soon as the diagnosis is made, or certainly prior to therapy, and again 2 years after therapy, and a booster every 6 years thereafter
- Autologous bone marrow transplantation may be efficacious in those children who have achieved a second remission with chemotherapy, and should be considered for this group of patients

PATIENT SATISFACTION/LIFESTYLE PRIORITIES

- Elderly patients are unlikely to develop Hodgkin's disease but those who do should be offered the full range of possible therapies, as the response to therapies and the prognosis are good in elderly patients
- Patients with pre-existing disability should be considered for all the possible therapeutic and diagnostic options. When recommending patients for staging laparotomy, the risks of potential morbidity must be considered
- Prognosis is best for patients aged 45 years or less

SUMMARY OF THERAPEUTIC OPTIONS

Choices

Radiation therapy, chemotherapy, or combined therapies are the treatments used in managing Hodgkin's disease. Both chemotherapy and radiation therapy increase the risk of developing secondary solid tumors (e.g. cancers of the lung, breast, and stomach).

- Radiation therapy can be localized to groups of lymph nodes: mantle field – neck, chest, and axillary nodes; abdominal field – para-aortic and splenic pedicle nodes; pelvic nodes. These three fields together constitute total nodal irradiation. Combined abdominal and pelvic fields are called an inverted Y
- Chemotherapy is effective but carries an increased risk of leukemia. The peak in risk is seen about 5 years after the initiation of chemotherapy. The risk is higher in patients who undergo splenectomy and who have advanced disease; the risk is unaffected by concomitant radiation therapy. Chemotherapy is normally based on the certain combinations: ABVD – doxorubicin, bleomycin, vinblastine, dacarbazine; ABV – same as ABVD but without dacarbazine; MOPP – mechlorethamine, vincristine, procarbazine, prednisone; Stanford V – doxorubicin, vinblastine, mechlorethamine, vincristine, bleomycin, etoposide, prednisone
- Granulocyte-colony stimulating factor (G-CSF) are a class of drugs that stimulate the production of granulocytic series (G-CSF) and granulocytic and macrophages series (GM-CSF). Both have been used in supportive care of patients with Hodgkin's disease

- Counseling: all patients will benefit from careful counseling about the treatment options and the prognostic uncertainties
- Vaccinations: polyvalent pneumococcal vaccine and other vaccines should be given prophylactically to all patients before splenectomy or splenic pedicle irradiation
- Sperm and oocyte harvesting: this should be considered and offered to all patients who wish to undertake these procedures, especially young adults with no children

The choice of treatment will depend on the stage of the disease and the histologic subtype and favorable prognostic factors.

Stage IA:

- Radiation therapy alone can achieve a cure of 90% or more
- Favorable prognostic factors include an ESR <50, patients aged <50 years, lymphocyte-predominant or nodular sclerosing histology, lack of B symptoms, and no bulky adenopathy
- Chemotherapy regimens alone or with radiation therapy may prove to be equally effective. The ultimate choice of therapy will then depend on short-term and long-term toxic effects

Stage IB:

These patients with B symptoms must receive combined therapy (radiation + chemotherapy), because those who undergo a laparotomy are upstaged and there is a high risk of relapse in those receiving chemotherapy alone.

Stage IIA:

- Radiation therapy alone can achieve a cure of 80% or more
- Patients with early-stage disease and favorable prognostic features can undergo radiation therapy, without needing laparotomy, after a careful clinical staging

Stage IIB:

Combination radiation with chemotherapy.

Stage IIIA:

- Combined chemotherapy with or without radiation therapy
- New dose-intensive, time-condensed regimens are under clinical evaluation

Stage IIIB:

- First-choice treatment is combined chemotherapy with or without radiation therapy to site of bulky disease – chemotherapy used: ABVD, ABV/MOPP hybrid or ABVD alone for 6–8 months; Stanford V regimen repeated 3 times can also be used
- A meta-analysis of 14 trials found no differences in 10-year survival when comparing chemotherapy alone vs chemotherapy plus radiation
- New dose-intensive, time-condensed regimens are under clinical evaluation

Stage IVA and B:

- Combination therapy is the first choice. Radiation therapy may be used to areas of bulky disease involvement or sites of initial disease – chemotherapy used: ABVD, ABV/MOPP hybrid or ABVD alone for 6–8 months; Stanford V regimen repeated 3 times can also be used
- New dose-intensive, time-condensed regimes are under clinical evaluation Chemotherapy with bone marrow transplantation is under trial

Never

- Never assume persistent lymphadenopathy is due to a self-limited viral cause, even in the presence of the relevant serology
- Never omit to ask about possible B symptoms and perform a thorough examination in all patients with persistent lymphadenopathy

FOLLOW UP

Follow up should be with oncologists who are experienced in the management of Hodgkin's disease. Most oncologists will perform an intensive follow up; relapsed patients are suitable for rescue.

Plan for review

Patients should be reviewed whenever new symptoms appear or previous symptoms recur or worsen, or as outlined below:

- After completion of treatment, a comprehensive post-treatment restaging is indicated, including all imaging studies that were positive at the initial staging
- History and examination: every 2–3 months for the first 2 years, then every 3–4 months for years 3–4, then every 6 months for year 5, annually for life thereafter
- Laboratory studies: CBC, platelets, ESR, chemistry profile every 2–3 months for the first 2 years, then every 3–4 months for years 3–4, then every 6 months for year 5, annually for life thereafter; thyroid-stimulating hormone (TSH) every 6 months if the patient received radiotherapy to the neck
- Chest imaging: chest X-ray every 3 months for the first 2 years, every 6 months up to the 5th year, annually thereafter; CT scans every year for the first 3 years or when abnormalities are found on chest X-ray
- Abdominopelvic imaging: plain X-rays on each visit until all the contrast has gone, if previous lymphangiography has been carried out; CT scan or gallium scan annually for the first 5 years (stages I–II of the disease), every 6 months for 3 years, then annually for years 4–5 for all other stages
- Mammograms: annually if the patient has received radiation therapy above the diaphragm. Initiate 8–10 years post-therapy if age <30 years at time of initial therapy; initiate at age 40 for all other women
- Counseling: reproduction, psychosocial, cardiovascular, breast self-examination, skin cancer risk, leukemic risk
- All stages: after completion of therapy, restage and image all previous positive areas plus bone marrow biopsy if initially positive. Depending on the response, further courses of chemotherapy are required (ABVD, MOPP/ABVD, or Stanford V) with or without further radiotherapy

Patients receiving radiation therapy or chemotherapy may well be immunocompromised and should seek prompt medical attention for even trivial-seeming symptoms or fever as soon as it is apparent, or with any malaise or nonspecific lack of wellbeing.

Information for patient or caregiver

- Treatments are effective but long-term follow up post-treatment of every patient is essential
- There are risks of developing secondary cancers many years after the first treatment
- There are risks of infertility especially after chemotherapy and subdiaphragmatic radiotherapy, so the options of sperm and oocyte storage should be discussed

DRUGS AND OTHER THERAPIES: DETAILS

Drugs

DOXORUBICIN

A cytotoxic antibiotic given by intravenous infusion. Dexrazoxane is approved by the Food and Drug Administration (FDA) to protect against the cardiotoxicity of this drug.

Dose

Between 30 and 50mg/m^2/ infusion. Total dose delivered must not exceed 450mg/m^2.

Efficacy

High when used in combination with other cytotoxic drugs.

Risks/Benefits

Risks:

- Use caution in hepatic impairment
- Specialist supervision required

Benefit: prolongs life and disease-free interval when given as part of a combination (ABVD, ABV, or Stanford V)

Side-effects and adverse reactions

- Cardiovascular system: cardiotoxicity
- Gastrointestinal: nausea, vomiting
- Metabolic: bone marrow suppression
- Skin: alopecia, local severe skin necrosis

Interactions (other drugs)

■ **Cyclosporin (increased toxicity)** ■ **Stavudine (inhibited action of stavudine)**

Contraindications

■ **Patients with cardiomyopathy and/or diminishment of cardiac ejection fraction have absolute contraindication to the use of doxorubicin** ■ **Hypersensitivity to doxorubicin** ■ **Pregnancy**

Acceptability to patient

Benefits of increased survival rates outweigh the toxic effects of nausea, vomiting, myelosuppression, alopecia, and mucositis.

Follow up plan

- Doxorubicin is largely excreted by the biliary tract and an elevated bilirubin concentration is an indication to reduce the dose; serum bilirubin should therefore be monitored
- It can also cause myelosuppression, so frequent CBCs are needed
- Higher cumulative doses can result in cardiomyopathy – sequential echocardiogram and radionucleotide ejection fractions may assist in safely limiting total dosage
- ABVD is usually given for 6–8 months, and MOPP/ABVD also for 6–8 months; Stanford V is usually given for 3 months

Patient and caregiver information

Patients should seek urgent medical attention with any intercurrent fever or illness even if seemingly trivial, such as a sore throat.

BLEOMYCIN

A cytotoxic antibiotic given by intravenous infusion.

Dose

Usually 10–15 U/m^2.

Efficacy

High when used in combination with other cytotoxic drugs.

Risks/Benefits

Risks:

- Use caution in poor circulation
- Expensive treatment
- Specialist supervision required

Benefit: prolongs life and disease-free interval when given as part of a combination (ABVD or ABV)

Side-effects and adverse reactions
- Gastrointestinal: nausea, vomiting
- Metabolic: bone marrow suppression
- Skin: pain, burning at site of injection, coldness, paleness of fingers, rash, pruritus, nail loss, alopecia

Interactions (other drugs)
None listed.

Contraindications
- Patients with marked myelosuppression
- Pregnancy
- Hypersensitivity to bleomycin

Acceptability to patient
- Benefits of increased survival rates outweigh the toxic effects: dermatologic, increased pigmentation and mucositis
- Long-term pulmonary fibrosis may occur

Follow up plan
Frequent checks of the respiratory system are needed – an increase in breathlessness, basal crepitations or suspicious chest X-ray changes are an indication to cease use of this drug.

Patient and caregiver information
- Hypersensitivity reactions manifested by chills and fevers commonly occur a few hours after administration and may be prevented by the simultaneous administration of corticosteroids
- Patients who have received extensive (>100,000U) treatment with bleomycin may be at risk of developing respiratory failure if a general anesthetic is given using high-inspired oxygen concentrations. Anesthesiologists should be warned if a patient has ever received bleomycin

VINBLASTINE
A vinca alkaloid given by intravenous injection.

Dose
5–10mg/m^2.

Efficacy
High when used in combination with other cytotoxic drugs.

Risks/Benefits
- Risk: specialist supervision required
- Benefit: prolongs life and disease-free interval when given as part of a combination (ABVD, ABV, or Stanford V)

Side-effects and adverse reactions
- Gastrointestinal: nausea, vomiting
- Metabolic: bone marrow suppression
- Skin: pain, burning at site of injection, coldness, paleness of fingers, rash, pruritus, nail loss, alopecia

Interactions (other drugs)
None listed.

Contraindications

- Hypersensitivity to vinblastine
- Pregnancy

Acceptability to patient

Benefits of increased survival rates outweigh the toxic effects, which include toxic neuropathy (peripheral paresthesia, abdominal pain and constipation, motor weakness), myelosuppression, and reversible alopecia.

Follow up plan

Examine the nervous system and reduce the dose or stop vinblastine therapy if there are signs or symptoms of neuropathy.

Patient and caregiver information

- Patients should seek urgent medical attention with any intercurrent fever or illness even if seemingly trivial, such as a sore throat
- Alopecia is usually reversible
- Patients should report any weakness, numbness, or constipation. Peripheral neurologic toxicity from vinblastine will recover slowly but completely

DACARBAZINE

An antineoplastic drug given intravenously.

Dose

150mg/m^2 infusion.

Efficacy

High when used in combination with other cytotoxic drugs.

Risks/Benefits

- Risk: specialist supervision required
- Benefit: prolongs life and disease-free interval when given as part of the ABVD combination

Side-effects and adverse reactions

- Gastrointestinal: nausea, vomiting
- Metabolic: bone marrow suppression
- Skin: pain, burning at site of injection, coldness, paleness of fingers, rash, pruritus, nail loss, alopecia

Interactions (other drugs)

None listed.

Contraindications

- Hypersensitivity to dacarbazine
- Pregnancy

Acceptability to patient

Benefits of increased survival rates outweigh the toxic effects, and appropriate care to these effects can diminish them.

Patient and caregiver information

- The nausea and vomiting may be intense and very unpleasant but will be transient
- Patients should seek urgent medical attention with any intercurrent fever or illness even if seemingly trivial, such as a sore throat

MECHLORETHAMINE

- An antineoplastic drug given by fast-running intravenous infusion
- Formerly known as nitrogen mustard

Dose

The dosage of mechlorethamine HCl varies with the clinical situation, the therapeutic response, and the magnitude of hematologic depression. A total dose of 0.4mg/kg of body weight for each course usually is given either as a single dose or in divided doses of 0.1–0.2mg/kg/day. Dosage should be based on ideal dry body weight.

Efficacy

High when used in combination with other cytotoxic drugs.

Risks/Benefits

- Risk: specialist supervision required
- Benefit: prolongs life and disease-free interval when given as part of the MOPP combination

Side-effects and adverse reactions

- Gastrointestinal: nausea, vomiting
- Metabolic: bone marrow suppression
- Skin: pain, burning at site of injection, coldness, paleness of fingers, rash, pruritus, nail loss, alopecia

Interactions (other drugs)

None listed.

Contraindications

- Hypersensitivity to meclorethamine
- Pregnancy

Acceptability to patient

Benefits of increased survival rates outweigh the toxic effects: mainly severe vomiting.

Patient and caregiver information

The nausea and vomiting may be intense and very unpleasant, but will be transient.

VINCRISTINE

Vincristine is a vinca alkaloid given by intravenous injection.

Dose

0.5–1mg/treatment.

Efficacy

High when used in combination with other cytotoxic drugs.

Risks/Benefits

Risks:

- Specialist supervision required
- Doses above 2mg/m^2 can cause a diminishment of intestinal movements leading to abdominal cramps and nausea
- In extreme cases it can simulate an acute abdomen, with acute lymphocytic leukemia characteristics, clinical and radiologic, that reverses with clinical treatment and no surgery is needed

Benefit: prolongs life and disease-free interval when given as part of the MOPP combination

Side-effects and adverse reactions

- Cardiovascular system: cardiotoxicity
- Gastrointestinal: nausea, vomiting
- Metabolic: bone marrow suppression
- Skin: alopecia, local severe skin necrosis

Interactions (other drugs)

Itraconazole (increased neurotoxicity).

Contraindications

- Hypersensitivity to vincristine
- Pregnancy

Acceptability to patient

Benefits of increased survival rates outweigh the toxic effects, which include toxic neuropathy (peripheral paresthesia, abdominal pain and constipation, motor weakness, myelosuppression, and alopecia).

Follow up plan

Examine the nervous system and reduce the dose or stop vincristine therapy if there are signs or symptoms of neuropathy.

Patient and caregiver information

- Patients should seek urgent medical attention with any intercurrent fever or illness even if seemingly trivial, such as a sore throat
- Alopecia is usually reversible
- Patients should report any weakness, numbness, or constipation
- Peripheral neurologic toxicity from vinblastine will recover slowly but completely

PROCARBAZINE

An oral antineoplastic agent derived from monoamine oxidase inhibitors.

Dose

50–300mg/day.

Efficacy

High when used in combination with other cytotoxic drugs.

Risks/Benefits

- Risk: specialist supervision required
- Benefit: prolongs life and disease-free interval when given as part of the MOPP combination

Side-effects and adverse reactions

- Cardiovascular system: cardiotoxicity
- Gastrointestinal: nausea, vomiting
- Metabolic: bone marrow suppression
- Skin: alopecia, local severe skin necrosis

Interactions (other drugs)

Concomitant alcohol intake can cause unpleasant feeling, disulfiram-like and must be avoided.

Contraindications

- Hypersensitivity to procarbazine
- Pregnancy

Acceptability to patient

Benefits of increased survival rates outweigh the toxic effects, which include nausea, myelosuppression, and a hypersensitivity rash precluding further use of the drug.

Patient and caregiver information

- Must be stopped if the patient develops a hypersensitivity rash
- Alcohol ingestion may cause a disulfiram-like reaction, so alcohol should not be taken

PREDNISONE

A systemic glucocorticosteroid.

Dose

5–60mg/day taken orally.

Efficacy

High when used in combination with cytotoxic drugs.

Risks/Benefits

Risks:

- Use caution in congestive heart failure, diabetes mellitus, and osteoporosis
- Use caution in hypertension (ophthalmic) and glaucoma
- Use caution in renal disease, ulcerative colitis, and peptic ulcer
- Use caution in the elderly
- Prednisone taken in doses higher than 7.5mg for a period of 3 weeks or longer may lead to clinically relevant suppression of the pituitary-adrenal axis

Side-effects and adverse reactions

- Side-effects are minimized by short duration of therapy
- Cardiovascular system: hypertension, thromboembolism
- Central nervous system: insomnia, euphoria, depression, psychosis, seizures
- Endocrine: adrenal suppression, impaired glucose tolerance, growth suppression in children
- Eyes, ears, nose, and throat: cataract, glaucoma, blurred vision
- Gastrointestinal: dyspepsia, peptic ulceration, esophagitis, oral candidiasis
- Musculoskeletal: proximal myopathy, osteoporosis
- Skin: delayed healing, acne, striae, fragile skin

Interactions (other drugs)

■ Aminoglutethimide (increased clearance of prednisone) ■ Diuretics (effects inhibited) ■ Antidiabetics (hypoglycemic effect inhibited) ■ Antihypertensives (effects inhibited) ■ Barbiturates (increased clearance of prednisone) ■ Cardiac glycosides (toxicity increased) ■ Cholestyramine, colestipol (may reduce absorption of corticosteroids) ■ Ketoconazole ■ Clarithromycin, erythromycin, troleandomycin (may enhance steroid effect) ■ Rifampin (may inhibit hepatic clearance of prednisone) ■ Cyclosporine (may increase levels of both drugs; may cause seizures) ■ Isoniazid (reduced plasma levels of isoniazid) ■ Nonsteroidal anti-inflammatory drugs (increased risks of bleeeding) ■ Warfarin (alters clotting time) ■ Oral contraceptives (enhanced effects of corticosteroids) ■ Salicylates (increased clearance of salicylates)

Contraindications

■ Systemic infection ■ Avoid live virus vaccines in those receiving immunosuppressive doses ■ History of tuberculosis ■ Cushing's syndrome ■ Recent myocardial infarction

Acceptability to patient

- Benefits on increased survival rates outweigh the toxic effects: central nervous system (CNS) depression, seizures, thromboembolism, weight gain, thinning of the skin, gastrointestinal hemorrhage, adrenal suppression, and osteoporosis
- Patients tend to be very cautious about corticosteroid use because of fear of side-effects and misinformation and confusion about anabolic corticosteroids
- It is worthwhile explaining the benefits and potentially life-saving effects of corticosteroids and that they are different from the anabolic corticosteroids renowned for their misuse in sports

Follow up plan

- All patients taking long-term corticosteroids should be monitored
- The dose should be kept to a minimum
- Monitor serum potassium and glucose

Patient and caregiver information

- Patients need accurate and clear information about the benefits and risks of long-term oral corticosteroids
- Patients should be warned not to stop taking corticosteroids suddenly because of the risks of adrenal suppression
- Adrenal insufficiency can occur up to one year after cessation of oral corticosteroid therapy
- Adrenal insufficiency can present with fatigue, depression, anorexia, weight loss, weakness, and dizziness

ETOPOSIDE

An oral or intravenous antineoplastic drug related to the vinca alkaloids.

Dose

120–240mg/m^2/day for 5 days. These doses can increase if high-dose chemotherapy/bone marrow transplantation are performed.

Efficacy

High when used in combination with other cytotoxic drugs.

Risks/Benefits

- Risk: specialist supervision required
- Benefit: prolongs life and disease-free interval when given as part of the Stanford V combination

Side-effects and adverse reactions

- Cardiovascular system: cardiotoxicity
- Gastrointestinal: nausea, vomiting
- Metabolic: bone marrow suppression
- Skin: alopecia, local severe skin necrosis

Interactions (other drugs)

None listed.

Contraindications

- Hypersensitivity to etoposide
- Pregnancy

Acceptability to patient

Benefits of increased survival rates outweigh the toxic effects, which include alopecia, myelosuppression, nausea, and vomiting.

Patient and caregiver information

Patients should seek urgent medical attention with any intercurrent fever or illness even if seemingly trivial, such as a sore throat.

GRANULOCYTE-COLONY STIMULATING FACTOR

G-CSF are a class of drugs that stimulate the production of granulocytic series (G-CSF) and granulocytic and macrophages series (GM-CSF). Both have been used in supportive care of patients with Hodgkin's disease.

Dose

Efficacy

- G-CSF stimulates leukocyte production following suppression of that production by irradiation or chemotherapy
- Can be given with or after such therapy

Risks/Benefits

Risks:

- Use caution when administered simultaneously with cytotoxic chemotherapy and radiotherapy
- Risk of maligant cell growth

Benefit: reduces leukopenia and therefore reduces the risk of overwhelming sepsis and treatment-related death

Side-effects and adverse reactions

- Cardiovascular system: transient hypotension, cutaneous vasculitis, deep vein thrombosis
- Central nervous system: headache, fever
- Gastrointestinal: diarrhea, nausea, vomiting
- Genitourinary: dysuria
- Hematologic: thrombocytopenia, anemia
- Metabolism: disturbances in liver enzymes and serum uric acid, proteinuria, hematuria, transient decrease in blood glucose, splenic enlargement, hepatomegaly
- Musculoskeletal: pain, osteoporosis, exacerbation of rheumatoid arthritis
- Respiratory: adult respiratory distress syndrome
- Skin: alopecia, rash

Interactions (other drugs)

Drugs that potentiate neutrophil release.

Contraindications

- **Known hypersensitivity to *Escherichia coli*-derived proteins** ■ **Known hypersensitivity to filgrastim or lenograstim**

Acceptability to patient

High as its use in some situations can diminish the myelosupression with few side-effects.

Radiation therapy

RADIATION THERAPY

- Has been successfully used in the management of Hodgkin's disease for more than 40 years
- Is the first-choice treatment used alone for treating early-stage disease, and is used together with chemotherapy in nearly all other cases

Efficacy
- Very high
- Can be used as the sole therapy in early stage without massive mediastinal involvement, and as combination therapy with chemotherapy at all other stages
- When used as sole therapy in stage IA/IIA patients, cure rates of >90% can be expected
- Given at low doses to uninvolved sites and at higher doses to regions of initial nodal involvement

Risks/Benefits
Risks:
- Early side-effects include skin burning at the site of irradiation
- Late side-effects include sclerosis of coronary arteries if mediastinal irradiation is used, and subsequent ischemic heart disease
- Late systemic side-effects include an increased risk of subsequent solid tumors, especially cancers of the bone, breast, lung, thyroid, and colon. At 15-year follow-up, the risk of second tumors is 13%; 75% of second tumors occur within radiation ports

Benefit: overall, the benefits far outweigh the risks – radiation therapy may effect cure rates of >90%

Acceptability to patient
High as long-term efficacy is high.

Follow up plan
Patients should be followed up for life because of the risks of recurrent disease and of subsequent solid tumors.

Patient and caregiver information
The high risks of later developing subsequent solid tumors must be discussed before commencing therapy.

Other therapies

VACCINATIONS
The following prophylactic vaccinations should be given to all patients undergoing splenectomy or splenic pedicle irradiation:
- Polyvalent pneumococcal vaccine
- *Haemophilus influenzae* vaccine
- Influenza vaccine
- Meningococcal vaccine

Efficacy
All have high efficacy.

Risks/Benefits
- Risk: there is an increased risk of sepsis from encapsulated organisms in splenectomized patients
- Benefit: the relevant vaccinations are known and established effective preventive agents against the relevant organisms

Acceptability to patient
High – have few side-effects and offer protection against potentially fatal diseases.

Follow up plan

- Influenza vaccines should be given annually – the vaccine used should be the preparation advised by the relevant health authorities for that year, and will depend on the particular strains of influenzavirus predicted to be prevalent for the near future
- Pneumococcal vaccine – titers of antipneumococcal antibody should be measured every 3 years after vaccination, and revaccination offered if the titers are low or falling; the initial dose should ideally be given 2 weeks before splenectomy or the start of chemotherapy
- *H. influenzae* vaccine – a single dose ideally 2 weeks before splenectomy is required and no revaccination is necessary
- Meningococcal vaccine – a single dose of meningitis C vaccine is required

Patient and caregiver information

- Side-effects tend to be minor and transient
- Does not preclude the need to seek urgent medical attention if signs of fever or seemingly trivial infections occur

EFFICACY OF THERAPIES

- Hodgkin's disease is a curable disease in close to 80% of cases – the treatment options, prognosis, and disease-free survival depend heavily on the staging of the disease and prognostic factors of each individual
- Chemotherapy and/or radiotherapy are the cornerstone of treatment
- In cases of relapse, high-dose chemotherapy and stem cell support can be used

Review period

- Patients on active treatment should initially be reviewed weekly, then every 2 weeks once stable for 1–3 months, then monthly for the first 6 months, and annually thereafter for life
- Patients who have received any active treatment will need lifelong surveillance to detect any secondary tumors or cardiovascular problems

PROGNOSIS

- The improvement in 5-year survival is unmatched in the US by any other cancer over the last 40 years
- Newly diagnosed patients have an overwhelming likelihood of being cured provided that the most appropriate therapy is selected and administered
- Cure rates have increased to such an extent that the overriding treatment considerations often relate to long-term toxicity, especially for patients with early- or intermediate-stage disease
- Even for advanced disease, there are still impressive cure rates
- Cure rates of 80% for early stage disease are usual
- Cure rates may be less for more advanced disease but are higher in children
- Even after recurrence, cure rates may approach 80%
- Effective drug combinations can produce prolonged disease-free survival in most patients who have recurrent disease when radiation therapy was the initial treatment
- Patients whose disease recurs following combination chemotherapy may be salvaged when treated with another regimen
- Is the main cause of death over the first 15 years after treatment
- By 15–20 years after therapy, the cumulative mortality from a second malignancy will exceed the cumulative mortality from Hodgkin's disease
- The International Prognosis Index is useful for stratifying patients as it provides a good estimate of the event-free survival at 5 years
- Special attention must be given to the possibility of second tumors even after 10–15 years after the end of therapy

Therapeutic failure

- For patients who relapse with stage IV disease and massive mediastinal involvement, autologous stem cell (or bone marrow) transplantation can be considered
- The patient's bone marrow is harvested and the patient then receives massive total body radiation before receiving an intravenous autologous transfusion of his or her bone marrow

Recurrence

- Recurrence is usually first discovered by the patient (55%), by physical examination in asymptomatic patients (14%), by chest X-ray (23%), by abdominal X-ray (7%), or by laboratory studies in 1%
- Patients who may have relapsed should undergo biopsy and the relapse must be confirmed histologically
- Management of relapse is similar to management of the initial disease, and will depend on the anatomical site(s) of the relapse, its staging, and its histologic features

Terminal illness

- Symptomatic relief of pain (opiates may be needed) and anemia (blood transfusions may help)
- Nutritional supplementation, counseling, and emotional support should always be offered
- Night sweats and pruritus can be disabling and resistant to many conventional therapies

COMPLICATIONS

- Leukemia, especially acute nonlymphocytic, may occur in patients treated with chemotherapy or combined chemotherapy and radiotherapy – after MOPP (mechlorethamine, vincristine, procarbozine, prednisone), there is a peak incidence at 5–9 years after commencement of chemotherapy and an overall risk of 3%; after ABVD (doxorubicin, bleomycin, vinblastine, dacarbazine), the 10-year risk of developing leukemia is less than 1%
- Second solid tumors, especially of the colon, lung, bone, breast, and thyroid, can occur in patients who received radiation therapy with or without chemotherapy. The overall risk is 13% at 15 years. The risk of lung cancer in patients whose Hodgkin's disease was treated with chemotherapy is increased if the patient smokes. Breast cancer follows more commonly in women treated before age 30 years
- Risk of nonHodgkin's lymphoma also increases but is not related to type or extent of treatment
- Other complications of irradiation include hypothyroidism and cardiovascular disease
- Other complications of chemotherapy include male and female infertility
- Fatigue is a commonly reported symptom of patients who have completed chemotherapy and usually lasts up to 6 months after completion of radiotherapy

CONSIDER CONSULT

Refer any patient who has the following even after treatment:

- Any sign or symptom of their Hodgkin's disease
- Any sign or symptom that may possibly be due to the development of any of the secondary tumors associated with the treatment
- Any sign or symptom of cardiac or thyroid disease

PREVENTION

- Hodgkin's disease is probably caused by a combination of environmental and genetic factors along with a susceptible immune system
- Exact triggers and factors are not known
- Although there is an association with Epstein-Barr virus infection, this factor is not invariably present
- There are no preventive measures that are or might be effective
- It is not known whether mass immunization against the Epstein-Barr virus would reduce the incidence of Hodgkin's disease

PREVENT RECURRENCE

Beyond vigorous management of the initial presentation and ensuring complete elimination of the tumor, there are no other means available that have been shown to reduce recurrences.

RESOURCES

ASSOCIATIONS

The Leukemia and Lymphoma Society
1311 Mamaroneck Avenue
White Plains, NY 10605–5221
Tel: (914) 949-5213 or (80) 955-4572
www.leukemia-lymphoma.org

National Cancer Institute
NCI Public Inquiries Office
Building 31, Room 10A03
31 Center Drive, MSC 2580
Bethesda, MD 20892–2580
Tel: (800) 422 6237 or (800) A-CANCER
www.nci.nih.gov

National Comprehensive Cancer Network (NCCN)
50 Huntingdon Pike, Suite 200
Rockledge, PA 19046
Tel: (215) 728-4788
Patient information service tel: (88) 909-NCCN
www.nccn.org

American Cancer Society
1599 Clifton Road NE
Atlanta, GA, 30329–4257
Tel: (404) 320-3333 or (800) ACS-2345
www.cancer.org

KEY REFERENCES

- NCCN Practice Guidelines for Hodgkin's Disease. Version 2000. Available from www.nccn.org
- Torrey PJ, Poen C, Hoppe RT. Detection of relapse in early-stage Hodgkin's disease: role of routine follow-up studies. J Clin Oncol 1997;17:253–61
- Leopold KA, Canellos GP, Rosenthal D, et al. Stage IA-11B Hodgkin's disease: staging and treatment of patients with large mediastinal adenopathy. J Clin Oncol 1989;7:1059–65
- Leoffler M, Brosteanu O, Hasenclever D, et al. Meta-analysis of chemotherapy versus combined modality treatment trials in Hodgkin's disease. J Clin Oncol 1998;16:818–29
- Longo DL, Russo A, Duffey PL, et al. Treatment of advanced-stage mediastinal Hodgkin's disease: the case for combined modality treatment. J Clin Oncol 1991;9:227–35
- Cannellos GP, Anderson JR, Propert KJ, et al. Chemotherapy of advanced Hodgkin's disease with MOPP, ABVD or MOPP alternating with ABVD. New Engl J Med 1992;327:1478–84
- Duggan D, Petroni G, Johnson J, et al. MOPP/ABV versus ABVD for advanced Hodgkin's disease. Proceed Am Soc Clin Oncol 1996;415:A-1271
- Bonfante V, Santaro A, Viviani S, et al. ABVD in the treatment of Hodgkin's disease. Sem Oncol 1992;19:38–45
- Fabian CJ, Mansfield CM, Dahlberg S, et al. Low-dose involved field radiation after chemotherapy in advanced Hodgkin's disease: a Southwest Oncology Group randomized study. Ann Int Med 1994;120:903–12
- Viviani S, Belladonna G, Santoro A, et al. Alternating versus hybrid MOPP and ABVD combinations in advanced Hodgkin's disease: ten-year results J Clin Oncol 1996;14:1421–30
- Longo DL, Glastein E, Duffey PL, et al. Alternating MOPP and ABVD chemotherapy plus mantle-field radiation therapy on patients with massive mediastinal Hodgkin's disease. J Clin Oncol 1997;15:3338–46
- Connors JM, Klimo P, Adams G, et al. Treatment of advanced Hodgkin's disease with chemotherapy: comparison of MOPP/ABV hybrid regime with alternating courses of MOPP and ABVD: a report from the National Cancer Institute of Canada Clinical Trials Group. J Clin Oncol 1997;15:1638–45
- Bartlett NL, Rosenberg SA, Hoppe RT, et al. Brief chemotherapy, Stanford V, and adjuvant radiotherapy for bulky or advanced-stage Hodgkin's disease: a preliminary report. J Clin Oncol 1995;13:1080–88

- Horning SJ. Eastern Cooperative Oncology Group: Phase III randomized study of doxorubicin, bleomycin, vinblastine, and dacarbazine (ABVD) versus doxorubicin, vinblastine, vincristine, bleomycin, mechlorethamine, etoposide and prednisone (Stanford V) with or without radiotherapy in patients with locally extensive or advanced stage Hodgkin's Disease with 0–2 risk factors (summary last modified 11/2000), E-2496, clinical trial, active 5/01/2000
- The Advisory Committee on Immunization Practices (ACIP): Recommendations of the Advisory Committee on Immunization Practices (ACIP): use of vaccines and immune globulins for persons with altered immunocompetence. Morbid Mortal Wkly Rep 1993;42 (RR-4):1–18
- Ng AK, Mauch PM. Radiation therapy in Hodgkin's lymphoma. Seminars in Hemat 1999;36:290–302
- Tarbell NJ, Thompson L, Mauch P. Thoracic irradiation in Hodgkin's disease: disease control and long term complications. Int J Radiat Biol Physics 1990;18:275–81
- Sears JD, Greven KM, Ferree CR, et al. Definitive irradiation in the treatment of Hodgkin's disease: analysis of outcome, prognostic factors and long term complications. Cancer 1997;79:145–51
- Gobbi PG; Cavalli C; Gendarini A, et al. Re-evaluation of prognostic significance of symptoms in Hodgkin's disease. Cancer 1985;15;56:2874–80
- A prognostic score for advanced Hodgkin's disease. International Prognostic Factors Project on Advanced Hodgkin's Disease Hasenclever D; Diehl V N Engl J Med 1998;19;339:1506–14

FAQS

Question 1

If a fine-needle aspiration (FNA) product shows a Reed-Sternberg cell, is it still necessary to perform a biopsy?

ANSWER 1

Most of the time yes. The product of FNA cannot usually be used to classify the disease.

Question 2

Which patients should be spared laparotomy?

ANSWER 2

Hodgkin's patients should be spared a laparotomy if possible due to its association with many complications. Its use should be restricted only to those with clinical stage Ia/IIa and without good prognosis signs.

Question 3

How long should a patient who had Hodgkin's disease be followed?

ANSWER 3

After 5 years, the patient may visit the doctor annually, but there are no strict rules. Most recurrences are detected by the patient rather than the doctor.

Question 4

Are the unpleasant side-effects of chemotherapy manageable?

ANSWER 4

Yes. With the development of new drugs, few patients have major problems with it, and the treatment is usually performed on an outpatient basis. Mainly, the inhibitors of serotonin receptors (ondansetron and similar) and CSF have been shown to be of crucial importance in the management of these patients. Only a few have heavy side-effects and need more intensive care.

CONTRIBUTORS

Gordon H Baustian, MD
Otavio A Clark, MD
Januario E Castro, MD

IDIOPATHIC THROMBOCYTOPENIC PURPURA

SUMMARY INFORMATION

DESCRIPTION

- Low platelet count, usually <100,000/mm^3 (<100x10^9/L)
- Purpura, bleeding from mucous membranes, and prolonged bleeding time
- More than 90% of children have acute onset, often preceded by a viral illness, and the condition resolves on its own
- In adults it is most often chronic, with insidious onset of easy bruising or minor bleeding
- Hemorrhage represents the most serious complication, and intracranial hemorrhage is the most frequent cause of death, occurring in 1–2% of patients diagnosed with idiopathic thrombocytopenic purpura

URGENT ACTION

Patients who bleed and/or have platelet count of <10,000/mm^3 (<10x10^9/L) should be transferred to the emergency department because of the serious risk of morbidity and mortality from bleeding, particularly intracranial hemorrhage or if patients are actively bleeding.

KEY! DON'T MISS!

Acute onset in an adult usually signals a more rapid and severe course, and should alert the physician to the possibility of serious hemorrhage.

ICD9 CODE
287.3 Primary thrombocytopenia.

SYNONYMS
- Immune thrombocytopenic purpura
- Primary autoimmune thrombocytopenic purpura
- Autoimmune thrombocytopenic purpura
- ITP
- Werlhof's disease
- Postinfectious thrombocytopenia

CARDINAL FEATURES
- Low platelet count, <100,000/mm^3 (<100x10^9/L)
- Purpura, bleeding from mucous membranes, and prolonged bleeding time
- Diagnosis of exclusion, in which thrombocytopenia exists in the absence of any obvious causative factors, such as disease or drugs
- Two clinical pictures: acute idiopathic thrombocytopenic purpura (ITP) and chronic ITP. Acute ITP often follows a viral infection and resolves spontaneously within 3 months. Chronic ITP typically presents with an insidious onset of easy bruising or minor bleeding over a number of months, with no antecedent infection, and persists for longer than 6 months
- More than 90% of children who present with ITP have the acute form
- Most adults who present with ITP have the chronic form
- Hemorrhage represents the most serious complication, and intracranial hemorrhage is the most frequent cause of death, occurring in 1–2% of patients diagnosed with ITP
- Secondary immune thrombocytopenic purpura presents as ITP, but as a result of a disease process (e.g. HIV infection and systemic lupus erythematosus), or in association with drugs (e.g. heparin and alcohol)

CAUSES
Common causes
ITP:
An abnormal autoantibody (immunoglobulin G) binds to the platelet membrane, causing their removal by the spleen.

Secondary immune thrombocytopenic purpura:
- HIV infection
- Collagen vascular diseases, such as systemic lupus erythematosus
- Lymphoproliferative disorders, such as chronic lymphocytic leukemia
- Drug-induced immune thrombocytopenic purpura (e.g. alcohol, heparin, quinine/quinidine, sulfonamides)

Rare causes
Secondary immune thrombocytopenic purpura:
- Herpes group infections
- Acute hepatitis
- Tuberculosis
- Hodgkin's disease

Serious causes
ITP: if platelet count drops below 20,000/mm^3 (20x10^9/L), then the disease may become serious.

Contributory or predisposing factors

- Acute viral illness (in children)
- Recent live virus immunization (in children)
- Age
- Cardiopulmonary bypass
- Hypersplenism
- Antiphospholipid antibody syndrome

EPIDEMIOLOGY

Incidence and prevalence

Many cases of acute ITP, particularly in children, are mild and self-limiting, and as such may not come to the attention of a clinician.

INCIDENCE

It has been estimated that the total incidence of ITP among adults in the US may be as high as 114/million/year.

Demographics

AGE

- Can affect individuals of any age; however, the peak incidence occurs in children aged 2–5 years and adults aged 20–50 years
- Onset in a patient older than 60 years is rare; thrombocytopenia is more likely to be due to myelodysplastic syndromes, acute leukemia, and myelophthisis (marrow infiltration)
- Approx. 40% of diagnoses are made in children under 10 years old
- Spontaneous remission occurs in more than 80% of children, but is uncommon in adults

GENDER

- Children: males and females affected equally
- Adults: females affected more often than males (3:1)

DIFFERENTIAL DIAGNOSIS

Thrombotic thrombocytopenic purpura

Thrombotic thrombocytopenic purpura is a potentially life-threatening hemolytic anemia; the precise cause is unknown.

FEATURES

- Thrombocytopenia with petechiae and purpura, especially on the lower extremities
- Fever
- Microangiopathic hemolytic anemia
- Neurologic dysfunction
- Renal injury

Hemolytic uremic syndrome

Hemolytic uremic syndrome is a systemic illness that usually occurs in children under 4 years, and causes renal failure.

FEATURES

- Usually preceded by gastroenteritis or upper respiratory tract infection
- Sudden onset
- Irritability, pallor, weakness, and lethargy
- Oliguria
- Dehydration
- Edema
- Hepatosplenomegaly
- Microangiopathic hemolytic anemia
- Thrombocytopenia, with petechiae
- Acute renal failure

Myelodysplastic syndromes

Myelodysplastic syndromes (MDS) form a group of acquired hematopoietic stem cell disorders.

FEATURES

- Anemia: fatigue, shortness of breath, lightheadedness, angina
- Leukopenia: fever, infection
- Thrombocytopenia with epistaxis and purpura
- Skin infiltrates

Disseminated intravascular coagulation

Disseminated intravascular coagulation (DIC) is a systemic illness with simultaneous clotting and bleeding.

FEATURES

- Often associated with sepsis, and occasionally with disseminated cancers
- Can produce widespread organ damage, including to the brain and kidneys
- Thrombocytopenia is common, with purpura

Acute leukemias

Acute leukemias are caused by proliferation and accumulation of abnormal blasts in the bone marrow and other tissues.

FEATURES

- Fever
- Bleeding, including petechiae, easy bruising, or oozing
- Bone pain, pallor, and fatigue
- Splenomegaly
- Hepatosplenomegaly
- Lymphadenopathy
- Gingival swelling
- May involve the central nervous system, presenting with symptoms of increased intracranial pressure

Pre-eclampsia

Pre-eclampsia is a pregnancy-related condition that occurs during the last 20 weeks of pregnancy.

FEATURES

- Hypertension
- Edema
- Proteinuria
- Rapid excessive weight gain
- Epigastric pain
- Headache
- Thrombocytopenia

Thrombocytopenia secondary to sepsis

Any multisystem inflammatory response to overwhelming infection should be considered in the differential diagnosis, including thrombocytopenia seconday to sepsis.

FEATURES

- Fever, chills, rigors, myalgias
- Tachycardia, tachypnea, and hypotension
- Altered mental status
- Signs and symptoms related to site of primary infection
- Signs and symptoms related to end-organ failure
- Occasionally accompanied by thrombocytopenia

Thrombocytopenia following blood transfusion

A decrease in the number of platelets may occur following blood transfusion.

FEATURES

- Significant thrombocytopenia (platelets 50,000–100,000/mm^3 (50–100x10^9/L)) may occur in patients receiving >15 units of blood (in an average-sized adult)
- Severe thrombocytopenia (platelets <50,000/mm^3 (<50x10^9/L)) is most common in patients receiving >20 units of blood
- Post-transfusion purpura can be caused by the transfusion of mismatched platelets (in rare individuals who have PI-A1 antigen-negative platelets and received PI-A1 positive platelets; classic scenario – multiparous woman who received a red blood cell transfusion about one week ago during routine surgery)

Pseudothrombocytopenia

Pseudothrombocytopenia is a laboratory artifact of ex vivo platelet clumping. This condition is commonly caused by EDTA when used as an anticoagulant.

FEATURES

- Absence of clinical bleeding
- Platelet clumping on the peripheral smear

Gestational thrombocytopenia

Gestational thrombocytopenia, also known as gestational benign thrombocytopenia (rarely present with platelets <70,000/mm^3 (<70x10^9/L)), is a difficult entity to diagnose, and can be confused with thrombotic thrombocytopenic purpura, hemolytic uremic syndrome, and more commonly with idiopathic thrombocytopenic purpura (ITP) . The clinical picture constitutes the best way to make the diagnosis: usually, this entity presents in a woman with no prior history of thrombocytopenia, resolves after delivery, and does not produce thrombocytopenia in the fetus. Some authors have reported that antiplatelet antibodies can help to make the diagnosis; nevertheless, the value of this test is controversial.

FEATURES

- New presentation of thrombocytopenia during pregnancy, with resolution after delivery
- Does not induce fetal thrombocytopenia

Drug-induced thrombocytopenia

- Diagnosis requires an exhaustive interrogation of the patient. Apart from the use of regular medications, the patient should be ask about the consumption of over-the-counter (OTC) medications, 'health products', and herbs
- Multiple medications can cause thrombocytopenia. The more common ones are quinidine, quinine, rifampin, trimethoprim-sulfamethoxazole, methyldopa, acetaminophen, digoxin, aspirin, vancomycin, cimetidine, tamoxifen, lithium, and nitroglycerine. A very complete list of medications that can induce thrombocytopenia has been formulated (Database for Drug-Induced Thrombocytopenia: An Update. Available on the University of Oklahoma Health Sciences website)
- Most typically the thrombocytopenia resolves after the medication is discontinued. The detection of specific antiplatelet antibodies induced by drugs cannot always be performed, delays the diagnosis, and does not always correlate with the presence of drug-induced thrombocytopenia

FEATURES

- History of the use of a new drug, OTC preparation, or herbs
- Resolves after the medication is discontinued

Hypersplenism

Usually present in patients with history of cirrhosis in the context of portal hypertension. Splenomegaly is usually found on physical examination, as well as other signs of liver failure and/or portal hypertension. Removal of the spleen in order to decrease the pooling of platelets is usually required. Low levels of thrombopoietin can be found in patients with cirrhosis, and this has been added as a confounding factor associated with thrombocytopenia in patients who have hypersplenism.

FEATURES

- History of chronic liver disease or portal hypertension
- Palpable spleen on examination

SIGNS & SYMPTOMS

Signs

- In childhood, typically an abrupt onset (acute ITP) and spontaneous resolution
- In adults, typically gradual onset (chronic ITP); waxing and waning course with few spontaneous remissions

- Petechiae: minute, red to purple hemorrhages that range in size from pinpoint to pinhead; nonpalpable; do not blanch on pressure; appear and regress, usually in crops, over a period of days
- Petechiae occur mostly in dependent regions or areas subjected to constrictions, such as from belts or stockings, and skin surfaces over bony prominences
- Ecchymosis (bruising)
- Purpuric lesions (petechiae and ecchymosis) are painless, flat, nonpuritic, and nonerythematous
- Hemorrhagic bullae on mucous membranes/buccal mucosa
- Gingival bleeding
- Mucocutaneous bleeding including recurrent epistaxis
- Menorrhagia
- Gastrointestinal bleeding, usually manifested by darkening of feces by blood or occasionally by vomiting blood
- Genitourinary bleeding
- Menometrorrhagia
- Retinal hemorrhages, small and numerous; occasionally subconjunctival hemorrhage
- Slow persistent oozing after minor trauma, such as scratches or razor nicks
- Excessive bleeding after tooth extractions, tonsillectomy, or other operations or injuries
- Spontaneous bleeding at platelet count below 20,000/mm^3 (20x10^9/L)
- Neurologic symptoms such as headaches, blurred vision, somnolence, or loss of consciousness secondary to intracerebral bleeding
- Nonpalpable spleen; splenomegaly is rare, as in the healthy population
- Absence of hepatosplenomegaly and remarkable lymphadenopathy

Symptoms

- Petechial rash, typically of the lower legs
- Bruising tendency
- Prolonged bleeding time
- Gingival bleeding
- Recurrent epistaxis
- Menorrhagia
- Blood in feces, vomit, or urine
- Neurologic symptoms secondary to intracerebral bleeding

KEY! DON'T MISS!

Acute onset in an adult usually signals a more rapid and severe course, and should alert the physician to the possibility of serious hemorrhage.

CONSIDER CONSULT

Consultation with a hematologist is appropriate for assistance in confirming a diagnosis of ITP.

INVESTIGATION OF THE PATIENT

Direct questions to patient

- Q **Have you been experiencing headaches, blurred vision, somnolence, or loss of consciousness?** Check for signs or symptoms of intracranial hemorrhage
- Q **Have you been bleeding anywhere for a sustained period of time?** Check for signs of major volume depletion
- Q **Do you have a history of easy bruising, bleeding into a joint, very heavy periods, or abnormally heavy bleeding with dental work or surgery?** These suggest the presence of a bleeding problem

- **Have you ever had to have a blood transfusion?** History of a transfusion requirement after minor trauma or surgery when such transfusion would ordinarily not be required suggests a bleeding problem
- **Do you have gingival bleeding or nosebleeds?** Both are common in ITP
- **Have you had blood in your urine, darkening of feces, or have you vomited blood?** Genitourinary or gastrointestinal bleeding may occur in ITP. Menorrhagia may be the only symptom of ITP
- **How long have you had unusual bleeding/purpuric lesions? Did they start gradually or suddenly?** Determine whether the condition is acute or chronic
- **Is bruising or bleeding a recurrent problem? How often does it occur?** Determine the severity of the bleeding
- **After injury, do you have immediate or delayed bleeding? Is it transient or prolonged? Is it superficial (into skin and mucous membranes) or deep (into tissues or viscera)?** Bleeding that is transient, superficial, and spontaneous or immediately after injury suggests a platelet problem such as ITP. Bleeding that is deep, delayed, and prolonged suggests a serious clotting factor problem
- **Are you on or have you been taking any medication, including OTC drugs?** Many drugs are associated with secondary immune thrombocytopenic purpura, some proven and some circumstantial. The most commonly implicated agents include heparin, gold salts, quinine/quinidine, sulfa drugs, histamine H_2 receptor antagonists, rifampin, carbamazepine, and valproic acid. Aspirin can also cause secondary immune thrombocytopenic purpura. In patients with low platelet counts all drugs that can safely be withdrawn should be; withdrawal of an offending drug is generally followed by recovery
- **How much alcohol do you drink?** Acute and chronic alcohol consumption is associated with secondary immune thrombocytopenic purpura. In chronic liver disease, thrombocytopenia sometimes presents with hypersplenism
- **Do you have or think you may have HIV infection?** Thrombocytopenia can occur in the acute antiretroviral syndrome of HIV infection, it can be an early indication of symptomatic HIV infection, and it may be a manifestation of AIDS
- **Do you have a fever?** Fever is considered a cardinal feature of thrombotic thrombocytopenic purpura, and can help in differentiating thrombotic thrombocytopenic purpura from ITP
- **Are you pregnant?** Gestational thrombocytopenia is a possible complication of pregnancy. It is usually mild (>80,000/mm^3) and asymptomatic, and is not associated with hemostatic impairment in the infant. However, ITP during pregnancy does need special consideration

Contributory or predisposing factors

- **Have you/your child had a recent illness?** Acute viral illness (in children) usually precedes ITP
- **Have you/your child had a recent immunization?** Recent live virus immunization (in children) occasionally precedes ITP
- **Have you had a cardiopulmonary bypass?** ITP can occasionally be a complication following cardiopulmonary bypass
- **Do you have hypersplenism?** Hypersplenism can predispose to ITP

Family history

- **Do you have a family history of abnormal bleeding?** This would suggest a hereditary bleeding problem rather than ITP.

Examination

- **Check the vital signs.** Hypertension and bradycardia may be signs of increased intracranial pressure associated with intracranial hemorrhage. Pre-eclampsia may be an alternative diagnosis in pregnant women

- **Check for neurologic signs.** Pupils should be equal in size and have intact extraocular muscles and symmetrical eye movements. Balance and gait should be intact. Any asymmetric finding can indicate an intracranial hemorrhage
- **Does the patient appear well?** ITP is primarily an illness occurring in an otherwise healthy person. Signs of chronic disease, infection, wasting, and poor nutrition indicate that the patient has another illness
- **Examine the eyes.** Numerous small hemorrhages may be seen in the retina with ITP; however, these may also suggest increased intracranial pressure associated with intracranial hemorrhage
- **Look for and examine any skin lesions.** Bruises that occur on the limbs and are <3cm in diameter are likely to be harmless and caused by unnoticed trauma. Bruises occurring spontaneously on the trunk or measuring >3cm in diameter on the limbs is more likely to suggest a bleeding problem. Failure to blanch helps to differentiate petechiae from nonpurpuric skin lesions. Shining a light tangentially onto the skin is a sensitive means of detecting elevated lesions, which may be confirmed by careful palpation. Purpuric lesions associated with ITP are painless, flat, nonpruritic, and nonerythematous
- **Examine the mucous membranes.** Signs of bleeding may be apparent in ITP. Hemorrhagic vesicles or bullae are probably the result of severe acute thrombocytopenia, rather than being a specific feature of ITP
- **Percuss the Traube space and palpate the spleen.** Splenomegaly should prompt a search for an alternative diagnosis; splenomegaly occurs with ITP only as frequently as it does in the population at large
- **Examine the abdomen.** Hepatosplenomegaly indicates that the patient has another illness
- **Examine the lymph nodes.** Remarkable lymphadenopathy indicates that the patient has another illness

Summary of investigative tests

- Complete blood count (CBC) from a blood sample sent to laboratory should be obtained to assess for the presence and degree of thrombocytopenia, and repeated as required to assess response to therapy
- Examination of the peripheral blood smear should be carried out to assist with diagnosis
- HIV antibody testing from a blood sample sent to laboratory should be carried out in all patients with risk factors for HIV infection, with the agreement of the patient. During the acute phase of HIV retroviral syndrome, HIV antibody testing may be negative, and testing for HIV infection can be carried out by polymerase chain reaction (PCR) for HIV DNA, using the proviral DNA PCR assay, from a blood sample sent to laboratory
- Bone marrow aspiration, normally performed by a specialist, should be carried out in certain circumstances: in patients over 60 years to help in the differential diagnosis of ITP vs myelodysplastic syndromes; to establish the diagnosis in patients considering splenectomy; in children with persistent thrombocytopenia lasting more than 6–12 months; and in children unresponsive to intravenous immune globulin (IVIg). It should not be performed in order to establish diagnosis before initiating therapy. ITP causes no characteristic bone marrow changes
- Abdominal computed tomography (CT) scan or ultrasound examination of children with suspected splenomegaly on initial physical examination. The spleen may be enlarged due to hematoma caused by ITP, or from other causes not related to ITP
- Preoperative thyroid function testing should be done before elective splenectomy
- Liver function testing may be done in pregnant women; this is normally performed by a specialist
- Brain imaging by ultrasound in newborns of mothers with ITP, with counts <50,000/mm^3, is normally performed by a specialist

DIAGNOSTIC DECISION

The diagnosis is based on the findings from the following:

- History
- Physical examination
- CBC
- Peripheral smear

In the absence of findings that are atypical or suggest another diagnosis, further diagnostic studies are not indicated, except in the following circumstances:

- Patients with risk factors for HIV infection: testing for HIV antibody or proviral DNA is appropriate
- Patients over 60 years of age: bone marrow aspiration is indicated to differentiate ITP from myelodysplastic syndromes
- Patients for whom splenectomy is considered: bone marrow aspiration is indicated to confirm the diagnosis. Preoperative thyroid function testing is appropriate to rule out occult hyperthyroidism and hypothyroidism before elective splenectomy
- Children with persistent thrombocytopenia lasting longer than 6–12 months: bone marrow aspiration is indicated to confirm the diagnosis
- Children unresponsive to IVIg: bone marrow aspiration is indicated to confirm the diagnosis. However, it should not be performed in order to establish diagnosis before initiating therapy

Guidelines

Idiopathic thrombocytopenic purpura: a practice guideline developed by explicit methods for the American Society of Hematology [7]. Available from the National Guidelines Clearinghouse

CLINICAL PEARLS

- A bone marrow aspirate/biopsy is not indicated in a typical case of ITP (e.g. young female with normal CBC and with no lymphadenopathy/splenomegaly)
- Careful history regarding HIV risk factors should be taken in all patients, and particularly in young males. If patient is homosexual and presents with thrombocytopenia, then HIV tests should be ordered

THE TESTS

Body fluids

COMPLETE BLOOD COUNT

Description

Venous blood sample.

Advantages/Disadvantages

Advantages:

- Easy to obtain
- Inexpensive

Normal

- Platelets: 156,000–352,000/mm^3 (156–352x10^9/L)
- Red blood cells (RBC): 4.3–5.7x10^6/mm3 (4.3–5.7x10^{12}/L)
- White blood cells (WBC): 3400–11,000/mm^3 (3.4–11.0x10^9/L)
- Neutrophils: 1900–7800/mm^3 (1.9–7.8x10^9/L)
- Lymphocytes: 1100–3100/mm^3 (1.1–3.1x10^9/L)
- Monocytes: 200–900/mm^3 (0.2–0.9x10^9/L)
- Eosinophils: 30–530/mm^3 (0.03–0.53x10^9/L)
- Basophils: 10–100/mm^3 (0.01–0.11x10^9/L)
- Mean corpuscular volume: 76–100mcm^3 (76–100fL)

Abnormal

- Platelet count of <100,000/mm^3 (<100x10^9/L)
- Isolated thrombocytopenia is the hallmark of ITP; other values are typically normal unless severe hemorrhage has occurred, when the WBC count and hemoglobin will be abnormal
- Keep in mind the possibility of a false-positive result
- Anemia out of proportion to blood loss suggests that cytopenia(s) may be due to thrombotic thrombocytopenic purpura, or an initial manifestation of acute leukemia, MDS, myelophthisic processes, or aplastic anemia

Drugs, disorders and other factors that may alter results

- A large number of drugs can cause thrombocytopenia, including heparin, gold salts, quinine/quinidine, sulfa drugs, H_2 receptor antagonists, rifampin, carbamazepine, and valproic acid
- Thrombocytopenia is a common finding in many disorders
- Pseudothrombocytopenia is a laboratory phenomenon that may result in the reporting of a low platelet count based on measurement by an automated counter, and is caused by the EDTA anticoagulant in the tube of blood. A new blood sample should be obtained in either heparinized or citrated blood, and a second automated platelet count performed. Manual examination of the peripheral blood smear will clarify the diagnosis

EXAMINATION OF PERIPHERAL BLOOD SMEAR

Description

Microscopic examination of the appearance of platelets.

Advantages/Disadvantages

Advantages:

- Easy to obtain
- Inexpensive

Normal

- The morphology of red blood cells and leukocytes is normal in ITP
- The morphology of platelets is typically normal in ITP

Abnormal

- Abnormalities in platelet size, both large and small, and an increased variation in size and shape may occur in ITP
- Megathrombocytes, or stress platelets, may be present in some cases of acute ITP, reflecting the early release of megakaryocytic fragments into the circulation
- Pseudothrombocytopenia is suggested if there are clumps of platelets on a peripheral smear prepared from blood using EDTA anticoagulant. This can be confirmed if the platelet count is normal when repeated on a blood sample using heparin or citrate anticoagulant
- If the majority of platelets are large (similar in diameter to RBC), or if they have abnormal color or lack granules, consider an inherited platelet disorder
- The presence of schistocytes suggests that the thrombocytopenia may be associated with a microangiopathic process
- Schistocytes and coagulation abnormalities suggest thrombocytopenia resulting from DIC
- Changes in leukocytes not attributable to either hemorrhage or complicating infection suggest acute leukemia, MDS, myelophthisic processes, or aplastic anemia

HIV ANTIBODY TESTING

Description

Enzyme-linked immunosorbent assay (ELISA) with positive results confirmed by Western blot assay. Both from a blood sample.

Normal
Nonreactive ELISA.

Abnormal
- Repeatedly reactive ELISA
- Positive Western blot, defined by the Centers for Disease Control and Prevention as the presence of any two of the gp24, gp41, and gp120/160 bands
- Indeterminate Western blot, defined as the presence of reactive bands that do not meet the criteria for a positive test
- Keep in mind the possibility of a false-positive result. All positive ELISAs should be confirmed by Western blot. Keep in mind the possibility of a false-positive Western blot

Cause of abnormal result
- Presence of HIV antibodies as a result of infection by HIV (repeatedly reactive ELISA followed by positive Western blot)
- Possible presence of HIV antibodies as a result of infection by HIV (repeatedly reactive ELISA followed by indeterminate Western blot)

Drugs, disorders and other factors that may alter results
ELISA:
- Hemophilia
- Autoimmune disorders
- Multiple myeloma
- Alcoholic hepatitis
- Hemodialysis
- A reactive plasmin reagin test
- Human error

Western blot:
- Hyperbilirubinemia
- Connective tissue disorders
- Polyclonal gammopathies

PROVIRAL DNA POLYMERASE CHAIN REACTION ASSAY
Description
PCR for HIV DNA from a blood sample.

Advantages/Disadvantages
- Advantage: sensitive detection of proviral DNA in adults
- Disadvantage: not US Food and Drug Administration (FDA)-approved for HIV testing

Normal
Negative: no proviral DNA detected.

Abnormal
- Positive: proviral DNA detected
- Keep in mind the possibility of a false-positive result
- All positive results should be confirmed by a second test using a blood sample taken on a different day, and/or by HIV antibody testing after 3–6 months

Cause of abnormal result
Presence of HIV infection.

Drugs, disorders and other factors that may alter results
- Low proviral DNA copy number
- Human error
- Sequence variation in the primer binding sites

Tests of function

THYROID FUNCTION TESTS

Description
- It is important to know the thyroid function because some patients with autoimmune thrombocytopenia can have other autoimmune diseases such as pernicious anemia and Addison's disease, including thyroiditis, and this can generate complications during the time of the surgery
- Cuffed venous blood sample

Normal
- Serum thyroxine T4: 4–11mcg/dL (51–142nmol/L)
- Serum T3 resin uptake: 25–35% (0.25–0.35)
- Serum T3: 75–220ng/dL (1.2–3.4nmol/L)
- Free T4: 0.9–2.0ng/dL (12–26pmol/L)
- Free T3: 0.2–0.52ng/dL (3–8pmol/L)

Abnormal
- Parameters outside the normal range
- Keep in mind the possibility of a falsely abnormal result

Imaging

COMPUTED TOMOGRAPHY SCAN

Description

Abdominal CT scan to examine the spleen.

Advantages/Disadvantages

Advantages:
- Readily available
- More easily performed in children than magnetic resonance imaging (MRI), which necessitates the patient lying still

Disadvantages:
- Involves exposure to radiation
- Less informative than MRI

Normal

Normal spleen or enlarged spleen of normal appearance.

Abnormal
- Hematoma on the spleen
- A mass in the spleen
- A mass around the spleen

Cause of abnormal result
- Hematoma may be caused by ITP or by injury
- A mass will need further investigation to elicit cause

CONSIDER CONSULT

- Hospitalization is appropriate for patients with severe, life-threatening bleeding, regardless of the platelet count, and for patients with platelets <20,000/mm^3 (<20x10^9/L) who have significant mucous membrane bleeding or who are inaccessible or noncompliant. Hospitalization is inappropriate for patients with platelet counts >20,000/mm^3 (>20x10^9/L) who are either asymptomatic or have only minor purpura. Indications for hospitalization under intermediate conditions are less clear [1]
- Consultation with a hematologist may be appropriate before initiating therapy
- Referral to a specialist is indicated for pregnant women with idiopathic thrombocytopenic purpura (ITP) with a platelet count of <50,000/mm^3 (<50x10^9/L) or who are bleeding

IMMEDIATE ACTION

In the event of severe hemorrhage:

- Provide oxygen
- Control hemorrhage
- Initiate intravenous fluids to maintain hemodynamic stability
- Transfer to emergency room

MANAGEMENT ISSUES

Goals

- Treat severe thrombocytopenia promptly to accelerate the increase in platelet count in order to avoid a serious hemorrhage, and to allow the patient to live a normal life while awaiting spontaneous or treatment-induced remission
- Monitor all patients while awaiting remission
- Consider splenectomy for severe, refractory cases
- Advise patients to avoid drugs that are known to cause thrombocytopenia and activities that carry a high risk of injury

Management in special circumstances

Patients with very low platelet count or significant bleeding symptoms are at risk of serious morbidity and mortality from hemorrhage and should be hospitalized.

COEXISTING DISEASE

HIV infection and AIDS:

- Immune thrombocytopenic purpura can be the first manifestation of HIV infection
- Generally the prevalence of thrombocytopenia increases with disease progression, although this may not be true in individual cases
- Thrombocytopenia occurs in 30–60% of adults and children with AIDS
- Life-threatening bleeding is rare, except in HIV-infected patients with hemophilia and thrombocytopenia
- There is no single treatment of thrombocytopenia due to HIV infection that is consistently successful
- The decision to initiate treatment should be based on the clinical consequences of thrombocytopenia in conjunction with the platelet count, and not on the platelet count alone, as for adults with ITP
- Rh(D) immune globulin (anti-D) has been reported to be successful in treating HIV-related thrombocytopenia if the patient is Rh(D)-positive; however, anti-D induces immune hemolysis, and should not be used if the patient has a hemoglobin concentration <8g/dL (80g/L)
- Zidovudine (AZT or ZDV) often increases the platelet count of patients with thrombocytopenia, but should only be used as part of a highly active antiretroviral therapy (HAART) regimen

- Didanosine (ddI) has also been reported to increase the platelet count of patients with thrombocytopenia, but should only be used as part of a HAART regimen
- The first-line therapy for ITP – glucocorticoids (prednisone and methylprednisolone) – does not generally produce a sustainable increase in platelet count in those with HIV-related thrombocytopenia, and poses a real risk of further compromising the immune status
- Splenectomy (surgical or laparoscopic) is controversial; although it has a sustained success rate of 40–60% it has been suggested that it may accelerate the progression of HIV infection to AIDS, although this is not substantiated

Systemic lupus erythematosus (SLE):

- 5–15% of patients with ITP fulfill the criteria for diagnosis of SLE at the time of presentation
- A small number of patients with ITP will develop SLE within a few years
- SLE is a chronic and fatal disease and early diagnosis is vital
- Patients with secondary immune thrombocytopenic purpura and SLE should be treated the same as those with ITP

COEXISTING MEDICATION

- Drug-induced secondary immune thrombocytopenic purpura is associated with many drugs, some circumstantially
- The following list comprises drugs for which evidence exists for the presence of drug-induced platelet antibodies: acetaminophen, acetazolamide, allopurinol, alprenolol, amiodarone, ampicillin, amrinone, antazoline, aspirin, carbamazepine, cephalexin, cephalothin, chlorothiazide, chlorpheniramine, chlorthalidone, cimetidine, diazepam, desipramine, digitoxin, diltiazem, diphenylhydantoin, furosemide, gentamicin, gold salts, heparin, imipramine, iopanoic acid, lidocaine, meprobamate, methicillin, methyldopa, minoxidil, morphine, novobiocin, para-aminosalicylic acid, penicillin, phenylbutazone, procainamide, quinidine, quinine, ranitidine, rifampin, spironolactone, sulfisoxazole, trimethoprim-sulfamethoxazole, valproic acid, and vancomycin
- The most common drug precipitants of secondary immune thrombocytopenic purpura are heparin, gold salts, quinine, quinidine, rifampin, carbamazepine, valproic acid, sulfa drugs, and histamine H_2 receptor antagonists
- It takes at least 6 days to initiate a primary immune response when taking a drug for the first time, but a patient who has been sensitized may develop thrombocytopenia, which can be severe, within hours
- Patients presenting with ITP should stop taking all drugs that are not essential
- Once the precipitating drug is stopped, the platelet count will usually normalize within 2–3 weeks
- Thrombocytopenia induced by gold salts will take longer to normalize, usually a few weeks or months, because gold remains in the tissues

SPECIAL PATIENT GROUPS

Pregnant women:

- In a large study of mothers and their infants, the incidence of infants with platelet counts $<50,000/mm^3$ ($<50x10^9/L$) born to mothers with ITP was 8.7%, whereas the incidence of infants with platelet counts $<50,000/mm^3$ ($<50x10^9/L$) born to mothers with gestational thrombocytopenia was 0.01%
- The highest incidence of neonatal thrombocytopenia exists in infants born to mothers with normal platelet count following splenectomy for ITP, and in infants born to mothers with circulating platelet antibodies
- Both the maternal and infant health should be considered in treatment decisions
- The platelet count of the mother during pregnancy does not correlate with the fetal platelet count. This is also true for changes in the mother's platelet count as a result of treatment

- Pregnant women with platelet counts >50,000/mm^3 (>50x10^9/L) and those with platelet counts of 30,000–50,000/mm^3 (30–50x10^9/L)who are in the first or second trimester do not routinely require treatment
- Pregnant women with platelet counts <10,000/mm^3 (<10x10^9/L) and those with platelet counts of 10,000–30,000/mm^3 (10–30x10^9/L) who are in the second or third trimester or are bleeding, do require treatment
- First-choice treatment is intravenous immune globulin (IVIg)
- Second-choice treatment is prednisone
- Therapy should be at the lowest dose possible to maintain a maternal platelet count of 50,000–60,000/mm^3 (50–60x10^9/L)
- In refractory patients, splenectomy (surgical or laparoscopic) can be considered if the patient is symptomatic and has a platelet count <10,000/mm^3 (<10x10^9/L)
- Splenectomy during pregnancy has higher complication rates
- The fetal platelet count should be obtained if the mother has a platelet count <40,000–50,000/mm^3 (<40–50x10^9/L), if she has previously delivered a baby with neonatal thrombocytopenia, or if she has had a splenectomy
- Delivery by cesarean section is recommended when the fetal platelet count is <50,000/mm^3 (<50x10^9/L)
- Mothers with ITP should not be discouraged from breast-feeding

Children:
- Children with platelet counts >30,000/mm^3 (>30x10^9/L) who are asymptomatic or who have only minor purpura do not routinely require treatment
- Children with platelet counts <20,000/mm^3 (<20x10^9/L) with significant mucous membrane bleeding do require treatment
- Children with platelet counts <10,000/mm^3 (<10x10^9/L) and minor purpura do require treatment
- Therapeutic options are as for adults

The elderly:
- ITP is less common in the elderly than in other age groups
- Older patients (>60 years) tend to be more refractory to therapy and have a higher incidence of hemorrhage than do other age groups

Guidelines

Idiopathic thrombocytopenic purpura: a practice guideline developed by explicit methods for the American Society of Hematology [1]. Available from the National Guideline Clearinghouse

PATIENT SATISFACTION/LIFESTYLE PRIORITIES

Patients should limit their medication to essential drugs and avoid activities that might precipitate injury/bleeding.

SUMMARY OF THERAPEUTIC OPTIONS

Choices

When to initiate treatment:
- The decision to initiate treatment should be made on the basis of clinical consequences of thrombocytopenia in conjunction with the platelet count, and not the platelet count alone
- Patients with a platelet count <20,000/mm^3 (<20x10^9/L) who have mucous membrane bleeding require hospitalization
- Patients with significant mucous membrane bleeding or severe bleeding require hospitalization, regardless of their platelet count
- Patients with a platelet count of 20–50,000/mm^3 (20–50x10^9/L) and no significant mucous membrane bleeding or severe bleeding can be treated as an outpatient

- Patients with a platelet count >50,000/mm^3 (>50x10^9/L) who are asymptomatic or have minor purpura do not require treatment, but should remain under observation
- Consider treating at higher platelet counts, particularly in symptomatic patients, if there are additional risk factors for increased bleeding, such as hypertension, peptic ulcers, recent aspirin ingestion, and activities in which injury is common

Therapeutic options:

- First-choice therapy is glucocorticoids, either oral prednisone or intravenous methylprednisolone
- Second-choice therapy is IVIg
- Alternatively, if the patient is Rh(D)-positive, then Rh(D) immune globulin (anti-D) may be used; however, anti-D induces immune hemolysis and should not be used if the patient has a hemoglobin concentration <8g/dL (80g/L)
- After 6 months, if the platelet count cannot be maintained at a safe level, or if it cannot be maintained at a safe level without serious treatment-related toxicity, the consider surgical splenectomy or laparoscopic splenectomy
- In the event of a splenectomy, adults and children over 2 years should be immunized with polyvalent *Streptococcus pneumoniae* vaccine and quadrivalent meningococcal polysaccharide vaccine preoperatively. If elective splenectomy is planned, then adults and children should be immunized with *Haemophilus influenzae* type b vaccine at least 2 weeks before surgery

Guidelines:
Idiopathic thrombocytopenic purpura: a practice guideline developed by explicit methods for the American Society of Hematology [1]. Available from the National Guideline Clearinghouse

Clinical pearls

- Platelet transfusions are not useful in ITP because their half-life is measured in hours (normal: 7–10 days)
- Low platelets does not represent a contraindication to splenectomy: as soon as a surgeon clamps the splenic artery, platelets significantly increase in the circulation
- 80% response to splenectomy should be expected within 3–4 days; if the response is not seen within a week, then rule out accessory spleen
- If patient did not respond to steroids (prednisone or methylprednisolone) and splenectomy, then he/she is considered to have refractory ITP. Such patients may have poor prognosis and their treatment has not been standardized

FOLLOW UP

Plan for review

- Monitor platelet count and clinical status daily to weekly, depending on the severity and treatment used
- Review treatment regularly as some improvements are not sustained

Information for patient or caregiver

Patients should not use aspirin.

DRUGS AND OTHER THERAPIES: DETAILS

Drugs

PREDNISONE

Dose

- Adult dose 0.5–2mg/kg/day (typically 1mg/kg/day) by mouth for 2–4 weeks, then taper
- Pediatric dose 4–8mg/kg/day by mouth for 2–4 weeks, then taper
- May require repetition in chronic ITP

Efficacy

- Glucocorticoids can achieve early responses (mostly transient) in adult patients
- Increase in platelet count of >50,000/mm^3 (>50x10^9/L) occurs in 65–85% of patients
- Sustained responses after discontinuation of therapy occurs in 25% or less of patients (long-term ranges from as low as 3% to as high as 50%)
- Long-term steroid use is associated with significant morbidity

Risks/Benefits

Risks:

- Use caution in congestive heart failure, renal disease, diabetes mellitus, glaucoma, ulcerative colitis, or peptic ulcer
- Use caution in the elderly
- Prednisone taken in doses higher than 7.5mg for 3 weeks or longer may lead to clinically relevant suppression of the pituitary-adrenal axis

Side-effects and adverse reactions

- Side-effects are minimized by short duration of therapy
- Cardiovascular system: hypertension, thromboembolism
- Central nervous system: insomnia, euphoria, depression, psychosis, seizures
- Endocrine: adrenal suppression, impaired glucose tolerance, growth suppression in children
- Eyes, ears, nose, and throat: cataract, glaucoma, blurred vision
- Gastrointestinal: dyspepsia, peptic ulceration, esophagitis, oral candidiasis
- Musculoskeletal: proximal myopathy, osteoporosis
- Skin: delayed healing, acne, striae, fragile skin

Interactions (other drugs)

■ Aminoglutethimide (increased clearance of prednisone) ■ Warfarin (alters clotting time) ■ Antidiabetics (hypoglycemic effect inhibited) ■ Antihypertensives (effects inhibited) ■ Barbiturates (increased clearance of prednisone) ■ Cardiac glycosides (toxicity increased) ■ Cholestyramine, colestipol (may reduce absorption of corticosteroids) ■ Ketoconazole ■ Clarithromycin, erythromycin, troleandomycin (may enhance steroid effect) ■ Cyclosporine (may increase levels of both drugs; may cause seizures) ■ Diuretics (effects inhibited) ■ Isoniazid (reduced plasma levels of isoniazid) ■ Nonsteroidal anti-inflammatory drugs (NSAIDs; increased risks of bleeding) ■ Oral contraceptives (enhanced effects of corticosteroids) ■ Rifampin (may inhibit hepatic clearance of prednisone) ■ Salicylates (increased clearance of salicylates)

Contraindications

■ Systemic infection ■ Avoid live virus vaccines in those receiving immunosuppressive doses ■ History of tuberculosis ■ Cushing's syndrome ■ Recent myocardial infarction

Evidence

- Initial treatment of ITP with prednisone is appropriate in adult patients with platelet counts <30,000/mm^3 (<30x10^9/L), and for those with platelets <50,000/mm^3 (<50x10^9/L) plus clinically significant bleeding or risk factors for bleeding [1] *Level C*
- Prednisone is an appropriate treatment for children with platelets <50,000/mm^3 (<50x10^9/L) and severe bleeding, those with mucosal bleeding and platelets <20,000/mm^3 (<20x10^9/L), and those with purpura and platelets <10,000/mm^3 (<10x10^9/L) [1] *Level C*

Acceptability to patient

Patients are often concerned about the long-term use of steroids due to the large number of common side-effects.

Follow up plan

Follow up for side-effects of medication, and to ensure patient compliance.

Patient and caregiver information

- Glucocorticoids should not be stopped abruptly
- Take with food if there is associated gastrointestinal upset
- Inform patient of the short- and long-term side-effects

METHYLPREDNISOLONE

Dose

- Adult loading dose 125–250mg intravenously; maintenance dose 0.5–1mg/kg every 6h for up to 5 days
- Pediatric loading dose 2mg/kg intravenously; maintenance dose 0.5–1mg/kg every 6h for up to 5 days

Efficacy

- Glucocorticoids can achieve early responses (mostly transient)
- Long-term steroid use is associated with significant morbidity
- Safety for use during pregnancy has not been established

Risks/Benefits

Risks:

- Overwhelming septicemia if patient has an infection
- Loss of control of blood glucose in those with diabetes
- Use caution in elderly due to risk of diabetes and osteoporosis
- Use caution in patients with psychosis, seizure disorders, or myasthenia gravis
- Use caution in congestive heart failure, hypertension, ulcerative colitis, peptic ulcer, or esophagitis
- Prolonged use causes adrenal suppression

Side-effects and adverse reactions

- Side-effects are minimized by short duration of therapy
- Cardiovascular system: hypertension, thromboembolism
- Central nervous system: insomnia, euphoria, depression, psychosis, seizures
- Endocrine: adrenal suppression, impaired glucose tolerance, growth suppression in children
- Eyes, ears, nose, and throat: cataract, glaucoma, blurred vision
- Gastrointestinal: dyspepsia, peptic ulceration, esophagitis, oral candidiasis, nausea, vomiting
- Musculoskeletal: proximal myopathy, osteoporosis
- Skin: delayed healing, acne, striae

Interactions (other drugs)

- **Aminoglutethimide** ■ **Antidiabetics** ■ **Barbiturates** ■ **Cholestyramine** ■ **Troleandomycin** ■ **Clarithromycin, erythromycin** ■ **Colestipol** ■ **Cyclosporine** ■ **Isoniazid** ■ **Ketoconazole** ■ **NSAIDs** ■ **Oral contraceptives** ■ **Rifampin** ■ **Salicylates**

Contraindications

- **Systemic infection** ■ **Avoid live virus vaccines in those receiving immunosuppressive doses**

Evidence

Methylprednisolone (high-dose parenteral glucocorticoid therapy) is appropriate for hospitalized patients with severe bleeding (regardless of the platelet count) [1] *Level C*

Acceptability to patient

Patients are often concerned about the long-term use of steroids due to the large number of common side-effects.

Follow up plan
Follow up for side-effects of medication, and to ensure patient compliance.

Patient and caregiver information
- Glucocorticoids should not be stopped abruptly
- Take with food if there is associated gastrointestinal upset
- Inform patient of the short- and long-term side-effects

INTRAVENOUS IMMUNOGLOBULIN
Dose
Adult dose: 1g/kg intravenously administered over 1–2 days.

Efficacy
- Can temporarily increase platelet count, and is useful if the situation requires a rapid rise in platelet count
- May be useful for children who are unresponsive to steroids and other treatments
- Approx. 75% of chronic ITP adult patients may have an increase in platelet count, but this effect is usually temporary

Risks/Benefits
Risk: allergic responses to gamma-globulin are extremely rare; any inflammation is due to localized chemical tissue irritation

Benefits:
- The rapid increase in platelet count in response to IVIg makes it useful for the treatment of patients with life-threatening bleeding, or prior to surgery
- Preferred first-line therapy in pregnancy

Side-effects and adverse reactions
- Central nervous system: chills, fever, lethargy
- Gastrointestinal: nausea
- Muskuloskeletal: muscle stiffness, tenderness at injection site
- Skin: urticaria, angioedema, myalgia

Interactions (other drugs)
Do not administer live virus vaccines within 3 months of immunoglobulin (Ig) administration.

Contraindications
■ Allergic response to IgA or gamma-globulin ■ Allergic response to thimerosal ■ Isolated IgA deficiency

Evidence
- IVIg is an appropriate initial treatment for adult patients with severe bleeding and platelet counts <50,000/mm^3 (<50x10^9/L) [1] *Level C*
- In children with ITP, initial treatment with IVIg is appropriate if there is severe bleeding (regardless of platelet count), and for children with platelets <10,000/mm^3 (<10x10^9/L) with minor purpura, or <20,000/mm^3 (<20x10^9/L) and mucous membrane bleeding [1] *Level C*

Patient and caregiver information
Inform patient of side-effects.

RH(D) IMMUNE GLOBULIN

Dose

- Specialist advice on dosage required
- Recommended adult and pediatric dosage, by intramuscular route only: 50mcg/kg as a single dose or in two divided doses over 2 days

Efficacy

- Effective in increasing platelet count in children with acute or chronic ITP, adults with chronic ITP, and ITP secondary to HIV infection
- Children respond better than do adults
- Nonsplenectomized patients respond better than do splenectomized patients

Risks/Benefits

Risks:

- Must not be injected intravenously
- Before administering treatment, all diagnostic laboratory criteria must be met

Side-effects and adverse reactions

Central nervous system: fever.

Interactions (other drugs)

None listed.

Contraindications

Pregnancy category C.

Evidence

- There is insufficient evidence to recommend the use of anti-D in the management of adult patients with ITP [1] *Level C*
- It is not appropriate for children with platelet counts above 30,000/mm^3 (30x10^9/L) to be treated initially with anti-D [1] *Level C*
- A prospective trial (no control group) studied intravenous anti-D therapy in nonsplenectomized children and adult patients with classic ITP and HIV-related thrombocytopenia. Anti-D provided a hemostatic platelet increase in >70% of Rh-positive nonsplenectomized patients. The effect lasted 21 days in 50% of the responders [2] *This study does not meet the criteria for level P*

Surgical therapy

SPLENECTOMY

Vaccines against encapsulated bacteria should be administered to any patient diagnosed with ITP before emergent splenectomy.

Efficacy

- Often recommended by experts when other therapies have failed
- Approx. two-thirds of adult patients achieve normal platelet counts
- Thrombocytopenia may recur with longer follow up

Risks/Benefits
Risks:
- Anesthesia
- Major surgery
- Infection
- Lifelong susceptibility to infection by encapsulated bacteria

Benefit: if successful, enables patients with severe ITP refractory to treatment to lead a normal life

Evidence
Splenectomy may be indicated for adult patients with bleeding and platelet counts remaining below 30,000/mm^3 (30x10^9/L) after 4–6 weeks of medical treatment [1] *Level C*

Acceptability to patient
May be accepted by patients for whom other options have failed.

Follow up plan
Relapses may occur, but these can respond to drug therapy.

Patient and caregiver information
Patients must be informed of the need to seek medical advice immediately if they become unwell with a fever.

Endoscopic therapy

LAPAROSCOPIC SPLENECTOMY

Efficacy
Laparoscopic splenectomy appears feasible and safe in the treatment of hematologic diseases.

Risks/Benefits
Risk: splenosis resulting from capsular fractures

Benefits:
- Shorter postoperative stay than open splenectomy
- More rapid return to full activity than open splenectomy

Acceptability to patient
May be accepted by patients for whom other options have failed.

Follow up plan
Patients must be monitored as relapses can occur following successful splenectomy.

Patient and caregiver information
Patients must be informed of the need to seek medical advice immediately if they become unwell with a fever.

OUTCOMES

EFFICACY OF THERAPIES

- The outcome is better in children than adults
- There is variability from treatment to treatment, in general the efficacy varies from 30 to 90%

Evidence

PDxMD are unable to cite evidence which meets our criteria for evidence for the management of idiopathic thrombocytopenic purpura in adults.

Review period

- Monitor platelet count and clinical status daily to weekly, depending on the severity, for both treated and untreated patients
- Review treatment regularly as some improvements are not sustained

PROGNOSIS

Acute idiopathic thrombocytopenic purpura (ITP):

- 80–85% completely recover within 2 months
- 15% proceed to chronic ITP

Chronic ITP:

- 10–15% recover spontaneously
- 60–90% respond to treatment with prednisone, or prednisone and Rh(D) immune globulin or intravenous immunoglobulin
- Spontaneous remissions and relapses occur in 5%
- Of those requiring splenectomy, approx. 60% have a sustained response and 10–15% have a partial response

Clinical pearls

In most patients ITP has benign course and does not affect life expectancy. However, in patients with platelet counts <30,000/mm^3 (<30x10^9/L), life expectancy may be compromised.

Therapeutic failure

Referral to a hematologist is appropriate in the event of therapeutic failure. Those patients who failed steroids and splenectomy are considered to have refractory ITP. Before you make the diagnosis of refractory ITP, make sure to rule out accessory spleens. Therapeutic options exist but there are no randomized controlled trials to support their use. The most evidence consists of small case series. Options include:

- Azathioprine: adult dose 2mg/kg daily by mouth or intravenously; no established pediatric dose. Can be used on its own, or in conjunction with prednisone to reduce prednisone dose in patients experiencing side-effects or to delay splenectomy

- Cyclophosphamide: adult dose 2mg/kg daily by mouth
- Danazol: adult dose 200–600mg/day by mouth. Reported to increase platelet counts in 40–50% of patients, particularly postmenopausal women
- Combined chemotherapy (e.g. CVP – cyclophosphamide, vincristine, prednisone)
- Vinca alkaloids
- High-dose dexamethasone
- Colchicines
- Cladribine
- Alfa-interferon
- X-ray therapy of spleen (if splenectomy was contraindicated)
- Ascorbic acid
- Autologous peripheral blood stem cell transplant
- Rituxamab
- Recent studies suggest eradication of *Helicobacter pylori* may normalize platelets

For most of the treatments listed above, the American Society of Hematology has provided data on outcomes. The choice of any of the treatments listed is not optimized and is mostly based on personal experience of a physician with a given treatment. The benefit:risk ratios of these competing treatments have not been determined. It is more frequent in patients failing prednisone to use high doses of steroids such as dexamethasone 40mg/day for 4 days and repeated every 4 weeks.

Recurrence

If a previous episode of ITP has been successfully treated then that treatment can be used again.

COMPLICATIONS

Hemorrhage:

- Mortality due to intracranial hemorrhage occurs in 1% of cases of ITP
- Severe blood loss due to hemorrhage can occur

Bacterial infection:

Patients who have had a splenectomy have a decreased natural defense against acute bacterial infection.

CONSIDER CONSULT

Referral to a hematologist is indicated for patients with refractory ITP.

PREVENTION

RISK FACTORS

- Heroin: heroin use is associated with secondary immune thrombocytopenic purpura
- Alcohol: alcohol use is associated with secondary immune thrombocytopenic purpura
- Prescribed medication: a number of drugs are associated with secondary immune thrombocytopenic purpura
- Over-the-counter medications: aspirin is associated with secondary immune thrombocytopenic purpura
- HIV infection: secondary immune thrombocytopenic purpura is a common manifestation of HIV infection and AIDS

MODIFY RISK FACTORS

Lifestyle and wellness

ALCOHOL AND DRUGS

- Drug use: heroin use can directly cause idiopathic thrombocytopenic purpura (ITP), needle sharing is a risk factor for HIV infection, and heavy drug use may contribute to sexual risk taking, which is also a risk factor for HIV infection. Advise all patients using intravenous drugs never to share needles. Clinicians must then assess the individual's readiness to change this practice, and provide patient education and support directed at recovery. Patients should be advised to stop using drugs and to enter a substance-abuse treatment program with relapse prevention
- Acute and chronic alcohol consumption can cause ITP. Heavy alcohol use may contribute to sexual risk taking. All patients should be advised to limit alcohol consumption to the equivalent of 30mL (men) or 15mL (women) ethanol per day
- Alcoholics giving up drinking will require a special program

SEXUAL BEHAVIOR

All patients should be advised to use latex condoms during sexual intercourse to reduce the risk of HIV transmission.

DRUG HISTORY

Care should be taken when prescribing the following drugs:

- Acetaminophen
- Acetazolamide
- Allopurinol
- Alprenolol
- Amiodarone
- Ampicillin
- Amrinone
- Antazoline
- Aspirin
- Carbamazepine
- Cephalexin
- Cephalothin
- Chlorothiazide
- Chlorpheniramine

- Chlorthalidone
- Cimetidine
- Diazepam
- Desipramine
- Digitoxin
- Diltiazem
- Diphenylhydantoin
- Furosemide
- Gentamicin
- Gold salts
- Heparin
- Imipramine
- Iopanoic acid
- Lidocaine
- Meprobamate
- Methicillin
- Methyldopa
- Minoxidil
- Morphine
- Novobiocin
- Para-aminosalicylic acid
- Penicillin
- Phenylbutazone
- Procainamide
- Quinidine
- Quinine
- Ranitidine
- Rifampin
- Spironolactone
- Sulfisoxazole
- Trimethoprim-sulfamethoxazole
- Valproic acid
- Vancomycin

SCREENING

Screening for ITP is not realistic because of the rarity of the disorder. Also, there are no screening tests available.

PREVENT RECURRENCE

Avoid drugs that are known to precipitate ITP.

Reassess coexisting disease

INTERACTION ALERT

Trimethoprim-sulfamethoxazole, used as a treatment and prophylaxis for opportunistic infections associated with HIV infection and AIDS, may cause recurrence of ITP.

RESOURCES

ASSOCIATIONS

National Organization of Rare Disorders
PO Box 8923
New Fairfield, CT 06812–8923
Tel: (203) 746-6518
Toll-free: (800) 999-6673
Fax: (203) 746-6481
www.rarediseases.org

American Society of Hematology
1900 M. Street, NW
Suite 200
Washington, DC 20036
Tel: (202) 776-0544
Fax: (202) 776-0545
www.hematology.org

KEY REFERENCES

- Anonymous. Diagnosis and treatment of idiopathic thrombocytopenic purpura: recommendations of the American Society of Hematology. The American Society of Hematology ITP Practice Guideline Panel. Ann Intern Med 1997;126:319–26
- George JN, Woolf SH, Raskob GE, et al. Idiopathic thrombocytopenic purpura: a practice guideline developed by explicit methods for the American Society of Hematology. Blood 1996;88:3–40
- Donini A, Baccarani U, Terrosu G, et al. Laparoscopic vs open splenectomy in the management of hematologic disease. Surg Endosc 1999;13:1220–5
- Katkhouda N, Hurwitz MB, Rivera RT, et al. Laparoscopic splenectomy: outcome and efficacy in 103 consecutive patients. Ann Surg 1998;228:568–78
- Godeau B, Caulier MT, Decuypere L, et al. Intravenous immunoglobulin for adults with autoimmune thrombocytopenic purpura: results of a randomized trial comparing 0.5 and 1 g/kg b.w. Br J Haematol 1999;107:716–9
- Scaradavou A, Woo B, Woloski BM, et al. Intravenous anti-D treatment of idiopathic thrombocytopenic purpura: experience in 272 patients. Blood 1997;89:2689–700
- Portielje JE, Westendorp RG, Kluin-Nelemans HC, Brand A. Morbidity and mortality in adults with idiopathic thrombocytopenic purpura. Blood 2001;97:2549–54
- Schwartz KA. Gestational thrombocytopenia and immune thrombocytopenias in pregnancy. Hematol Oncol Clin North Am 2000;14:1101–16

Evidence reference and guidelines

1 George JN, Woolf SH, Raskob GE, et al. Idiopathic thrombocytopenic purpura: a practice guideline developed by explicit methods for the American Society of Hematology. Blood 1996;88:3–40

2 Scaradavou A, Woo B, Woloski BM, et al. Intravenous anti-D treatment of idiopathic thrombocytopenic purpura: experience in 272 patients. Blood 1997;89:2689–700

FAQS

Question 1

Is bone marrow aspirate/biopsy mandatory test to establish the diagnosis of idiopathic thrombocytopenic purpura (ITP)?

ANSWER 1

No. In most patients the diagnosis of ITP can be made without bone marrow biopsy/aspirate and by excluding other causes of thrombocytopenia on clinical grounds.

Question 2

Is ITP a 'benign' disease?

ANSWER 2

Yes. Most patients with chronic ITP may expect to have normal life expectancy (particularly those with platelets >30,000/mm^3 (>30x10^9/L)). Acute ITP is usually a self-limited disorder.

Question 3

Should every patient with ITP be treated?

ANSWER 3

No. Asymptomatic patients with platelet count >50,000/mm^3 (>50x10^9/L) may be observed without treatment. Withholding treatment is considered inappropriate for patients with a platelet count <20,000/mm^3 (<20x10^9/L), regardless of their symptoms, and for patients with a platelet count <50,000/mm^3 (<50x10^9/L) who present with significant mucous membrane bleeding, or who have risk factors for bleeding, such as hypertension, peptic ulcer disease, or vigorous lifestyle.

Question 4

What is considered standard sequence of treatment for chronic ITP?

ANSWER 4

Based on the established experience, most physicians use steroids followed by splenectomy. Those patients who fail splenectomy should be encouraged to participate in investigative trials for 'refractory ITP'.

CONTRIBUTORS

Mary Jo Groves, MD
Benjamin Djulbegovic, MD, PhD
Januario E Castro, MD

IRON-DEFICIENCY ANEMIA

SUMMARY INFORMATION

DESCRIPTION

- Anemia due to decreased iron stores caused by inadequate iron intake, poor absorption, or blood loss
- Most often seen in women with heavy menses and during pregnancy; cause in men is usually gastrointestinal bleeding
- Skin and conjunctival pallor may be present but otherwise physical examination may be normal
- Rarely, glossitis, koilonychia, angular stomatitis are present
- Treatment includes increasing dietary iron, and oral or intravenous iron replacement

URGENT ACTION

Red blood cell transfusion is indicated if anemia is life-threatening, depending on patient's hematocrit, rate of blood loss, and comorbid conditions such as angina or other cardiac decompensation. Ferritin, serum iron, and total iron-binding capacity should be drawn prior to transfusion to help clarify diagnosis once patient is stable.

ICD9 CODE

- 280.0 Iron-deficiency anemia due to chronic blood loss
- 280.1 Iron-deficiency anemia due to inadequate dietary intake
- 280.8 Other specified iron-deficiency anemia
- 280.9 Unspecified
- 648.2 Iron-deficiency anemia complicating pregnancy

SYNONYMS

- Anemia of chronic blood loss
- Hypochromic, microcytic anemia
- Chlorosis

CARDINAL FEATURES

- Most common form of anemia in general practice and clinical hematology
- Patients may be asymptomatic with a normal physical examination
- Fatigue, dizziness, exertional dyspnea may be reported by patient
- Conjunctival and skin pallor may be present
- Koilonychia – spoon-shaped fingernails that are flat and thin
- Triad of dysphagia (web of mucosa between hypopharynx and esophagus), angular stomatitis, and lingual abnormalities including glossitis if the cause is malabsorption
- Pagophagia – ingestion of abnormal amounts of ice
- Pica – ingestion of dirt, clay as well as 'food pica': ingestion of abnormal amounts of a specific food, usually crunchy like potato chips, carrots, celery, raw potatoes
- Low hemoglobin – often<8g/dL
- Reduced mean corpuscular volume and mean corpuscular hemoglobin
- Exaggeration of central pallor of red blood cells on peripheral blood smear
- Reduced serum iron concentration, transferrin saturation, and serum ferritin
- Increased total iron-binding capacity

CAUSES

Common causes

In adults:

- Diet – rare causes of iron deficiency; more common in developing countries where poverty, war, agricultural practices, or religious and social customs favor diet low in heme iron
- Gastrointestinal blood loss (common cause) – may be occult with steady loss of blood or frank and can be caused by colon or gastric cancer, diverticulosis, angiodysplasia, gastritis, peptic ulcer disease, inflammatory bowel disease, nonsteroidal anti-inflammatory drugs, *Helicobacter Pylori* and *H. pylori*-related gastritis; and parasitic infections, including hookworm infestation (*Necator americanus* or *Ancylostoma duodenale*)
- Menstrual bleeding (most common cause in women)
- Regular blood donation
- Alveolar hemorrhage – hemoptysis may not be evident; patients may swallow sputum-tinged blood leading to occult blood in stools and diagnostic confusion
- Long-distance runners – mild hemolysis, hematuria of unclear origin, and gastrointestinal bleeding caused by stress, jarring motion, or ischemia
- Nosocomial blood loss – phlebotomy for diagnostic tests in hospitalized patients
- Chronic renal failure treated with hemodialysis – due to dialysis process and laboratory evaluation
- Pregnancy and lactation causing increased demand for iron

- Impaired absorption – achlorhydria with impaired absorption of inorganic iron. Whether histamine H_2 inhibitors or proton pump inhibitors increase this risk remains controversial. Although some iron-deficient animal models have demonstrated a decrease in iron absorption rates, it is unknown if this holds true for conditions in humans with higher iron absorption requirements such as iron-deficiency anemia. Some consider it more important to follow vitamin B12 than iron levels in patients taking chronic antiacid therapy. In general, it is recommended that patients take iron supplements at least 2h before, or 4h after, antacids
- Pica – ingestion of dirt, clay, laundry starch, ice, or other unusual food substances; may be cultural
- Postgastric or small bowel surgery – due to loss of gastric acidity; increased transit time for food and decreased absorption of iron

In infants:

- Decreased total body iron at birth – linear relation between body iron and bodyweight
- Low birth weight
- Prematurity
- Twins
- Early clamping of umbilical cord – up to 100mL blood left in the placenta; delayed clamping may increase red blood cell volume by 58%
- Fetomaternal hemorrhage
- Inadequate diet – iron in human milk more accessible than in cow's milk
- Blood loss – may be caused by early introduction of cow's milk into infant's diet

Rare causes

- Factitious anemia: self-induced blood letting
- Hereditary hemorrhagic telangiectasia: recurrent hemorrhage from the nose, gastrointestinal tract, and other sites
- Intravascular hemolysis – such as paroxysmal nocturnal hemoglobinuria

Serious causes

Gastrointestinal bleeding: may be occult and indicative of gastric or colon cancer. May increase risk of life-threatening hemorrhage, such as with peptic ulcer disease or diverticular bleeding.

Contributory or predisposing factors

- Infants and menstrual-aged women are predisposed to iron-deficiency anemia due to increased demand

- Peptic ulcer disease and its treatment – antiacid therapy may decrease iron absorption rate in cases of iron deficiency
- *H. pylori* and *H. pylori*-related gastritis
- Crohn's disease
- Celiac disease

EPIDEMIOLOGY

Incidence and prevalence

Most common form of anemia seen in general medical and clinical hematology practice.

PREVALENCE

- 50/1000 adult men
- 140/1000 adult women
- 470/1000 children between 12 and 24 months

FREQUENCY

Prevalence in low-income pregnant women 9, 14, and 37% in first, second, and third trimesters, respectively.

Demographics

AGE

- More common in infants with unsupplemented milk diets
- Common in women during reproductive years (menses, pregnancy)

GENDER

- Adults: female>male
- Infants: female=male

RACE

Slightly greater incidence in African-American women.

SOCIOECONOMIC STATUS

Prevalence higher in those living in chronic poverty.

DIAGNOSIS

DIFFERENTIAL DIAGNOSIS

Anemia of chronic disease

Anemia of chronic disease is present in chronic inflammation such as rheumatoid arthritis, Crohn's disease (may also cause iron-deficiency anemia), and cancer.

FEATURES

- Characterized by decreased iron, decreased total iron-binding capacity, increased ferritin, and increased marrow iron stores, red cells that are slightly hypochromic and microcytic, hemoglobin that is normally 7–11g/dL, rarely <7g/dL
- Symptoms are those of the underlying disease

Sideroblastic anemia

Sideroblastic anemia includes a heterogeneous group of disorders. It is characterized by ferric phosphate and ferric hydroxide deposits in the erythroblast mitochondria.

FEATURES

- Signs and symptoms of anemia
- Congenital (rare, X-linked) and acquired (most commonly idiopathic) forms of the disease present
- Severe forms recognized in childhood
- Mild hepatosplenomegaly
- Cardiac arrhythmias, congestive heart failure
- Impaired growth and development in infants and children
- Acquired form may be treated with high-dose pyridoxine

Thalassemia trait

Inherited disorder that affects synthesis of alpha- or beta-hemoglobin. Thalassemia trait is most commonly seen in the Mediterranean region, Middle East, and Southeast Asia.

FEATURES

- Mild anemia with microcytosis and hypochromia and poikilocytosis
- Hemoglobin electrophoresis is diagnostic

SIGNS & SYMPTOMS

Signs

- Patient may have no signs
- Skin and conjunctival pallor
- Koilonychia
- Angular stomatitis
- Glossitis

Symptoms

- Fatigue
- Dizziness
- Exertional dyspnea
- Anorexia
- Pagophagia
- Pica
- Melena
- Hematochezia
- Hemoptysis

CONSIDER CONSULT

- If gastrointestinal blood loss suspected, consider referral to a gastroenterologist
- If bone marrow aspirate needed, refer to hematologist

INVESTIGATION OF THE PATIENT

Direct questions to patient

- Q **Have your eating habits changed in the last year?** Loss of appetite, change of diet to exclude heme iron-containing foods, fad dieting, cultural changes may contribute to iron deficiency
- Q **Do you crave unusual amounts of crunchy foods or eat dirt, clay, laundry starch, or more than one ice cube tray of ice per day?** While overt pica includes dirt, clay, starch, and ice, it has been reported that some patients with iron-deficiency anemia crave crunchy foods
- Q **Is there a history of heavy menstrual periods?** Use of more than four pads/day or bleeding that cannot be controlled with tampons alone signals excessive menstrual periods
- Q **Is there a history of gastric or bowel surgery?** Possible loss of gastric acidity; increased transit time for food and decreased absorption of iron
- Q **Has there been a change in stool color or odor?** May indicate gastrointestinal blood loss
- Q **Do you take aspirin or nonsteroidal anti-inflammatory drugs (NSAIDs) for arthritis or other conditions?** Possible cause of occult gastrointestinal blood loss
- Q **Have you experienced a cough?** Signals the need to investigate possibility of alveolar hemorrhage even if patient has not noticed hemoptysis. (This would be a very rare cause of iron-deficiency anemia)
- Q **Are you a long-distance runner?** Signals the need to investigate occult gastrointestinal blood loss, hematuria, hemolysis
- Q **What is the color of your urine? Have you noticed blood in your urine?** Signals possible blood loss/hematuria, hemoglobinuria (e.g. paraxoxysmal nocturnal hemoglobinuria)

Contributory or predisposing factors

- Q **Are you pregnant?** Increased demand of fetus for iron may cause iron deficiency in mother
- Q **Are you being treated for chronic renal failure with hemodialysis?** Treatment and laboratory monitoring can both contribute to iron-deficiency anemia combined with anemia of chronic disease
- Q **Do you suffer from a chronic disease?** Chronic diseases such as rheumatoid arthritis and Crohn's disease can lead to anemia of chronic disease, or iron-deficiency anemia
- Q **Is the patient an infant in the first year of life?** Dramatic growth causes increased demand for iron
- Q **Have you had gastric surgery?** Iron-deficiency anemia is a potential complication of gastric surgery

Family history

- Q **Is there a history of iron deficiency in the family?** While not a genetic disorder, it does tend to run in the family due to customs and cultural associations with food intake.

Examination

- **Physical examination** is often normal
- **Inspect skin, conjunctiva, mucosa** for pallor, blue sclerae
- **Inspect oral cavity** for glossitis, angular stomatitis
- **Inspect fingernails** for koilonychia – spoon-shaped fingernails that are flat and thin
- **Auscultate heart** for tachycardia, arrhythmia
- **Perform a rectal examination and a hemoccult test** to determine if rectal bleeding (occult or frank blood) is the cause of possible anemia. A mass may be felt
- **Pelvic examination** may reveal uterine cause of excess bleeding
- **Urine analysis,** to rule out hematuria/hemoglobinuria

Summary of investigative tests

- Complete blood cell count (CBC)
- Hemoglobin and hematocrit are used to confirm anemia
- Red blood cell (RBC) indices – low mean corpuscular volume (MCV) confirms microcytic anemia
- Serum ferritin concentration – low serum ferritin is the most specific indicator of low iron stores
- Total iron-binding capacity reflects the availability of iron-binding sites on transferring, which is increased in iron deficiency
- Serum iron concentration measures the total amount of iron in the serum, which is decreased in iron deficiency
- Bone marrow biopsy is rarely needed for the diagnosis of iron-deficiency anemia, but would typically show absent iron stores
- Erythrocyte protoporphyrin concentration increases when there is insufficient iron for hemoglobin production
- Serum transferrin receptor concentration – increases in iron-deficiency anemia, reflects index of tissue needs; this is no longer recommended since it is less sensitive and less specific than ferritin

DIAGNOSTIC DECISION

- Diagnosis is suspected on the basis of the history and examination
- Laboratory testing confirms the diagnosis
- Mean cell volume is an indicator of hypochromic microcytic anemia (a hallmark of iron-deficiency anemia)
- Anisocytosis and increased red cell distribution width (RDW) are the earliest signs of iron deficiency

Guidelines

Centers for Disease Control and Prevention. Recommendations to prevent and control iron deficiency in the United States [1].

CLINICAL PEARLS

- If ferritin is low (<12ng/mL), it is virtually certain that the patient has iron-deficiency anemia
- In male or nonmenstruating woman, assume gastrointestinal bleeding as a cause of anemia until proven otherwise

THE TESTS

Body fluids

COMPLETE BLOOD COUNT

Description

- Venous blood sample taken for laboratory analysis
- Measures RBCs, hemoglobin/hematocrit, RBC indexes, white blood cells (WBCs), and platelet count, but specifically interested in hemoglobin concentration (information provided for hemoglobin only here)

Advantages/Disadvantages

Advantages:

- Widely available
- Specimen easy to obtain
- Rapid results
- Confirms anemia
- Test can be run on capillary tube of blood

Disadvantages:

- Late indicator of iron deficiency
- Not diagnostic of the cause of the anemia

Normal

- Newborn: 15.0–24.0g/dL
- 1–23 months: 10.5–14.0g/dL
- 2–9 years: 11.5–14.5g/dL
- 10–17 years (male): 12.5–16.1g/dL
- 10–17 years (female): 12.0–15.0g/dL
- >18 years (male): 13.5–18.0g/dL
- >18 years (female): 12.5–16.0g/dL

Abnormal

- Newborn: <15.0g/dL
- 1–23 months: <10.5g/dL
- 2–9 years: 11.5–14.5g/dL
- 10–17 years (male): <12.5g/dL
- 10–17 years (female): <12.0g/dL
- >18 years (male): <13.5g/dL
- >18 years (female): <12.5g/dL

Cause of abnormal result

Inadequate production or excessive loss of blood.

Drugs, disorders and other factors that may alter results

- Acute blood loss (hemoglobin/hematocrit and RBC morphology changes may lag acute blood loss)
- NSAIDs
- Aspirin

HEMATOCRIT

Description

Peripheral blood sample.

Advantages/Disadvantages

Advantages:

- Widely available
- Specimen easy to obtain
- Rapid results
- Test can be run on capillary tube of blood

Disadvantage: late indicator of iron deficiency

Normal

- Newborn: 44–70%
- 1–23 months: 32–42%
- 2–9 years: 33–43%
- 10–17 years (male): 36–47%
- 10–17 years (female): 35–45%
- >18 years (male): 42–52%
- >18 years (female): 37–47%

Abnormal

- Newborn: <44%
- 1–23 months: <32%
- 2–9 years: <33%

- 10–17 years (male): <36%
- 10–17 years (female): <35%
- >18 years (male): <42%
- >18 years (female): <37%
- Keep in mind possibility of a false-positive result

Cause of abnormal result
Decreased hemoglobin or increased plasma volume.

Drugs, disorders and other factors that may alter results
- Acute blood loss (hemoglobin/hematocrit and RBC morphology changes may lag acute blood loss
- NSAIDs
- Aspirin

RED BLOOD CELL INDICIES
Description
Peripheral blood sample.

Advantages/Disadvantages
Advantages:
- Specimen easily obtained
- Low MCV indicates iron deficiency
- Can be calculated by manual methods if automated instruments not available

Disadvantages:
- Nonspecific to disorder
- Mean corpuscular hemoglobin concentration is poor indicator of iron-deficiency anemia as decrease occurs only when anemia severe

Normal
- MCV: 82–92mcm^3 82–92fL (hematocrit divided by RBC count)
- Mean corpuscular hemoglobin (MCH): 27–31pg (hemoglobin divided by RBC count)
- Mean corpuscular hemoglobin concentration (MCHC) 32–36mg/dL (320–360mg/L) (hemoglobin divided by hematocrit)

Abnormal
- Degree of change related to duration and severity of anemia
- MCV: <80mcm^3 <80fL
- MCH: <27pg
- MCHC: <32mg/dL (<320mg/L)
- Keep in mind the possibility of a false-positive result

Cause of abnormal result
Changes of intracellular hemoglobulin concentration relative to RBC size.

Drugs, disorders and other factors that may alter results
- Acute blood loss (hemoglobin/hematocrit and RBC morphology changes may lag acute blood loss)
- NSAIDs
- Aspirin

SERUM FERRITIN CONCENTRATION

Description

Peripheral blood sample.

Advantages/Disadvantages

Advantages:

- Single best indicator of iron storage
- Specimen easily obtained
- Test widely available
- Can be used to measure compliance with therapy

Disadvantage: not sensitive – normal value does not rule out iron deficiency

Normal

- Newborns: 25–200ng/mL (25–200mcg/L)
- One month: 200–600ng/mL (200–600mcg/L)
- 2–5 months: 50–200ng/mL (50–200mcg/L)
- 6 months to 15 years: 7–142ng/mL (7–142mcg/L)
- Adult male: 20–300ng/mL (20–300mcg/L)
- Adult female: 12–120ng/mL (12–120mcg/L)

Abnormal

- Newborns: <25ng/mL (<25mcg/L)
- One month: <200ng/mL (<200mcg/L)
- 2–5 months: 50–200ng/mL (50–200mcg/L)
- 6 months to 15 years: <7ng/mL (<7mcg/L)
- Adult male: <20ng/mL (<20mcg/L)
- Adult female: <12ng/L (<12mcg/L)

Cause of abnormal result

Decrease is indicative of iron-deficiency anemia.

Drugs, disorders and other factors that may alter results

Increase can be seen in acute and chronic liver disease, alcoholism, infection and inflammation, iron overload, other anemias, end-stage renal disease.

TOTAL IRON-BINDING CAPACITY

Description

Peripheral blood sample.

Advantages/Disadvantages

Advantage: test is widely available and specimen easily obtained

Disadvantages:

- Not useful alone in diagnosing iron deficiency
- May be elevated in liver damage

Normal

250–450mcg/dL (45–81mcmol/L).

Abnormal

- >450mcg/dL (>81mcmol/L)
- Keep in mind the possibility of a false-positive result due to factors outlined below

Cause of abnormal result

Lack of functional iron.

Drugs, disorders and other factors that may alter results

- Elevated in liver disease, acute and chronic blood loss, late pregnancy, use of progesterone birth control pills
- Decreased in hemochromatosis, cirrhosis of liver, thalassemia, anemia related to infection, anemia of chronic disease, nephrosis, hyperthyroidism

ERYTHROCYTE PROTOPORPHYRIN

Description

Peripheral blood sample.

Advantages/Disadvantages

Advantages:

- This test is not frequently performed but can be very helpful. The red cell zinc protoporphyrin level is increased in both iron deficiency and the anemia of chronic disease in which iron is present but trapped in macrophages and, therefore, not 'available' for heme synthesis. Red cell zinc protoporphyrin is also elevated in lead poisoning. Thus, measurement of zinc protoporphyrin may be doubly useful in screening pediatric populations for both iron deficiency and lead poisoning
- Determines availability of iron for heme synthesis

Disadvantages:

- Not specific
- Sensitivity and specificity for iron deficiency in adults are significantly less than serum ferritin
- Most laboratories do not have a hematofluorometer with which to conduct test

Abnormal

- >10mcg/dL packed RBCs
- Keep in mind the possibility of a false-positive result

Cause of abnormal result

Lack of iron for last step in heme synthesis.

Drugs, disorders and other factors that may alter results

- Chronic infections
- Noninfectious inflammation
- Malignancies
- Chronic liver disease
- Moderate or severe hemolytic anemias

SERUM IRON

Description

Venous blood sample.

Advantages/Disadvantages

Advantages:

- Test is widely available
- Specimen easily obtained
- A measure of the amount of iron bound to transferrin

Normal

60–170mcg/dL.

Abnormal

Results below the normal reference range.

Cause of abnormal result

Lack of functional iron.

TREATMENT

CONSIDER CONSULT

- Consider referral to gastroenterologist for treatment of underlying gastrointestinal lesions
- Refer to oncologist for diagnosis/treatment of suspected colon, esophageal, or other gastrointestinal cancer

IMMEDIATE ACTION

Iron-deficiency anemia is rarely life-threatening but blood transfusion may occasionally be needed, especially in patients with cardiac decompensation or in the elderly.

PATIENT AND CAREGIVER ISSUES

Patient or caregiver request

What is the cause of iron-deficiency anemia? The most common mistake is to treat iron-deficiency anemia without explaining its etiology.

Health-seeking behavior

- **Have you been treated for iron-deficiency anemia in the past?** This may indicate poor compliance with therapy or recurrent disorder
- **Have you self-medicated?** Patient may be taking vitamin supplements for self-diagnosis of 'iron-poor blood'. These preparations may, or may not, contain iron
- **Have you visited a walk-in clinic or emergency room?** Symptoms may lead patients to seek ambulatory care outside of primary care setting. Unless followed up with primary care physician (PCP), underlying cause of anemia may be missed

MANAGEMENT ISSUES

Goals

- Replenish iron stores
- Identify underlying causes for iron deficiency

Management in special circumstances

COEXISTING DISEASE

- Management of peptic ulcer disease with agents that decrease acidification of gastric secretions may increase malabsorption of iron
- Additional iron supplements may be required

COEXISTING MEDICATION

Medications that block acidification of gastric secretions.

SPECIAL PATIENT GROUPS

- In pregnant women, iron supplementation should begin at first trimester to avoid depletion of iron stores
- Lactating mothers have same requirements for iron as menstruating women due to iron loss with nursing
- Infants (first year of life) and children (11–14 years) may need iron supplementation during growth spurts; dose of iron is based on weight – infants will need liquid supplementation
- Elderly people with memory deficiencies may require 'pill count' monitoring to ensure compliance with therapy

PATIENT SATISFACTION/LIFESTYLE PRIORITIES

- Noncompliance with iron supplement regimen is a problem in asymptomatic patient
- Constipation must be addressed if it affects wellbeing or compliance
- Pill counts at follow up may help assess compliance with regimen

SUMMARY OF THERAPEUTIC OPTIONS

Choices

- First choice for therapy is oral ferrous sulfate but this preparation may not be well tolerated due to gastrointestinal side-effects
- Second choice for therapy is oral ferrous gluconate. This preparation has lower elemental iron than ferrous sulfate and is better tolerated but requires a longer duration of therapy
- Third choice for therapy is parenteral iron dextran

Guidelines

- Centers for Disease Control and Prevention. Recommendations to prevent and control iron deficiency in the United States [1]
- The American Academy of Family Physicians have produced information on anemia: [2]

Clinical pearls

- The response rate to oral iron is similar to the response rate to parenteral treatment
- Anemia should be accurately diagnosed prior to initiating iron supplementation
- The ultimate proof of the diagnosis is a response to treatment – if the patient does not respond to iron supplementation, suspect the accuracy of the diagnosis. The most common mistake it to treat patients with anemia of chronic disease or thalassemia with iron

Never

If the patient had anaphylactic reaction to parenteral iron, iron supplementation should not be attempted.

FOLLOW UP

Regular follow up is important to determine compliance with therapy and to assess for recurrence.

Plan for review

- Hematocrit and hemoglobin should be rechecked periodically to ensure return to normal
- Make sure that the underlying cause is adequately treated, if possible
- Regular follow up to assess for recurrence

Information for patient or caregiver

- Iron replacement therapy is best absorbed on an empty stomach but if gastrointestinal upset, take with food
- Liquid iron supplements should be taken through a straw to avoid staining teeth
- Therapy is typically recommended until 3 months after hemoglobin has returned to normal (this is usually measured by normal ferritin level)
- Iron supplements may turn stools black or dark green

DRUGS AND OTHER THERAPIES: DETAILS

Drugs

FERROUS SULFATE

Oral iron supplement indicated in iron-deficiency anemia.

Dose

- Each tablet contains 160mg dried ferrous sulfate, equivalent to 50mg elemental iron
- Adult: one or two tablets daily or as recommended by a physician. Maximum of four tablets daily may be taken
- Child: one tablet daily. Tablets must be swallowed whole

Efficacy

- Rapid subjective improvement
- Pagophagia resolved within one week
- Normal hemoglobin reached at about 2 months

Risks/Benefits

Risks:

- The treatment of any anemic condition should be under the advice and supervision of a physician. As oral iron products interfere with absorption of oral tetracycline antibiotics, these products should not be taken within 2h of each other
- Accidental overdose of iron-containing products is a leading cause of fatal poisoning in children under 6 years

Side-effects and adverse reactions

Gastrointestinal: nausea, vomiting, bloating, abdominal discomfort, black stools, diarrhea, constipation (leading to colic), anorexia.

Interactions (other drugs)

- **Alkalinizers** ■ **Antacids** ■ **Calcium carbonate** ■ **Chloramphenicol** ■ **Pancreatic enzymes** ■ **Cimetidine** ■ **Doxycycline** ■ **Famotidine** ■ **Levodopa** ■ **Methyldopa** ■ **Penicillamine** ■ **Nizatidine** ■ **Quinolones** ■ **Ranitidine** ■ **Tetracycline** ■ **Vitamin E**

Contraindications

- **Hemosiderosis** ■ **Hemochromatosis** ■ **Hemolytic anemia** ■ **Regional enteritis** ■ **Hypersensitivity to iron or any component of treatment** ■ **Ulcerative colitis**

Acceptability to patient

Gastrointestinal side-effects may cause compliance problems and indicate need to switch to alternative supplementation.

Follow up plan

- Periodic hemoglobin and hematocrit until return to normal. Time interval is variable and depends on the clinical condition of the patient. In the ambulatory setting, follow up every 3–4 weeks would be appropriate
- Regular follow up to assess for compliance and recurrence. Significant hemoglobin increase at 3–4 weeks and normalization of hemoglobin at 2–4 months should occur with adequate iron replacement. If these changes do not happen, compliance of patient should be determined or another cause of anemia should be sought

Patient and caregiver information

Therapy typically extends until 3 months after normalization of hematocrit, in order to fully replenish iron stores. However, there are no clear guidelines as to how long therapy should be continued. Some physicians stop when the hemoglobin level becomes normal (which helps as a marker of occult blood loss when it would be expected to see a recurrent decline in hemoglobin after a period of successful replenishment), while others believe it wise to treat for about 6 months after the hemoglobin normalizes (in order to completely replenish iron stores).

FERROUS GLUCONATE

Indicated in iron-deficiency anemia for replacement of iron.

Dose

- Adult: 100–200mg/day orally in three divided doses
- Child aged 2–12 years: 3mg/kg/day orally in three to four divided doses
- Infants: 10–25mg/day orally in three to four divided doses

Efficacy

- Subjective improvement in one week of therapy
- Longer to reach normal hemoglobin due to decreased dose of iron

Risks/Benefits

Risk: use caution in patients with elevated serum ferritin levels

Benefits:

- Preparation is well tolerated
- Subjective improvement is seen quickly

Side-effects and adverse reactions

Gastrointestinal: nausea, vomiting, bloating, black stools, constipation.

Interactions (other drugs)

■ Alkalinizers ■ Antacids ■ Calcium carbonate ■ Doxycycline ■ Cimetidine ■ Levodopa ■ Famotidine ■ Methyldopa ■ Nizatidine ■ Penicillamine ■ Quinolones ■ Ranitidine ■ Tetracycline ■ Pancreatic enzymes ■ Chloramphenicol ■ Vitamin E

Contraindications

■ Hypersensitivity to any iron-containing supplement ■ Hemochromatosis ■ Hemosiderosis ■ Pregnant women and nursing mothers should not use more than RDA (recommended daily allowance) amounts (30 and 15mg/day, respectively)

Acceptability to patient

- Oral preparation is acceptable to patients – few side-effects if taken with food
- If gastrointestinal side-effects persist, compliance may be a problem

Follow up plan

- Periodic hemoglobin and hematocrit until return back to normal
- Regular follow up to assess for compliance and recurrence

Patient and caregiver information

Therapy needs to be taken for at least 12 months to replace iron stores.

IRON DEXTRAN

- Intravenous iron preparation for replacement of iron stores
- Refer to an hematologist for administration because of possible side-effects including life-threatening anaphylactic reactions

Dose

- Periodic hematologic determination (hemoglobin and hematocrit) is a simple and accurate technique for monitoring hematologic response, and should be used as a guide in therapy
- Preparation containing 50mg iron/mL solution
- To calculate a patient's weight in kg when lb are known: patient's weight in lb ÷ 2.2 = weight in kg
- Requires test dose which may be unacceptable to patient

Adults and children over 15kg (33 lb):

- Dose can be calculated using following: dose (mL) = 0.0442 (Desired Hb – Observed Hb) x LBW + (0.26 x LBW)

Based on:

- Desired hemoglobin (Hb) = the target Hb in g/dL
- Observed Hb = the patient's current Hb in g/dL
- LBW = lean bodyweight in kg. A patient's lean bodyweight (or actual bodyweight if less than lean bodyweight) should be utilized when determining dosage
- For males: LBW = 50kg + 2.3kg for each inch of patient's height over 5ft
- For females: LBW = 45.5kg + 2.3kg for each inch of patient's height over 5ft

Children 5–15kg (11–33 lb):

- Total dose may be calculated:
- Dose (mL) = 0.0442 (Desired Hb – Observed Hb) x W + (0.26 x W)

Based on:

- Desired Hb = the target Hb in g/dL (normal Hb for children 15kg or less is 12g/dL)
- W = weight in kg

Efficacy

Subjective improvement in one week of therapy.

Risks/Benefits

Risks:

- Risk of severe and fatal anaphylactic reactions (epinephrine should be immediately available in the event of acute hypersensitivity reactions)
- Use caution in patients with history of significant allergies and/or asthma
- Patients with rheumatoid arthritis may have an acute exacerbation of joint pain and swelling following the administration of iron dextran
- Intramuscular iron dextran in neonates has been associated with an increased incidence of Gram-negative sepsis, primarily due to *Escherichia coli*

Side-effects and adverse reactions

- Cardiovascular: chest pain, chest tightness, shock, cardiac arrest, hypotension, hypertension, tachycardia, bradycardia, flushing, arrhythmias
- Central nervous system: convulsions, seizures, syncope, headache, weakness, unresponsiveness, paresthesia, febrile episodes, chills, dizziness, disorientation, numbness, unconsciousness

- Gastrointestinal: abdominal pain, nausea, vomiting, diarrhea
- Genitourinary: hematuria
- Hematologic: leucocytosis, lymphadenopathy
- Musculoskeletal: arthralgia, arthritis, brown skin and/or underlying tissue discoloration (staining), soreness or pain at or near intramuscular injection sites; cellulitis; swelling; inflammation; local phlebitis at or near intravenous injection site
- Respiratory: respiratory arrest, dyspnea, bronchospasm, wheezing, respiratory difficulty and/or cardiovascular collapse
- Skin: urticaria, pruritus, purpura, rash, cyanosis

Interactions (other drugs)

- **Angiotensin-converting enzyme (ACE) inhibitors** ■ **Chloramphenicol**

Contraindications

- **Pregnancy** ■ **Safety and efficacy have not been established in infants under 4 months**
- **Hypersensitivity to iron**

Acceptability to patient

- Flu-like side-effects may make therapy unacceptable to patient
- Lack of gastrointestinal side-effects may make this therapy more acceptable to some patients
- Requires test dose which may be unacceptable to patient

Follow up plan

- Weekly hemoglobin and hematocrit until return to normal
- Regular follow up to assess for compliance and recurrence

Patient and caregiver information

- Therapy needs to be taken for at least 4 months to replace iron stores but can take for up to one year
- Requires test dose to rule out allergic reaction
- Most side-effects are transient and relieved by slowing infusion
- Parenteral route does not replenish iron stores faster than oral preparations

OUTCOMES

EFFICACY OF THERAPIES

- Supplemental iron therapy is generally successful in replenishing iron stores that are low in iron-deficiency anemia
- It is important to find the underlying cause of iron-deficiency anemia to ensure adequate treatment

Review period

- Periodic hemoglobin and hematocrit until return to back to normal
- Regular follow up to assess for compliance and recurrence

PROGNOSIS

Curable with iron therapy, and if underlying condition can be discovered and treated.

Clinical pearls

Prognosis depends on the underlying cause.

Therapeutic failure

- Failure to respond to iron replacement is usually related to misdiagnosis, noncompliance, inadequate treatment, continuing iron loss, or malabsorption
- Parenteral iron therapy may be considered if oral therapy fails

Recurrence

- Recurrence is usually due to noncompliance with therapy or recurrence of underlying condition
- Consider referral to hematologist for further investigation of source of anemia
- Consider referral to gastroenterologist for evaluation of gastrointestinal bleeding

Deterioration

- If anemia falls to life-threatening level, blood transfusion may be life-saving but will not correct iron-deficiency anemia without other supplementation
- Consider specialty referral for further investigation of source of anemia

Terminal illness

Patient is unlikely to become terminally ill from this disorder.

COMPLICATIONS

Complications are usually related to underlying disease.

CONSIDER CONSULT

Refer to hematologist if refractory to oral and intravenous iron preparations.

RISK FACTORS

- Blood loss: related to peptic ulcer disease, gastric or colon cancer, trauma, diverticulosis, angiodysplasia, gastritis, inflammatory bowel disease
- Poor iron intake: lack of heme iron in diet, poverty, pica
- Poor iron absorption: gastritis, peptic ulcer, disease treatment, gastric surgery, malabsorption (e.g. celiac disease)
- Increased demand: growth in infancy, adolescence, pregnancy
- Hookworm infestation: competition with host for iron
- Long-distance runner: mild hemolysis, hematuria of unclear origin, and gastrointestinal bleeding caused by stress, jarring motion, or ischemia

MODIFY RISK FACTORS

Lifestyle and wellness

DIET

- Inclusion of dietary sources of iron including meat, beans, leafy green vegetables
- Limit milk to one pint daily in adults
- Eliminate pica

PHYSICAL ACTIVITY

In runners, decrease distance or switch to different physical exercise.

DRUG HISTORY

- Use of antacids to treat peptic ulcer disease may contribute to decreased iron absorption and may indicate possible cause of gastrointestinal blood loss
- Nonsteroidal anti-inflammatory drug use may predispose to gastrointestinal blood loss

CHEMOPROPHYLAXIS

Prophylactic iron supplementation in pregnancy.

Cost/efficacy

- Ferrous sulfate 325mg = $1.50–$4.83 for 100 tablets
- Ferrous gluconate 300mg = $2.13–$4.43 for 100 tablets
- May prevent low hemoglobin at birth and at 6 weeks postpartum although there is little information on pregnancy outcomes for mother or baby

SCREENING

Screening is recommended for:

- Pregnant women at their first prenatal visit
- High-risk infants, preferably at 6–12 months of age

High-risk infants include:

- Infants living in poverty, African-Americans, native Americans, native Alaskans
- Infants living in and/or immigrating from developing countries
- Preterm and low birth weight infants
- Infants whose major dietary intake is unfortified cow's milk

HEMOGLOBIN AND HEMATOCRIT

May be measured from capillary tube sample but venous blood more accurate.

Cost/efficacy

Normal values for hemoglobin and hematocrit are well published; efficacy for establishing presence of anemia is high.

SERUM FERRITIN

Sensitive indicator for assessing body stores of iron.

Cost/efficacy

Best sensitivity and specificity for detecting iron deficiency in anemic patients.

PREVENT RECURRENCE

Recurrence is usually related to noncompliance with treatment or recurrence of underlying disorder.

Reassess coexisting disease

Gastric surgery may contribute to malabsorption of iron.

INTERACTION ALERT

Treatment for peptic ulcer disease may interfere with iron absorption and contribute to recurrent iron-deficiency anemia.

PATIENT SATISFACTION/LIFESTYLE PRIORITIES

Long-distance runners who continue in their sport after treatment for iron-deficiency anemia risk recurrence of disease – discontinuing sport may be difficult for some patients.

ASSOCIATIONS

The American Society of Hematology
1900 M Street, NW, Suite 200
Washington, DC 20036
Tel: (202) 776-0544
Fax: (202) 776-0545
E-mail: ASH@hematology.org
www.hematology.org

Centers for Disease Control and Prevention
1600 Clifton Road
Atlanta, GA 30333
Tel: (404) 639-3311
www.cdc.gov

KEY REFERENCES

- Bridges KR. Iron deficiency. In: Rakel RE, ed. Latest approved methods of treatment for the practicing physician. Philadelphia (PA): WB Saunders, 2000, p356–8
- Center for Disease Control. Guidelines for diagnosis of iron deficiency anemia in infants, children and women of child-bearing age. Morb Mortal Wkly Rep 1998;47(RR-3):1–36
- Duffy TP. Microcytic and hypochromic anemias. In: Goldman L, Bennett JC, eds. Cecil textbook of medicine, 21st edn. Philadelphia (PA): WB Saunders, 2000, p855–7
- Frewin R, Henson A, Provan D. ABC of clinical haematology: iron-deficiency anemia. BMJ 1997;314:360
- Guyatt GH, Oxman AD, Mahmoud A, et al. Laboratory diagnosis of iron-deficiency anemia: an overview. J Gen Int Med 1992;7:143–53
- Lee GR. Iron deficiency and iron-deficiency anemia. In: Lee GR, Forrester J, Lukens J, et al, eds. Wintrobe's clinical hematology, 10th edn. Baltimore (MD): Williams & Wilkins, 1999, p979–1010, 1022–4
- National Kidney Foundation – Dialysis Outcomes Quality Initiative (KF-DOQI). Clinical practice guidelines for the treatment of anemia of chronic renal failure. New York: National Kidney Foundation, 1997
- Ravel R. Factor deficiency anemia. In: Ravel R, ed. Clincial application of laboratory data, 6th edn. St Louis (MO): Mosby, 1995, p22–34
- Wallach J, ed. Interpretation of diagnostic tests. Philadelphia (PA): Lippincott, Williams & Wilkins, 2000, p6, 8, 327, 333, 363–4

Evidence references and guidelines

1. Centers for Disease Control and Prevention. Recommendations to prevent and control iron deficiency in the United States. MMWR 1998/47(RR-3);1–36
2. The American Academy of Family Physicians have produced information on anemia: Little DR. Ambulatory management of common forms of anemia. Am Fam Physician 1999;59:1598–604

FAQS

Question 1

In women who are heavily menstruating, what are the odds of developing iron-deficiency anemia?

ANSWER 1

About 80% or higher. Young females who aren't at risk for other diseases that can cause iron-deficiency anemia can be treated by iron replacement therapy with no additional workup.

Question 2
What are common gastrointestinal causes of iron-deficiency anemia?

ANSWER 2
Common abnormalities in the upper gastrointestinal tract are gastritis and peptic ulceration, often due to nonsteroidal anti-inflammatory drugs. Colon cancer and diverticulosis are common causes for lower gastrointestinal bleeding.

Question 3
If the workup detects one bleeding gastrointestinal lesion, should it be extended to look for other sites of gastrointestinal bleeding?

ANSWER 3
This depends on the character of the bleeding and the consistency of the pathologic finding with the clinical presentation. Also, presence of a colon polyp increases the risk of others being found and warrants complete lower endoscopy.

Question 4
If upper endoscopy and colonoscopy are negative, should more extensive workup be undertaken?

ANSWER 4
Over one-third of the patients may have no detectable lesions in gastrointestinal tract. Further gastrointestinal follow up may be indicated to detect lesions in the small intestine. This gastrointestinal follow up is especially required if no other sources of bleeding (urinary, pulmonary, gynecologic, iatrogenic) or other reasons for iron-deficiency anemia (e.g. poor absorption) are found.

Question 5
What are the major complications of intravenous iron?

ANSWER 5
Reactions may be expected in 26% of patients. 5% may experience serious reactions, 1% may have serum sickness, and 0.6% may develop life-threatening anaphylactoid reaction.

CONTRIBUTORS
Eric F Pollack, MD, MPH
Benjamin Djulbegovic, MD, PhD
Naixi N Chen, MD

LUNG MALIGNANCIES

SUMMARY INFORMATION

DESCRIPTION

- Primary malignancies arising from lung tissue
- Epithelial cancers arising from the bronchial surface epithelium or bronchial mucous glands
- 12 types of primary lung malignancies
- All the primary lung malignancies except small cell cancers behave similarly
- Crucial difference is between small cell carcinoma and non-small cell carcinoma
- The therapeutic approaches and prognoses are therefore based on this important grouping, and differ between the two groups
- Lung cancer is the leading cause of death from cancer in men and women in the world
- It has high mortality and low cure rates, but recent therapeutic advances have led to improvements in survival
- Majority of cases occur in people who smoke or have smoked cigarettes for many years

URGENT ACTION

Arrange immediate admission if:

- There is massive hemoptysis
- There are symptoms and signs of respiratory distress, or of acute severe pneumonia
- If a primary lung malignancy is suspected or confirmed, urgent referral to a respiratory specialist is mandatory

Patients presenting with complications require immediate referral including:

- Hypercalcemia
- Superior vena cava syndrome
- Pericardial effusion or tamponade
- Spinal cord compression

KEY! DON'T MISS!

- The development of a new cough, if persistent, in a smoker should alert the clinician to a possible diagnosis of primary lung malignancy
- Cough with hemoptysis, weight loss, or systemic symptoms in a smoker should alert the clinician to a possible primary lung malignancy, and warrants urgent investigation and possible referral
- Lung cancer that presents with a paraneoplastic lesion

ICD9 CODE

162.9 Malignant neoplasm of bronchus and lung, unspecified.

SYNONYMS

- Bronchogenic carcinoma
- Lung carcinoma
- Lung cancer
- Bronchial cancer
- Carcinoma of the bronchus
- Cancer of the bronchus

CARDINAL FEATURES

- Primary lung malignancies are carcinomas arising from the bronchial epithelium or bronchial mucous glands
- Untreated, lung cancer is always fatal and has a poor prognosis
- The presenting features are nonspecific and heterogeneous, including cough and hemoptysis; dyspnea or wheezing; malaise, anorexia, and weight loss; fever; and chest, bone, or shoulder pain
- Primary lung malignancies occur most commonly in people who smoke or smoked and are aged over 40 years
- Presentation can be insidious and gradual or by dramatic hemoptysis or sudden severe dyspnea
- Common presentations are also those of lobar pneumonia, which may fail to resolve clinically or radiologically despite conventional therapy, or as a chance finding on chest X-ray
- Although 12 types of primary lung malignancies have been described, in practice the important distinction is between nonsmall cell cancers, which have a better prognosis, and small cell cancers. Prognosis also depends on the stage: stage IV nonsmall cell lung cancer has a worse prognosis than limited small cell lung cancer
- Treatment is based on the cellular type of the cancer and by staging (the size of the primary tumor and the presence of local spread to lymph nodes and of metastases)
- Metastases are common and include the following sites: brain, bone, liver, and adrenal glands

The characteristics of the most common types of primary lung malignancies are as follows.

Small cell carcinomas:

- They are distinguished from all other types of primary lung malignancy, and their management and prognosis differs from all the other types
- Also known as oat cell carcinomas
- 20% of all primary lung malignancies
- High cavitation rate
- Central location
- Tend to metastasize through lymphatics
- Associated with lesion of the short arm of chromosome 3

The following are all classified as nonsmall cell carcinomas. They share similar prognoses and are all managed in the same way.

Adenocarcinoma:

- 35% of all primary lung malignancies
- Frequently peripheral or located in mid lung
- Metastasizes to lymphatics, at least initially

Squamous cell carcinoma:
- 20–30% of all primary lung malignancies
- Also known as epidermoid carcinomas
- Central location
- Metastasizes by local invasion
- Frequently cavitates and causes bronchial obstruction or collapse

Large cell carcinoma:
- 15–20% of all primary lung malignancies
- Metastasizes to the mediastinum and central nervous system
- Usually peripheral
- Rapid growth rate and early metastases

Bronchoalveolar carcinoma:
- 5% of all primary lung malignancies
- Metastasize initially through the lymphatics, blood, and local invasion
- Frequently peripheral
- May be bilateral
- Rarely cavitate
- The only type of primary lung malignancy not associated with cigarette smoking

Staging of primary lung malignancies determines its management and prognosis. Nonsmall cell lung cancer is staged using the tumor, nodes, and metastases (TNM) classification.

Stage definition 5-year survival rate (%):
- 1: T1–2, N0, M0 55–75
- 2: T1–2, N1, M0 25–50
- 3A: T3, N0–1, M0 20–40 or T1–3, N2, M0
- 3B: T4, any N, M0 <10 or any T, N3, M0
- 4: any M <10

Tumor (T):
- T1: Tumor <3cm diameter
- T2: Tumor <3cm diameter has associated atelectasis-obstructive pneumonitis extending to the hilar region
- T3: Tumor with direct extension into the chest wall, diaphragm, mediastinal pleura or pericardium
- T4: Tumor invades the mediastinum or the presence of malignant pleural effusions

Regional lymph nodes (N):
- N0: No nodes involved
- N1: Metastasis to peribronchial or ipsilateral hilar nodes
- N2: Metastasis to ipsilateral mediastinal or subcarinal nodes
- N3: Metastasis to contralateral hilar or mediastinal nodes or to any supraclavicular or scalene nodes

Distant metastasis (M):
- M0: No known distant metastasis
- M1: Distant metastasis present

Small cell cancer is staged as follows:
- Limited stage disease: tumor confined to the one side of the chest and regional lymph nodes (mediastinal, contralateral hilar and usually ipsilateral supraclavicular). Partly this stage relates to whether the tumor can be encompassed within a radiation port
- Extensive stage disease: defined as disease extending beyond the limited stage

CAUSES

Common causes

- Cigarette smoking: >80% of primary lung malignancies are associated with and probably caused by cigarette smoking; this is by far the most important cause. Potential carcinogens in tobacco smoke include aromatic hydrocarbons, nitrosamines, nitrosonormiatine, polarium, and arsenic; passive smoking, especially if exposure is prolonged and heavy, may account for a proportion of lung cancers in lifelong nonsmokers
- High levels of pollution, radiation (especially radon exposure), and asbestos exposure will also increase the risk, especially in smokers

Rare causes

- Cooks, firefighters, and chemists may also have an increased risk of developing primary lung malignancies, presumably as a result of frequently inhaling carcinogens, especially if they also smoke
- Heavy or prolonged exposure to industrial agents, especially in smokers, has also been implicated as cause of primary lung malignancies. Such agents include coal dust, ionizing radiation, asbestos, nickel, uranium, vinyl chloride, chromium, formaldehyde, and arsenic

Serious causes

Cigarette smoking: >80% of primary lung malignancies are associated with and probably caused by cigarette smoking. It is by far the most important cause. Stopping smoking reduces the risk of developing primary lung cancer; the rate falls to that of nonsmokers within 10–15 years of giving up.

Contributory or predisposing factors

Genetic predisposition for primary lung malignancies may occur as not all smokers will be affected; any genetic component is subtle and as yet not well understood.

EPIDEMIOLOGY

Incidence and prevalence

Primary lung malignancies are the leading cause of death in men and women in the US.

INCIDENCE

- The overall incidence is about 1/1000
- The incidence in men is about 0.7/1000 and in women about 0.22/1000

PREVALENCE

- 100,000 men and 80,000 women are affected in the US each year
- 40,000 men and women are affected in the UK each year

FREQUENCY

- Primary lung malignancies account for 14% of all new cancers in men and 13% in women
- 33% of cancer deaths in males and 23% in females are due to primary lung malignancies

Demographics

AGE

- 70% of deaths occur in patients aged 55–74
- Most cases occur in people aged >50 years
- 4% of cases of primary lung malignancies occur in people aged <40 years
- There is a small recent trend of increasing incidence and mortality in younger age groups

GENDER

- Men are more likely to develop primary lung malignancies than women, but as the ratio of men to women smokers is steadily increasing, the number of men and women affected will tend to equilibrate

- Primary lung malignancies are the leading cause of cancer deaths in men, accounting for 14% of all new cancers and 33% of all cancer deaths
- In women, the figures are 13% and 24%, respectively
- In women, primary lung malignancies are becoming more common and result in more deaths than breast cancer
- As the proportion of male to female smokers declines in North America and Europe, there will be concomitant increase in the ratio of female to male incidences of primary lung malignancies over the next 30–50 years
- The risk of developing primary lung malignancy is 10 times greater in male smokers than nonsmokers and 3–5 times greater in female smokers

RACE

Highest in African-Americans, lowest in Native Americans in the US.

GENETICS

- Small cell carcinomas are associated with a lesion on the short arm of chromosome 3, but this characteristic is not directly inherited
- Lung cancers may have 10 or more acquired genetic lesions
- Early detection of asymptomatic cases may be of value in the future, especially of the early occurring loss of 3p and 9p

GEOGRAPHY

- The incidence of primary lung cancers is determined mainly by smoking habits in any population. The proportion of smokers in the US and Europe has been declining since the late 20th century, and rates of primary lung cancers there are beginning to fall and will continue to do so
- The proportion of smokers in many other parts of the world, especially in China, southern and southeastern Asia and sub-Saharan Africa is increasing, and there are expected to be significant increases in the rates of primary lung malignancies in these parts of the world over the first half of the 21st century
- In the US, the areas with the highest incidences include northeastern urban areas and southern Atlantic and Gulf areas, particularly in communities where there are paper, petrochemical, and shipbuilding industries

SOCIOECONOMIC STATUS

- The incidence of primary lung cancers is highest in people with the lowest income and educational status, reflecting the higher proportion of such people who smoke or are exposed to heavy industrial pollution
- Especially high rates of primary lung malignancies occur in coal miners and asbestos workers who also smoke heavily

DIAGNOSIS

DIFFERENTIAL DIAGNOSIS

- There are many conditions which need to also be considered in a patient who may have a primary lung malignancy, including pneumonia, tuberculosis, chronic obstructive pulmonary disease (COPD), metastatic lung disease, lung abscess, sarcoidosis, mycobacterial and fungal lung disease, granulomatous disease, benign solitary pulmonary nodule, and endocrine diseases
- Primary lung malignancy may develop in patients with pre-existing respiratory disorders, and especially in smokers with COPD
- Chest X-ray is mandatory for the differential diagnosis of clubbing, neurologic, and endocrine presentations, especially in smokers

Pneumonia

Pneumonias are common and occur more commonly in patients with such smoking-related disorders as COPD. Lobar collapse or consolidation may occur secondary to a primary lung malignancy of a bronchus. All cases of pneumonia should be followed up clinically and radiologically to exclude an underlying primary lung malignancy, especially in patients who are aged over 40 and who smoke or smoked cigarettes.

FEATURES

- Pneumonias usually present with the following: an acute episode of dyspnea, cough, and discolored sputum: fever and malaise; localized signs of lung consolidation (crackles, bronchial breath sounds, and coarse crepitations); and characteristic changes on the chest X-ray
- Pneumonia may occur as a result of a previously undiagnosed primary lung malignancy
- Radiologic changes of acute or resolving pneumonia may obscure or mask the radiologic features of a primary lung malignancy

Pulmonary tuberculosis

Pulmonary tuberculosis is a common primary infection of the lung caused by the bacterium *Mycobacterium tuberculosis*. Its peak incidence is in infancy, teenage years, pregnancy, and old age, and it is not related to smoking.

FEATURES

- Like primary lung malignancies, pulmonary TB can result in weight loss, cough and hemoptysis, fever and night sweats, wasting and cachexia; chest examination is often normal
- Chest X-ray and sputum culture and cytology will usually distinguish the two conditions
- Bronchoscopy, pleural or bronchial biopsies, and computed tomography (CT) scans of the chest may be needed
- Primary lung malignancies occur mainly in smokers or ex-smokers aged over 40 years
- Pulmonary TB can occur at any age and is not related to smoking

Chronic obstructive pulmonary disease

(COPD) occurs commonly in middle or old age in people with a current or past smoking history. Primary lung malignancies also occur in this group of people, and the two conditions can arise in the same patient, causing diagnostic confusion and possible delay in treatment.

FEATURES

- Cough and breathlessness on exertion occurring in middle or old age in smokers or ex-smokers
- There may be morning sputum, and cachexia in the later stages
- Hemoptysis and clubbing do not occur in primary and uncomplicated COPD
- Both primary lung malignancies and COPD may initially present with acute pneumonia

- COPD is a slowly progressive disorder over many years
- Chest X-ray, spirometry, and sputum cytology and culture will all help distinguish the two conditions, as will the relatively slow progression and deterioration in COPD

Metastatic carcinoma to the lung

Many cancers spread to the lungs, including breast cancer, bone cancer, prostate cancer, stomach cancer, renal cancer, colon cancer, and melanoma. Many cancers will occur in middle-aged or elderly smokers.

FEATURES

- The symptoms and signs are as for primary lung malignancies, and there may be symptoms and signs from the underlying primary cancer
- Occasionally the lung metastasis will be the first presenting feature of a cancer
- Chest X-ray and CT scans of the lungs may be needed to distinguish primary lung malignancies from metastatic lung cancers
- Metastatic cancers are usually multiple, rather than solitary
- The location of the lesions may also help to differentiate the two
- Additionally, bronchoscopy with biopsies, mediastinoscopy or open lung biopsy are needed in order to obtain tissue for histologic confirmation of the cancer and its type

Lung abcess

Lung abscesses may occur as a result of bronchial obstruction and distal lobar or lobular collapse, followed by infection (usually bacterial) of the collapsed part of the lung. Lung abscesses may occur as a result of lung cancers.

FEATURES

- The patient is usually acutely ill with fever and malaise
- There are signs of consolidation over the affected lobe or lobule
- Chest X-ray will confirm the presence of a lung abscess
- Follow up is mandatory
- The possibility of a primary lung malignancy being the cause of a lung abscess must always be excluded

Sarcoidosis

Sarcoidosis is a chronic systemic granulomatous disease of unknown cause.

FEATURES

- Its characteristic histologic feature is the presence of nonspecific, noncaseating granuloma
- It occurs most commonly in people aged 20–40
- Not related to cigarette smoking
- It can present with similar symptoms and signs to those of primary lung malignancies
- Chest X-ray and CT scanning will help distinguish sarcoidosis from primary lung malignancies

Mycobacterial and fungal lung diseases

Fungi and nontuberculous mycobacteria are common organisms which can infect the lungs and respiratory tract. Infections often occur in the immunocompromised. No predilection for smokers.

FEATURES

- Occurrence especially with an underlying chronic lung disease, or persistent hypersensitivity reactions
- Aspergillosis can result in an acute hypersensitivity pneumonitis, the symptoms and signs of which include cough, dyspnea, and malaise
- Invasive aspergillosis presents as a necrotizing bronchopneumonia with fever, cough, and dyspnea

- Aspergillomas commonly cause hemoptysis, and usually occur in patients with chronic lung disease such as pulmonary tuberculosis, sarcoidosis or emphysema
- Mycobacterial diseases can also cause a variety of respiratory symptoms, including cough, hemoptysis, and dyspnea as well as weight loss and cervical or axillary lymphadenopathy (which may be unilateral)
- Chest X-ray changes as a result of mycobacterial and fungal lung diseases may show a variety of features ranging from cavitation and lobar consolidation or collapse to small patchy infiltrates
- Definitive diagnosis is confirmed by *Aspergillus* serum precipitating antibodies, positive sputum cultures for *Aspergillus* or mycobacteria, and, if there is still uncertainty, by lung biopsies

Granulomatous diseases

Granulomatous lung diseases include:

- Wegener's granulomatosis
- Lymphomatoid granulomatosis
- Churg-Strauss syndrome
- Necrotizing sarcoid granulomatosis
- Bronchiocentric granulomatosis
- Sarcoidosis
- They mostly occur in people aged 30–50 years and are not related to smoking

FEATURES

- All the granulomatous lung diseases can present with cough, pleurisy, dyspnea, malaise, and hemoptysis
- Chest X-rays in any of the above conditions may show opacities and possible cavitation
- CT scans and even lung biopsies may be needed for definitive diagnosis

Benign solitary pulmonary nodule

The finding of a single pulmonary nodule on a chest X-ray should always be carefully followed up as such a nodule may be a primary lung malignancy.

FEATURES

- An incidental finding of an asymptomatic solitary pulmonary nodule is not uncommon
- If the nodule has been present and has not changed for months or years, or if it shows radiologic evidence of calcification, it can be considered benign and ignored
- In all other cases, the nodule should be biopsied if the patient is fit enough for the procedure, and the nodule resected if necessary. Subsequent management will depend on the histology
- If the patient is unfit for surgery, the nodule should be monitored by repeat chest X-rays every 3–4 months; if there is no change after 1–2 years, consider the nodule benign, otherwise reconsider biopsy and resection
- All cases of a finding of a solitary pulmonary nodule should be referred to a pulmonologist for opinion

Endocrine disorders

The most common endocrine disorders associated with primary lung malignancies are adrenocorticotropic hormone (ACTH) production and inappropriate antidiuretic hormone (ADH) secretion. These disorders may occur independently of lung cancer.

FEATURES

- Ectopic ACTH production results in a syndrome of: hypertension; central obesity with peripheral wasting: hirsutism, skin pigmentation, and fragility; menstrual irregularities; psychiatric symptoms; weakness and muscle wasting; and malaise and fatigue
- Causes of raised ACTH production include iatrogenic (excess glucocorticoids), pituitary disease, adrenal neoplasms, and ectopic production from primary lung malignancies, pancreatic cancer, thyroid cancer, thymus cancer, and renal cancer

- Ectopic ACTH from primary lung malignancies tends to result only in weakness and malaise
- Inappropriate secretion of ADH results in delirium, lethargy and malaise
- The syndrome results in hyponatremia and if severe can lead to seizures and death

The following conditions are associated with inappropriate secretion of ADH:
- Neoplasms (primary lung malignancies, pancreas cancer, brain tumors, bladder cancer, prostatic cancer, and thymus cancers, mesotheliomas and lymphomas)
- Pulmonary disorders (TB, emphysema, bronchiectasis, pneumonia)
- Intracranial pathology (trauma, neoplasia, infections)
- Postoperative stress, anesthesia, surgery
- Drugs (chlorpromaxine, thiazides, oxytocin, phenothiazines, tricyclic antidepressants, nicotine, narcotics, chemotherapeutic agents)
- Guillain-Barré syndrome, myxedema, psychosis, ACTH deficiency, delirium tremens)

SIGNS & SYMPTOMS

Signs

Respiratory signs:
- Lobar consolidation
- Localized wheezing
- Pleural effusion (dull percussion note and absent breath sounds)
- Tracheal shift or tug
- Stridor if there is tracheal obstruction

Generalized signs:
- Cachexia
- Lymphadenopathy, especially cervical and axillary
- Hepatomegaly, ascites
- Clubbing
- Muscle weakness and wasting

Signs from associated syndromes:
- Muscle wasting and weakness, especially the proximal groups
- Ptosis, pupillary constriction, dry ipsilateral face
- Hoarse voice
- Dilated neck and thoracic veins
- Horner's syndrome (ptosis, constricted pupil, anhidrosis of the face)
- Ectopic ACTH syndrome – usually results only in weight loss and weakness but the following may rarely occur: thin skin, wasted extremities, central obesity, hirsutism, menstrual irregularities, hypogonadism, bruising, and acne

Symptoms

Respiratory symptoms:
- Cough: usually dry, persistent (common)
- Dyspnea with or without wheezing (common)
- Hemoptysis: may be small and recurrent or sudden and massive
- Symptoms of acute pneumonia (that is slow to resolve)

Generalized symptoms (occur in about 30% of cases of primary lung malignancies):
- Weight loss (common)
- Anorexia
- Fatigue
- Chest pains, pains in the shoulder, bone pains
- Muscle weakness, focal or regional, or muscle pains
- Confusion, memory loss, depression, co-ordination problems

Rarer symptoms (occur in 12–20% of cases of primary lung malignancies):
- Dysphagia
- Hoarse or husky voice (from recurrent laryngeal nerve involvement)
- Superior vena cava syndrome (headache, nausea, dizziness, visual changes, syncope, respiratory distress)
- Eaton-Lambert syndrome (proximal myopathies causing weakness)

Endocrine manifestations (occur in 12–20% of cases of primary lung malignancies):
- Hypercalcemia – renal colic, constipation, abdominal pains
- Inappropriate secretion of antidiuretic hormone – delirium, lethargy

Metastatic spread of primary lung malignancies is likely to cause:
- Tracheal obstruction with stridor and dyspnea
- Dysphagia
- Hoarseness
- Horner's syndrome
- Superior vena cava syndrome
- Pleural effusions
- Respiratory failure

ASSOCIATED DISORDERS

The following paraneoplastic syndromes may occur as a result of primary lung malignancies:
- Eaton-Lambert syndrome – proximal muscle group wasting
- Endocrine abnormalities – inappropriate ADH secretion, ectopic ACTH secretion, hypercalcemia
- Neurologic – peripheral neuropathies, cerebellar degeneration, degeneration of the cerebral cortex, pseudodementia
- Musculoskeletal – clubbing, hypertrophic pulmonary osteoarthropathy, polymyositis
- Vascular – anemia, thrombocytosis, thrombocytopenia, migratory thrombophlebitis, marantic thrombosis
- Cutaneous – dermatomyositis, acanthosis nigricans
- Pulmonary – pleural effusions, pneumonias
- Superior vena cava syndrome – primary lung malignancies or their metastases may block the venous return of the superior vena cava, causing dizziness, syncope, headache, nausea, and respiratory distress. The neck veins are distended and there is facial edema, plethora, and cyanosis
- Horner's syndrome (ptosis, constricted pupil, anhidrosis of the face), caused by spinal cord damage between C8 and T1 from a superior sulcus tumor
- Pancoast's tumor describes a superior sulcus tumor with ipsilateral Horner's syndrome and shoulder pain

Primary lung malignancies can also result in pleural space fluid leading to the following symptoms and signs:
- Breathlessness and respiratory distress
- Cough and chest pains
- Tachypnea and tachycardia
- Absent breath sounds and stony dull percussion note over the pleural space fluid

KEY! DON'T MISS!

- The development of a new cough, if persistent, in a smoker should alert the clinician to a possible diagnosis of primary lung malignancy
- Cough with hemoptysis, weight loss, or systemic symptoms in a smoker should alert the clinician to a possible primary lung malignancy, and warrants urgent investigation and possible referral
- Lung cancer that presents with a paraneoplastic lesion

CONSIDER CONSULT

- Any patient with respiratory symptoms for which there is no clear diagnosis, and which persist, should be investigated and referred
- Any patient presenting with features which may suggest any of the syndromes or complications associated with primary lung malignancies should be referred
- Any patient with a new pulmonary nodule on chest X-ray should be referred

INVESTIGATION OF THE PATIENT

Direct questions to patient

- Q **Have you ever smoked, and if so, how many cigarettes a day and for how long?** Primary lung malignancies are nearly always associated with a smoking history of at least 20 pack-years (one pack-year is equivalent to 20 cigarettes a day for one year). The only type of primary lung malignancy which is not smoking-related is bronchoalveolar carcinoma (5% of all primary lung malignancies)
- Q **How long have you had your current respiratory problems and symptoms?** Symptoms and problems from primary lung malignancies usually begin insidiously but fairly rapidly; long-standing symptoms of several months or years, which are not changing, make the diagnosis of primary lung malignancy less likely. New respiratory or generalized symptoms arising in a smoker or ex-smoker with pre-existing respiratory problems or symptoms should be considered as being due to primary lung malignancies until proved otherwise
- Q **Have you experienced hemoptysis, shortness of breath, chest pain, or a new and persistent cough?** These are typical symptoms, which warrant further investigation
- Q **Do you have any generalized symptoms such as fatigue, weight loss, and weakness as well as having respiratory symptoms?** Primary lung malignancies often cause systemic symptoms either as nonspecific accompanying symptoms from the primary malignancy, or secondary to local spread, lymph node enlargement or to one or other of the syndromes associated with primary lung malignancies
- Q **Has your voice changed?** A hoarse voice is a common finding in patients with primary lung malignancies, and is usually due to laryngeal nerve involvement

Contributory or predisposing factors

- Q **Do you smoke, or did you smoke in the past?** An accurate smoking history is essential in diagnosing possible primary lung malignancies
- Q **Are you aged over 40 years?** Primary lung malignancies occur rarely in younger patients, and occur most commonly in the 50- to 65-year age group
- Q **What is your current and past employment?** Primary lung malignancies occur more commonly in people exposed to asbestos, radon, and coal dust, for example, and increase the cumulative risk of developing primary lung malignancies in smokers

Examination

- **Is the patient clubbed?** Primary lung malignancies are an important cause of finger clubbing
- **Are there signs of focal consolidation or collapse of the lung?** Such changes may be secondary to a primary lung malignancy
- **Is there any evidence of tracheal tug or stridor?** This may indicate local spread of disease
- **Is there acute respiratory distress?** Primary lung malignancies will not cause this but secondary infection, lobar collapse, or pleural effusions can do so
- **Are the cervical or axillary lymph nodes enlarged?** Such lymphadenopathy suggests possible local spread from a primary lung malignancy and adversely affects the prognosis. Finding enlarged nodes should prompt a search for the definite diagnosis of their cause, and may require biopsy or excision of the suspect nodes
- **Are there signs of peripheral wasting, central obesity, edema, or cachexia?** The presence of these features in a patient who smokes or smoked and who also has respiratory symptoms implies a possible diagnosis of primary lung malignancy complicated by an endocrine or other syndrome

- **Is Horner's syndrome present?** If so, one of the most important and common reasons for the syndrome is primary lung malignancy

Summary of investigative tests

Imaging is the main first-line investigation:

Chest X-ray is the most important initial investigation as it will reveal the following: the size and extent of any tumor; local spread; complications such as lymphadenopathy or pleural effusion; secondary lobar collapse; and hilar or mediastinal lymph node enlargement. Should be done in anteroposterior and lateral views using a high voltage (>125kV) to ensure adequate penetration through the tumor and the mediastinum. Review of a prior X-ray is essential if possible. The lesion may have been present for several years, and not changed in size, making the diagnosis less likely to be malignant.

Blood tests should routinely be ordered as part of the work-up to evaluate the patient's overall fitness:

- Complete blood count may reveal anemia or leukocytosis if there is secondary infection. Thrombocytosis or throbocytopenia may be part of a paraneoplastic syndrome
- Liver function tests may be abnormal if there are metastases to the liver
- Renal function test should routinely be ordered as part of the workup to evaluate the patient's overall fitness
- Calcium group tests may reveal hypercalcemia secondary to malignancy
- Cytology of sputum may reveal cancer cells; these are diagnostic if found, although negative cytology does not rule out primary lung malignancies

A specialist normally performs the following scans and biopsies:

- CT scan is often necessary to evaluate mediastinal or pleural spread of suspected tumors and to assess intrathoracic lymph node involvement. CT is recommended as a staging procedure for patients with nonsmall cell carcinoma. If there is evidence of disease in the mediastinum or contralateral chest, further investigation and treatment will be affected
- Magnetic resonance imaging (MRI) has no advantage over CT scanning for evaluation of enlarged lymph nodes. MRI is not useful in routine staging, but can help to clarify the extent of tumor invasion in the mediastinum, root of neck, chest wall, and diaphragm if CT scanning results are equivocal
- Positron emission tomography (PET): accurate imaging investigation for possible intrathoracic lymph node involvement. It is best used in conjunction with CT scanning for accurate localization and interpretation
- Enhanced MRI scans of the brain and isotope bone scans may detect asymptomatic occult metastases in many patients
- When CT scanning the thorax it seems sensible to include views of the liver and adrenal glands
- Bronchoscopy and bronchial washings, brushings and biopsy: histologic confirmation of any suspicion of primary lung malignancies is essential to accurately diagnose the malignancy, ascertain its cell type and to plan the relevant treatment and predict the prognosis. Bronchoscopy is usually performed by a specialist, although some primary care physicians, especially in isolated areas, may offer this investigation. Transbronchial needle aspiration can be used to sample mediastinal masses or paratracheal lymph nodes
- Percutaneous needle biopsy: needle biopsy of a peripheral suspicious lesion, often under CT scanning guidance. It is useful for patients who are unfit for surgery; it has a high diagnostic success rate but a negative biopsy should not necessarily exclude cancer
- Mediastinoscopy or mediastinotomy: an invasive procedure allowing endoscopic or direct views of the mediastinum. It is useful in evaluating the true extent of a mediastinal lymph node involvement. It is usually omitted if there is no evidence of mediastinal lymph node involvement, particularly if the tumor is peripheral, although a proportion of patients may have microscopic lymph node metastases

- Thoracoscopy and thoracentesis: an invasive endoscopic procedure allowing views of the pleura and pleural spaces, and aspiration of any pleural space fluid. It is useful in differentiating malignant pleural effusions from those secondary to consolidation distal to an obstruction lesion
- Biopsy of lymph nodes or pleura: surgical resection of axillary or cervical lymph nodes, or of the pleura, or percutaneous biopsies of them, may be needed in cases of diagnostic doubt or to assess local spread
- Cytology of sputum, bronchial washings, or pleural space fluid: cancer cells are diagnostic if found; negative cytology does not rule out primary lung malignancies

DIAGNOSTIC DECISION

- Accurate diagnosis and assessment of primary lung malignancies is important to determine the staging, operability, suitability for radiotherapy, chemotherapy or palliation
- Accurate histologic proof of malignancy, its type and its staging are needed
- Histologic proof requires biopsies of the affected bronchi or other affected tissue, or positive cytology from bronchial brushings or washings, pleural space fluid or sputum. Histologic proof should always be sought unless there are overwhelming, explicit reasons not to (e.g. a moribund patient)
- Early diagnosis is desirable
- Primary lung malignancies can be detected in their presymptomatic phase by radiologic evidence (lesions of 5–10mm in diameter are visible) or by sputum cytology
- About 5% of diagnoses of primary lung malignancies are made in their presymptomatic phase, usually as incidental chest X-ray findings or as cytologic or radiologic findings during workups for unrelated conditions

CLINICAL PEARLS

Determination of stage (resectability) is the key aspect of the diagnostic process in nonsmall cell lung cancer.

THE TESTS

Body fluids

COMPLETE BLOOD COUNT

Description

Cuffed venous sample sent for laboratory analysis.

Advantages/Disadvantages

Advantages:

- Useful as a nonspecific indicator of the patient's general fitness and nutritional state
- Simple test

Normal

- Hemoglobin: male, 13.6–17.7g/dL (8.4–11.0mmol/L); female, 12–15g/dL (7.4–9.3mmol/L)
- White cell count: 4.0–11.0x10^9/L
- Platelets: 150–400x10^9/L

Abnormal

- Results outside the normal reference range
- There may be an iron deficiency anemia or thrombocytosis
- White cell count will be raised if there is an infection due to bronchial obstruction
- Keep in mind the possibility of a false-positive result

Cause of abnormal result

- Normochromic, normocytic anemia may be secondary to malignancy
- Platelet count may be affected due to a paraneoplastic syndrome
- White cell count will be raised if there is an infection due to bronchial obstruction

LIVER FUNCTION TESTS

Description

Cuffed venous sample sent for laboratory analysis.

Advantages/Disadvantages

Advantages:

- Useful as nonspecific markers of the patient's overall fitness
- Simple test

Disadvantage: normal results do not exclude a diagnosis of primary lung malignancy

Normal

- Alkaline phosphatase (ALP): 30–300 IU/L
- Aspartate transaminase (AST): 5–35 IU/L
- Alanine aminotransferase (ALT): 5–35 IU/L
- Gamma-glutamyl transpeptidase (GGT): 7–51 IU/L
- Bilirubin: 0.25–1.5mg/dL (3–17mcmol/L)

Abnormal

- Results outside normal reference range
- Keep in mind the possibility of a false-positive result

Cause of abnormal result

May imply hepatic metastases.

Drugs, disorders and other factors that may alter results

- Many drugs and disorders can alter liver function tests
- Examples include cirrhosis, alcohol excess, cholelithiasis, phenothiazines, anticonvulsants

CALCIUM GROUP BLOOD TESTS

Description

Venous uncuffed sample sent for laboratory analysis.

Advantages/Disadvantages

- Advantage: useful as nonspecific markers of the patient's overall fitness
- Disadvantage: normal results do not exclude a diagnosis of primary lung malignancy

Normal

Total calcium 2.12–2.65mmol/L.

Abnormal

- Results outside normal reference range
- Keep in mind the possibility of a false-positive result

Cause of abnormal result

Deranged calcium, alkaline phosphatase, or phosphate levels imply bony metastases.

Drugs, disorders and other factors that may alter results

Low serum protein levels are markers of nonspecific illness or poor nutritional states. Calcium level should be adjusted for the albumin level.

TESTS OF RENAL FUNCTION

Description

Cuffed venous sample sent for venous laboratory analysis.

Advantages/Disadvantages

- Advantage: useful as nonspecific markers of the patient's overall fitness
- Disadvantage: normal results do not exclude a diagnosis of primary lung malignancy

Normal

- Blood urea nitrogen: 8–18mg/dL (3–6.5mmol/L)
- Serum creatinine: 0.6–1.2mg/dL (50–110mcmol/L)

Abnormal

- Results outside normal reference range
- Keep in mind the possibility of a false-positive result

Cause of abnormal result

- Elevated blood urea nitrogen (BUN) or creatinine, or biochemical evidence of disordered acid-base balance imply secondary spread of a primary lung malignancy
- Such changes are not seen from primary lung malignancies without metastases

Biopsy

BRONCHOSCOPY AND BRONCHIAL BIOPSY, BRUSHINGS, AND WASHINGS

Description

- Endoscopic means of investigating the respiratory tract by direct vision, using a rigid or flexible bronchoscope via the mouth and larynx
- Usually performed under sedation with local anesthesia
- Biopsies of suspicious areas can be taken either by punch biopsy, fine-needle biopsy, bronchial brushings, or aspiration of bronchial washings

Advantages/Disadvantages

Advantages:

- Allows direct visual inspection of the vocal cords and vocal cord function
- Allows direct vision of the traches, carina, main and larger bronchi
- Allows biopsies to be taken of suspicious areas
- Accessible lymph nodes can also be biopsied by using fine needle transbronchial aspiration

Disadvantages:

- An invasive process with risk of infection, hemorrhage, perforation
- Requires local or even general anesthesia with the subsequent risks especially of post-procedure aspiration

Normal

The whole of the visible respiratory tract appears normal and bronchial brushings and washings are cancer-negative.

Abnormal

- There are areas of suspicious looking tissues with local lymphadenopathy and cancer-positive cells on subsequent histologic or cytology examination
- False-positive results are unusual
- False-negative inspection and biopsy results can occur

Cause of abnormal result

Malignancy of the respiratory tract.

Drugs, disorders and other factors that may alter results
The procedure is more hazardous in moribund patients or in those with other concomitant disorders such as COPD, heart failure, or AIDS.

Imaging

CHEST X-RAY

Description
- Chest X-rays are essential for the diagnosis of primary lung malignancies
- Posteroanterior and lateral views should be requested, and the X-rays should be taken at high voltage (>125kV)
- Review of a prior X-ray is essential if possible. The lesion in question may have been present for several years, and not changed in size, making the diagnosis less clear

Advantages/Disadvantages
Advantages:
- Shows the size and extent of any tumor
- Shows any collapse of the lung and any pleural effusion
- Shows hilar or mediastinal enlargement, which may well indicate enlarged lymph nodes
- Safe, quick, easy to perform, and cheap

Disadvantage: radiation exposure

Abnormal
- Any focal or diffuse changes in the chest X-ray of any patient aged 40 years or over who smokes or smoked should be assumed to be secondary to primary lung malignancy unless proved otherwise
- The radiologic appearances will vary with the cell type: small cell carcinomas tend to be central; non-small cell carcinomas tend to be peripheral (adenocarcinoma, large cell or bronchoalveolar) or central (squamous cell carcinoma)
- Pleural effusion, lobar atelectasis and mediastinal lymphadenopathy can accompany any cell type

Cause of abnormal result
Chest X-ray changes can be produced by primary lung malignancies and also by benign lesions or conditions.

Drugs, disorders and other factors that may alter results
- Lobar atelectasis: TB, pneumonia, allergic bronchopulmonary aspergillosis, chronic inflammatory disease
- Multiple pulmonary nodules: Wegener's granulomatosis, sarcoidosis, fungal disease, septic emboli
- Mediastinal enlargement or lymphadenopathy: lymphoma, sarcoidosis, TB, fungal infections, silicosis, pneumoconiosis
- Pleural effusion: congestive heart failure, pneumonia with effusions, TB, viral pneumonitis, ascites, pancreatitis, collagen-vascular disease

COMPUTED TOMOGRAPHIC SCANS

Description
- Computerized radiologic scan which allows a three-dimensional picture of the area scanned to be assembled and displayed
- CT scans of the thorax should also include the upper abdomen and adrenals, and request forms should include these areas
- Contrast enhancement makes it easier for inexperienced observers to interpret the CT findings
- Spiral CT scanning allows optimal contrast enhancement and should be used when practicable

Advantages/Disadvantages

Advantages:

- Identifies enlarged mediastinal lymph nodes and allows determination of the best approach for biopsy or aspiration of the appropriate node or nodes, especially in nonsmall cell carcinomas
- Determines the T stage of nonsmall cell carcinomas and whether resection is an option
- Accurately identifies metastases in the chest and in the adrenals and upper abdomen if included in the areas to be scanned
- May rule out the need for further testing if there is mediastinal or contralateral involvement

Disadvantages:

- Expensive
- Large dose of radiation
- Needs trained and experienced personnel to perform the procedure and to interpret the results accurately
- The accuracy of CT scanning for N staging is poor (sensitivity and specificity of approximately 60–65% and 60–70%, respectively)
- Will demonstrate spread of any tumor as well as identifying any intrathoracic lymph node enlargement. Nodes with a maximum short axis diameter of over 10mm are suspicious and warrant biopsy or aspiration
- Preoperative CT scanning has been shown to overstage or understage the cancer when compared to operative findings in about 40% of patients. In patients in whom the only contraindication for surgery is lymph node enlargement on the CT scan, histologic or cytologic confirmation of intrathoracic lymph node involvement is required before a decision not to intervene surgically is made

Abnormal

Films consistent with primary lung malignancy, with or without spread to the lymph nodes, mediastinum, chest wall, or adrenal glands.

Cause of abnormal result

Malignant disease of the lung.

Special tests

CYTOLOGY

Description

Microscopic examination and analysis of cells from sputum, bronchial washings, or bronchial brushings.

Advantages/Disadvantages

Advantage: a positive result is nearly always diagnostic

Disadvantages:

- The cellular content of any fluid may be scanty
- Positive results rely on the skill and experience of the microscopist
- A negative result does not exclude a diagnosis of primary lung malignancy
- Sputum samples are easily obtained, noninvasive but more likely to yield false-negative results; several samples should be submitted for examination
- Bronchial brushings or washings will reveal fewer false negatives, but again negative results do not disprove a diagnosis of primary lung malignancy
- Bronchial specimens require bronchoscopy, an invasive and potentially hazardous procedure

Abnormal

Presence of malignant cells: a positive result is nearly always diagnostic.

Cause of abnormal result

Tumor in the respiratory tract which is shedding malignant cells.

Drugs, disorders and other factors that may alter results

- Intercurrent infection may contaminate the specimen with leukocytes, organisms, or other cells
- Sputum samples can be difficult to obtain in some patients, who may produce salivary samples instead (which are rarely useful in diagnosing primary lung malignancy)

TREATMENT

CONSIDER CONSULT

- Refer all patients with radiographic or other evidence of a diagnosis of possible primary lung malignancy to a respiratory physician for an opinion about future investigations and management
- It may be more efficient to organize investigations while awaiting a specialist opinion
- Referral to an experienced cardiothoracic surgeon is required if surgery is indicated
- Respiratory physicians, thoracic surgeons, primary care physicians, and radiologists should collaborate to organize a service with minimal delays

IMMEDIATE ACTION

Hemoptysis (massive) or acute respiratory distress warrants immediate admission to the emergency room.

PATIENT AND CAREGIVER ISSUES

Impact on career, dependants, family, friends

- The prognosis of primary lung malignancies is generally poor
- The diagnosis is usually devastating for the patient, family, and friends, and should be communicated rapidly, with adequate and appropriate back-up from medical, nursing, and counseling staff
- A management plan should accompany the diagnosis, which should be discussed and agreed with the patient
- Active management and palliation are usually incompatible with maintaining employment or careers

Patient or caregiver request

- Public perception of primary lung malignancies is that they are untreatable, painful, and rapidly fatal
- Full and frank discussions with education are necessary
- All patients should receive advice about their management plan from their respiratory physician
- Such plans may include further investigation and treatment plans after consultation with other specialists, including cardiothoracic surgeons, oncologists, and palliative medicine physicians

MANAGEMENT ISSUES

Goals

- To cure the disease
- To prolong life
- To improve quality of life
- To provide palliation of symptoms
- To have minimum adverse affects of treatments

Management in special circumstances

COEXISTING DISEASE

Pulmonary disease:

- Many patients with primary lung malignancies smoke or smoked, and may also have smoking-related chronic obstructive pulmonary disease (COPD)
- If a lobectomy is being considered, patients should have an FEV_1 of >1.5L
- If a pneumonectomy is being considered, patients should have an FEV_1 of >2.0L, providing there is no interstitial lung disease or unexpected disability due to breathlessness
- The management of patients with FEV_1 values below these levels should include full respiratory function tests and discussion between a respiratory physician, thoracic surgeon, and oncologist, since there are no absolute FEV values which exclude patients from potentially curative surgeries

Cardiovascular disease:

- Pre-existing coronary artery disease increases the risk of nonfatal myocardial infarction or death within 30 days of noncardiac surgery
- Patients who have had a myocardial infarction should not be considered for surgery within 6 weeks
- Previous coronary artery bypass operations are not a contraindication for lung surgery
- The guidelines from the American College of Cardiology and the American Heart Association should be used as a basis for assessing the perioperative cardiovascular risk of patients undergoing lung resection
- If the patient has major risks, they should undergo full cardiovascular assessment and their management discussed at a multidisciplinary meeting. A few patients may need to undergo coronary artery bypass surgery before lung resection
- Patients with minor cardiovascular risk should not normally be considered to be at greater than average risk for postoperative complications

General condition:

- A history of recent weight loss, poor nutritional status, and poor performance status (World Health Authority or Eastern Cooperative Oncology Group scales) have all been independently associated in lung cancer with advanced disease and a poor overall prognosis

SPECIAL PATIENT GROUPS

- Perioperative morbidity increases with advancing age
- Careful preoperative assessment of comorbidity is needed in all patients, especially the elderly
- Lobectomy or wedge resection is not contraindicated even in the very old
- Pneumonectomy is associated with a higher mortality in the elderly and age should be a factor in deciding suitability for pneumonectomy

PATIENT SATISFACTION/LIFESTYLE PRIORITIES

- All patients, regardless of age, should be thoroughly assessed and investigated to determine which may benefit form active medical or surgical treatment, unless there are compelling and explicit reasons to the contrary
- All patients should be offered the most active treatment appropriate for their disease and its staging irrespective of age and other disabilities, unless the overall fitness of the patient is such that active intervention is likely to cause more harm than benefit

SUMMARY OF THERAPEUTIC OPTIONS

Choices

Treatments of primary lung malignancies are:

- Surgery
- Chemotherapy: cisplatin, carboplatin, etoposide, doxorubicin, docetaxel, cyclophosphamide, vincristine, have all been used; newer agents include: gemcitabine, paclitaxel, vinorelbine, and irinotecan
- Radiotherapy
- Photodynamic therapy is advocated for the treatment of nonsmall cell cancer in patients unable to tolerate surgery or radiotherapy. Multiple other complementary therapies are being tried; however, none is licensed, none has been shown to be efficacious, and no formal clinical trials have been published

Surgery:

- Surgical resection is indicated for patients with limited nonsmall cell cancer (not involving the ribs, pleura, mediastinal nodes or distant sites). This represents 15–30% of diagnosed cases
- Surgery is not indicated in small cell cancers, however resection of a solitary nodule prior to accurate diagnosis is acceptable even if it is small cell
- Pneumonectomy or lobectomy may be carried out

- Preoperative evaluation of nutritional, cardiovascular, and pulmonary states will help predict which patients can most benefit from surgical intervention
- Preoperative chemotherapy should be considered in patients with more advanced disease (stage IIIA)
- Resection of isolated metastasis in nonsmall cell lung cancer (e.g. in brain) may result in prolongation of survival

Chemotherapy:
- Combination or monotherapy with chemotherapeutic agents has been shown to be of benefit in managing both small cell and nonsmall cell cancers
- Regimens based on cisplatin are effective for nonsmall cell cancers
- Other promising new treatments require further evaluation
- Chemotherapy plus thoracic irradiation is associated with improved survival compared with radiotherapy alone in patients with unresectable stage 3 nonsmall cell cancers
- Cisplatin chemotherapy regimens compared to best supportive care in patients with stage IV nonsmall cell cancers results in improved survival, and may improve quality of life
- Docetaxel may improve survival of patients with stage IIIB or IV nonsmall cell cancer who had previously received cisplatin-based chemotherapy
- For patients with small cell cancers, standard chemotherapy is usually etoposide plus cisplatin. There is no evidence that other regimens are any more effective
- In patients with extensive small cell carcinoma, treatment with oral etoposide showed reduced survival rates when compared to combination chemotherapy. Because of its low toxicity, oral etoposide may be indicated in frail patients with extensive disease or in patients with a poor prognosis
- Chemotherapy will be prescribed by an oncologist, and usually is administered as an inpatient (day stay)

Radiotherapy:
- In unresectable nonsmall cell cancers, radiotherapy can be used alone or in combination with chemotherapy
- It is used primarily for the treatment of central nervous system (CNS) and skeletal metastases, superior vena cava syndrome, and obstructive atelectasis
- It is used for treating stage III nonsmall cell cancers, with limited effect on survival rates
- In patients with small cell cancers, adding thoracic irradiation improves survival. The best timing, dose, and fractionation remain uncertain
- Prophylactic cranial irradiation in patients with limited stage small cell cancers who are in complete remission reduces the incidence of brain metastases with a small improvement in survival but uncertain effects on neurophysiologic function

The treatment approach to patients with primary lung malignancies depends on the type of carcinoma.

Nonsmall cell cancers:
(Resectable – stages I, II, IIIa and some T3 and N1 lesions)
- Surgery
- Radiotherapy for patients considered unfit for surgery
- Postoperative radiotherapy for N2 disease

(Nonresectable – N2 and M1)
- Confined to chest – high-dose radiotherapy plus chemotherapy; consider adjuvant chemotherapy followed by surgery
- Extrathoracic – radiotherapy to symptomatic local sites; chemotherapy

Small cell cancers:
- Limited stage: chemotherapy plus chest radiotherapy
- Extensive stage (good performance status): chemotherapy
- Complete tumor responders: prophylactic cranial radiotherapy
- Poor performance status (all patients): modified dose chemotherapy plus palliative radiotherapy

All patients:
- Radiotherapy: for brain metastases, spinal cord compression, weight-bearing lytic bony lesions, symptomatic local lesions (e.g. hemoptysis, nerve paralysis, obstructed airways)
- Emotional and psychologic support and care
- Nutritional support
- Encouragement to stop smoking

Clinical pearls
Surgery may result in cure in early stages of lung cancer.

FOLLOW UP
Plan for review
During treatment:
- At least weekly when having active treatment
- Thereafter, monthly or more frequently if symptomatic or problems have arisen, for 6 months
- If still in remission, 3-monthly for 2 years, then at least annually for life
- Each review should include a thorough history, examination of the chest, lymph nodes, and liver
- Chest X-rays should be repeated if there are any new or worsening symptoms or signs

Information for patient or caregiver
- An accurate diagnosis is needed which should be shared with the patient or caregiver
- A management plan should accompany the diagnosis and be discussed and agreed with the patient
- Any prognosis should be guarded until staging is complete
- The patient or caregiver should have access to written information appropriate to his or her case

DRUGS AND OTHER THERAPIES: DETAILS
Surgical therapy
SURGICAL RESECTION OF THE LUNG

Surgical resection of lung cancer may be performed by a variety of operative procedures within an escalating hierarchy of complexity and extent of pulmonary resection:
- Sublobar resection – wedge or segmental
- Major pulmonary resection – lobectomy, bilobectomy, pneumonectomy
- Bronchoplastic resection – sleeve resection, cardinal resection
- In addition, the method of intraoperative management of mediastinal lymph nodes can be by sampling (opportunistic or systematic) and by clearance

Efficacy

Surgery has a good chance of being curative in early-stage disease:
- Sublobar resection is recommended in patients with impaired pulmonary reserve; there is a higher local recurrence rate than with lobectomy and survival is decreased by 5–10%
- Systematic lymph node dissection at the time of lung resection is essential for accurate staging
- Radical lymphadenectomy is of uncertain value

Risks/Benefits

- Risk: the perioperative mortality and morbidity need to be weighed against the increased survival rates in those who have undergone surgery
- Benefit: cure is impossible without surgery

Acceptability to patient

Generally high but decreased in patients with low levels of general fitness or who have complicating concomitant diseases or disorders.

Follow up plan

All patients need follow up for life.

Patient and caregiver information

The perioperative risks (infection, hemorrhaging) and potential need for potent analgesia need explaining.

Complementary therapy

PHOTODYNAMIC THERAPY

- Advocated for the treatment of nonsmall cell cancer in patients unable to tolerate surgery or radiotherapy
- A photosensitive dye, Porfimer sodium, is injected intravenously and, 50min later, the malignant cells have taken up the dye
- Fiberoptic laser therapy can then be applied to these cells via a bronchoscope

Efficacy

Uncertain – there have been no clinical trials that have demonstrated its efficacy.

Risks/Benefits

Risk: its use may preclude more effective therapies

Patient and caregiver information

Patients and caregivers must be made aware that such therapy is not licensed.

Radiation therapy

- Radiotherapy has an important part to play in the management of primary lung malignancies
- Continuous, hyperfractionated, accelerated radiotherapy (CHART) has recently been introduced in an attempt to improve the efficacy of radiotherapy. Radiotherapy is given at a rate of two or more fractions a day, each of smaller dose than conventionally fractionated doses. The number of fractions a week is gradually increased to shorten overall duration of therapy

RADIOTHERAPY

The role of radiotherapy in the management of primary lung malignancies will depend on the type and stage of the cancer. It is indicated in the following circumstances.

Nonsmall cell cancers considered resectable:

- Patients unfit for surgery
- Postoperatively for patients with N2

Nonsmall cell cancers considered nonresectable:

- If the tumor is confined to the chest, radiotherapy combined with chemotherapy
- If the tumor is extrathoracic, radiotherapy should be focused on symptomatic local sites

Small cell cancers:
- Limited stage – chemotherapy and radiotherapy combined
- Complete tumor responders – prophylactic cranial radiotherapy
- Poor performance status – chemotherapy and palliative radiotherapy

All patients with:
- Brain metastases
- Spinal cord compression
- Weight-bearing lytic bony lesions
- Symptomatic local lesions such as hemoptysis, atelectasis, or nerve damage

Efficacy
- Radiotherapy used alone may provide palliation of symptoms and improve the quality of the remainder of the life of patients with primary lung malignancies
- Combined with chemotherapy or surgery, will improve survival rates and quality of life in selected patients

Risks/Benefits
Risk: the side-effects, especially of nausea, vomiting, and diarrhea, need to be weighed against the potential palliation of other symptoms, or the potential increased life expectancy

Acceptability to patient
- Treatments can only be given in radiotherapy centers, so many patients may have to travel frequently
- Treatments often continue for 4–6 weeks
- A balance of benefit in terms of survival vs quality of remaining life must be made

Follow up plan
All patients should be followed up for life.

Patient and caregiver information
Treatment should be completed, however prolonged, for maximum efficacy.

Chemotherapy

CISPLATIN
- Cisplatin is a platinum compound used in the treatment of small cell and nonsmall cell cancers
- It is rarely used alone in the US; most often in a combination with other chemotherapeutic agents
- It is given intravenously
- Dose is based on body surface area calculation

Efficacy
- Improves survival by months in patients with stage IIIA, IIIB, and IV nonsmall cell cancer
- Improves quality of life in stage IV nonsmall cell cancer compared to best supportive care
- In patients with limited stage small cell cancer, combining radiotherapy with cisplatin improves survival
- Cisplatin is more effective but more toxic than etoposide in patients with small cell cancer

Risks/Benefits
Risks:
- Must be administered under specialist supervision
- Should not be used in patients with hearing impairment

- Should not be used in myelosuppressed patients
- Use caution with renal impairment
- Peripheral blood counts should be monitored weekly

Benefits:
- Can be given in a day-care setting
- Improves survival if given preoperatively in patients with stage IIIA nonsmall cell cancer
- Combined with radiotherapy, its use leads to improved survival compared to radiotherapy alone in patients with unresectable stage III nonsmall cell cancer and with limited-stage small cell cancer

Side-effects and adverse reactions
- Central nervous system: fatigue
- Eyes, ears, nose, and throat: ototoxicity
- Gastrointestinal: nausea, vomiting, anorexia
- Genitourinary: sexual dysfunction
- Hematologic: bone marrow suppression
- Metabolic: renal toxicity
- Skin: alopecia

Interactions (other drugs)
Pyridoxine plus hexmethylmelamine (may affect response duration).

Contraindications
- Hypersentivity to cisplatin or platinum-containing preparations
- Renal impairment

Acceptability to patient
Side-effects may make treatment less acceptable.

Follow up plan
Careful follow-up is needed.

Patient and caregiver information
- Decreased quality of life may be short-term, and the benefits of therapy may be long-term
- If possible, try to complete any course of therapy that is started

CARBOPLATIN
A platinum analog.

Efficacy
There is no convincing evidence that any other combinations of chemotherapeutic agent are superior to cisplatin-based regimens.

Risks/Benefits
The small increase in survival rates needs to be balanced against any adverse affects on quality of life.

Risks:
- Must be administered under specialist supervision
- Will typically cause nausea, vomiting, tiredness, fall in white cell count, hair loss, and neuropathy
- Bone marrow suppression is dose-related and may be severe, resulting in infection and/or bleeding. Anemia may be cumulative and may require transfusion support

- Should not be employed in patients with severe bone marrow depression or significant bleeding
- Bone marrow suppression is increased in patients who have received prior therapy, especially regimens including cisplatin
- Carboplatin has limited nephrotoxic potential, but concomitant treatment with aminoglycosides has resulted in increased renal and/or audiologic toxicity

Side-effects and adverse reactions
- Cardiovascular system: bradycardia, hypotension
- Central nervous system: infections, peripheral neuropathy, ototoxicty, asthenia
- Gastrointestinal: diarrhea, nausea, vomiting, mucositis
- Hematologic: neutropenia, leukopenia, thrombocytopenia, anemia
- Musculoskeletal: arthralgia, myalgia
- Skin: alopecia

Interactions (other drugs)

Nephrotoxic compounds (may potentiate renal effects of these compounds).

Contraindications

■ Patients with a history of severe allergic reactions to cisplatin or other platinum-containing compounds, or mannitol ■ Breast-feeding ■ Safety and efficacy in pediatric patients have not been established ■ Pregnancy category D

Acceptability to patient
- Myelosuppressium, hypersensitivity reactions, nausea, vomiting, fluid retention, and rashes may all limit the acceptability of these therapies to patients.
- Many agents must be given by intravenous injection or infusion, or require prior hydration, necessitating day care or even inpatient hospital stays.

Follow up plan

Careful follow up of all patients treated with chemotherapy is needed, for life.

Patient and caregiver information
- Decreased quality of life may be short-term, and the benefits of therapy may be long-term
- If possible, try to complete any course of therapy that is started

GEMCITABINE

An antimetabolite.

Efficacy

There is no convincing evidence that any other combinations of chemotherapeutic agent are superior to cisplatin-based regimens.

Risks/Benefits

The small increase in survival rates needs to be balanced against any adverse affects on quality of life.

Risks:
- Use caution with renal or hepatic impairment
- Safety and efficacy not established in children
- Should not be used during pregnancy and breast-feeding
- Patients should be monitored for myelosuppression

Side-effects and adverse reactions

- Cardiovascular system: myocardial infarction, cerebrovascular accident, arrhythmia, hypertension
- Central nervous system: fever
- Gastrointestinal: nausea, vomiting
- Hematologic: myelosuppression
- Metabolism: proteinuria, hematuria
- Respiratory: dyspnea, bronchospasm
- Skin: alopecia, rash, pruritus

Interactions (other drugs)

None listed.

Contraindications

■ Hypersensitivity to gemcitabine ■ Should not be used during pregnancy and breast-feeding ■ Safety and efficacy not established in children

Acceptability to patient

- Myelosuppressium, hypersensitivity reactions, nausea, vomiting, fluid retention, and rashes may all limit the acceptability of these therapies to patients.
- Many agents must be given by intravenous injection or infusion, or require prior hydration, necessitating day care or even inpatient hospital stays.

Follow up plan

Careful follow up of all patients treated with chemotherapy is needed, for life.

Patient and caregiver information

- Decreased quality of life may be short-term, and the benefits of therapy may be long-term
- If possible, try to complete any course of therapy that is started

PACLITAXEL

A taxane.

Efficacy

There is no convincing evidence that any other combinations of chemotherapeutic agent are superior to cisplatin-based regimens.

Risks/Benefits

The small increase in survival rates needs to be balanced against any adverse affects on quality of life.

Risks:

- Must be administered under specialist supervision
- Should not be used in patients with solid tumors who have baseline neutrophil counts of <1500 cells/mm^3 or in patients with AIDS-related Kaposi's sarcoma with baseline neutrophil counts of <1000 cells/mm^3
- Anaphylaxis and severe hypersensitivity reactions characterized by dyspnea and hypotension requiring treatment, angioedema, and generalized urticaria
- Bone marrow suppression (primarily neutropenia) is dose-dependent and is the dose-limiting toxicity
- Risk of severe conduction abnormalities
- Must not be used during pregancy
- Hypotension, bradycardia, and hypertension have been observed during administration

- Peripheral neuropathy is frequent; the development of severe symptomatology is unusual and requires a dose reduction of 20% for all subsequent courses
- Toxicity of paclitaxel is enhanced in patients with elevated liver enzymes

Side-effects and adverse reactions
- Cardiovascular system: bradycardia, hypotension
- Central nervous system: infections, peripheral neuropathy
- Gastrointestinal: diarrhea, nausea, vomiting, mucositis
- Hematologic: neutropenia, leukopenia, thrombocytopenia, anemia
- Musculoskeletal: arthralgia, myalgia
- Skin: alopecia

Interactions (other drugs)
■ Cisplatin (decreases paclitaxel clearance) ■ Doxorubicin (may cause increased doxorubicin levels) ■ Substrates or inhibitors of the cytochrome P-450 isoenzymes CYP2C8 and CYPA4 (may affect metabolism of paclitaxel) ■ Substrates of CYP3A4 and protease inhibitors (possible interactions)

Contraindications
■ Patients who have a history of hypersensitivity reactions to paclitaxel or other drugs formulated in Cremophor EL (polyoxyethylated castor oil) ■ Pregnancy category D ■ The safety and efficacy in pediatric patients have not been established ■ Breast-feeding

Acceptability to patient
- Myelosuppressium, hypersensitivity reactions, nausea, vomiting, fluid retention, and rashes may all limit the acceptability of these therapies to patients.
- Many agents must be given by intravenous injection or infusion, or require prior hydration, necessitating day care or even inpatient hospital stays.

Follow up plan
Careful follow up of all patients treated with chemotherapy is needed, for life.

Patient and caregiver information
- Decreased quality of life may be short-term, and the benefits of therapy may be long-term
- If possible, try to complete any course of therapy that is started

DOXORUBICIN
A cytotoxic antibiotic.

Efficacy
There is no convincing evidence that any other combinations of chemotherapeutic agent are superior to cisplatin-based regimens.

Risks/Benefits
The small increase in survival rates needs to be balanced against any adverse affects on quality of life.

Risks:
- Must be administered under specialist supervision
- Will typically cause nausea, vomiting, tiredness, fall in white cell count, hair loss, and neuropathy
- Special attention must be given to the cardiotoxicity induced by doxorubicin
- Cardiomyopathy and/or congestive heart failure may be encountered several months or years after discontinuation of doxorubicin therapy

Side-effects and adverse reactions

- Cardiovascular system: cardiotoxicity, phlebosclerosis
- Central nervous system: acute nausea and vomiting, mucositis, peripheral neurotoxicity
- Eyes, ears, nose, and throat: conjunctivitis, lacrimation
- Hematologic: secondary acute myeloid leukemia
- Hypersensitivity reactions: fever, chills, urticaria
- Genitourinary: red coloration to the urine for 1–2 days after administration
- Skin: severe cellulitis, vesication and tissue necrosis

Interactions (other drugs)

■ Paclitaxel ■ Progesterone ■ Verapamil ■ Cyclosporine

Contraindications

■ Marked myelosuppression induced by previous treatment with other antitumor agents or by radiotherapy ■ Previous treatment with complete cumulative doses of doxorubicin, daunorubicin, idarubicin, and/or other anthracyclines and anthracenes ■ Pregnancy category D ■ Breast-feeding

Acceptability to patient

- Myelosuppressium, hypersensitivity reactions, nausea, vomiting, fluid retention, and rashes may all limit the acceptability of these therapies to patients.
- Many agents must be given by intravenous injection or infusion, or require prior hydration, necessitating day care or even inpatient hospital stays.

Follow up plan

Careful follow up of all patients treated with chemotherapy is needed, for life.

Patient and caregiver information

- Decreased quality of life may be short-term, and the benefits of therapy may be long-term
- If possible, try to complete any course of therapy that is started

VINORELBINE

An antimetabolite.

Efficacy

There is no convincing evidence that any other combinations of chemotherapeutic agent are superior to cisplatin-based regimens.

Risks/Benefits

Risks:

- Specialist supervision required
- Administration of vinorelbine tartrate is contraindicated in patients with pretreatment granulocyte counts <1000 cells/mm^3
- Risk of acute shortness of breath and severe bronchospasm
- Risk of fatal interstitial pulmonary changes and acute respiratory distress syndrome (ARDS)
- May cause severe constipation
- Use caution with bone marrow suppression

Side-effects and adverse reactions

- Central nervous system: asthenia
- Gastrointestinal: nausea, vomiting, constipation, diarrhea
- Hematologic: granulocytopenia, leukopenia, thrombocytopenia, anemia
- Skin: alopecia

Interactions (other drugs)

■ Drugs known to inhibit drug metabolism by hepatic cytochrome P-450 isoenzymes in the CYP3A subfamily ■ Anticancer vinca alkaloids

Contraindications

■ Administration of vinorelbine tartrate is contraindicated in patients with pretreatment granulocyte counts <1000 cells/mm^3 ■ Pregnancy category D ■ Breast-feeding ■ Safety and effectiveness in pediatric patients have not been established

Acceptability to patient

- Myelosuppressium, hypersensitivity reactions, nausea, vomiting, fluid retention, and rashes may all limit the acceptability of these therapies to patients.
- Many agents must be given by intravenous injection or infusion, or require prior hydration, necessitating day care or even inpatient hospital stays.

Follow up plan

Careful follow up of all patients treated with chemotherapy is needed, for life.

Patient and caregiver information

- Decreased quality of life may be short-term, and the benefits of therapy may be long-term
- If possible, try to complete any course of therapy that is started

DOCETAXEL

A taxane.

Efficacy

There is no convincing evidence that any other combinations of chemotherapeutic agent are superior to cisplatin-based regimens.

Risks/Benefits

Risks:

- Specialist supervision required
- Risk of severe hypersensitivity reactions characterized by hypotension and/or bronchospasm, or generalized rash/erythema

Side-effects and adverse reactions

- Cardiovascular system: hypotension
- Gastrointestinal: stomatitis, nausea, vomiting, diarrhea
- Hematologic: leukopenia, neutropenia, thrombocytopenia, febrile neutropenia
- Musculoskeletal: myalgia, arthralgia
- Skin: alopecia
- Other: infection

Interactions (other drugs)

Drugs that induce, inhibit or are metabolized by cytochrome P-450 3A4.

Contraindications

■ History of severe hypersensitivity reactions to docetaxel or to other drugs formulated with polysorbate 80 ■ Docetaxel therapy should not be given to patients with neutrophil counts of <1500 cells/mm^3 ■ Pregnancy category D ■ Breast-feeding ■ The safety and effectiveness of docetaxel in pediatric patients have not been established

Acceptability to patient

- Myelosuppressium, hypersensitivity reactions, nausea, vomiting, fluid retention, and rashes may all limit the acceptability of these therapies to patients.
- Many agents must be given by intravenous injection or infusion, or require prior hydration, necessitating day care or even inpatient hospital stays.

Follow up plan

Careful follow up of all patients treated with chemotherapy is needed, for life.

Patient and caregiver information

- Decreased quality of life may be short-term, and the benefits of therapy may be long-term
- If possible, try to complete any course of therapy that is started

CYCLOPHOSPHAMIDE

An immunosupressant.

Risks/Benefits

Risks:

- Use caution with radiation therapy
- The risks of bone marrow suppression and hepatoxicity must be weighed against the limited evidence for real therapeutic benefit in established renal involvement in Henoch-Schoenlein purpura

Benefit: prognosis has improved dramatically with institution of this therapy

Side-effects and adverse reactions

- Cardiovascular system: cardiotoxicity (at high doses)
- Central nervous system: dizziness, headache
- Gastrointestinal: nausea, vomiting, diarrhea
- Genitourinary: amenorrhea, azoospermia, ovarian fibrosis, sterility, hematuria, hemorrhagic cystitis, neoplasms
- Hematologic: leukopenia, myelosuppression, pancytopenia, thrombocytopenia
- Metabolic: bone marrow supression
- Respiratory: fibrosis
- Skin: alopecia, dermatitis

Interactions (other drugs)

■ Allopurinol (increased cyclophosphamide toxicity) ■ Clozapine (may cause agranulocytosis) ■ Digoxin (decreased digoxin absorption from tablet form) ■ Pentostatin (increased toxicity with high-dose cyclophosphamide) ■ Phenytoin (reduced absorption of phenytoin) ■ Succinylcholine (prolonged neuromuscular blockade) ■ Suxamethonium (enhanced effect of suxamethonium) ■ Warfarin (inhibits hypoprothrombinemic response to warfarin)

Contraindications

■ Serious infections, including chickenpox and herpes zoster ■ Myelosuppression

VINCRISTINE

Antineoplastic.

Risks/Benefits

Risks:

- This preparation is for intravenous use only. It should be administered by individuals experienced in the administration of vincristine sulfate

- Risk of acute uric acid nephropathy
- Acute shortness of breath and severe bronchospasm have been reported
- Care must be taken to avoid contamination of the eye with concentrations of vincristine sulfate used clinically

Side-effects and adverse reactions
- Central nervous system: neuritic pain
- Eyes, ears, nose, and throat: blurred or double vision
- Gastrointestinal: constipation
- Central nervous system: headache, paresthesias
- Other: peripheral neuropathy, leukopenia
- Skin: alopecia

Interactions (other drugs)
Oral or intravenous administration of phenytoin (may reduce blood levels of the anticonvulsant)

Contraindications
■ Patients with the demyelinating form of Charcot-Marie-Tooth syndrome should not be given vincristine sulfate ■ Pregnancy category D ■ Breast-feeding

ETOPOSIDE
Related to the vinca alkaloids.

Efficacy
There is no convincing evidence that any other combinations of chemotherapeutic agent are superior to cisplatin-based regimens.

Risks/Benefits
Risks:
- Specialist supervision required
- Patients being treated with etoposide must be frequently observed for myelosuppression
- Risk of anaphylactic reaction manifested by chills, fever, tachycardia, bronchospasm, dyspnea, and hypotension

Side-effects and adverse reactions
- Hematologic: anemia, thrombocytopenia, leukopenia
- Gastrointestinal: nausea, vomiting, abdominal pain, anorexia, stomatitis
- Skin: alopecia

Interactions (other drugs)
None listed.

Contraindications
■ Hypersentivity to etoposide ■ Safety and effectiveness in pediatric patients have not been established ■ Pregnancy category D

Acceptability to patient
- Myelosuppressium, hypersensitivity reactions, nausea, vomiting, fluid retention, and rashes may all limit the acceptability of these therapies to patients.
- Many agents must be given by intravenous injection or infusion, or require prior hydration, necessitating day care or even inpatient hospital stays.

Follow up plan

Careful follow up of all patients treated with chemotherapy is needed, for life.

Patient and caregiver information

- Decreased quality of life may be short-term, and the benefits of therapy may be long-term
- If possible, try to complete any course of therapy that is started

ISOFOSFAMIDE

An alkylating agent.

Efficacy

There is no convincing evidence that any other combinations of chemotherapeutic agent are superior to cisplatin-based regimens.

Risks/Benefits

Risks:

- Must be administered under specialist supervision
- Risks of hemorrhagic cystitis, confusion, and coma
- Should not be used with severely depressed bone marrow function
- Use caution with renal impairment

Side-effects and adverse reactions

- Cardiovascular system: cardiotoxicity, hypotension, hypertension
- Central nervous system: toxicity, somnolence, confusion, hallucinations, coma, fever
- Gastrointestinal: nausea, vomiting, anorexia, constipation
- Genitourinary: urotoxic side-effects, hemorrhagic cystitis
- Hematologic: severe myelosuppression, hematuria
- Metabolic: renal impairment, liver impairment
- Skin: alopecia, dermatitis, delayed wound healing

Interactions (other drugs)

None listed.

Contraindications

■ Known hypersensitivity to isofosfamide ■ Safety and efficacy in children have not been established ■ Severely depressed bone marrow function ■ Pregnancy and breast-feeding

Acceptability to patient

- Myelosuppressium, hypersensitivity reactions, nausea, vomiting, fluid retention, and rashes may all limit the acceptability of these therapies to patients.
- Many agents must be given by intravenous injection or infusion, or require prior hydration, necessitating day care or even inpatient hospital stays.

Follow up plan

Careful follow up of all patients treated with chemotherapy is needed, for life.

Patient and caregiver information

- Decreased quality of life may be short-term, and the benefits of therapy may be long-term
- If possible, try to complete any course of therapy that is started

IRINOTECAN

A topoisomerase I inhibitor.

Efficacy

There is no convincing evidence that any other combinations of chemotherapeutic agent are superior to cisplatin-based regimens.

Risks/Benefits

Risks:

- Specialist supervision required
- Early diarrhea (occurring during or shortly after infusion of irinotecan hydrochloride) may be accompanied by cholinergic symptoms of rhinitis, increased salivation, miosis, lacrimation, diaphoresis, flushing, and intestinal hyperperistalsis that can cause abdominal cramping
- Risk of fatal myelosuppression

Side-effects and adverse reactions

- Central nervous system: fever, chills
- Gastrointestinal: nausea, vomiting, diarrhea, anorexia, constipation, abdominal cramps
- Hematologic: leukopenia, neutropenia, anemia
- Musculoskeletal: asthenia, pain
- Skin: alopecia, rash

Interactions (other drugs)

- Dexamethasone
- Other antineoplastic agents
- Prochlorperazine

Contraindications

- Known hypersensitivity to irinotecan
- Pregnancy category D
- Breast-feeding
- Safety and effectiveness of irinotecan in pediatric patients have not been established

Acceptability to patient

- Myelosuppressium, hypersensitivity reactions, nausea, vomiting, fluid retention, and rashes may all limit the acceptability of these therapies to patients.
- Many agents must be given by intravenous injection or infusion, or require prior hydration, necessitating day care or even inpatient hospital stays.

Follow up plan

Careful follow up of all patients treated with chemotherapy is needed, for life.

Patient and caregiver information

- Decreased quality of life may be short-term, and the benefits of therapy may be long-term
- If possible, try to complete any course of therapy that is started

Other therapies

STOPPING SMOKING

- Continued smoking will continue to reduce the body's immune system, accelerate the age-related decline in lung function, and decrease overall fitness
- Continued smoking will increase the risks of recurrence of primary lung malignancies
- Smoking cessation is important for all patients with primary lung malignancies, especially for those with the best prognoses
- Quitting smoking is very difficult for many patients, and requires support

Risks/Benefits

Benefit: the health benefits from quitting are potentially huge, especially in patients whose primary lung malignancy carries a more favorable prognosis

Acceptability to patient
Some patients may perceive the vague future benefits outweighed by the immediate difficulties in quitting, especially if their prognosis is poor.

Follow up plan
Most patients will benefit from help, support, and follow up in quitting smoking.

Patient and caregiver information
Perseverance is needed.

LIFESTYLE

- For patients with primary lung malignancies, good general fitness will reduce the perioperative risks from surgery and increase the likelihood of surgical or more radical nonsurgical options being offered
- Fitness can be improved by paying attention to nutritional status, obesity, excess alcohol intake, and quitting smoking

ACCEPTABILITY TO PATIENT
Usually low.

EFFICACY OF THERAPIES

- Untreated primary lung malignancies are fatal
- With treatment the overall 5-year survival rate is 10–12%
- Over 50% of patients will have metastatic cancers at the time of diagnosis

Nonsmall cell carcinoma:

- Surgery will lead to an improvement in 5-year survival rate to about 50% in patients with localized disease at the time of diagnosis
- Preoperative chemotherapy significantly improves survival
- For patients with initially unresectable nonsmall cell cancer, combined chemotherapy and radiotherapy followed by surgery results in only modest improvements in 5-year survival

Small cell carcinoma:
Patients with limited stage disease who receive chemotherapy and mediastinal irradiation have a median survival of 18–24 months.

PROGNOSIS

- The overall 5-year survival rate for primary lung malignancy is 10–12%
- The best prognosis is for patients with nonsmall cell cancer that is resectable and localized (stage I)
- The prognosis declines with local spread of the disease and the presence of distant metastases

Clinical pearls

A new lung lesion in a patient previously treated for lung cancer may not be a metastasis, but a new primary lesion. This can be treated with curative intent.

Therapeutic failure

Recurrence in the chest of the primary lung malignancy is the major cause of first treatment failure and carries an extremely poor prognosis.

Recurrence

Recurrence is usually treated with radiotherapy to any symptomatic lesions, although radical radiotherapy is probably more effective. Other active therapies have proved ineffective.

Deterioration

Palliative radiotherapy may be needed for symptomatic local or metastatic disease.

Terminal illness

- Domiciliary oxygen may be needed for symptomatic relief of dyspnea
- Potent analgesia may be required, especially for pleural involvement or bony metastases
- Antitussives are generally ineffective
- Hyoscine or its derivatives may help reduce troublesome bronchial secretions

COMPLICATIONS

Paraneoplastic syndromes:

- Eaton-Lambert syndrome: proximal muscle group myopathies
- Endocrine syndromes: SIADH (syndrome of inappropriate antidiuretic hormone secretion), ectopic ACTH (adrenoconticotropic hormone) production
- Musculoskeletal complications include clubbing, hypertrophic pulmonary osteoarthropathy, polymyositis

- Hematologic and vascular syndromes include anemia, thrombocytopenia, thrombocytosis, migratory thrombophlebitis
- Peripheral neuropathies, cortical or cerebellar degeneration
- Dermatomyositis, acanthosis nigricans

Chest problems:
- Pleural effusions and pleuritic pain
- Distal atelectasis and recurrent or persistent pneumonias

Intrathoracic complications:
- Recurrent laryngeal nerve palsy causing hoarseness
- Horner's syndrome: constricted pupil, anhidrosis, ptosis
- Pancoast's tumor: Horner's syndrome plus shoulder pain
- Superior vena cava obstruction

Extrathoracic metastases:
- Brain
- Bone
- Liver
- Adrenal glands
- Bone marrow

CONSIDER CONSULT

Refer every patient who has previously received treatment for primary lung malignancy to a respiratory physician in the first instance if:
- There are any local or systemic symptoms to suggest recurrence (persistent cough, hemoptysis, weight loss, malaise, bone pain, prolonged fatigue)
- If there are any relevant physical or radiologic findings (any new change on a chest X-ray, lymphadenopathy, cachexia, new neurologic or endocrine findings)

PREVENTION

- The most important cause of primary lung malignancies is cigarette smoking
- Helping all smokers to quit and stopping all nonsmokers from starting are the most important ways of preventing primary lung malignancies
- Reduction in exposure to the effects of passive smoking is also important, but passive smoking poses a much smaller risk than actively smoking
- Improved environmental protection is also important, especially in reducing the exposure of people to asbestos, ionizing radiation, nickel, uranium, arsenic, chromium and coal dust, and to natural radon (found in many rocks such as granite)

MODIFY RISK FACTORS

Lifestyle and wellness

TOBACCO

- Helping all smokers to quit and stopping all nonsmokers from starting are the most important ways of preventing primary lung malignancies
- Reduction in exposure to the effects of passive smoking is also important, but passive smoking poses a much smaller risk than actively smoking

ENVIRONMENT

Improved environmental protection is also important, especially in reducing the exposure of people to asbestos, ionizing radiation, nickel, uranium, arsenic, chromium and coal dust, and to natural radon (found in many rocks such as granite).

SCREENING

Primary lung malignancies fail to fulfil the criteria for successful screening:

- The natural history is not one of a long incubation period
- Many primary lung malignancies metastasize early
- Early detection has not been proven to improve outcome

CHEST X-RAYS

- Chest X-rays are neither specific nor accurate in the early diagnosis of primary lung malignancies
- There is variation in interpreting changes on an X-ray
- Chest X-rays will only show masses that have attained a certain size; if malignant, they have usually metastasized

Cost/efficacy

- To be effective, chest X-rays would need to be taken frequently (every 6–12 months)
- This would be prohibitively expensive and cause problems to administer

COMPUTED TOMOGRAPHY SCANS

Computed tomography (CT) scans are more specific and accurate than chest X-ray in the early diagnosis of primary lung malignancies.

Cost/efficacy

- To be effective, scans would need to be taken frequently (every 6–12 months)
- This would be prohibitively expensive and cause problems to administer
- The risks from the radiation of the annual or twice-yearly CT scans would be considerable, and may lead to an increase in incidence and mortality from primary lung malignancies

PREVENT RECURRENCE

Quitting smoking is the most important factor.

Reassess coexisting disease

PATIENT SATISFACTION/LIFESTYLE PRIORITIES

To maximize life expectancy but to have maximum quality in whatever life is left.

ASSOCIATIONS

American Lung Association
1740 Broadway
New York, NY 10019
Tel: (212) 315-8700
Toll free: (800) 586-4872
www.lungusa.org

National Cancer Institute
NCI Public Enquiries Office
Building 31 Room 10A03
31 Center Drive MSC 2580
Bethesda, MD 20892
Tel: (301) 405-3848
Toll free: (800) 4-CANCER
www.nci.nih.gov

Alliance for Lung Cancer Advocacy, Support and Education
PO Box 849
Vancouver, WA 98666
Tel: (360) 696-2436
Toll free: (800) 298-2436
www.alcase.org

American Cancer Society
Toll free: (800) ACS-2345
www.cancer.org

American Society of Clinical Oncology
225 Reinekers Lane Suite 650
Alexandria, VA 22314
Tel: (703) 299-0150
www.asco.org

KEY REFERENCES

- Non-Small cell Cancer Collaborative Study Group. Chemotherapy for non-small cell lung cancer (Cochrane Review). In: The Cochrane Library, 1, 2001 Oxford: Update Software
- Elderly Lung Cancer Vinorelbine Study Group. Effects of vinorelbine on quality of life and survival of elderly patients with nonsmall cell lung cancer. J Natl Cancer Inst 1999;91:66–72
- Anderson H, Hopwood P, Stephens RJ, et al. Gemcitabine plus best supportive care (BSC) versus BSC in inoperable nonsmall cell lung cancer in a randomised trial with quality of life as the prime outcome. Br J Cancer 2000;83:447–53. Medline
- Roszkowski K, Pluzanska A, Krakowski M, et al. A Muticenter, randomised phase III study of docetaxel plus best supportive care versus best supportive care in chemo-naive patients with metastatic or nonresectable localised non-small cell lung cancer (NSCLC). Lung Cancer 2000;27:145–57. Medline
- Ranson M, Davidson N, Nicholson M, et al. Randomised trial of paclitaxel plus supportive care versus supportive care for patients with advanced non-small cell lung cancer. J Natl Cancer Inst 2000;92:1047–80. Medline
- Lilenbaum RC, Langenberg P, Dickersin K. Single agent versus combination chemotherapy n patients with advanced non-small cell lung cancer a meta-analysis of response, toxicity and survival. Cancer 1998;82:116–26. Medline

- Keller SM, Adak S, Wagner H, et al. A randomized trial of postoperative adjuvant therapy in patients with completely resected stage II or stage IIIA non-small cell lung cancer. N Engl J Med 2000;343:1217–22
- Non-Small Cell Lung Cancer Collaborative Group. Chemotherapy in non-small cell lung cancer: a meta-analysis using update individual patient data from 52 randomised clinical trials. BMJ 1995;311:899–909
- Goss P, Paszat L, Newman T, et al. Use of preoperative chemotherapy with or without postoperative radiotherapy in technically resctable stage IIIA non-small cell lung cancer. Cancer Prev Control 1998;2:32–9
- Feld R, Rubinstein L, Thomas PA. Lung Cancer Study Group. Adjuvant chemotherapy with cyclophosphamide, doxorubicin and cisplatin in patients with completely resected stage I nonsmall cell lung cancer. J Natl Cancer Inst 2993;85:299–306

CONTRIBUTORS

Joseph E Scherger, MD, MPH

Benjamin Djulbegovic, MD, MPH

Ted Turnquest, MD

MEGALOBLASTIC ANEMIA

SUMMARY INFORMATION

DESCRIPTION

- Characterized by megaloblasts in the bone marrow (erythroblasts that have delayed nuclear maturation because of impaired DNA synthesis)
- Anemia is usually present and may be severe
- Mean corpuscular volume is usually increased
- Commonly seen in vitamin B12 deficiency (caused by an autoimmune mechanism, inadequate dietary intake, or malabsorption) or folate deficiency (caused by inadequate dietary intake, excess alcohol intake, chronic hemolytic anemia or malabsorption syndromes)
- Other circumstances in which megaloblastic anemia is seen include myelodysplasia and treatment with drugs that interfere with DNA synthesis; megaloblastic anemia may also be congenital

URGENT ACTION

- Severe anemia (hematocrit <25%) in the elderly or those with compromised cardiac status, or neurologic symptoms related to vitamin B12 deficiency should be treated immediately after blood samples (to determine vitamin B12 and folate levels) are obtained to avoid further complications
- Treatment consists of administering vitamin B12 and folate, and in some cases blood transfusions (exceedingly rarely; most patients start feeling better after several doses of vitamin B12/folate) to immediately correct anemia

KEY! DON'T MISS!

Because megaloblastic anemias due to vitamin B12 and folate deficiency are hematologically indistinguishable, clinical presentation is important in determining next diagnostic steps.

ICD9 CODE
- 281.0 Pernicious anemia
- 281.1 Vitamin B12 deficiency
- 281.2 Folate deficiency
- 281.3 Vitamin B12 with folate deficiency
- 281.4 Protein or amino acid deficiency
- 281.8 Nutritional
- 281.9 Megaloblastic anemia

SYNONYMS
- Pernicious anemia
- Folate deficiency
- Vitamin B12 deficiency
- Cobalamin deficiency

CARDINAL FEATURES
In megaloblastic anemia due to vitamin B12 deficiency:
- Low serum vitamin B12; normal folate levels (red blood cell folate may be low in up to 60% of cases secondary to low intestinal folate absorption, which occurs in B12 deficiency)
- Onset gradual (over years) if due to dietary deficiency; more rapid onset if due to malabsorption
- Mucosal pallor
- Glossitis
- Peripheral sensory neuropathy in early stages
- Absent reflexes in advanced cases

In megaloblastic anemia due to folate deficiency:
- Low folate levels in serum and red blood cells; normal vitamin B12 levels (in 10–20% of cases serum vitamin B12 may be falsely low)
- Mucosal pallor
- Glossitis
- No abnormal neurologic findings

CAUSES
Common causes
Vitamin B12 deficiency, which may be due to:
- Autoimmune causes: antibodies against gastric parietal cells, intrinsic factor in the presence of atrophic gastric mucosa (pernicious anemia)
- Strict vegetarian or vegan diets that excludes all dietary animal protein
- Abnormality in small bowel lumen with abnormal or absent transfer of cobalamin to intrinsic factor (e.g. in pancreatic insufficiency)
- Binding of vitamin B12 by bacteria instead of intrinsic factor, as occurs in stagnant bowel syndromes (e.g. diverticulosis, strictures, fistulas, anastomoses), slowed bowel motility (scleroderma, pseudo-obstruction) or hypogammaglobulinemia and as may be caused by *Diphyllobothrium latum*
- Abnormal ileal architecture causing malabsorption from Crohn's disease, gluten enteropathy, ileal resection, tropical or nontropical sprue, lymphoma, or amyloidosis
- Deficiency of intrinsic factor molecules: caustic destruction (as with lye), total or partial gastrectomy
- Gastric carcinoma
- Pancreatic insufficiency causing deficiency of pancreatic proteases necessary for cobalamin absorption

Folate deficiency, which may be due to:

- Inadequate dietary intake
- Increased demand, as in pregnancy, lactation, and infancy
- Increased demand caused by pathologic conditions such as chronic hemolytic anemia, malaria, sickle cell anemia, thalassemia, hereditary spherocytosis, paroxysmal nocturnal hemoglobinopathy, leukemia, lymphoma, myelodysplastic syndrome, agnogenic myeloid metaplasia with malignant disease, or psoriasis
- Malabsorption syndromes that affect the small bowel, such as gluten enteropathy, tropical or nontropical sprue, or Crohn's disease
- Medications that act as folate antagonists (methotrexate)
- Drugs that affect folate metabolism: alcohol, sulfasalazine, triamterine, pyrimethamine, trimethoprim-sulfamethoxazole, diphenylhydantoin, barbiturates, nitrous oxide
- Congenital folate malabsorption
- Familial aplastic anemia
- Exposure to arsenic or chlordane

Rare causes

Megaloblastic anemia due to defective cobalamin transport or metabolism:

- Congenital transcobalamin deficiency or defective transcobalamin receptors
- Inborn enzyme errors that affect the metabolism of vitamin B12

Disorders of DNA synthesis, which may be:

- Congenital (e.g. orotic aciduria, Lesch-Nyhan syndrome, congenital dyserythropoietic anemia)
- Acquired (e.g. thiamine-responsive megaloblastosis, erythroleukemia, refractory sideroblastic anemias)
- Caused by exposure to antineoplastic drugs that inhibit DNA synthesis

Serious causes

- Lymphoma: infiltration of gut by lymphoma can cause vitamin B12 deficiency due to malabsorption
- Amyloidosis: infiltration of the bowel with amyloid deposits can cause B12 deficiency due to malabsorption
- Caustic destruction (ingestion of lye) of gastric mucosa causes reduction of intrinsic factor production
- Crohn's disease: may cause B12 deficiency, especially if the terminal ileum is involved

Contributory or predisposing factors

Megaloblastic anemia caused by vitamin B12 deficiency:

- Age: more common in elderly
- Autoimmune diseases: Crohn's disease, idiopathic diabetes mellitus, Graves' disease, and Addison's disease have been associated with vitamin B12 deficiency of autoimmune origin
- Chronic gastritis: involves loss of gastric secretions including intrinsic factor

Megaloblastic anemia caused by folate deficiency:

- Strict vegetarian diets, 'fad' diets
- Age: more common in elderly people with chronic illness or who are in residential homes or institutions, where cooking methods may destroy folate
- Chronic alcoholism: poor eating habits and abnormal folate metabolism including excessive excretion in urine, trapping of folate in liver, and inhibition of folate absorption
- Poverty: poor dietary intake

EPIDEMIOLOGY
Incidence and prevalence
- Megaloblastic anemia due to vitamin B12 deficiency is most common in African-American women over 60 years of age
- Megaloblastic anemia due to folate deficiency is most common in vegetarians and the elderly

INCIDENCE
Greater incidence in women and elderly patients.

PREVALENCE
Megaloblastic anemia due to vitamin B12 deficiency:
- 0.9% in those over 60 years of age
- Higher in women (2.7%)
- Highest in African-American women (4.3%)
- 0.13–0.20% of Scandinavian, English, and Irish ancestry have the disease

FREQUENCY
2500 births/year involving neural tube defects due to folate deficiency in maternal diet.

Demographics
AGE
Megaloblastic anemia due to vitamin B12 deficiency is rarely diagnosed before the age of 35.

GENDER
- Megaloblastic anemia due to vitamin B12 deficiency is more common in women than men
- Megaloblastic anemia due to folate deficiency is equally common in both sexes

RACE
Megaloblastic anemia due to vitamin B12 deficiency:
- Incidence higher in African-American women
- High-risk groups include those of Scandinavian, English, and Irish ancestry
- As common in Native Americans as in Caucasians

Megaloblastic anemia due to folate deficiency:
More common in strict vegetarians.

GENETICS
Megaloblastic anemia due to vitamin B12 deficiency:
- Rarer, congenital form is probably autosomal recessive
- No substantial evidence for relationship between congenital and adult forms of megaloblastic anemia
- Multiple occurrences of adult form is common in same family (20 times the prevalence is found in children, siblings, parents, and parents' siblings than that of population at large)
- Relatives of patients with pernicious anemia are predisposed to make antibodies to gastric parietal cells
- Pattern of inheritance of the more common adult form is unclear
- Weak association between histocompatibility antigen HLA-B7 and pernicious anemia in Caucasians; stronger evidence for HLA- DW2, DW5, and DR2

GEOGRAPHY

Megaloblastic anemia due to vitamin B12 deficiency:

- Most common in African-American women and those of Scandinavian, English, or Irish ancestry
- Reported in South African Bantu, and in the Far East and Arabic nations

Megaloblastic anemia due to folate deficiency:
India and other areas that are predominantly Hindu (strict vegetarians).

SOCIOECONOMIC STATUS

- Megaloblastic anemia due to vitamin B12 deficiency, when caused by a diet that is insufficient in cobalamin, is more common in low-income populations
- Megaloblastic anemia due to folate deficiency, when caused by a diet that is insufficient in folate, is more common in low-income populations

DIFFERENTIAL DIAGNOSIS

Myelodysplastic syndrome

Abnormal hematopoietic maturation of unknown etiology, resulting in peripheral cytopenias with bone marrow erythroid megaloblastoid change and peripheral macrocytosis. The vitamin B12 level is usually normal to increased.

FEATURES

Clinical features may include:

- Splenomegaly (can also be a feature of pernicious anemia)
- Skin pallor
- Mucosal bleeding
- Ecchymosis
- Fatigue
- Fever
- Infection
- Dyspnea

Hematologic features:

- Anemia with a normal or increased mean corpuscular volume (MCV)
- Reduced reticulocyte count
- Hypogranular or agranular neutrophils
- Hypercellular bone marrow

Aplastic anemia

Aplastic anemia is bone marrow failure that causes stem cell destruction or suppression with resulting pancytopenia. It is usually caused by immunologically mediated bone marrow failure (e.g. as a result of toxins, drugs, radiation, infection – especially acute viral hepatitis) and may be inherited (Fanconi's anemia). The vitamin B12 level is usually normal to increased.

FEATURES

Clinical features may include:

- Pallor
- Ecchymoses, petechiae, retinal hemorrhages
- Fever
- Oral ulcers

Hematologic features:

- Pancytopenia
- Macrocytic anemia
- Toxic granulation of neutrophils

Hypothyroidism

Hypothyroidism may be seen in up to 25% of patients with pernicious anemia.

FEATURES

- Dry hair and dry, coarse skin with loss of the outer third of the eyebrows
- Nonpitting edema in the skin of the eyelids and hands
- Dulled facial expression
- Thickened tongue
- Bradycardia
- Slowed mentation and poor memory

- Hearing impairment
- Peripheral neuropathy
- Disordered thyroid function tests
- May cause erythroid macrocytosis
- Often accompanies vitamin B12 deficiency due to pernicious anemia

Hemolysis causing reticulocytosis

Hemolysis leads to increased red cell production, which can result in increased numbers of reticulocytes (which are larger than mature erythrocytes) in the peripheral blood. Hemolytic anemia may be inherited or acquired.

FEATURES

- Reticulocytosis
- Anemia may or may not be present (depending on the severity of the hemolysis)
- Morphologic abnormalities of the erythrocytes, depending on the cause of the hemolysis
- Raised serum bilirubin and excess urinary urobilinogen

Megaloblastic anemia associated with leukemia

Megaloblastic anemia may occur in acute leukemia or in chronic myeloid leukemia. Rapidly dividing leukocyte precursors may deplete folic acid stores, resulting in megaloblastic anemia.

FEATURES

- Macrocytic anemia
- Blood picture of underlying leukemia

Megaloblastic anemia of pregnancy

Pregnancy or the puerperium may be associated with a temporary megaloblastic anemia, although this is less common than iron-deficiency anemia during pregnancy. Coexistence of megaloblastic anemia and iron-deficiency anemia may occur. The mechanism is assumed to be increased demand for folic acid or (less commonly) vitamin B12. The condition is usually avoided if folic acid supplements are taken during pregnancy.

FEATURES

- Macrocytic anemia
- Dimorphic blood picture if megaloblastic anemia and iron-deficiency anemia coexist

SIGNS & SYMPTOMS

Signs

Megaloblastic anemia due to vitamin B12 deficiency:

- Generalized weakness
- Glossitis
- Pale mucosa
- Splenomegaly, hepatomegaly
- Paresthesias (in early disease)
- Absent reflexes (in advanced disease)
- Loss of joint position sense
- Delirium
- Dementia

Megaloblastic anemia due to folate deficiency:

- Weakness
- Glossitis
- Pale mucosa
- Splenomegaly, hepatomegaly

Symptoms

Megaloblastic anemia due to vitamin B12 deficiency:

- Triad of weakness, sore tongue, and paresthesia is classic clinical presentation although initial symptoms may vary widely
- Gait disturbance
- Confusion
- Memory loss

Megaloblastic anemia due to folate deficiency:

- Generalized weakness
- Sore tongue

ASSOCIATED DISORDERS

Megaloblastic anemia due to vitamin B12 deficiency:

- Idiopathic diabetes mellitus type 1 or type 2
- Graves' disease
- Addison's disease
- Hashimoto's thyroiditis
- Primary hypoparathyroidism
- Primary ovarian failure
- Myasthenia gravis
- Vitiligo
- Gastric carcinoma

KEY! DON'T MISS!

Because megaloblastic anemias due to vitamin B12 and folate deficiency are hematologically indistinguishable, clinical presentation is important in determining next diagnostic steps.

CONSIDER CONSULT

Refer to gastroenterologist for endoscopy at diagnosis to rule out gastric carcinoma.

INVESTIGATION OF THE PATIENT

Direct questions to patient

- Q **Do you have a sore tongue?** Glossitis is a key physical finding of both vitamin B12 and folate deficiencies
- Q **Are you experiencing generalized weakness?** This symptom is often reported along with mental functioning changes
- Q **Are you experiencing difficulty walking?** Loss of joint position sense may indicate advanced vitamin B12 deficiency but is not usually present in folate deficiency
- Q **Are you experiencing changes in mental functioning?** Memory loss, depression and dementia may be present in vitamin B12 deficiency
- Q **Are you currently being treated for cancer?** Many antineoplastic drugs inhibit DNA synthesis and may contribute to folate deficiency
- Q **Do you drink alcohol?** Chronic ethanol consumption may contribute to both vitamin B12 and folate deficiency
- Q **Are you being treated for Crohn's disease, tuberculosis, lymphoma, or amyloidosis?** All of these disorders may affect ileal mucosal receptors and absorption of vitamin B12
- Q **Are you being treated for sickle cell anemia, thalassemia, leukemia, or myelodysplastic syndrome?** These disorders and their treatment may increase folate requirements that are not met by diet alone
- Q **Have you recently been on a weight-loss or any other special diet?** May indicate a nutritional deficiency of vitamin B12 or folate

Contributory or predisposing factors

- Q **Does the patient have a diagnosis of any autoimmune disorder?** Crohn's disease, diabetes mellitus type 1 or type 2, Graves' disease, Addison's' disease, primary hypoparathyroidism, primary ovarian failure, myasthenia gravis, and vitiligo have all been associated with megaloblastic anemia due to vitamin B12 deficiency (pernicious anemia)
- Q **Is the patient a strict vegetarian?** Vegetarians who do not supplement their diets may experience deficiency in both vitamin B12 and folate
- Q **What is the patient's drinking pattern?** Chronic alcoholism is associated with both vitamin B12 and folate deficiencies due to poor diet and altered metabolism
- Q **Is the patient elderly and/or institutionalized?** Cooking methods in institutions may contribute to destruction of folate in foods. Chronic disease may contribute to poor dietary habits of elderly who live alone

Family history

- Q **Are there any family members with megaloblastic anemia?** This may indicate a cultural diet or habit that would cause a deficiency of vitamin B12 or folate.

Examination

- **Examine the oropharynx.** Mucosal pallor and glossitis are common findings in both vitamin B12 and folate deficiencies
- **Examine the abdomen.** Splenomegaly and/or hepatomegaly may be present
- **Weigh the patient.** Significant weight loss in short periods of time may indicate fad dieting
- **Observe the patient's gait.** Gait disturbance may be an indicator of loss of joint position sense. This may indicate advanced vitamin B12 deficiency
- **Examine patient's reflexes.** Loss of reflexes may be present in advanced vitamin B12 deficiency
- **Perform a mental status examination.** Mental status changes, dementia, and memory loss may indicate advanced vitamin B12 deficiency

Summary of investigative tests

Tests useful in all megaloblastic anemias include:

- Complete blood count (CBC), which is useful to determine the extent of anemia, and red blood cell (RBC) indices performed with the CBC reveal elevated MCV in both folate and vitamin B12 deficiency
- Reticulocyte count, which indicates the level of RBC production and may be first indication of successful treatment
- Peripheral blood smear, which reveals hypersegmented neutrophils (>5 nuclear segments per neutrophil) in pernicious anemia and macrocytic red cells in both cobalamin and folate deficiencies
- Serum vitamin B12 level
- Serum folate level
- RBC folate level, which gives a more accurate result than serum folate and represents folate used in production of RBCs
- A Schilling test can distinguish between low vitamin B12 levels that are due to lack of intrinsic factor and low vitamin B12 levels that are due to malabsorption
- Serum lactate dehydrogenase is elevated in 85% or more of patients with megaloblastic anemia
- Serum and urinary methylmalonic acid is increased in megaloblastic anemia caused by cobalamin deficiency, even if vitamin B12 levels are normal. It remains normal in megaloblastic anemia caused by folate deficiency
- Total homocysteine level is elevated in both vitamin B12 and folate deficiency
- Intrinsic factor antibody
- Antiparietal antibody test is more sensitive but less specific than intrinsic-factor antibody and is usually ordered by the consulting specialist

DIAGNOSTIC DECISION

- Megaloblastic anemia is a primary indication of vitamin B12 or folate deficiency but may also be seen in a variety of other conditions. Search for cause will be dictated by other clinical features
- Diagnosis is considered to be adequately documented and vitamin B12 replacement should begin if one of the following conditions exists: low serum vitamin B12 with or without megaloblastic anemia; low or normal serum vitamin B12 and increased methylmalonic acid in serum or urine with evidence of macrocytic anemia or symptoms suggesting B12 deficiency
- Diagnosis is considered to be adequately documented and folate replacement should begin if one of the following conditions exists: low serum folate level; low RBC folate level (but avoid giving folate alone without making sure the vitamin B12 level is normal)

CLINICAL PEARLS

- A patient with low vitamin B12 levels and positive anti-intrinsic factor antibody has megaloblastic anemia until proven otherwise
- In patients with aleukemic leukemia or myelodysplastic syndrome, always try to rule out vitamin B12/folate deficiency (once in a while this results in avoiding life-threatening treatment with poor prognosis)

THE TESTS

Body fluids

COMPLETE BLOOD COUNT WITH RETICULOCYTE COUNT

Description

Peripheral blood sample.

Advantages/Disadvantages

Advantages:

- Specimen easily obtained
- Results may be obtained in minutes to hours
- Specifies degree of anemia
- May reveal other cytopenias
- Increase of reticulocyte count is an early sign of successful treatment

Disadvantages:

- Does not specify type of anemia
- Reticulocyte count is nonspecific
- Specimen may need to be sent out of office for analysis

Normal

- White blood cell (WBC) count (adult): $4.0–10.5x10^3/mm^3$ ($4.0–10.5x10^9/L$)
- RBC count (adult male): $4.7–6.0x10^6/mm^3$ ($4.7–6.0x10^{12}/L$)
- RBC count (adult female): $4.2–5.4x10^6/mm^3$ ($4.2–5.4x10^{12}/L$)
- Hemoglobin (adult male): 13.5–18.0g/dL (135–180g/L)
- Hemoglobin (adult female): 12.5–16.0g/dL (125–160g/L)
- Hematocrit (adult male): 42–52%
- Hematocrit (adult female): 37–47%
- MCV (adult): $78–100mcm^3$ (78–100fL)
- Mean corpuscular hemoglobin (MCH) (adult): 27–31pg/cell
- Mean corpuscular hemoglobin concentration (MCHC): 32–36g/dL (320–360g/L)
- Red cell distribution width (adult): 11.5–14.0%
- Platelet count: $150–450x10^3/mm^3$ ($150–450x10^9/L$)
- Reticulocyte count: 0.5–1.85% of erythrocytes
- Absolute reticulocyte count: $28–87x10^9/L$

Abnormal
- Results outside the normal reference range
- Keep in mind the possibility of a false-positive result

Cause of abnormal result
- Decreased WBC count: secondary abnormalities of myeloid elements that is caused by deficiency in vitamin B12 or folate; present in advanced megaloblastic anemia
- Decreased RBC count: late event in megaloblastic anemias and does not correlate with neurologic symptoms in vitamin B12 deficiency. Caused by vitamin B12 and folate deficiencies
- Decreased hemoglobin and hematocrit due to effect of vitamin B12 and folate deficiencies on bone marrow
- Elevated MCV due to effect of vitamin B12 and folate deficiencies on bone marrow
- Elevated MCHC due to vitamin B12 or folate deficiency
- Increased red cell distribution width due to marked anisocytosis or poikilocytosis
- Decreased platelet count due to abnormalities of megakaryocytic elements in bone marrow

Drugs, disorders and other factors that may alter results
- Exposure to antineoplastic agents may decrease WBC, RBC, and platelet counts as well as hemoglobin, hematocrit
- Viral infection may cause decrease in WBC count
- Acute blood loss may cause decrease in red cell count, hemoglobin, hematocrit
- Drugs that cause hemolysis may cause decrease in red cell count, hemoglobin, hematocrit

Reticulocyte count may be affected by:
- Blood loss or increased RBC destruction
- Iron therapy for iron-deficiency anemia
- Polycythemia
- Metastatic cancer in bone marrow
- Di Guglielmo's disease

MCV increased in:
- Oral contraceptives
- Anticonvulsants
- Antineoplastics
- Orotic aciduria
- Di Guglielmo's disease
- Alcoholism
- Liver disease
- Anemia of hypothyroidism
- Hemolytic anemia
- Hemorrhage
- Myelodysplastic syndromes
- Postsplenectomy

MCHC increased in:
- Sickle cell anemia
- Hereditary spherocytosis
- Some autoimmune hemolytic anemias
- Disorders with cold agglutinins
- Disorders with severe lipemia of serum
- High heparin concentration

PERIPHERAL BLOOD SMEAR

Description

Peripheral blood sample.

Advantages/Disadvantages

Advantages:

- Easy to obtain
- Allows study of RBC morphology
- Requires only microscope and light

Disadvantages:

- Requires expertise in interpretation
- Does not differentiate between vitamin B12 and folate deficiency

Normal

- RBCs are round and uniform with pale centers and diameters of 7.2–7.9mcm
- WBCs seen in a normal smear include neutrophils, eosinophils, basophils, monocytes, and lymphocytes
- Platelets are small blue cytoplasmic fragments 1–2mcm in diameter and widely varied in shape

Abnormal

- Decreased number of RBCs
- Larger than normal RBCs 'macrocytes' that are oval in shape
- Decreased number WBCs
- Morphology of WBCs reveals hypersegmentation (over 5% WBC with more than five segments)
- Decreased number of platelets
- Interpretation of blood smears requires experienced examiner
- Keep in mind the possibility of a false-positive result

Cause of abnormal result

- Decreased numbers of RBCs, WBCs, and platelets may be due to lack of vitamin B12 or folate for DNA synthesis
- Larger than normal RBCs and abnormal WBC morphology may be due to lack of vitamin B12 or folate that interferes with normal marrow function

Drugs, disorders and other factors that may alter results

- Decreased numbers of WBCs, RBCs, and platelets may be the result of exposure to antineoplastic drugs or other drugs that can cause pancytopenia
- Decreased number of WBCs may be result of viral infection

SERUM VITAMIN B12

Description

- Peripheral blood sample
- Blood should be collected before blood transfusion or other therapy is initiated

Advantages/Disadvantages

Advantages:

- Specimen easily obtained
- Helps differentiate between vitamin B12 and folate deficiencies

Disadvantages:

- Does not identify source of deficiency
- Vitamin B12 deficiency is not reflected for months, so is not an early indicator of disorder

Normal
- 190–900ng/L
- By seventh decade decreased by 60–80%

Abnormal
- <190ng/L in megaloblastic anemia
- Keep in mind the possibility of a false-positive result

Cause of abnormal result
- Decreased intrinsic factor
- Strict vegetarian diet
- Increased demand in pregnancy, lactation
- Malabsorption

Drugs, disorders and other factors that may alter results
- Malabsorption due to gastrectomy, atrophic gastritis, or gastric irradiation
- Small bowel disease
- Primary hypothyroidism
- Parasites
- Blind loop syndrome

SERUM FOLATE LEVEL

Description
- Peripheral blood sample
- Blood should be collected before blood transfusion or other therapy is initiated

Advantages/Disadvantages

Advantages:
- Specimen easy to obtain
- Differentiates between combined folate and vitamin B12 deficiency and folate deficiency alone
- Falls quickly, so is early indicator of disorder

Disadvantages:
- Does not indicate source of disorder
- Indicates only negative folate balance not deficiency – need RBC folate to determine true deficiency

Normal

3.5–20mcg/L.

Abnormal
- <3.5mcg/L
- Keep in mind the possibility of a false-positive result

Cause of abnormal result
- Dietary deficiency
- Age (infancy, elderly)
- Increased demand (pregnancy)
- Chronic disease

Drugs, disorders and other factors that may alter results
- Alcoholism
- Hyperthyroidism
- Hemolytic anemias

- Cancer
- Use of folic acid antagonists
- Inadequate specimen storage

RED BLOOD CELL FOLATE

Description

Peripheral blood sample.

Advantages/Disadvantages

Advantages:

- Specimen easily obtained
- More reliable indicator of tissue folate deficiency because it reflects folate status at time RBCs were produced
- Not affected by daily variation in diet

Disadvantages:

- RBC folate does not fall below normal until body stores are depleted
- Not reliable indicator of megaloblastic anemia alone; must be drawn with serum folate and vitamin B12 levels

Normal

5–15ng/mL.

Abnormal

<5ng/mL.

Cause of abnormal result

Depletion of folate from body stores of folate due to:

- Chronic, strict vegetarianism
- Alcoholism
- Infancy, elderly
- Chronic disease
- Hemodialysis
- Anorexia nervosa
- Increased demand: pregnancy, hyperthyroidism
- Malabsorption

Drugs, disorders and other factors that may alter results

- Folic acid antagonists: methotrexate, trimethoprim, pyrimethamine
- Anticonvulsants
- Oral contraceptives
- Aspirin
- Improper specimen storage

SERUM LACTATE DEHYDROGENASE

Description

Peripheral blood specimen.

Advantages/Disadvantages

Advantages:

- Specimen easily obtained
- Results available in hours

Disadvantage: nonspecific

Normal
50–150U/L (0.82–2.66mckat/L).

Abnormal
>150U/L (>2.66mckat/L).

Cause of abnormal result
Elevated due to ineffective production and destruction of erythroid precursors in bone marrow.

Drugs, disorders and other factors that may alter results
- Blood transfusion reaction
- Any drug that causes hemolysis

METHYLMALONIC ACID
Description
Serum and urine specimens.

Advantages/Disadvantages
Advantages:
- Can be performed on same serum sample as vitamin B12 levels and folate levels
- Test is widely available through many laboratories, including national reference laboratories in the US
- Combined cost of this test and total homocysteine is equal to that of the Schilling test
- Most useful follow up test for distinguishing between vitamin B12 and folate deficiencies

Disadvantages:
- Not performed in most offices – specimen needs to be sent to a laboratory
- If patient on broad-spectrum antibiotics, result may be false-negative

Normal
- Plasma: 70–270nmol/L
- Urine: <8mmol/mol creatinine

Abnormal
- Plasma: >270nmol/L, with values as high as 2,000,000nmol/L, seen in megaloblastic anemia caused by vitamin B12 deficiency
- Urine: <50mmol/moL creatinine
- Remains normal in megaloblastic anemia caused by folate deficiency

Cause of abnormal result
- Vitamin B12 deficiency
- Keep in mind the possibility of a false-positive result

Drugs, disorders and other factors that may alter results
- Renal failure
- Intravascular volume depletion

TOTAL HOMOCYSTEINE LEVEL
Description
Serum sample.

Advantages/Disadvantages

Advantages:

- Can be performed on serum that remains after vitamin B12 levels and folate
- Test widely available through many laboratories including national reference laboratories in the US

Disadvantages:

- Not performed in most offices – specimen needs to be sent to a laboratory
- If patient on broad-spectrum antibiotics, result may be false-negative

Normal

<12mcmol/L.

Abnormal

- >14mcmol/L
- Elevated in both vitamin B12 and folate deficiency
- Keep in mind the possibility of a false-positive result

Cause of abnormal result

Lack of vitamin B12 and folate.

Drugs, disorders and other factors that may alter results

- Renal failure
- Intravascular volume depletion

INTRINSIC FACTOR ANTIBODY

Description

Serum sample.

Advantages/Disadvantages

Advantages:

- Diagnostic for pernicious anemia
- Specimen easily obtained

Disadvantage: test must be sent to outside laboratory

Normal

No intrinsic factor antibodies in the serum.

Abnormal

- Presence of intrinsic factor antibodies in the serum
- Keep in mind the possibility of a false-positive result

Cause of abnormal result

Pernicious anemia (highly specific for this disorder).

Drugs, disorders and other factors that may alter results

None known; test is very specific for pernicious anemia.

Tests of function

SCHILLING TEST

Description

- Performed in patients who have low vitamin B12 levels
- Fasting patient is given oral vitamin B12 tagged with ^{58}Co and vitamin B12 tagged with ^{57}Co bound to intrinsic factor
- In 1–2h, a flushing dose of 1mg nonradioactive vitamin B12 is injected to saturate vitamin B12-binding sites
- 24-h urine specimen collected

Advantages/Disadvantages

Advantage: differentiates between lack of intrinsic factor and gastrointestinal absorption problems as a cause of vitamin B12 deficiency

Disadvantages:

- Complete 24-h urine collection may be difficult
- Patient must have normal renal function for results to be valid

Normal

Both types of tagged vitamin B12 are normally absorbed and excreted.

Abnormal

- In pernicious anemia, ^{58}Co in urine is low, but ^{57}Co is normal
- In intestinal malabsorption, both ^{58}Co and ^{57}Co are low but become normal if underlying cause is treated
- Keep in mind the possibility of falsely abnormal result

Cause of abnormal result

- Lack of intrinsic factor
- Malabsorption of vitamin B12

Drugs, disorders and other factors that may alter results

Abnormal renal function.

CONSIDER CONSULT

Refer to hematologist if there is any suspicion that the underlying cause of megaloblastic anemia is anything other than vitamin B12 of folate deficiency. Try to explain reasons for low vitamin B12/folate.

IMMEDIATE ACTION

- If anemia is life-threatening or patient is elderly or has cardiac complications, blood transfusion may be lifesaving. Draw peripheral blood samples for vitamin B12 and folate levels prior to transfusion
- However, blood transfusion is exceedingly rarely appropriate. Avoid blood transfusion in megaloblastic anemia, as it can precipitate acute pulmonary edema. Anemia develops insidiously and most patients are able to tolerate very low levels of hemoglobin. Start with vitamin replacement, which will lead to rapid improvement even in these patients

PATIENT AND CAREGIVER ISSUES

Health-seeking behavior

- **Has the patient been treated for megaloblastic anemia in the past?** Lifelong nature of treatment may be difficult for patients to tolerate and this episode may be related to recurrent anemia
- **Has the patient self-medicated?** Patient may be taking vitamin supplements for self-diagnoses 'iron poor blood'. These preparations may or may not contain iron and/or vitamin B12
- **Has the patient visited a walk-in clinic or emergency room?** Severe symptoms such as painful tongue/mouth and neurologic deficits may lead patients to seek emergency medical care. Unless followed up with primary care physician (PCP), underlying cause of anemia may be missed

MANAGEMENT ISSUES

Goals

- Replace stores of deficient vitamin
- Treat any underlying disease
- Prevent progression of neurologic abnormalities (vitamin B12 deficiency)
- Prevent neurologic deficits in infants of nursing mothers with vitamin B12 deficiency

Management in special circumstances

- Patients with cardiac decompensation may require treatment for cardiac failure and blood transfusion prior to definitive diagnosis and treatment for megaloblastic anemia
- Folate must be administered before pregnancy to avoid neural tube defects and cleft palate in infants

COEXISTING DISEASE

Management choices for megaloblastic anemia are not affected by coexisting diseases.

COEXISTING MEDICATION

Management choices for megaloblastic anemia are not affected by coexisting medications.

SPECIAL PATIENT GROUPS

- Folic acid should be given before pregnancy to prevent neural tube defects and cleft palate
- Vitamin B12 and folic acid should be given to nursing mothers with deficiencies in these vitamins to prevent megaloblastic anemia and neurologic deficits in nursing infants

PATIENT SATISFACTION/LIFESTYLE PRIORITIES

- Lifelong therapy may be difficult for patients to maintain, especially if asymptomatic
- Patients with impaired vision, neurologic deficits, or memory loss due to age or other abnormality or learning deficits may have difficulty with self-injection of vitamin B12

SUMMARY OF THERAPEUTIC OPTIONS

Choices

- First choice for treatment of megaloblastic anemia due to vitamin B12 deficiency is cyanocobalamin
- First choice for treatment of megaloblastic anemia due to folic acid deficiency is folic acid
- Up to one-third of patients have concurrent iron deficiency, which needs to be corrected at the same time to avoid therapeutic failure

Clinical pearls

The diagnosis of multiple sclerosis, amyotrophic lateral sclerosis, and diabetic neuropathy should not be accepted without first ruling out vitamin B12 deficiency.

FOLLOW UP

- Monitor serum potassium for first 4 days of therapy and give supplemental potassium to patients receiving diuretics for cardiac failure
- Weekly hemoglobin and red blood cell (RBC) counts until return to normal
- Determine underlying cause while correcting the anemia

Plan for review

- Daily serum potassium for 4 days
- Weekly complete blood count (CBC) until return to normal
- If underlying cause determined to be pernicious anemia, surveillance for gastric carcinoma may be warranted

Information for patient or caregiver

- Therapy for megaloblastic anemia due to vitamin B12 deficiency is usually lifelong even if symptoms are not present
- When major medical problems (unplanned surgery) come up, it is not unusual for chronic vitamin B12 or folic acid therapy to be forgotten. It is important to continue therapy for megaloblastic anemia with other treatments

DRUGS AND OTHER THERAPIES: DETAILS

Drugs

CYANOCOBALAMIN (VITAMIN B12)

Indicated in megaloblastic anemia due to vitamin B12 deficiency.

Dose

Pernicious anemia:

- A dose of 100mcg/day for 6 or 7 days by intramuscular injection
- If there is clinical improvement and if a reticulocyte response is observed, the same amount may be given on alternate days for 7 doses, then every 3–4 days for another 2–3 weeks
- This regimen should be followed by 100mcg monthly for life

Patients with normal intestinal absorption:

- Initial treatment similar to that for patients with pernicious anemia may be indicated, depending on the severity of the deficiency
- Compliant patients who do not like monthly injection may be treated with oral therapy after blood count and vitamin B12 levels are restored

Gel for intranasal administration:
- Intranasal cyanocobalamin may be used once blood count and vitamin B12 levels are restored with intramuscular injections
- The recommended initial dose of cyanocobalamin gel is 500mcg administered intranasally once weekly

Efficacy
- Increase in wellbeing noted before hematologic improvement
- Anemia is reversible with continued therapy
- Neurologic deficits present at diagnosis may not be reversible with therapy

Risks/Benefits

Risks:
- Should not be used in patients with Leber's optic atrophy
- Hypokalemia and sudden death may occur in severe megaloblastic anemia which is treated intensively with vitamin B12

Benefits:
- Effect of therapy is seen early after the start of treatment
- Intranasal therapy avoids monthly injections

Contraindications
- Hypersensitivity to vitamin B12
- Optic nerve atrophy

Acceptability to patient

Prospect of lifelong injections for deficiency may not be acceptable to some patients; alternative therapy with intranasal vitamin B12 may be more acceptable.

Follow up plan
- Daily serum potassium for 4 days
- Weekly CBC, vitamin B12 levels until return to normal then monthly CBC
- In compliant patients with normal CBC, yearly CBC and RBC indices is adequate follow up
- If underlying cause determined to be pernicious anemia, surveillance for gastric carcinoma may be warranted
- With intranasal route, dose should be increased if vitamin B12 levels drop. If this continues, return to intramuscular treatment may be appropriate

Patient and caregiver information

Therapy must be lifelong to prevent neurologic complications.

FOLIC ACID

Indicated for the treatment of megaloblastic anemia due to folate deficiency.

Dose

Adults and children >4 years:
- 1mg/day orally (preferred route), intravenously, intramuscularly, or subcutaneously until clinical symptoms have subsided and the blood picture has become normal
- 0.4mg/day for maintenance dose

Children <4 years
- 1mg/day orally (preferred route), intravenously, intramuscularly, or subcutaneously until clinical symptoms have subsided and the blood picture has become normal
- 0.1–0.3mg/day for maintenance dose

Efficacy

Tissue stores are replenished after a few weeks of therapy.

Risks/Benefits

- Risk: use caution in patients with undiagnosed anemia
- Benefit: oral preparation well tolerated

Side-effects and adverse reactions

- Respiratory: bronchospasm (rare)
- Skin: itching and rash

Interactions (other drugs)

- **Anticonvulsants** ■ **Cholestyramine** ■ **Colestipol** ■ **Colchicine** ■ **Fluoxetine** ■ **Lithium** ■ **Lometrexol** ■ **Metformin** ■ **Methotrexate** ■ **Phenobarbital** ■ **Phenytoin** ■ **Pyrimethamine** ■ **Nonsteroidal anti-inflammatory drugs** ■ **Sulfasalazine**

Contraindications

Hypersensitivity to folic acid.

Acceptability to patient

- Oral preparation is particularly acceptable to patients
- Duration of therapy may be lifelong if cause of deficiency is not correctable; this may be difficult for patient to accept

Follow up plan

Weekly CBC and measurement of folate level until they return to normal; then monthly CBC.

Patient and caregiver information

If cause of folate deficiency is chronic then therapy will be lifelong.

EFFICACY OF THERAPIES

- In megaloblastic anemia caused by vitamin B12 deficiency, administration of cyanocobalamin allows hemoglobin and red blood cell (RBC) counts to return to normal in 6–12 weeks
- In megaloblastic anemia caused by folic acid deficiency, administration of folic acid replenishes folate stores within weeks

Review period

- Weekly complete blood count (CBC), vitamin B12 or folate levels until return to normal, then monthly CBC
- In compliant patients on vitamin B12 therapy, yearly CBC and RBC indices are acceptable follow up

PROGNOSIS

With appropriate replacement of either vitamin B12 or folic acid, megaloblastic anemia resolves with in weeks.

Therapeutic failure

- Return of anemia in compliant patients indicates another cause of anemia
- Referral to hematologist is appropriate
- Up to one-third of patients have concurrent iron deficiency, which causes therapeutic failure if not replaced at the same time
- Empiric treatment of megaloblastic anemia with folate may correct macrocytosis but not prevent neurologic damage related to underlying B12 deficiency

Recurrence

Referral to hematologist is appropriate if anemia recurs on therapy.

Terminal illness

- While megaloblastic anemia is very treatable, it has a mortality rate of 4% in hospitalized patients
- More that 50% of fatalities occur within first week of hospitalization and one-third of these are sudden and unexpected
- Most of these patients (75%) have evidence of congestive heart failure, and therapy for congestive heart failure should be initiated if recognized
- Blood transfusions may be lifesaving for severely anemic patients but may exacerbate congestive heart failure unless diuretics are given. Transfusions are rarely needed

COMPLICATIONS

- Hypokalemia in first week of treatment with vitamin B12
- Subacute combined degeneration of the spinal cord may occur in severe vitamin B12 deficiency. Physical therapy should be started as soon as possible. Replacement of vitamin B12 will prevent further neurologic degeneration. Slow improvement in neurologic degeneration present at diagnosis may be seen but further improvement after 5 months is unusual
- Pulmonary and urinary infections may be seen. Trimethoprim-sulfamethoxazole should be avoided in untreated patients with megaloblastic anemia secondary to vitamin B12 deficiency, due to its interference with folate. These patients will require higher doses of vitamin B12

CONSIDER CONSULT

- Referral to hematologist is appropriate if anemia recurs on therapy
- Refer to cardiology if cardiac decompensation does not respond to initial treatment

PREVENTION

RISK FACTORS

- Vegetarian diet without vitamin B12 supplementation: more common in strict vegetarians (vegans, Hindus from India), breast-fed children of mothers with megaloblastic anemia
- Gastrectomy: removes all intrinsic factor-secreting cells
- Gastric bypass surgery for morbid obesity: intrinsic factor is secreted but exposed to pepsin and trypsin before binding to vitamin B12
- Blind loop syndrome: anatomic abnormalities (diverticuli, anastomoses, fistulas) that allow bacterial overgrowth and thus vitamin B12 deficiency
- Ileal bypass, resection, or diseases localized to ileum: vitamin B12 absorbed in the ileum; malabsorption has been noted with removal of as little as 1ft of ileum
- Zollinger-Ellison syndrome: impaired vitamin B12 absorption due to low pH of intestinal contents
- Fish tapeworm infestation: *Diphyllobothrium latum* is parasite of freshwater fish found widely, but megaloblastic anemia (malabsorption of vitamin B12) seems to occur only Finland, Baltic states, or Russia and is caused by competition between the worm and host for vitamin B12
- Malabsorption syndromes: tropical sprue and celiac disease
- Drug-induced megaloblastic anemia: oral calcium-chelating drugs, para-aminosalicylic acid (when consumed for more than 6 weeks), biguanides
- Chronic pancreatitis: causes impaired absorption of vitamin B12
- Hemodialysis
- HIV infection: especially in patients receiving zidovudine therapy
- Alcoholism: alcohol alters absorption of vitamin B12

MODIFY RISK FACTORS

Lifestyle and wellness

ALCOHOL AND DRUGS

Limit alcohol intake.

DIET

- Ensure that diet contains vitamin B12 (protein from animal sources) and folate
- If strict vegetarian, monitor for vitamin B12 and folate deficiencies

DRUG HISTORY

Avoid oral calcium-chelating drugs, para-aminosalicylic acid, biguanides, or, if necessary to take, monitor for vitamin B12 deficiency.

CHEMOPROPHYLAXIS

- Folate supplementation during pregnancy improves hemoglobin levels and may prevent neural tube defects and cleft palate in infants born to deficient mothers but must be started prior to pregnancy to be effective
- Megaloblastic anemia due to vitamin B12 deficiency has been seen in infants breast-fed by mothers with deficiency; supplementation for mother will correct

Cost/efficacy

- Folate: US$0.89–15.65 for 100 1mg tablets
- Vitamin B12 (cyanocobalamin): 1000mcg injection US$0.10–0.47
- Both are effective in treating condition

PREVENT RECURRENCE

Compliance with replacement therapy is the chief way to prevent recurrence.

Reassess coexisting disease

Treatment for megaloblastic anemia may be inadvertently discontinued when patient is unexpectedly hospitalized, causing recurrence of disease.

ASSOCIATIONS

The American Society of Hematology
1900 M Street, NW, Suite 200
Washington, DC 20036
Tel: (202) 776-0544
Fax: (202) 776-0545
E-mail: ASH@hematology.org
www.hematology.org

March of Dimes Birth Defects Foundation
1275 Mamaroneck Avenue
White Plains, NY 10605
Tel: (888) MODIMES (663-4637)
www.modimes.org

KEY REFERENCES

- The College of Physicians and Surgeons of Manitoba (Canada): The diagnosis and management of vitamin B_{12} deficiency: Available online: http://www.umanitoba.ca/colleges/cps/Guidelines_and_Statements/326.html
- Little DR. Ambulatory management of common forms of anemia. Am Fam Physician 1999;59(6):1598–604
- Kuzminski AM, Del Giacco EJ, Allen RH, et al. Effective treatment of cobalamin deficiency with oral cobalamin. Blood 1998;92:1191–8
- Pruthi RK, Tefferi A. Pernicious anemia revisited. Mayo Clin Proc 1994;69:144–50
- Slot WB, Merkus FW, Van Deventer SJ, Tytgat GN. Normalization of plasma vitamin B12 concentration by intranasal hydroxocobalamin in vitamin B_{12} -deficient patients. Gastroenterology 1997;113:430–3
- Smith DL. Anemia in the elderly. Am Fam Physician 2000;62:1565–72
- Stabler SP. Vitamin B_{12} deficiency in older people: improving diagnosis and preventing disability. J Am Geriatr Soc 1998;46:1317–9
- Swain R. An update of vitamin B_{12} metabolism and deficiency states. J Fam Pract 1995;41:595–600

FAQS

Question 1

What is the mean corpuscular volume (MCV) result in patients with thalassemia/iron-deficiency anemia and folate/vitamin B12 deficiency?

ANSWER 1

In both of these conditions, MCV will tend to be normal. Concomitant thalassemia (usually alpha-thalassemia) and B12 deficiency is relatively commonly seen in young individuals of African ancestry.

Question 2

Can vitamin B12/folate deficiency explain severe pancytopenia?

ANSWER 2

Yes. After replacement treatment, it takes about 7–14 days to correct white blood cell/platelet counts but up to 6–8 weeks to correct anemia. If the diagnosis is correct, a brisk reticulocyte response is usually seen within 1–3 days.

Question 3

What is the role of a Schilling test?

ANSWER 3

The Schilling test is not done to diagnose vitamin B12 deficiency. It is performed to determine the etiology of vitamin B12 deficiency (i.e. pernicious anemia vs gastrointestinal malabsorption).

Question 4

Is gastrointestinal workup necessary to diagnose pernicious anemia?

ANSWER 4

No. Patients with low levels of vitamin B12 and anti-intrinsic factor antibody are assumed to have pernicious anemia.

Question 5

Can patients with normal methylmalonic acid and homocysteine levels have vitamin B12 deficiency?

ANSWER 5

No. Clinically significant vitamin B12 deficiency is virtually ruled out by normal levels of these metabolites.

CONTRIBUTORS

Fred F Ferri, MD, FACP
Benjamin Djulbegovic, MD, PhD
Naixi N Chen, MD

MULTIPLE MYELOMA

SUMMARY INFORMATION

DESCRIPTION

- Neoplasm of mature and immature plasma cells
- Most common primary bone cancer
- Symptoms result from marrow replacement, bone destruction, and production of monoclonal antibodies or antibody fragments
- Typically presents with recurrent bacterial infections, anemia, osteolytic lesions, and renal insufficiency
- Chemotherapy is standard treatment but is not curative
- Roles of allogeneic or autologous bone marrow or peripheral blood stem cell rescue are promising and are still being evaluated

URGENT ACTION

Refer urgently if:

- Cord compression suspected
- Hypercalcemia present
- Transfusion necessary
- Pathologic fracture suspected
- In renal failure
- Symptoms are severe, particularly pain

KEY! DON'T MISS!

- Hypercalcemia (common in myeloma; it causes constipation, confusion, and dehydration, and responds to rehydration and bisphosphonates)
- Renal stones – secondary to hypercalciuria
- Cord compression, which is a radiotherapeutic emergency; 5% of patients present with paralysis secondary to cord compression by extradural plasma cell mass
- Pathologic fracture as an additional cause of bone pain – requires stabilization
- Remember to consider prostatic cancer in men presenting with bone pain and hypercalcemia

BACKGROUND

ICD9 CODE
203.0 Multiple myeloma.

SYNONYMS
- Plasma cell myeloma
- Myeloma
- Myelomatosis
- Kahler's disease

CARDINAL FEATURES
- Malignancy of single plasma cell line
- Presents with an excessive production of monoclonal immunoglobulins by malignant cells, which appears as an M-spike (or monoclonal band) in serum protein electrophoresis
- Osteolytic lesions are caused by the rapid growth of the malignant plasma cells and by excessive osteoclast activation, and they result in bone pain, pathologic fractures, and hypercalcemia
- Usually affects multiple bony sites
- High monoclonal antibody levels cause hyperviscosity syndromes: blurred vision, dizziness, and altered consciousness
- 55% produce immunoglobulin (Ig) G paraprotein, 21% IgA, 22% light chain only, and 2% others (IgD, IgE)
- A small number of malignant plasma cells are found in the circulation but most are in the bone marrow
- Light chain fragments may be excreted in the urine as Bence Jones protein (found in 75%)
- Bone marrow replacement causes anemia, thrombocytopenia, and immunosuppression leading to fatigue, bruising, and chronic infections
- Monoclonal antibody fragments and hypercalcemia, as much as secondary amyloidosis, may cause chronic renal failure

CAUSES
Common causes
Etiology usually unknown.

Contributory or predisposing factors
- Predisposing factors usually unknown
- Because peak age is among the elderly it is thought that susceptibility may increase with the aging process, with reduction in immune surveillance, and a lifelong accumulation of toxic insults or antigenic challenges
- Agricultural workers, petroleum workers, workers in leather industries, and cosmetologists with exposure to herbicides, insecticides, petroleum products, heavy metals, plastics, and various dusts including asbestos have been considered to be potentially at an increased risk developing multiple myeloma, although the risk is ill-defined and has not been quantified
- People exposed to large amounts of radiation (such as survivors of the atomic bomb explosions in Japan) have an increased risk
- Human herpesvirus 8 (HHV-8), a new human herpesvirus, has been found in the nonmalignant bone marrow dendritic cells of patients with myeloma. The role of HHV-8 needs to be determined
- May be preceded by solitary plasmacytoma or monoclonal gammopathy of undetermined significance (MGUS) – a significant percentage of these patients go on to develop myeloma

EPIDEMIOLOGY

Incidence and prevalence

INCIDENCE

- Annual incidence: 4 per 100,000
- In African-Americans: twice as common
- More than 13,000 new cases are diagnosed each year in the US
- The actual incidence has probably not changed over the past 5 decades
- The apparent increase in incidence is probably related to the increased availability and use of medical facilities, and to better diagnostic techniques

Demographics

AGE

- Predominantly age 40–80 years
- Peak incidence in seventh decade
- Median age: 69 years (men), 71 years (women)
- Only 18% of sufferers are <50 years
- Only 3% of sufferers are <40 years

GENDER

More commonly affects males (1.5 times).

RACE

- African descent individuals are affected twice as frequently as Caucasians
- Asian individuals are affected half as often as Caucasians
- One of the top 10 leading causes of cancer death among African-Americans

GENETICS

- Abnormal karyotypes are present in 30–40% of patients but there is no specific karyotypic abnormality
- Chromosome abnormalities are present in about 50% of patients
- Monosomy 13 and trisomy or tetrasomy for chromosome 9 are the most common numerical abnormalities
- Poor prognosis: loss of 13, translocation of 11q, translocation of 1q
- Good prognosis: trisomy of 6, 9, and 17
- Occasional familial occurrence suggests recessive heredity
- Slight increased risk among children and siblings of those with myeloma

DIFFERENTIAL DIAGNOSIS

Metastatic carcinoma

Metastatic cancer can produce lytic lesions and plasmacytosis and may have an associated, unrelated monoclonal gammopathy.

FEATURES

- Small M component
- <10% of plasma cells in bone marrow
- Bone pain is less related to movement, and usually more severe at night
- Signs and symptoms relating to primary cancer

Lymphoma

Lymphoma is a solid tumor of the lymphoreticular system and is subdivided into Hodgkin's and nonHodgkin's disease by cell type. NonHodgkin's lymphoma is the sixth most common neoplasm in the US. Hodgkin's lymphoma has roughly the same incidence as multiple myeloma. Usually intermediate- to high-grade.

FEATURES

- Commonly presents with lymphadenopathy alone
- Fever and night sweats
- Weight loss
- Recurrent infection due to immunosuppression
- Pruritus
- Hepatosplenomegaly may be present
- Median age: 50 years for nonHodgkin's lymphoma, increasing with age
- Hodgkin's disease peaks at 15–34 years and again at >50 years
- When associated with HIV, brain lymphoma predominates

Primary neoplasm of bone and cartilage

Invasive, anaplastic tumors that can metastasize. Examples include osteosarcoma, chondrosarcoma, and Ewing's sarcoma.

FEATURES

- Pain and swelling in an otherwise well patient
- Osteosarcoma usually arises at long bone metaphysis, usually 10–20 years; 50% are around the knee
- Chondrosarcoma usually involves the pelvis, upper femur, or shoulder; usually >40 years
- Ewing's sarcoma causes painful soft-tissue mass and usually affects midshaft of long bone; peak age 10–15 years

Monoclonal gammopathy of undetermined significance

Occurs in approx. 0.2% of patients aged 25–49 years, 2% of those aged 50–79 years, and 10% of those aged 80–90 years. It is a common condition where a monoclonal protein is present, other criteria for myeloma diagnosis are absent, and no cause can be identified. One study reported that 16% of cases of monoclonal gammopathy of undetermined significance (MGUS) develop into multiple myeloma during long-term follow up of 30 years or more. No laboratory tests are currently available that can predict which patients with MGUS will progress to multiple myeloma.

FEATURES

It presents in asymptomatic patients with:

- M component of <3g/dL
- <10% bone marrow plasma cells
- Absence of osteolytic lesions, anemia, hypercalcemia, or renal insufficiency
- No or only small amounts of M protein in the urine (Bence Jones protein)

The serum and urinary M protein should be periodically measured, and clinical and other laboratory features should be re-evaluated, to determine whether other lymphoproliferative disorders have developed.

Plasmacytoma

Rare solid tumors, which may predispose to myeloma.

FEATURES

Solitary plasmacytoma:

- Usually located in the spine or long bones of the extremities
- Diagnosis is based on histologic evidence of a plasma cell tumor
- Complete skeletal radiographs must show no other lesions
- Bone marrow aspirate must contain no evidence of multiple myeloma
- No M protein on urine or serum
- Overt multiple myeloma develops in approx. 55% of patients
- New bone lesions or local recurrence develop in about 10%
- Progression usually occurs within 3–4 years

Extramedullary plasmacytoma:

- Plasma cell tumor that arises outside the bone marrow
- In 80% of cases it is located in the upper respiratory tract (nasal cavity, sinuses, nasopharynx, and larynx)
- May also occur in the gastrointestinal tract, central nervous system, urinary bladder, thyroid, breast, testes, parotid gland, and lymph nodes
- There is a predominance of immunoglobulin (Ig)A M protein
- Diagnosis is based on the finding of a plasma cell tumor in an extramedullary location and the absence of multiple myeloma on bone marrow examination, radiography, and appropriate studies of serum and urine
- Treatment consists of radiotherapy
- Prognosis is favorable
- Regional recurrences develop in approx. 25% of patients
- Development of typical multiple myeloma is uncommon

Idiopathic Bence Jones proteinuria

Small traces of Bence Jones proteinuria are common. Patients excrete only small amounts of this protein (60mg/L) – only 2–3% of these patients excrete greater quantities. In most patients who excrete >1g Bence Jones protein in 24h without evidence of malignant plasma cell proliferation, multiple myeloma or amyloidosis will eventually develop (but it may not occur for up to 20 years).

FEATURES

Bence Jones protein is excreted in urine by approx.:

- 70% of myeloma patients
- 30% of patients with Waldenstrom's macroglobulinemia
- 20% of patients with lymphoproliferative malignancy
- 10% of patients with so-called benign (secondary and idiopathic) monoclonal gammopathy

If Bence Jones proteinuria is the only abnormality, this is not indicative of malignancy but careful follow up is needed.

Sarcoidosis

Sarcoidosis is a chronic systemic granulomatous disease of unknown cause. Nonspecific caseating granulomas are characteristic.

FEATURES

- Fatigue, weight loss, anorexia, malaise
- Hypercalcemia leading to bone pain, renal stones
- Hypergammaglobulinemia (usually nonmonoclonal)
- Blurred vision, ocular discomfort, uveitis
- Skin papules and macules, erythema nodosum
- Arrhythmias, cardiomyopathy
- Hepatosplenomegaly
- Cranial nerve palsies
- Pulmonary manifestations – dry cough, dyspnea
- Diabetes insipidus
- Parotid enlargement

Tuberculosis

Tuberculosis is an infection caused by the bacterium *Mycobacterium tuberculosis*, causing systemic symptoms which may resemble those of myeloma. Extrapulmonary tuberculosis may affect bone and, therefore, may have further features in common with myeloma.

FEATURES

- Weight loss
- Night sweats
- Fever
- Cough and dyspnea
- Large joint arthritis with effusion
- Spondylitis of spine, often lower thoracic
- Parasinous abscess
- Cord compression

Aplastic anemia

A primary bone marrow failure characterized by stem cell destruction or suppression. Aplastic anemia is usually immunologically mediated. Etiology is unknown in >50% of patients but common etiologic factors include toxins (e.g. benzene, insecticides), drugs, ionizing irradiation, and infections (e.g. HIV). It may be inherited (Fanconi's anemia).

FEATURES

- Anemia
- Thrombocytopenia
- Immunosuppression
- Pancytopenia on complete blood count (CBC)
- Reticulocytopenia
- No monoclonal bands or Bence Jones proteins

Myelodysplastic syndromes

A group of acquired clonal disorders of hematopoiesis affecting stem cells. It is associated with abnormal hematopoeitic maturation, and bone marrow hypercellularity but peripheral blood cytopenia. 50–90% of cases are associated with chromosomal abnormalities.

FEATURES

- Fever
- Fatigue

- Recurrent infection
- Dyspnea
- Bruising
- Anemia
- Patients most commonly >65 years

Paget's disease of bone

Paget's disease is a nonmetabolic disease of bone. Osteolytic foci trigger excessive attempts at repair, resulting in heavy but weakened and distorted areas of the bone. It may be mono-ostotic or polyostotic; long bones, pelvis, and skull are commonly involved. 5–10% of patients develop bone sarcomas (osteosarcoma, malignant fibrous histiocytoma, or chondrosarcoma).

FEATURES

- Bone pain
- Bowing of long bones
- Pathologic fractures
- Headache
- Cranial nerve compression at exit foramina
- Cord compression due to vertebral involvement
- Increased heat over lesions
- Kyphoscoliosis
- Secondary osteoarthritis
- High output cardiac failure
- Raised serum alkaline phosphatase but normocalcemia

HIV

HIV is an RNA retroviral infection leading to depletion of T helper cells and severe immunodeficiency. Usually intermediate- to high-grade.

FEATURES

- Immunosuppression characterized by falling CD4 count
- Weight loss
- Night sweats
- Diarrhea
- May present with generalized lymphadenopathy
- May present with sore throat, headache, fever, and rash
- May present with recurrent infections typical of T cell immunodeficiency
- May present with lymphoma and other unusual tumors

SIGNS & SYMPTOMS

Signs

- Bone signs: bone tenderness (secondary to lytic lesions, hypercalcemia, and pathologic fractures); swellings on ribs, vertebrae, and other bones; pathologic fractures
- Skeletal survey may identify areas of impending fracture in weight-bearing bones prior to symptoms
- Signs due to marrow infiltration – pallor (in anemia), bruising, and epistaxis (in thrombocytopenia)
- Evidence of infections due to immunosuppression and leucopenia
- Confusion and dehydration, secondary to hypercalcemia
- Signs consistent with renal failure are found in 25% at presentation; etiology can be multifactorial: interstitial nephritis, hypercalcemia and hypercalciuria, prerenal azotemia, light chain deposition disease
- Motor weakness secondary to spinal cord compression
- Signs consistent with amyloidosis are present in 10–15% of patients at diagnosis

Symptoms

- 20% of patients are asymptomatic at diagnosis and picked up by blood test
- Bone symptoms – bone pain, typically in the back or thorax and described as wandering and intermittent, in 60% at presentation
- Symptoms caused by bone marrow infiltration symptoms – fatigue or weakness, palpitations, dyspnea, and poor wound healing due to normocytic, normochromic anemia (60% are anemic at presentation); epistaxis and easy bruising due to thrombocytopenia
- Recurrent infections (chest and urinary tract infection) due to deficiency of normal Igs
- Weight loss
- Low-grade fever, night sweats
- Symptoms caused by hypercalcemia (found in 20% of patients at diagnosis) and renal impairment (50%) – thirst, abdominal pain, nausea, and vomiting
- Symptoms caused by hyperviscosity, particularly with IgA syndromes – blurred vision, headache, confusion, breathlessness, and chest pain
- Symptoms of nerve root compression (paresthesiae, focal loss of function, pain (e.g. carpal tunnel syndrome), paralysis secondary to cord compression by extradural plasma cell mass (presentation in 5% of cases))
- Pain and numbness in the fingers and toes in cold weather – can be caused by cryoglobulinemia
- Anorexia

ASSOCIATED DISORDERS

- Amyloidosis presents in 10–15% of myeloma patients at diagnosis
- Occurs more often in patients whose plasma cells produce only light chains
- Symptoms may include low blood pressure, and kidney, heart, and liver failure
- Carpal tunnel syndrome, nephrotic syndrome, cardiac failure, and neuropathy can occur secondary to amyloid depositions
- In about 5% of patients at diagnosis, myeloma is static and may not progress for months or years. They have 'smoldering myeloma' (lower tumor burden) and are not troubled by the anemia, bone disease, renal failure, and frequent infections
- They are not treated with chemotherapy until disease progression, onset of symptoms, or development of new lytic bone lesions

KEY! DON'T MISS!

- Hypercalcemia (common in myeloma; it causes constipation, confusion, and dehydration, and responds to rehydration and bisphosphonates)
- Renal stones – secondary to hypercalciuria
- Cord compression, which is a radiotherapeutic emergency; 5% of patients present with paralysis secondary to cord compression by extradural plasma cell mass
- Pathologic fracture as an additional cause of bone pain – requires stabilization
- Remember to consider prostatic cancer in men presenting with bone pain and hypercalcemia

CONSIDER CONSULT

Referral for bone marrow biopsy is required in all cases to confirm diagnosis.

INVESTIGATION OF THE PATIENT

Direct questions to patient

Q **For how long have you been unwell?** Myeloma can range from indolent or smoldering symptoms to rapid onset and severe symptoms with poorer prognosis

Q **Have you lost any weight?** Weight loss when the patient has not been trying to lose weight is always a suspicious feature for malignancy

Q **Do you have any bone pain?** Bone pain associated with myeloma is usually worse on movement and gnawing in quality. Pathologic fractures may cause sudden onset, unremitting pain

- Q **Do you feel tired or short of breath?** Myeloma makes patients feel weary, short of breath, and easily fatigued on minimal exercise as a result of anemia
- Q **Do you suffer from palpitations?** These may signify anemia
- Q **Have you had any unusual bleeding?** This may signify thrombocytopenia
- Q **Do you bruise easily?** Easy bruising and epistaxis may signify thrombocytopenia
- Q **Have you been suffering from recurrent infections?** Consider marrow suppression and immunocompromise. Pneumonia and urinary tract infections are the most common recurrent infections reported
- Q **Have you noticed any blurring of your vision?** Hyperviscosity should be considered if vision is blurred
- Q **Have you recently been constipated?** Consider hypercalcemia if the patient responds positively
- Q **Have you experienced any numbness or tingling anywhere?** Consider nerve root compression if the patient responds positively
- Q **Have you 'gone off your feet'?** Consider cord compression if the patient answers positively
- Q **Are you passing water normally? Is there any blood or pain?** Consider renal stones, dehydration, or renal failure if blood is passed or pain is experienced
- Q **Do you feel sick?** If nausea is experienced, consider constipation, uremia, and hypercalcemia
- Q **What do you think might be causing these problems?** It is always important to find out what the patient thinks before proceeding with examination and investigation, and to make it clear to the patient if his or her hypothesis is likely or needs excluding
- Q **Would you like something for the pain?** Always remember to treat as well as to investigate

Contributory or predisposing factors

- Q **What job do/did you do?** Look for signs of exposure to radiation or petrochemicals that may suggest an industrial cause. Agricultural occupations, petroleum workers, workers in leather industries, and cosmetologists with exposure to herbicides, insecticides, petroleum products, heavy metals, plastics, and various dusts including asbestos seem to have a higher than average risk
- Q **Have you ever been exposed to radiation?** Individuals exposed to large amounts of radiation, such as survivors of the atomic bomb explosions in Japan, have an increased risk

Family history

- Q **Have you heard of a condition called myeloma? Have any of your relatives had this condition?** There is some evidence for autosomal recessive inheritance.

Examination

- **Perform a general inspection** looking for weight loss and cachexia, paleness, and bruising
- **Record the vital signs.** Increased respirations may be due to anemia; tachycardia may be due to sepsis or anemia. The patient may be febrile
- **Observe the patient's mental status.** Consider hypercalcemia and renal failure, both of which may cause sudden-onset confusion
- **Examine the hydration status.** Consider hypercalcemia but also infectious illness
- **Examine painful or lumpy areas on bone.** Lytic lesions will be tender; pathologic fractures will be extremely tender
- **Perform a neurologic examination** if the patient cannot weight-bear. A neurologic examination for a sensory level is mandatory when considering cord compression

Summary of investigative tests

- Complete blood count (CBC) to look for anemia, thrombocytopenia, or neutropenia. Useful in all tired patients or patients losing weight
- Erythrocyte sedimentation rate (ESR) is raised if there is significant monoclonal Ig secretion, very high in hyperviscosity. Usually very high in myeloma but nonspecific
- Blood urea nitrogen (BUN) and creatinine should be used to assess renal function

- Serum uric acid is raised in myeloma but is nonspecific
- Serum total protein is raised in myeloma
- Serum calcium level is required to detect hypercalcemia
- Serum alkaline phosphatase suggests pathologic fractures or alternative diagnosis when raised
- Serum lactate dehydrogrnase (LDH)
- 24-h excretion of protein and protein electrophoresis (PEP) and immunoelectrophoresis (IEP) of a concentrated specimen, and urine Bence Jones protein
- PEP, IEP, and quantitative Igs (QIG) – serum plasma protein immunoelectrophoresis for monoclonal bands is positive in >75% of patients, who also show decreased levels of normal Igs
- Plasma viscosity assesses level of disease and need for plasmapheresis
- Serum beta-2-microglobulin measures disease activity and is a guide to prognosis. Beta-2-microglobulin is a protein that is shed by B cells and correlates with myeloma cell mass. Levels >2.5mg/L are associated with a poorer prognosis
- Bone marrow aspirate and biopsy may demonstrate proliferating plasma cell line and is the most likely test to give definitive diagnosis. This is normally performed by a specialist. Samples are usually obtained from iliac crest, and then the number of plasma cells present is counted for diagnosis and staging. Plasma cell labeling index (PCLI) indicates the percentage of plasma cells that are actively dividing
- Complete skeletal survey by X-ray, including skull and long bones X-rays, is an essential part of staging and will show lytic lesions
- Technetium-99 bone scan is said to be of no benefit as lesions are lytic. Positive bone scans in myeloma usually indicate regions of fracture or arthritis – it should not be ordered as part of staging
- Order magnetic resonance imaging (MRI) of spinal cord if there is a paraspinal mass or signs of cord or nerve root compression

DIAGNOSTIC DECISION

Diagnostic criteria for multiple myeloma according to Durie–Salmon diagnostic criteria require a minimum of one major and one minor criterion (1+1 is not sufficient) or three minor criteria that must include 1+2.

Major criteria:

- Plasmacytoma on tissue biopsy
- Bone marrow plasmacytosis with >30% of plasma cells
- M protein – IgG >3.5g/L; IgA >2.0g/L, kappa or lambda chain excretion on urine electrophoresis >1g/24h in the absence of amyloidosis

Minor criteria:

- Bone marrow plasmacytosis with 10–30% plasma cells
- Detection of an M protein in serum or urine but less than levels defined above
- Lytic bone lesion
- Residual normal IgM <500mg/L, IgA <1g/L, or IgG <6g/L

Diagnostic decision for indolent multiple myeloma:

- Criteria as for myeloma with the following limitations
- Absent or only limited bone lesions (=3 lytic lesions), no compression fracture
- Paraprotein levels IgG <7.0g/dL, IgA <5.0g/dL
- No symptoms or associated disease features – hemoglobin >10mg/dL, serum creatinine <2mg/dL, normal serum calcium, and no infections

Diagnostic decision for smoldering myeloma:

- As for indolent multiple myeloma with additional constraints
- Bone marrow plasma cells 10–30%

- No bone lesions
- The recognition of this subset of patients is crucial because they should not be treated unless progression occurs

MGUS:
- Paraprotein levels IgG =3.5g/dL; IgA =2.0g/dL; Bence Jones protein =1.0g/24h
- Bone marrow plasma cells <10%
- No bone lesions
- No symptoms

Solitary plasmacytoma:
- Single plasma cell tumor
- No diagnostic criteria for systemic myeloma
- Little or no paraprotein after local therapy
- <10% plasma cells in the bone marrow

Clinical and laboratory evaluation of patients with monoclonal gammopathies:
- Serum and urine electrophoresis of high resolution is indicated for all patients suspected of having a plasma cell dyscrasia. The quantitative level of M protein should be defined precisely by densitometry
- Quantitation of 24h urine protein excretion to assess the presence, type, and daily excretion of monoclonal free light chains
- High-resolution electrophoresis assesses changes in level of a previously identified monoclonal protein in serum or urine at regular intervals that vary from every 1–2 months for patients being treated for multiple myeloma
- Hyperviscosity syndrome requires emergency plasma exchange with indications based on clinical features. Serum viscosity and serum protein electrophoresis are recommended prior to the first plasma exchange to correlate the level of M protein with symptoms in that patient. This correlation may be used to anticipate repeat plasma exchanges as the M protein approaches the level associated with hyperviscosity

Staging of multiple myeloma:
- Classification of Durie and Salmon is used for staging multiple myeloma
- This system correlates well with tumor mass and prognosis
- Stage is determined by level of M protein, number of lytic bone lesions, hemoglobin concentration, and serum calcium level
- Patients are further subdivided into classes A and B on the basis of the serum creatinine level

Stage I:
All of the following must be present:
- Hemoglobin >10g/dL
- Serum calcium =12mg/dL
- Normal bone structure or solitary plasmacytoma on radiographs
- Low M component
- IgG <5g/dL
- IgA <3g/dL
- Urine light chains <4g/24h

Stage II:
Not fitting stage I or III.

Stage III:
One or more of the following:
- Hemoglobin <8.5g/dL

- Serum calcium >12mg/dL
- Advanced lytic bone lesions – more than three sites of bone damage
- Hyper M component
- IgG >7g/dL
- IgA >5g/dL
- Urinary light chain excretion >12g/24h

Subclassification:
- A – serum creatinine <2.0mg/dL
- B – serum creatinine c.2.0mg/dL

CLINICAL PEARLS

- Serum interleukin (IL)-6 levels correlate with disease activity and tumor cell mass
- Increased IL-6 serum levels in almost all patients in terminal phase shows that this cytokine is an important factor in the progression the disease
- Early in the disease, *Streptococcus pneumoniae* is the most common pathogen, but infections with *Haemophilus influenzae* or other streptococci are also seen
- With disease progression and therapy, infections caused by *Staphylococcus aureus* predominate, accounting for 80% of all septic complications and most deaths related to infection

THE TESTS

Body fluids

COMPLETE BLOOD COUNT

Description

Venous blood sample.

Advantages/Disadvantages

Advantages:
- Minimally invasive test
- Good general screen for causes of tiredness and weight loss
- Investigates red cells, white cells, and platelets, and will also detect abnormal forms

Normal
- White blood cells: 3200–9800/mm^3 or 3.2–9.8x10^9/L
- Hemoglobin: males, 13.6–17.7g/dL (136–177g/L); females, 12–15g/dL (120–150g/L)
- Hematocrit: males, 39–49%; females, 33–43%
- Mean corpuscular volume: 76–100mcm^3
- Red cell distribution width index (RDW): 11.5–14.5%
- Platelet count: 130–400x10,000/mm^3 (130–400x10^9/L)

Abnormal
- Results outside the normal reference range
- Keep in mind the possibility of a false-positive result

Cause of abnormal result
- In myeloma, the red cell count and the platelet count are low, the white cell count is frequently normal until marrow replacement is extensive
- Lower values than these in all cell lines suggest marrow replacement or failure
- Normocytic normochronic anemia is usual in myeloma and is caused by replacement of the normal marrow by tumor cells and inhibition of hemopoiesis
- 67% of myeloma patients are anemic at presentation

Drugs, disorders and other factors that may alter results

Drugs that may suppress bone marrow include:

- Chemotherapeutic agents, e.g. cyclophosphamide
- Quinine
- Digitalis
- Nonsteroidal anti-inflammatory drugs (NSAIDs)
- Sulfa, penicillin, cephalosporins
- Phenytoin
- Other neoplasms
- Myelodysplastic syndromes

ERYTHROCYTE SEDIMENTATION RATE

Description

Blood test.

Advantages/Disadvantages

Advantages:

- Low invasiveness
- Cheap
- If suspicion of myeloma, ESR is considerably raised

Disadvantages:

- Poor specificity
- Only 5% of levels >100 are myeloma

Normal

- Male: 3–15mm/h
- Female: 3–20mm/h

Abnormal

- Above the normal range
- Hyperviscosity syndromes will tend to lower ESR
- Myeloma accounts for 5% of levels >100
- Raised in 90% of cases of myeloma at presentation

Cause of abnormal result

- ESR is raised in multiple myeloma due to an increase in globulins and the presence of paraproteins
- Fibrinogen is increased in malignancy, which raises ESR
- Anemia can raise the ESR

Drugs, disorders and other factors that may alter results

Steroids may lower ESR level.

BLOOD UREA NITROGEN AND CREATININE

Description

Blood test.

Advantages/Disadvantages

- Advantage: cheap and relatively noninvasive
- Disadvantage: nonspecific to renal failure or myeloma

Normal
- Urea nitrogen: 8–18mg/dL (3–6.5mmol/L)
- Creatinine: 0.6–1.2mg/dL (50–110mcmol/L)

Abnormal
- Raised urea nitrogen level
- Raised creatinine level
- Keep in mind the possibility of a false-positive result

Cause of abnormal result
- Renal failure (interstitial nephritis, hypercalcemia and hypercalciuria, prerenal azotemia, light chain deposition disease)
- Renal outflow obstruction
- Amyloidosis

Drugs, disorders and other factors that may alter results
- Urea nitrogen raised by: drugs e.g. aminoglycosides, diuretics, lithium, corticosteroids, anabolic steroid abuse
- Creatinine raised by: antibiotics (aminoglycosides, cephalosporins, hydantoin, diuretics, methyldopa)

SERUM URIC ACID
Description
Blood test.

Advantages/Disadvantages
Advantages:
- Easily included with other tests
- Relatively noninvasive

Disadvantage: nonspecific for myeloma

Normal
2–7mg/dL (120–420mcmol/L).

Abnormal
- Raised in myeloma
- Keep in mind the possibility of a false-positive result

Cause of abnormal result
Raised in:
- Renal failure
- Myeloproliferative disorders
- Cell lysis, e.g. with chemotherapy, radiotherapy

Drugs, disorders and other factors that may alter results
- High-protein or high-purine diet
- Diuretics
- Ethambutol
- Nicotinic acid
- Gout

- Addison's disease
- Active psoriasis
- Acidosis

SERUM TOTAL PROTEIN
Description
Blood test.

Advantages/Disadvantages
Advantages:
- Easily performed with other tests
- Relatively noninvasive and cheap
- Level may give a guide to tumor load

Disadvantage: nonspecific for myeloma

Normal
6–8g/dL (60–80g/L).

Abnormal
- Levels raised in myeloma
- Keep in mind the possibility of a false-positive result

Cause of abnormal result
Raised in:
- Dehydration
- Myeloma
- Waldenstrom's macroglobulinemia
- Sarcoidosis
- Collagen vascular diseases
- MGUS

Drugs, disorders and other factors that may alter results
Low-protein diet and malabsorption may falsely lower level.

SERUM CALCIUM LEVEL
Description
Blood test.

Advantages/Disadvantages
Advantages:
- Essential and useful if myeloma is suspected
- Performed with other tests
- Relatively cheap and noninvasive

Disadvantage: nonspecific to myeloma

Normal
- 8.8–10.3mg/dL (2.2–2.58mmol/L)
- If protein levels are abnormal, calcium levels need to be corrected for this. Local laboratory calibrations vary – local laboratory will advise but corrected calcium is higher if protein levels are lower

Abnormal

- Raised in myeloma due to increased osteoclast activity
- Keep in mind the possibility of a false-positive result

Cause of abnormal result

Bony lysis in multiple myeloma results in substantial mobilization of calcium from bone.

Drugs, disorders and other factors that may alter results

- Thiazides
- Lithium
- Toxic levels of theophylline
- Spurious due to tight cuff during phlebotomy
- Hypercalcemia

Hypercalcemia can be caused by:
(Common causes)

- Myeloma
- Leukemia
- Other malignancies (especially breast, prostate, lung, and kidney, but any tumor has potential)
- Neoplastic secretion of parathyroid hormone (PTH)-like substance
- Hyperparathyroidism

(Uncommon causes)

- Sarcoid
- Hyperthyroidism
- Immobilization
- Addison's disease
- Milk-alkali syndrome
- Vitamin D toxicity
- Diuretic phase of acute tubular necrosis

SERUM ALKALINE PHOSPHATASE

Description

Blood test.

Advantages/Disadvantages

Advantages:

- Easily performed with other tests
- Relatively cheap and noninvasive
- Helps differentiate myeloma from Paget's disease of bone

Disadvantage: nonspecific for myeloma

Normal

30–120U/L.

Abnormal

- May be raised in myeloma if fractures are present
- Normal in the absence of fractures or bone repair
- Keep in mind the possibility of a false-positive result

Cause of abnormal result

Raised in:

- Biliary disease
- Liver disease
- Paget's disease of bone
- Rickets
- Thyroid disease
- Ulcerative colitis
- Bony metastases
- Bone neoplasms
- Cytomegalovirus and mononucleosis
- Heart failure
- Hypernephroma
- Myelofibrosis
- Leukemia
- Myeloma if fractures or bone repair present

Drugs, disorders and other factors that may alter results

Raised by:

- Estrogens
- Albumin
- Erythromycin
- Phenothiazines
- Pregnancy

URINARY BENCE JONES PROTEIN

Description

Urine test for excreted light chain fragments.

Advantages/Disadvantages

Advantages:

- Simple to perform
- Relatively cheap
- Positive in about 70% of cases for light chains
- One of diagnostic criteria for myeloma if positive
- Negative urine immunelectrophoresis and negative serum immunoelectrophoresis exclude myeloma in 99% of cases

Disadvantages:

- Negative result does not exclude myeloma
- Positive result does not confirm myeloma alone
- Inconsistent results frequently hinder diagnosis

Normal

Normal result is negative but small amounts of monoclonal light chains (Bence Jones proteinuria) are not uncommon.

Abnormal

- Positive – when myeloma produces light chain immunoglobulin only (22% of cases), it is small enough to cross renal basement membrane and be excreted in the urine
- Keep in mind the possibility of a false-positive result

Cause of abnormal result
- Myeloma
- Idiopathic Bence Jones proteinuria

Bence Jones proteinuria:
- Bence Jones proteins are found in 70% of myeloma
- Bence Jones proteinuria is most frequently associated with multiple myeloma, primary amyloidosis, Waldenstrom's macroglobulinemia, or other lymphoproliferative disorders
- Bence Jones proteinuria may be 'benign'
- In most patients who excrete >1g Bence Jones protein in 24h without evidence of malignant plasma cell proliferation, multiple myeloma or amyloidosis will eventually develop
- This change may not occur for up to 20 years. Therefore, these patients are described as having idiopathic Bence Jones proteinuria

SERUM PROTEIN IMMUNOELECTROPHORESIS

Description

Blood test.

Advantages/Disadvantages

Advantages:
- Easy to perform
- Relatively noninvasive
- Can be sent to laboratory as part of primary care physician (PCP) investigation
- If positive, gives one of two required criteria for diagnosis
- Negative urine immunoelectrophoresis and negative serum immunoelectrophoresis exclude myeloma in 99% of cases

Normal

Serum proteins immunoelectrophoresis:
- Total protein – 6.00–8.30g/dL
- Alpha-2 – 0.38–0.84g/dL
- Albumin – 3.75–5.01g/dL
- Beta – 0.60–0.99g/dL
- Alpha-1 – 0.26–0.56g/dL
- Gamma – 0.72–1.46g/dL

Abnormal
- Paraprotein bands (M proteins)
- M spike in approx. 80% of patients with myeloma
- Keep in mind the possibility of a false-positive result

Cause of abnormal result
- The malignant plasma cells produce one specific protein, which is always exactly the same in one patient. M proteins show up as a 'spike': 50% are IgG protein, 20% IgA, 17% free monoclonal light chains
- Levels of functional Ig are depressed in individuals with multiple myeloma. It appears that the functional Ig made by existing normal plasma cells breaks down more quickly in patients with multiple myeloma than in healthy individuals
- Paraprotein bands may suggest myeloma but are also sometimes seen in: connective tissue disease, plasmacytoma, lymphoma, amyloidosis, chronic lymphatic leukemia, MGUS, Waldenstrom's macroglobulinemia, some solid tumors

PLASMA VISCOSITY

Description

Blood test.

Advantages/Disadvantages

Advantages:

- Simple to perform
- Relatively noninvasive
- Easily performed with other investigations

Normal

1.4–1.8 relative to water.

Abnormal

- Raised
- Symptoms likely to occur at levels >4.0
- Keep in mind the possibility of a false-positive result

Cause of abnormal result

Raised in:

- Monoclonal gammopathies – multiple myeloma, Waldenstrom's macroglobulinemia, MGUS; the incidence is highest in Waldenstrom's macroglobulinemia with IgM, followed by IgA myeloma, and the syndrome is observed usually when serum viscosity exceeds 4.0 centipoule (cp) units relative to normal serum
- Hyperfibrinogenemia

Imaging

X-RAY

Description

X-ray of areas of pain.

Advantages/Disadvantages

Advantages:

- Can be ordered by PCP
- Quick and relatively cheap
- May help point to diagnosis
- Finding of pathologic fracture may alter management

Disadvantage: radiation exposure

Abnormal

- Typical X-ray lesions: rounded punched out lytic lesions corresponding with pain site; in the ribs – osteolytic lesions with the appearance of diffuse mottling; in the spine – rarefaction, globular tumor formation, shortening and twisting of the vertebral column, and disappearance of intervertebral disks
- Skull often shows punched out lesions with no sclerotic or reactive border; these may be multiple, the so-called 'pepperpot skull'
- Periosteal reaction is uncommon
- Vertebral compression fractures are often seen
- 0.5–3.0% of the patients have mainly osteosclerotic lesions: sites – thoracic and lumbar spine, the tibia and fibula, the scapula, and sites of tendon and ligament insertions of the hands; X-ray appearance – irregular, fluffy, or spiculated; must be differentiated from metastases of breast or prostate carcinomas
- Occasionally, a mixture of lytic and sclerotic lesions is seen

Cause of abnormal result

- Myeloma
- Secondary tumor deposit from another primary. Prostate and breast secondaries usually cause sclerotic lesions but most others are lytic
- Osteoporosis
- Normal impact fracture: compare with history. Fracture with minimal or no force is usually pathologic

TREATMENT

CONSIDER CONSULT

- Refer all for consideration of treatment
- Most patients have symptomatic disease at diagnosis and require referral for cytotoxic therapy, but not all patients fulfilling the diagnostic criteria should be treated
- Patients should not be treated unless myeloma-related bone pain, anemia, hypercalcemia, renal impairment or recurrent bacterial infections develop
- If there is doubt about whether to begin chemotherapy, the oncologist is likely to re-evaluate the patient in 2 months and to delay therapy until progressive disease is evident. Primary care physicians (PCPs) in very rural areas may take this into account when considering referral times

IMMEDIATE ACTION

- Treat symptoms: analgesia for pain, intravenous fluids for dehydration, transfusion for anemia, rehydration and pamidronate for hypercalcemia, plasmapheresis for hyperviscosity
- For most PCPs and most patients, this will mean admitting the patient to hospital
- Bear in mind possible renal disease when prescribing analgesics – of the opiates, only fentanyl is metabolized via the liver rather than the kidneys
- In cord compression, give immediate high-dose oral dexamethasone (16mg) or prednisone (120mg) to reduce swelling then transfer urgently to unit offering radiotherapy. The longer cord compression persists, the worse the outcome – treatment must be begun within 24h

PATIENT AND CAREGIVER ISSUES

Forensic and legal issues

- Confused and disorientated patients may be unable to consent to treatment
- Elderly patients with pre-existing dementia may be unable to give consent
- There is an over-riding need to treat pain and distress
- Symptomatic treatment would not usually be ruled out by a 'Do not resuscitate' (DNR) order, or 'living will' or 'advance directive'
- The division between chemotherapy as palliation and chemotherapy as an attempted life-prolonging treatment with its own unpleasant side-effects is not very clear – in circumstances where patients cannot consent and an advance directive exists, careful discussion with relatives and caregivers as to the patient's likely wishes is important
- A mentally competent patient can refuse any treatment if he or she so wishes. This is not uncommon in patients who have had myeloma for some time and are requiring increasingly frequent transfusion or other treatment
- The mentally competent patient always has a right to call a halt to invasive treatment but it is important that relatives are aware and the decision is well documented so that when the patient deteriorates, treatment is not reinstated against his or her wish
- It is important to clarify with the patient rejecting further aggressive treatment whether symptomatic treatment of, for example, dehydration, hypercalcemia, or urinary tract infection is still wished for if he or she becomes confused
- Terminal palliative care can be difficult as pain and depression are sometimes difficult to control; patients may request heavy sedation and this needs to be discussed with caregivers and all medical staff, as early sedation may be perceived as hastening death

Impact on career, dependants, family, friends

- Chronic disease is exhausting and debilitating
- Symptoms are very unpleasant, often with severe generalized pain and even impaired mobility or paralysis
- Knowledge that they have a 'spreading' or infiltrating cancer is also very distressing for many elderly people
- Treatment may be unpleasant

- Extra help and support in the home is necessary, with early involvement of palliative care teams and day centers for symptomatic patients
- Asymptomatic patients with no lytic bone lesions have a median survival of 10 years but are at high risk of depression due to knowledge of the disease and expectation of progression

Patient or caregiver request

- Patients may have read publicity for recent trials of thalidomide for myeloma, which have been highly publicized in the US
- Patients may take their diagnosis as a death sentence but should be encouraged to have some hope, as prognosis can be good in selected patients
- Patients may have fears and preconceptions about chemotherapy
- Patients with bruising may fear that they will bleed to death and must be reassured that symptoms can be managed
- Patients frequently fear that increasing pain medication is addictive and dangerous – reassurance is important
- Patients may fear a painful death – while there are no guarantees, the patient and family need to feel that good palliative care is available and that pain medication will be increased whenever required
- Patients may ask about bone marrow transplant (BMT) and should be fully informed – best results are seen in younger, low-risk patients with a low tumor burden, and offer complete response in only 20–30% of this group. The mortality associated with BMT is high. Finding suitable donors for allogeneic transplant may be impossible

MANAGEMENT ISSUES

Goals

- For most individuals, meaningful prolongation of life with lasting relief of pain and other disease symptoms, and preservation of normal performance and quality of life for as long as possible
- The goal of some treatments may be complete remission, the definition of which is absence of M protein from serum or urine, absence of myeloma cells from the bone marrow, and absence of clinical symptoms or laboratory signs of myeloma
- Good doctor-patient relationship to aid future treatment decisions
- Understanding of patient's beliefs and expectations regarding disease and treatment
- Cure, if possible, with BMT
- Prolongation of symptom-free survival where cure is not possible
- Management and palliation of symptoms as they occur
- Dignified and pain-free death when treatment is no longer effective or desired

Management in special circumstances

Management is difficult and prognosis is poor where there is refractory renal failure.

COEXISTING DISEASE

- Patients with underlying disease may be less able to tolerate chemotherapeutic agents
- Patients with renal failure have particular difficulties – many analgesics are excreted by the kidney and can build up to toxic levels, and bone pain may prove difficult to control with coexisting renal failure
- Depression often coexists with myeloma and is often secondary to pain. Adequate pain management is essential
- Hypercalcemia also causes depression and pain, and vigilance is necessary to spare the patient from symptoms that can be easily treated

PATIENT SATISFACTION/LIFESTYLE PRIORITIES

- Predominantly a disorder of elderly patients
- Patients may be frail and may live alone

- Symptoms may have insidious onset and be exhausting to physical and mental health – extra help will be needed if the patient wishes to stay at home
- Symptoms of hypercalcemia may mimic those of the myeloma itself – it is important to be vigilant for the treatable part of the disease process
- Depression is common in the elderly infirm, particularly where there is pain. Myeloma can be particularly unpleasant to live with and antidepressant therapy, adequate analgesia, and emotional and practical support are necessary, particularly in older patients who live alone
- In late stages of the disease, 24-h nursing care is commonly necessary – families of patients living alone may need to be aware of this and plan for it

SUMMARY OF THERAPEUTIC OPTIONS

Choices

Treatment for symptoms and complications:

- Renal impairment – high fluid intake, and a high-carbohydrate and low-protein diet; allopurinol to prevent urate nephropathy
- Hypercalcemia – hyperhydration; bisphosphonates (reduce skeletal complications and bone pain, and also been shown to have some survival advantage). Zoledronic acid is in development
- Bone pain/fracture – analgesia, bisphosphonates (pamidronate), radiotherapy. Clodronate reduces the incidence of new lytic lesions and fractures; it is not US Food and Drug Administration (FDA)-approved for use in the US except in trials

Cord compression:

- Definitive diagnosis must be established immediately by computed tomography myelography or magentic resonance imaging
- The patient must be given high doses of dexamethasone (4–10mg intravenously every 6h)
- Surgical decompression must be undertaken within hours, usually followed by radiotherapy
- If spinal cord compression is imminent but no permanent damage has occurred, high-dose dexamethasone therapy combined with radiotherapy may be sufficient

Others:

- Hyperviscosity – plasmapheresis
- Anemia – epoetin alfa; if necessary, transfusion
- Infections – intravenous immunoglobulin therapy should be considered for life-threatening infections; antibiotics

Chemotherapeutic options – high-dose therapy with stem cell transplantation in newly diagnosed patients:

- Complete remission is obtained in up to 50% of patients
- Event-free survival is extended to more than 3 years
- Overall survival is extended to more than 5–6 years

Autologous peripheral stem cell transplantation:

- Patient should be <70 years
- Consider aggressive chemotherapy (vincristine, doxorubicin, dexamethasone (VAD)) with stem cell transplantation
- Peripheral stem cells should be collected before the patient is exposed to alkylating agents

Allogeneic (donor) BMT:

- Only 5–10% of patients can be candidates for allogeneic BMT
- There is a high transplant-related mortality ranging from 30 to 50%
- The complete remission rate is 40% but most patients relapse, and in the series with the longest follow up there was no survival plateau
- Only 10–20% of patients can be cured by allogeneic BMT

Chemotherapy – preferred initial treatment for overt, symptomatic multiple myeloma and in patients >70 years or in younger patients in whom transplantation is not feasible.

Melphalan and prednisone (MP):

- Standard treatment for the last 25 years
- Partial response (>50% reduction in monoclonal protein) has been observed in 50–60% of the patients
- 3–5% of patients achieve a complete remission

Other alkylating agent-based combinations:

- Vincristine, melphalan, cyclophosphamide, and prednisone (VMCP) alternating with carmustine (a drug also known as BCNU), vincristine, doxorubicin, and prednisone (VBAP) – VMCP/VBAP combination
- High-dose chemotherapy (HDCT)
- In the majority of studies it was shown that these combinations were equivalent to MP
- Patients with good risk prognostic variables seemed to fare better when treated with MP, whereas those with poor prognostic factors did better with combination chemotherapy
- VAD – provides quick response, effectiveness in hypercalcemia, quick relief of bone pain, applicability in patients with renal failure, and no cumulative bone marrow stem cell damage, allowing subsequent mobilization of stem cells
- Randomized trials between VAD and other chemotherapeutic agents failed to show any survival advantage

Plateau phase and maintenance treatment:

- There is no evidence that continued chemotherapy is of benefit after the attainment of a plateau phase
- The role of alpha-interferon maintenance is still controversial
- Chemotherapy must be reinstituted when relapse occurs. Most patients will respond to the reinstitution but the quality and duration of response is inferior to that of the initial response

Ongoing clinical trials for multiple myeloma are testing various combinations of chemotherapy drugs (including thalidomide and analogs), BMTs, immunotherapy, immunomodulatory drugs, and total-body irradiation.

Radiation:

- Usually limited to patients with severe and persistent pain from a localized lesion that does not respond to chemotherapy
- Can be used as palliative treatment for impending pathologic fracture and cord compression

Thalidomide:

- Can act in various ways including antiangiogenic activity, down-regulation of anti tumor necrosis factor (TNF)-alpha activity, immunomodulation, and changes in adhesion molecules
- Trials combining it with other traditional chemotherapeutic regimens are underway

In view of the rapid developments in treatment, patients may benefit from a treatment review by a center specializing in the treatment of multiple myeloma.

Clinical pearls

- Patients with monoclonal gammopathy of unknown significance (MGUS) or those with multiple myeloma who are classified as having smoldering multiple myeloma may remain stable for several years without treatment. However, virtually all patients with multiple myeloma eventually develop active symptomatic disease that requires treatment
- Prophylactic daily penicillin (orally) often benefits patients with recurrent streptococcal pneumonia infections

- Pneumococcal and influenza vaccine should be given to all patients despite their antibody response
- The median survival for patients with multiple myeloma is approx. 3 years

Never

Delay the diagnosis and treatment for patients with suspected cord compression, because it may compromise the prognosis.

FOLLOW UP

- Follow up is regular and life-long by an oncologist/hematologist
- While treatment is ongoing, regular review and blood tests will be necessary depending on the drug combination in use

Plan for review

- 3- to 6-monthly review with a repeat of blood tests for blood count, renal function, viscosity, and paraprotein levels may be sufficient if the patient is asymptomatic
- Patients should be advised to report any new symptoms that may develop
- Review when symptomatic will be determined by clinical status and need/wish for treatment

Information for patient or caregiver

- Patients should know which symptoms to look for, particularly: increased tiredness, aches and pains, constipation, confusion, urinary difficulties (stones and urinary tract infections), blurred vision, and dizziness
- Patients should also be aware that there is real prospect of a prolonged symptom-free course over many years
- Caregivers should be aware of significant risk of depression

DRUGS AND OTHER THERAPIES: DETAILS

Drugs

CYCLOPHOSPHAMIDE

Cyclophosphamide is an antineoplastic alkylating agent.

Dose

- 1–5mg/kg/day orally or 10–15mg/kg intravenously every 10 days
- Duration defined by clinical response

Risks/Benefits

Risk: use caution when administering with radiation therapy

Side-effects and adverse reactions

- Cardiovascular system: cardiotoxicity (at high doses)
- Central nervous system: dizziness, headache
- Gastrointestinal: nausea, vomiting, diarrhea
- Genitourinary: amenorrhea, azoospermia, ovarian fibrosis, sterility, hematuria, hemorrhagic cystitis, neoplasms
- Hematologic: leukopenia, myelosuppression, panycytopenia, thrombocytopenia
- Metabolic: bone marrow supression
- Respiratory: fibrosis
- Skin: alopecia, dermatitis

Interactions (other drugs)

■ Phenobarbital increases the metabolism rate and leukopenic activity of cyclophosphamide ■ Cyclophosphamide causes a marked and persistent inhibition of cholinesterase activity and potentiates the effect of succinylcholine chloride ■ If a patient has been treated with cyclophosphamide within 10 days of general anesthesia, the anesthesiologist should be alerted

Contraindications

■ Hypersensitivity to cyclophosphamide ■ Serious infections, including chicken pox and herpes zoster ■ Myelosuppression

Acceptability to patient

May cause a painful hemorrhagic cystitis, but that may be prevented with vigorous hydration and/or with the use of uroprotectants.

Patient and caregiver information

Patient should report dysuria or hematuria.

DOXORUBICIN

Doxorubicin is a cytotoxic anthracycline antibiotic obtained from a streptomyces mold.

Dose

- Usually 30–60mg/m^2
- Frequency and duration as defined by treatment schedule
- Maximum 450mg/m^2 (above this the risk of cardiac insufficiency increases markedly)

Risks/Benefits

Risks:

- Must be administered under specialist supervision
- Will typically cause nausea, vomiting, tiredness, fall in white cell count, hair loss, and neuropathy
- Special attention must be given to the cardiotoxicity induced by doxorubicin
- Cardiomyopathy and/or congestive heart failure may be encountered several months or years after discontinuation of doxorubicin therapy

Side-effects and adverse reactions

- Cardiovascular system: cardiotoxicity, phlebosclerosis
- Central nervous system: acute nausea and vomiting, mucositis, peripheral neurotoxicity
- Eyes, ears, nose, and throat: conjunctivitis, lacrimation
- Hematologic: secondary acute myeloid leukemia
- Hypersensitivity reactions: fever, chills, urticaria
- Genitourinary: red coloration to the urine for 1–2 days after administration
- Skin: severe cellulitis, vesication, tissue necrosis

Interactions (other drugs)

■ Paclitaxel ■ Progesterone ■ Verapamil ■ Cyclosporine

Contraindications

■ Hypersensitivity to doxorubicin ■ Marked myelosuppression induced by previous treatment with other antitumor agents or by radiotherapy ■ Previous treatment with complete cumulative doses of doxorubicin, daunorubicin, idarubicin, and/or other anthracyclines and anthracenes ■ Pregnancy category D ■ Breast-feeding

Acceptability to patient

Can cause myocarditis and pericarditis

Patient and caregiver information

Patient must report chest pain or shortness of breath.

VINCRISTINE

Vincristine is an antineoplastic alkaloid obtained from the periwinkle plant.

Dose

- Dosage should be decided by a specialist
- Duration as defined by treatment schedule
- This drug is fatal if given intrathecally

Risks/Benefits

Risks:

- This preparation is for intravenous use only. It should be administered by individuals experienced in the administration of vincristine sulfate
- Risk of acute uric acid nephropathy
- Acute shortness of breath and severe bronchospasm have been reported
- Care must be taken to avoid contamination of the eye with concentrations of vincristine sulfate used clinically

Side-effects and adverse reactions

- Central nervous system: neuritic pain, headache, paresthesias
- Eyes, ears, nose, and throat: blurred or double vision
- Gastrointestinal: constipation
- Other: peripheral neuropathyleukopenia
- Skin: alopecia

Interactions (other drugs)

- Serum levels of digoxin may be decreased
- Serum levels of phenytoin may be decreased
- Metoclopramide may reverse symptoms of paralytic ileus

Contraindications

- This drug is fatal if given intrathecally
- Pregnancy category D
- Breast-feeding

Acceptability to patient

Can cause severe neurologic side-effects, including paresthesias, neuritic pain, and motor disturbances.

Patient and caregiver information

Patients should be warned of the possible side-effects.

CARMUSTINE

Dose

150–200mg/m^2 intravenously every 6 weeks when used as single drug in previously untreated patients.

Risks/Benefits

Risks:

- Should be admistered by a specialist
- Thrombocytopenia and leukopenia may contribute to bleeding and overwhelming infections in an already compromised patient
- Blood counts should be monitored weekly for at least 6 weeks after a dose
- Pulmonary toxicity from carmustine appears to be dose related. Patients receiving >1400mg/m^2 cumulative dose are at significantly higher risk than those receiving less
- Delayed pulmonary toxicity can occur years after treatment, and can result in death, particularly in patients treated in childhood
- Nursing should be discontinued when starting treatment

Side-effects and adverse reactions

- Cardiovascular system: pulmonary toxicity
- Gastrointestinal: nausea, vomiting
- Hematologic: myelosuppression
- Metabolic: hepatoxicity
- Other: nephrotoxicity

Interactions (other drugs)

None listed.

Contraindications

- Hypersensitivty to carmustine
- Safety and efficacy in children have not been established
- Pregnancy category D

PAMIDRONATE

- Approved for the treatment of bone metastases
- Not another form of chemotherapy
- Intravenous pamidronate is also used to treat hypercalcemia
- Hydration with isotonic saline and administration of furosemide plus prednisone and pamidronate disodium is effective at lowering blood calcium

Dose

- In hypercalcemia: given intravenously in a dose titrated against the corrected calcium level 30–90mg over 24h
- Preventive pamidronate use: 90mg over 4h once a month

Risks/Benefits

Risk: use caution in renal dysfunction

Benefits:

- Effective palliation for hypercalcemia and bone pain
- Delays and reduces bone complications, such as fractures, and may reduce bone pain

Side-effects and adverse reactions

- Cardiovascular system: hypertension
- Central nervous system: headache, seizures
- Eyes, ears, nose, and throat: iritis
- Gastrointestinal: abdominal pain, anorexia, nausea, vomiting
- Metabolic: decrease in potassium, magnesium, and phosphate levels

Interactions (other drugs)

■ Aminoglycosides ■ Antacids ■ Calcium salts ■ Iron

Contraindications

■ Hypersensitivity to the drug ■ Pregnancy and breast-feeding

Acceptability to patient

Usually high.

Follow up plan

- Continue to monitor blood calcium levels with frequency depending on clinical condition
- Although rare, long-term use can affect the kidneys; therefore, kidney function is tested periodically (every 3–4 months) with standard tests of renal function, such as serum creatinine, blood urea nitrogen, and urine creatinine and protein

Patient and caregiver information

Patient needs to be aware that once it has been present hypercalcemia is likely to recur, and so they should be alert for signs and symptoms.

ZOLEDRONIC ACID

- A bisphosphonate in development for the treatment of tumor-induced hypercalcemia and for the prevention and treatment of bone metastases
- Zolendronate was recently given FDA approval for hypercalcemia of malignancy

Dose

- The maximum recommended 4mg dose must be diluted in 100mL sterile 0.9% sodium chloride, USP (United States Pharmacopeia), or 5% dextrose injection, USP. The dose must be given as a single intravenous infusion over no less than 15min
- Retreatment if calcium levels persist high; should await at least 7 days due to risk of renal failure
- Patients must be adequately rehydrated prior to administration of zoledronic acid. Loop diuretics should not be used until the patient is adequately rehydrated and should be used with caution in combination with zoledronic acid in order to avoid hypocalcemia
- If patients have a normal serum creatinine prior to treatment with zoledronic acid but have an increase of 0.5mg/dL within 2 weeks of their next dose, zoledronic acid should be withheld until the serum creatinine is at least within 10% of their baseline value
- If patients have an abnormal serum creatinine prior to treatment with zoledronic acid but have an increase of 1.0mg/dL within 2 weeks of their next dose, zoledronic acid should be withheld until the serum creatinine is at least within 10% of their baseline value

Efficacy

May be superior to pamidronate in the normalization of serum calcium, duration of complete response, and time to relapse, while demonstrating a similar safety profile: for patients with high serum calcium levels with cancer, zoledronic acid normalized calcium by day 10 in 90% of patients, compared with 70% with pamidronate.

Risks/Benefits

Risks:

- Single doses of zoledronic acid should not exceed 4mg and the duration of infusion should not be <15min (due to thr risk of serious renal deterioration)
- Standard hypercalcemia-related metabolic parameters, such as serum levels of calcium, phosphate, and magnesium, as well as serum creatinine, should be carefully monitored following initiation of therapy with zoledronic acid for injection

- In any patient requiring repeated administration of zoledronic acid for hypercalcemia of malignancy, serum creatinine must be evaluated prior to each dose
- Use caution in patients with aspirin-sensitive asthma
- Use caution when administering to nursing mothers

Benefits:
- May be superior to pamidronate in the normalization of serum calcium, duration of complete response, and time to relapse, while demonstrating a similar safety profile
- Treatment with zoledronic acid can be administered in an infusion of about 15min compared with a 2–4h infusion with pamidronate

Side-effects and adverse reactions
- Cardiovascular system: hypotension
- Central nervous system: fever, chills, insomnia, anxiety, confusion, agitation
- Eyes: conjunctivitis
- Gastrointestinal: nausea, vomiting, constipation, diarrhea, abdominal pain, anorexia
- Genitourinary: urinary tract infection
- Hematologic: anemia
- Metabolic: hypomagnesemia, hypophosphatemia, hypokalemia
- Musculoskeletal: bone pain and/or arthralgias, myalgia
- Respiratory: dyspnea, coughing
- Skin: swelling and redness at injection site, rash, pruritus
- Other: progression of cancer, moniliasis

Interactions (other drugs)

- Aminoglycosides - Loop diuretics

Contraindications

- Zoledronic acid for injection is contraindicated in patients with clinically significant hypersensitivity to zoledronic acid or other bisphosphonates, or any of the excipients in the formulation of zoledronic acid - Pregnancy category C - The safety and efficacy in pediatric patients have not been established

Acceptability to patient

First studies showed safe profile but one must be careful with renal function.

Follow up plan

Not yet known but likely to be similar to other bisphophonates.

Patient and caregiver information
- Need to be aware of signs and symptoms of hypercalcemia to watch for recurrence
- Need to be aware of signs and symptoms of renal function deterioration

CLODRONATE (ORAL)

Clodronate is not FDA-approved for use in the US except in trials.

Dose

Dosage should be decided by a specialist (1.6–3.2g/day by mouth in two divided doses have been used).

ALLOPURINOL
- Used as a treatment for hyperuricemia to prevent gout
- Allopurinol inhibits the conversion of hypoxanthine to uric acid

Dose
200–600mg/day orally, depending on severity – not to exceed 800mg/day.

Efficacy
Is effective for the prevention and treatment of hyperuricemia.

Risks/Benefits
Risks:
- Ensure adequate fluid intake during treatment
- Use caution in hepatic or renal impairment
- Treatment should be discontinued at first sign of allergic reaction, such as skin rash or other reaction
- There may be an acute attack of gout when first administered

Side-effects and adverse reactions
- Central nervous system: drowsiness, headache
- Gastrointestinal: nausea, abdominal pain, peptic ulceration, cholestatic jaundice, diarrhea, liver failure
- Genitourinary: renal failure
- Musculoskeletal: athralgia, myopathy
- Skin: rashes, alopecia, Stevens-Johnson syndrome

Interactions (other drugs)
- Angiotensin-converting enzyme (ACE) inhibitors
- Cyclophosphamide
- Mercaptopurine
- Antacids
- Azathioprine
- Oral anticoagulants
- Theophylline

Contraindications
Patients who have developed a severe reaction to allopurinol should not be restarted on the drug.

Acceptability to patient
Usually high.

Follow up plan
Usual follow up for myeloma, depending on progress of underlying disease.

EPOETIN ALFA
- Used to treat anemia
- Expensive

Dose
- Usual start dose 50–100U/kg three times weekly, subcutaneous or intravenous
- Dose may be increased or reduced according to response
- Maintenance dose at target hematocrit is usually 25U/kg three times weekly

Efficacy
Symptomatic anemia during the plateau phase is often benefited by the administration of erythropoietin.

Risks/Benefits
Risks:
- Risk of allergic reaction
- Risk of hypertensive reaction

- Use with caution in patients with known history of hematologic disorder
- Use with caution in patients with known history of seizure disorder
- Multidose preserved formulation contains benzyl alcohol which has been associated with an increased incidence of neurologic and other complications in premature infants, which are sometimes fatal

Benefits:
- Symptomatic improvement
- Reduces need for transfusion

Side-effects and adverse reactions
- Cardiovascular system: hypertension, tachycardia, edema
- Central nervous system: headache, seizures, fatigue
- Gastrointestinal: diarrhea, nausea, vomiting
- Metabolism: iron deficiency, hyperkalemia
- Musculoskeletal: arthralgia, myalgia
- Respiratory: shortness of breath
- Skin: stinging at injection site

Interactions (other drugs)
None known.

Contraindications
■ Uncontrolled hypertension ■ Hypersensititvity to albumin (human) ■ Hypersensitivity to mammalian-derived products or to human albumin

Acceptability to patient
Usually high.

Follow up plan
Monitoring of hematocrit is usually every 2 weeks during treatment.

THALIDOMIDE
- Considered by many to be the first new agent with major antimyeloma activity in >30 years
- How it works against multiple myeloma is unknown, although it suppresses angiogenesis in vitro and in animals
- Mechanism of action is probably multiple antiangiogenic activity, down-regulation of anti-TNF-alpha activity, immunomodulation, and changes in adhesion molecules
- It is still unclear whether thalidomide can change the natural history of myeloma or result in better outcomes than current best-available therapy
- This is an off-label indication

Dose
- In the trial, thalidomide was supplied in a 50mg capsule and was administered nightly at a dose of 200mg
- The dose was increased by 200mg every 2 weeks for 6 weeks so that the final dose was 800mg/day
- The duration of treatment ranged from 2–465 days (median 80 days)

Efficacy
An active agent against advanced, previously treated myeloma.

Risks/Benefits

Risks:

- Use caution in bradycardia
- Use caution in photosensitization

Side-effects and adverse reactions

- Central nervous system: dizziness, vertigo, headache, neuropathy, fatigue
- Gastrointestinal: nausea, vomiting, constipation, dry mouth
- Genitourinary: impotence
- Hematologic: leukopenia, anemia
- Metabolic: hypothyroidism
- Skin: rashes

Interactions (other drugs)

■ Alcohol ■ Barbiturates ■ Chlorpromazine ■ Reserpine ■ Drugs that interefere with oral contraceptives (HIV protease inhibitors, griseofulvin, rifampin, rifabutin, phenytoin, or carbamazepine)

Contraindications

■ Women of childbearing age ■ Pregnancy

Acceptability to patient

- Side-effects are not usually limiting
- Patients seem to tolerate well in trials

Follow up plan

Investigators recommend baseline and serial thyroid (thyroid-stimulating hormone) assessment during treatment with thalidomide. Thyroid replacement therapy can be used to improve thyroid deficiency.

Patient and caregiver information

Awareness of contraindication in pregnancy, although as the age group for myeloma does not usually overlap with that of pregnancy this is not really an issue.

DEXAMETHASONE OR METHYLPREDNISOLONE ALONE

Dose

- Dosage should be decided by a specialist
- Dexamethasone: variable, usually 4–9mg/day
- Methylprednisolone: 2g intravenously three times weekly for a minimum of 4 weeks

Efficacy

- Dexamethasone alone may decrease the M protein in approximately 40% of previously untreated patients and in 20–40% of patients who have not responded to primary treatment
- Methylprednisolone in a dosage of 2g intravenously 3 times weekly for a minimum of 4 weeks produced an objective response in 25% of patients refractory to alkylating agents

Risks/Benefits

Risks:

(Dexamethasone)

- Overwhelming septicemia if patient has an infection
- Loss of control of blood glucose in those with diabetes
- Use caution in renal disease, esophagitis, peptic ulcer, and ulcerative colitis
- Use caution in cerebral malaria, latent tuberculosis and AIDS

(Methylprednisolone)
- Overwhelming septicemia if patient has an infection
- Loss of blood glucose control in those with diabetes
- Use caution in elderly owing to risk of diabetes and osteoporosis
- Use caution in patients with psychosis, seizure disorders, or myasthenia gravis
- Use caution in congestive heart failure, hypertension
- Use caution in ulcerative colitis, peptic ulcer, or esophagitis
- Prolonged use causes adrenal suppression

Benefits: corticosteroids alone may be used in elderly patients and those who have impaired performance status. This is in contrast to the more usual treatment of steroids with melphalan

Side-effects and adverse reactions
Dexamethasone and methylprednisolone:
- Side-effects are minimized by short duration of therapy
- Cardiovascular system: hypertension, thromboembolism
- Central nervous system: insomnia, euphoria, depression, psychosis, headache
- Endocrine: adrenal suppression, impaired glucose tolerance, growth suppression in children
- Eyes, ears, nose, and throat: cataract, glaucoma, blurred vision
- Gastrointestinal: dyspepsia, peptic ulceration, esophagitis, oral candidiasis
- Musculoskeletal:: proximal myopathy, osteoporosis
- Skin: delayed healing, acne, striae

Interactions (other drugs)
Dexamethasone:
■ Aldesleukin ■ Aminoglutethimide ■ Antibiotics ■ Anticholinesterases ■ Anticoagulants ■ Antidiabetics ■ Antifungals ■ Barbiturates ■ Bismuth subsalicylate ■ Colestyramine ■ Colestipol ■ Diltiazem ■ Ephedrine ■ Estrogens ■ Formoterol ■ Imitanib mesylate ■ Insulin ■ Mifepristone ■ Nondepolarizing muscle relaxants ■ Phenytoin ■ Rifabutin ■ Oral contraceptives ■ Rifampin ■ Rifapentine ■ Salicylates ■ Troleandomycin ■ Verpamil ■ Xanthine derivatives

Methylprednisolone:
■ Aminoglutethamide ■ Antidiabetics ■ Barbiturates ■ Cholestyramine ■ Cyclosporine ■ Colestipol ■ Clarithromycin, erythromycin ■ Isoniazid ■ Ketoconazole ■ Troleandomycin ■ Oral contraceptives ■ Nonsteroidal anti-inflammatory drugs ■ Rifampin ■ Salicylates

Contraindications
Dexamethasone:
■ Lack of a definite diagnosis ■ Systemic infection ■ Avoid live virus vaccines in those receiving immunosuppressive doses

Methylprednisolone:
■ Systemic infection ■ Avoid live virus vaccines in those receiving immunosuppressive doses

Acceptability to patient
- Acceptable to most patients
- Occasionally sleeplessness, mania, and psychosis force immediate discontinuation

Follow up plan
As for the underlying disease, depending on clinical condition.

Radiation therapy

External beam radiotherapy is used to treat bony lesions.

RADIOTHERAPY

- Targeted external beam radiotherapy is used for localized bone pain and for pathologic fractures (where stabilization by pinning or traction is also essential for pain control as healing will not occur)
- Also used for cord compression, which is a radiotherapeutic emergency

Efficacy

Usually very effective treatment for pain due to lytic lesions or fracture.

Risks/Benefits

Risks:

- Radiation dose is high and cumulative, increasing risk of radiation-associated disease
- Risks depend on area irradiated: chest wall irradiation can cause radiation pneumonitis cardiomyopathy; pelvic irradiation may cause damage to pelvic structures including bladder and bowel; lumbar spine irradiation may cause chronic diarrhea

Benefit: effectively manages bone pain

Acceptability to patient

Patients often have a fear and dread of radiotherapy and may need reassurance.

Follow up plan

Review as appropriate to underlying disease.

Patient and caregiver information

Patients should be warned about the side-effects.

Chemotherapy

- The preferred initial treatment for overt, symptomatic multiple myeloma in patients >70 years or in younger patients in whom transplantation is not feasible
- Should be continued until the patient reaches a plateau state (consisting of a period of disease stability after chemotherapy lasting at least 4–6 months in which tumor progression does not occur)
- Conventional chemotherapy rarely results in complete remission but in different degrees of partial response
- Asymptomatic patients do not necessarily require treatment
- Standard treatment does not cure myeloma but aims to push the patient into a plateau phase – paraprotein levels fall until they reach a plateau that may last for weeks to years
- Duration of survival in patients who achieve disease stabilization is similar, irrespective of whether they fulfill the objective response criteria; patients who achieve a partial response should also be considered responders
- There is no evidence that continued chemotherapy is of benefit after the attainment of a plateau phase. In fact, continued chemotherapy may lead to a greater number of myeloma cells resistant to chemotherapy or to the development of myelodysplasia or acute leukemia

MELPHALAN

- Alkylating agent
- Given with prednisone, this is standard chemotherapy for multiple myeloma – prednisone suppresses cell growth. Produces response in 50–60% of cases
- Melphalan is usually administered for 6–9 months as an outpatient, with treatment continued if a response is ongoing

- Treatment with melphalan is usually stopped when the M protein (paraprotein) concentration decreases to a stable value called the plateau phase

Efficacy
- Not curative
- Aim is to bring down paraprotein levels and reduce symptoms until a plateau phase is reached when measured paraprotein levels have stopped falling
- Melphalan and prednisone have constituted standard therapy for patients with multiple myeloma for 25 years
- Overall response rate is 50–60%, and the median duration of survival ranges from 2–3 years
- Have been shown to be as effective as more intense regimens including VAD and vincristine, carmustine (BCNU), melphalan, cyclophosphamide, and prednisone (VBMCP), with less toxicity

Risks/Benefits

Risks:
- Myelosuppression is the dose-limiting toxic effect of melphalan
- Prednisone – usual hazards of high-dose long-term steroids
- Because of variability in the absorption of melphalan, this drug must be given while the patient is fasting, and the dose should be adjusted until midcycle cytopenia occurs

Acceptability to patient
- Acceptable if symptoms improve
- Side-effects, including nausea and vomiting, may be troublesome

Follow up plan
- Leukocyte and platelet counts must be determined at 3-week intervals, and the melphalan and prednisone regimen is repeated every 6 weeks
- Complete blood count and platelet check every 6 weeks thereafter

Patient and caregiver information

Need to attend for follow up blood tests.

ALPHA-INTERFERON
- The role of interferon alpha-2 (IFN alpha-2) maintenance on response duration and survival in patients responding to chemotherapy is still controversial
- Does not appear to prolong survival but may extend plateau phase
- Given with melphalan

Efficacy
- Five studies have shown a significant benefit from IFN alpha-2 maintenance with a gain in response duration ranging from 5–12 months
- Other trials have not shown a longer duration of response in patients maintained with IFN alpha-2
- A large meta-analysis, based on the data of each patient included in all the IFN alpha-2 maintenance trials by the Myeloma Trialists' Collaborative Group in Oxford, is being carried out
- The use of interferon as a single agent for refractory patients has been disappointing; response rates have ranged from 10–20%

Risks/Benefits

Risk: interferon is sometimes poorly tolerated, causing severe flu-like symptoms.

Acceptability to patient

May be difficult due to nausea, vomiting, and flu-like symptoms. It varies from patient to patient.

Follow up plan

Every 3 weeks, as with melphalan.

Patient and caregiver information

- Patient needs to attend for blood tests
- Attention to fever during chemotherapy; it may be a sign of neutropenia

VINCRISTINE, DOXORUBICIN, AND DEXAMETHASONE

- Patients with multiple myeloma who either fail to respond or who become refractory to the initial alkylating therapy have a low response rate to subsequent chemotherapy and a short survival
- Vincristine and doxorubicin are administered simultaneously and continuously as an infusion for 4 days. Dexamethasone is taken in tablet form for 4 days, which may be repeated twice, with 4-day rest intervals. VAD is repeated approx. every 28 days
- The antibiotic bactrim is taken during the VAD program to protect against a lung infection called *Pneumocystis carinii pneumonia*, which may occur in patients being treated with chemotherapy and corticosteroids. Additionally, ranitidine is taken to protect the stomach from ulceration
- VAD may be used in patients with acute renal insufficiency

Efficacy

Most effective in patients resistant to standard chemotherapy – second-line approach in these patients.

Risks/Benefits

Risk: the major shortcomings of VAD are that vincristine and doxorubicin are given by a central venous catheter; significant steroid toxicity is manifested by infection, myopathy, and gastrointestinal bleeding

Acceptability to patient

Side-effects of chemotherapy may be severe.

Follow up plan

- Regular blood counts during and before therapy are essential
- Follow up is determined by patient response and clinical condition

Patient and caregiver information

Need to be aware of need to call doctor if persistent fever or other severe symptoms develop – may indicate chemotherapy-induced neutropenia and require hospital admission.

HIGH-DOSE CHEMOTHERAPY: VMCP/VBAP

The usual protocol consists of vincristine, melphalan, cyclophosphamide, and prednisone (VMCP), or vincristine/BCNU/doxorubicin/prednisone (VBAP).

Efficacy

This produces an objective response in approx. 70% of patients, but the median duration of survival is not significantly different from that obtained with melphalan and prednisone.

Risks/Benefits

- Risk: less well tolerated than melphalan and prednisone, with increased toxicity
- Benefit: clear benefit in younger patients

Acceptability to patient

- More difficult for patient than melphalan and prednisone
- Patient may present with nausea, vomiting, alopecia, neutropenia
- Patients with heart disease need to be carefully followed because adriamycin is cardiotoxic

Follow up plan

- Regular blood counts during and before therapy are essential
- Follow up is determined by patient response and clinical condition

Patient and caregiver information

Patient should be aware of need to call doctor if persistent fever or other severe symptoms develop – may indicate chemotherapy-induced neutropenia and require admission.

HIGH-DOSE CHEMOTHERAPY

Involves treatment with vincristine, melphalan, cyclophosphamide, prednisone/vincristine, BCNU, doxorubicin, and prednisone. In a large study, treatment with VBMCP/VBAP produced significantly more objective responses than melphalan and a survival advantage.

Efficacy

Patients with good-risk prognostic variables (lower tumor load, younger, less severe symptoms) seemed to fare better when treated with melphalan and prednisone, whereas those with poor prognostic factors did better with combination chemotherapy.

Risks/Benefits

Risk: increased toxicity of regimen set against questionable benefit

Acceptability to patient

Difficult and complex chemotherapy with high rate of side-effects.

Follow up plan

- Regular review with frequent blood tests as determined by clinical status
- Patients chosen for this therapy will be more unwell and will require review at least three times weekly if not as inpatients

Other therapies

PLASMAPHERESIS

- Palliative treatment
- Hyperviscosity is characterized by oronasal bleeding, blurred vision, neurologic symptoms, and congestive heart failure
- Serum viscosity levels do not correlate well with the symptoms or the clinical findings
- Plasmapheresis promptly relieves the symptoms and should be done regardless of the viscosity level when the patient is symptomatic

Efficacy

Very effective.

Risks/Benefits

Risks:

- Invasive and time-consuming
- High risk of line infection

Acceptability to patient

- Patients often dislike this treatment as it is time-consuming
- Intravenous therapy may not be well tolerated

Follow up plan

Plasma viscosity review required every 3–6 weeks.

CHEMOTHERAPY WITH STEM CELL RESCUE

- High-dose therapy (HDT) followed by marrow or peripheral blood stem cell rescue is an alternative approach for patients with multiple myeloma
- If the patient is <65 years (some state 70 years), the physician should discuss the possibility of autologous peripheral blood stem cell transplantation. Ideally, this should be done as part of a prospective study
- Granulocyte colony-stimulating factor (G-CSF) is given to the stem cell donor to stimulate production and release of stem cells into the peripheral blood. Cells are then collected by apheresis for 2–4h for 2–3 days, frozen, and stored
- HDT is then administered and stem cells are infused within 1–2 days
- During the engraftment process, the infused stem cells find their way to the bone marrow where they begin to develop into new blood cells, red blood cells, white blood cells, and platelets. Engraftment usually takes about 2–4 weeks

Treatment 1:

- The patient is initially treated with VAD or a similar program for 3–4 months in order to reduce the number of tumor cells in the bone marrow and peripheral blood
- The patient then is given high-dose cyclophosphamide followed by G-CSF and peripheral stem cells are then collected
- One can proceed with a transplant in which the patient is given high-dose melphalan and total-body radiation followed by infusion of the peripheral blood stem cells

Treatment 2:

- Treat the patient with alkylating agents until reaching a plateau state and then maintain the patient with IFN alpha-2 or no therapy until early relapse
- When patient relapses, treat with high-dose melphalan and total-body radiation, and the previously collected peripheral blood stem cells are infused

Efficacy

- Not curative as patients own peripheral stem cells, but 20–30% response rate seen
- Stem cells transplanted after HDT replace the stem cells destroyed by HDT and make it possible for normal production of blood cells to begin again
- Myeloablative therapy is currently not recommended for patients who have resistant relapse because of the high toxicity related to the procedure and the short duration of response in responding patients
- Patients with stable disease after initial chemotherapy or even those with primary refractory disease appear to benefit from early myeloablative therapy followed by autotransplantation
- Although the complete remission rate is higher with intensive therapy, the median duration of response is relatively short and usually ranges from 18–36 months, with no plateau

Risks/Benefits

Risks:

- Procedure mortality (2–3%)
- Myeloablative therapy is currently not recommended for patients who have resistant relapse, because of both a high toxicity related to the procedure and a short duration of response in responding patients
- Transplant-related mortality (<2%)
- There are two major limitations – eradication of the malignant clone and the removal of myeloma cells and their precursors from the bone marrow or peripheral blood

Acceptability to patient

Variable.

Follow up plan
- Intensive monitoring during treatment
- Follow up of M protein levels for recurrence as for all plateau phase myeloma if plateau is achieved

ALLOGENEIC BONE MARROW TRANSPLANTATION
- A donor, such as a brother or sister, provides the stem cells for transplantation to a recipient
- Allogeneic transplants are more complex than autologous transplants, because a donor must be found who genetically closely matches the recipient to avoid graft-versus-host disease
- Should be considered in younger patients because mortality is high in patients >55 years, so few patients with myeloma will qualify
- Patient must be fit
- Stem cells transplanted after HDT replace the stem cells destroyed by HDT and make it possible for normal production of blood cells to begin again

Method:
- G-CSF is given to the stem cell donor to stimulate production and release of stem cells into the peripheral blood. They are collected by apheresis for 2–4h for 2–3 days, frozen, and stored
- When enough stem cells have been collected and stored, high-dose chemotherapy is administered. The stem cells are infused within 1–2 days
- During the engraftment process, the infused stem cells find their way to the bone marrow where they begin to develop into new blood cells, red blood cells, white blood cells, and platelets. Engraftment usually takes about 2–4 weeks

Efficacy
- Allogenic transplant has been performed for multiple myeloma for many years
- The proportion of patients who might be cured ranges from 10–20%
- Transplant-related mortality is 15–40%
- Results could be improved if the transplantation is performed earlier in the course of the disease and if the two main problems (transplant-related mortality and relapse) could be improved
- One approach to decrease the transplant-related mortality could be the use of peripheral stem cell allografts to speed engraftment
- Transplantation with allogeneic bone marrow has improved significantly during the last 5 years due to a significant improvement in survival, which was the result of a reduction in transplant-related mortality. Overall 4-year survival from transplant with autotransplantation was 46%, and with allotransplantation 31%

Risks/Benefits
Risks:
- High transplant-related mortality ranging from 15–40%, mainly due to bacterial and fungal infections, interstitial pneumonitis, and graft-versus-host disease
- Although the complete remission rate after allogeneic BMT is at least 40%, most patients have relapse, and in the series with the longest follow up there is no survival plateau

Benefits:
- The graft does not contain tumor cells that can subsequently lead to relapse
- Prospect of complete cure, which is prime treatment aim
- Can have a graft-versus-myeloma effect

Acceptability to patient
Often acceptable if there is prospect of cure but risks are high.

Follow up plan

Patient will be asked to attend closely to have blood tests performed and to adjust medication dosage.

Patient and caregiver information

- Patient and caregiver need to be aware of risk level
- Treatment of complications may be long and difficult

IMMUNOTHERAPY

- Experimental treatment in trial phase
- Current approaches in immunotherapy include: specific cells of the immune system, cytokines, and vaccines
- Results of early studies in patients with multiple myeloma provide information about the safety of certain immunotherapies. Additionally, the results may indicate the dosages required to achieve a response and give indications of which patients may benefit most from a particular immunotherapy. Currently, vaccines are being evaluated post-transplant and in early-stage multiple myeloma. Each additional study provides more answers

Efficacy

- Complete remission has been achieved in some patients receiving allogeneic stem cell transplantation and donor lymphocyte infusion. This is due to a graft-versus-myeloma response, which means that T cell lymphocytes in the donor lymphocyte infusion attack and destroy the myeloma tumor cells in the patient
- Interleukin (IL)-2 is a cytokine that is normally produced by a specific group of T cells and is involved in the induction of virtually every immune response in which T cells play a role. The role of IL-2 in controlling multiple myeloma and keeping it in a stable phase is being evaluated in a pilot study
- Idiotypic vaccine contains the idiotypic protein of the patient's monoclonal immunoglobulin, which induces a cytotoxic T cell response that in conjunction with other substances maximize the immune response. A series of immunizations are required to maintain this response and are typically given when the patient is in remission and minimal residual disease exists
- Gene-modified plasma cell vaccine uses a virus as a vehicle to carry specific genes into the patient's plasma cells
- DNA vaccines contain a fragment of the cancer cell DNA. The purpose of the DNA vaccine is to activate immunity against these tumor-specific antigens
- Preliminary results of these initial investigations are promising

LIFESTYLE

- Patients should be encouraged to be as active as possible because prolonged bedrest contributes to osteopenia and hypercalcemia
- Low-protein, high-calorie, and high-carbohydrate diet with good fluid intake to avoid dehydration is beneficial for hypercalcemia and renal failure
- Reduction in renal function occurs in one-quarter of patients initially and may develop insidiously or acutely. Maintenance of a high urine output (3L/day) is important for preventing renal failure in patients with Bence Jones proteinuria
- If creatinine clearance falls and edema develops, fluid restriction will be necessary

RISKS/BENEFITS

Risk: it may be difficult for patients to balance the advice to drink plenty (in order to avoid hypercalcemia) with concern regarding swelling due to renal failure

ACCEPTABILITY TO PATIENT

Usually not difficult if patient wants to comply.

FOLLOW UP PLAN

Regular review with PCP – every 3 months would be appropriate for asymptomatic patients, with open access if problems arise.

PATIENT AND CAREGIVER INFORMATION

The patient and caregiver need to understand that if significant edema develops, the patient should not stop drinking completely. The PCP should be contacted so the patient can be evaluated for a possible change in management.

Advice to the patient on dealing with fatigue:

- Have your hemoglobin checked regularly
- Eat a well-balanced diet with frequent, small meals
- Drink lots of water during the day
- Include short periods of rest and relaxation – take naps every day
- Start an exercise program (start slowly). Exercise can relieve fatigue
- Try to keep a regular daily routine that is reasonable
- Avoid caffeine in the evening
- Delegate chores and ask for help from others
- Try to avoid stresses in your life
- Join support groups and share your feelings
- Find activities/hobbies that are physically less demanding, such as reading
- Most importantly, let your doctors and nurses know that you feel fatigued. Don't hide it and don't accept it

OUTCOMES

EFFICACY OF THERAPIES

- Average survival times vary
- Median survival given variously as 24–40 months
- Significant numbers survive for much longer

Efficacy of cure:
- Only bone marrow transplant offers chance of total cure but with few suitable patients and high treatment mortality, with a 4- to 10-year survival of 3–6%
- Myeloma is generally not considered to be a curable disease
- Allogeneic or autologous peripheral blood or bone marrow stem cell rescue permits the use of high-dose chemotherapy (HDCT) and total-body irradiation. This approach produces greater tumor kill and longer remissions, but it is doubtful that it will cure many patients

Efficacy of palliation:
- Chemotherapy is not curative
- Radiotherapy is effective for localized bone pain
- Chronic bisphosphonate therapy may reduce bone pain and skeletal events
- Alpha-interferon may prolong the plateau phase
- Melphalan has a high success rate in achieving a plateau, which may last weeks to several years; 40–60% respond
- VAD (vincristine, duxorubicin, dexamethasone) is used for nonresponders
- HDCT with autologous stem cell transplantation improves response rate, event-free survival, and overall survival, with complete response in 20–30%: best in patients <50 years with beta2-microglobulin levels <-2.5mg/L
- Dexamethasone alone may be of benefit in those unable to tolerate other therapies
- Pamidronate reduces hypercalcemia successfully over 2–5 days
- Other treatments are symptomatic (including transfusion, erythropoeitin, rehydration, and plasmapheresis) and are titrated against effect

Review period

Dependent on disease stage, ongoing treatment, and patient's clinical state.

Solitary osseous plasmacytoma:
- Assess immunoglobulins and M proteins after treatment
- Annual bone survey
- Bone marrow biopsy as clinically indicated
- Paraprotein measurement every 3 months

Extraosseous solitary plasmacytoma:
- Paraprotein measurement every 3 months for four cycles then every 12 months
- Computed tomography or magnetic resonance imaging every 6 months for two cycles then as clinically indicated

Systemic stage II or III myeloma:
- Measure quantitative immunoglobulins and M protein with alternate cycles of therapy and every 3 months thereafter
- Complete blood count (CBC), differential, platelets, blood urea nitrogen (BUN), creatinine, calcium
- Bone survey annually or for symptoms
- Bone marrow biopsy as clinically indicated

PROGNOSIS

- For about 5% of patients at diagnosis, myeloma is static and may not progress for months or years. These patients usually have lower tumor burden (stage I disease) and are not troubled by the anemia, bone disease, renal failure, and frequent infections that characterize active multiple myeloma. This is referred to as 'smoldering myeloma' and can last some years before progression to active disease
- Autotransplantation improves survival and quality of life by slowing the rate of progression
- Response to drug treatment is usually good – most patients will enter a plateau phase during which they will be symptom-free
- Median survival on standard treatment is 24–40 months: 10-year survival in 3%, 5-year survival in 27%
- At stage I, 5-year survival in 25–40%
- At stage II, 5-year survival in 15–30%
- At stage III, 5-year survival in 10–25%

Factors reflecting the inherent proliferative capacity of the malignant clone:
- Labeling index
- Serum thymidine kinase
- Multidrug resistance phenotype
- Plasma cell morphology of the malignant clone

Factors reflecting tumor bulk:
- Beta-2-microglobulin
- Stage of disease

Factors affecting renal function:
- Creatinine
- Beta-2-microglobulin

Factors reflecting host-tumor interaction:
- C reactive protein
- Interleukin (IL)-6 and soluble IL-6 receptor level
- CD38-positive cells
- IL-2 levels

Clinical pearls

- Both clinically and biologically, the plateau phase is near the quiescent state observed in smoldering multiple myeloma or monoclonal gammopathy of undetermined significance (MGUS). However, the residual malignant cells lead to relapse in virtually all cases, whereas multiple myeloma or related disorders develop in only one-fourth of patients with MGUS
- In a patient with myeloma, if there is doubt about whether to begin chemotherapy, the most reasonable approach is to re-evaluate the patient in 2 months and to delay therapy until progressive disease is evident
- If a patient relapses, chemotherapy must be reinstituted. Most patients will respond to reinstitution of the initial chemotherapeutic regimen, but the duration and quality of response are usually inferior to those of the initial response

Therapeutic failure

- Relapse is associated with poorer response to chemotherapy
- Most patients will respond to reinstitution of the initial chemotherapeutic regimen, but the duration and quality of response are usually inferior to initial response
- Second-line chemotherapy (VAD) may be used in cases of nonresponse to melphalan

Recurrence

- Chemotherapy must be reinstituted when relapse occurs
- VBAP (vincristine, duxorubicin, prednisone) or VBAD given every 3–4 weeks produces an overall response in about one-third of patients and has a low toxicity
- High-dose dexamethasone can be tried for resistant or relapsing disease, or for patients unable to tolerate other therapies
- If the patient had pancytopenia or prefers not to take VAD, methylprednisolone is an alternative. Methylprednisolone in a dosage of 2g intravenously three times weekly for a minimum of 4 weeks produced an objective response in 25% of patients refractory to alkylating agents
- Cyclophosphamide 600mg/m^2/day intravenously for 4 days (days 1–4), plus prednisone 50mg orally twice daily for the same 4-day period followed by granulocyte colony-stimulating factor (G-CSF) has been a beneficial treatment in refractory patients with advanced disease
- In patients resistant to a rescue regimen with VAD or VBAD as well as those in whom these treatments are not feasible (poor performance status, severe pancytopenia, cardiac disorders), a conservative approach with alternate-day prednisone (50–100mg) and cyclophosphamide (150–300mg/m^2) orally weekly or along with pulse dose cyclophosphamide (800–1200mg intravenously) every 2–3 weeks. This approach is a palliative treatment that can temporarily control the disease with a very low toxicity
- Intravenously administered gamma-globulin may be helpful for patients with recurrent infections, but it is very expensive

Deterioration

- Second-line chemotherapy (VAD) may be used in case of nonresponse to melphalan
- Bone marrow transplantation (BMT) may be considered when primary treatment has failed
- Prompt and appropriate therapy for bacterial infections is essential
- Prophylactic daily penicillin (orally) often benefits patients with recurrent streptococcal pneumonia infections
- Pneumococcal and influenza vaccine should be given to all patients despite their suboptimal antibody response
- Intravenously administered gamma-globulin may be helpful for patients with recurrent infections, but it is very expensive

Terminal illness

Palliative care:

- Bone pain – it is partially opiate-responsive; fentanyl is excreted hepatically and does not accumulate where renal failure may cause toxicity with other opiates; nonsteroidal anti-inflammatory drugs (NSAIDs) are often helpful if the patient can tolerate them. Cover with proton pump inhibitor or misoprostol may be advisable. Beware of NSAIDs if the patient is also on steroids
- Erythropoeitin and transfusion for anemia, thrombocytopenia
- Plasmapheresis for hyperviscosity
- Bisphosphonates and intravenous fluids for hypercalcemia
- Dexamethasone 2–8mg may be helpful for appetite and general wellbeing
- Careful fluid monitoring for renal failure
- Anxiolytics/antidepressants for depression
- Terminal care is often difficult in myeloma as patients often have both generalized pains and confusion. Addition of small quantities of sedative, and delivery of medication by transdermal patch (fentanyl) and syringe driver (sedatives) may be helpful

- Nausea may be treated with haloperidol or methotrimeprazine, either of which may be sedative
- Small doses of steroids (dexamethasone 2mg daily) occasionally improve appetite and well-being
- 24h nursing care is often necessary in the final stages
- Most common causes of death are sepsis, hypercalcemia, hemorrhage, and renal failure

COMPLICATIONS

- Amyloidosis (about 15% have generalized amyloidosis at autopsy)
- Cord compression
- Stroke due to hyperviscosity
- Heart failure due to amyloid deposition
- Plasma cell leukemia
- Pathologic fracture
- Depression
- Renal failure: about 50% will develop kidney disease
- Hemodialysis is necessary in patients with symptomatic azotemia
- In one series, 6/20 patients with nonreversible renal failure who were undergoing chronic hemodialysis survived >3 years
- Plasmapheresis may be helpful in acute renal failure, but patients with severe myeloma cast formation or other irreversible changes are unlikely to benefit
- Severe renal failure is usually irreversible. Renal transplantation for myeloma kidney has been followed by prolonged survival
- Solitary plasmacytoma of bone

Plasma cell leukemia:

- May occur as a leukemic transformation of multiple myeloma
- Defined as the presence of >20% plasma cells in the peripheral blood and an absolute plasma cell count of $>2x10^9$/L. It is classified as primary when it presents de novo (60% of cases) and as secondary when it is a leukemic transformation of a previously recognized multiple myeloma (40%)
- Patients with plasma cell leukemia have more cytogenic abnormalities and higher levels of serum IL-6 than do patients with classic multiple myeloma
- Treatment of primary plasma cell leukemia is unsatisfactory and the duration of response is short
- Secondary plasma cell leukemia, which constitutes the terminal event in 1–2% of patients with myeloma, rarely responds to treatment

CONSIDER CONSULT

- Refer back to hospital if signs of renal failure develop: anorexia, nausea, vomiting, thirst, diarrhea, malaise, tiredness, fluid retention, dyspnea
- Urgent plasmapheresis is sometimes instituted for impending renal damage, and may alleviate symptoms and delay progression
- Refer for intravenous pamidronate if hypercalcemia develops or is suspected
- Refer if hospital inpatient care is needed to palliate symptoms
- Refer back for new areas of bone pain
- Refer back for refractory anemia
- Refer back if symptom control measures are failing

PREVENTION

No preventive measures can be taken as etiology is unknown.

SCREENING

- Not appropriate as the disease may have a long natural history or latent phase, and there is no evidence that early detection would improve outcome as treatment is in any case delayed until symptoms develop
- Nevertheless, patients with monoclonal gammopathy of unknown significance and other nonmyeloma gammopathy should be kept under regular review

PREVENT RECURRENCE

Currently no treatment successfully prevents relapse, although allogeneic bone marrow transplantation can sometimes offer cure.

ASSOCIATIONS

NCI Publication – What You Need To Know About Multiple Myeloma
Summary: This National Cancer Institute (NCI) booklet describes symptoms, diagnosis, and treatment of this type of cancer. http://www.cancer.gov/cancer_information/

American Cancer Society Inc
1599 Clifton Road NE
Atlanta, GA 30329
Tel: (800) ACS-2345
www.cancer.org

AMC Cancer Research Center
1600 Pierce Street
Denver, CO 80214
Tel: (303) 233-6501
Fax: (800) 321-1557
www.amc.org

Cancer Information Service
Tel: (800) 4-CANCER ((800) 422-6237)
http://cis.nci.nih.gov
This site also has information on ongoing trials at http://www.cancer.gov/clinical_trials/

Committee for Standards in Haematology has published UK guidelines on diagnosis and treatment on their website at www.ukmf.org.uk/guidelines.shtml

The Multiple Myeloma Research Foundation
3 Forest Street
New Canaan, CT 06840
Tel: (203) 972-1250
E-mail: themmrf@themmrf.org
Up-to-date information for patients and professionals, evidence, and ongoing research and trials
www.multiplemyeloma.org

KEY REFERENCES

- Attal M, Harousseau JL, Stoppa AM, et al. A prospective, randomized trial of autologous bone marrow transplantation and chemotherapy in multiple myeloma. Intergroupe Francais du Myeloma. N Engl J Med 1996;335:91
- Browman GP, Bergsagel D, Sicheri D, et al. Randomized trial of interferon maintenance in multiple myeloma: a study of the National Cancer Institute of Canada Clinical Trials Group. J Clin Oncol 1995;13:2354
- Boccadoro M, Marmont F, Tribalto M, et al. Multiple myeloma: VMCP/VBAP alternating combination chemotherapy is not superior to melphalan and prednisone even in high-risk patients. J Clin Oncol 1991;9:444
- Blade J, San Miguel JF, Alcala A, et al. Alternating combination VCMP/VBAP chemotherapy versus melphalan/prednisone in the treatment of multiple myeloma: a randomized multicentric study of 487 patients. J Clin Oncol 1993;11:1165
- Bloomfield DJ. Should bisphosphonates be part of the standard therapy of patients with multiple myeloma or bone metastases from other cancers? An evidence based review. J Clin Oncol 1998;16:1218–25
- Berenson JR, Lichtenstein A, Porter L, et al. Long-term pamidronate treatment of advanced multiple myeloma patients reduces skeletal events. J Clin Oncol 1998;16:593–602. Myeloma Aredia Study Group
- Garton JP, Gertz MA, Witzig TE, et al. Epoetin alfa for the treatment of the anemia of multiple myeloma. A prospective, randomized, placebo-controlled, double-blind trial. Arch Intern Med 1995;155:2069
- Singhal S, Mehta J, Desikan R, et al. Antitumor activity of thalidomide in refractory multiple myeloma. N Engl J Med 1999;341:1565–71

- Berenson JR, Lichtenstein A, Porter L, et al. Long-term pamidronate treatment of advanced multiple myeloma patients reduces skeletal events. J Clin Oncol 1998;16:593–602
- Myeloma Trialists' Collaborative Group. Combination chemotherapy versus melphalan plus prednisone as treatment for multiple myeloma: an overview of 6,633 patients from 27 randomized trials. J Clinical Oncol 1998:16:3832–42
- Pavlovsky S, Corrado C, Santarelli MT, et al. An update of two randomized trials in previously untreated multiple myeloma comparing melphalan and prednisone versus three- and five-drug combinations: an Argentine Group for the Treatment of Acute Leukemia study. J Clin Oncol 1988;6:769–75
- Blade J, San Miguel JF, Alcala A, et al. Alternating combination VCMP/VBAP chemotherapy versus melphalan/prednisone in the treatment of multiple myeloma: a randomized multicentric study of 487 patients. J Clin Oncol 1993;11:1165–71
- Oken MM, Harrington DP, Abramson N, et al. Comparison of melphalan and prednisone with vincristine, carmustine, melphalan, cyclophosphamide, and prednisone in the treatment of multiple myeloma: results of Eastern Cooperative Oncology Group Study E2479. Cancer 1997;79:1561–7
- Gertz MA, Lacy MQ, Lust JA, et al. Prospective randomized trial of melphalan and prednisone versus vincristine, carmustine, melphalan, cyclophosphamide, and prednisone in the treatment of primary systemic amyloidosis. J Clin Oncol 1999;17:262–7

FAQS

Question 1

Which are the minimal criteria for the diagnosis of multiple myeloma?

ANSWER 1

Bone marrow with >10% plasma cells or plasmacytoma plus one of the following:

- Monoclonal protein in serum (usually >3g/dL)
- Monoclonal protein in urine
- Lytic bone lesions

The patient must have the usual clinical features of multiple myeloma. Connective tissue disorders, metastatic carcinoma, lymphoma, leukemia, and chronic infections must be excluded.

Question 2

Which tests can the primary care physician (PCP) order to investigate differential diagnosis of multiple myeloma?

ANSWER 2

- Complete blood count and differential; peripheral blood smear
- Chemistry screen (including calcium and creatinine determinations)
- Serum protein electrophoresis, immunofixation, quantitation of immunoglobulins
- Serum viscosity if IgG value >6g/dL, IgA value >5g/dL, or symptoms of hyperviscosity are present
- Routine urinalysis, 24-h urine collection for electrophoresis and immunofixation
- Skeletal X-ray
- Beta-2-microglobulin, C-reactive protein, and lactate dehydrogenase determinations

Question 3

What is the impact of using bisphosphonates in a patient with multiple myeloma?

ANSWER 3

- The use of bisphosphonates significantly reduces pathologic fractures, bone pain, spinal cord compression, and the need for bone irradiation
- This was shown in a randomized, double-blind study in which patients with stage III myeloma received monthly intravenous pamidronate

Question 4

Is there any difference in the efficacy of the various schemes of chemotherapy concerning survival?

ANSWER 4

- A meta-analysis of studies comparing melphalan plus prednisone with drug combinations concluded that both forms of treatment were equally effective
- Randomized trials comparing combinations of alkylating agents and prednisone, given simultaneously or alternately, have not proven to be superior to therapy with melphalan and prednisone

CONTRIBUTORS

Russell C Jones, MD, MPH
Luciana G O Clark, MD
Sandeep Garg, MD

MYELOFIBROSIS

SUMMARY INFORMATION

DESCRIPTION

- A myeloproliferative clonal disorder of a multipotent hematopoietic progenitor cell associated with abnormal deposition of fibrotic material (usually collagen) in the bone marrow
- Characterized by abnormal growth of hematopoietic elements, the presence of bone marrow fibrosis, and myeloid metaplasia
- 90% are primary (idiopathic) and 10% are secondary as a consequence of another myeloproliferative disease
- Average life-span from diagnosis is 5–7 years

URGENT ACTION

May be required in cases of massive splenomegaly in which rupture could lead to severe complications.

ICD9 CODE

289.8 Myelofibrosis.

SYNONYMS

- Primary myelofibrosis
- Idiopathic myelofibrosis
- Agnogenic myeloid myelofibrosis
- Agnogenic myeloid metaplasia
- Myelofibrosis and myeloid metaplasia
- Osteosclerosis
- Myelosclerosis
- Myelofibrosis-osteosclerosis

CARDINAL FEATURES

- One-third of patients are asymptomatic at diagnosis
- 40% have constitutional symptoms including fever, weight loss, night sweats, pruritus, and bone pain
- Splenomegaly is present in 85–100% of cases and is massive in 10% of patients
- There is fibrosis of the bone marrow
- There may be severe, normochromic, normocytic anemia
- Philadelphia chromosome is absent
- There is BCL-ABL rearrangement in peripheral blood cells
- Megakaryocytes are often increased and there may be leukocytosis with a leftward shift
- Polychromasia, anisocytosis, and poikilocytosis may be present
- Nucleated red blood cells and circulating immature myeloid cells may be present in peripheral blood film

CAUSES

Common causes

- Stimulatory factors (signal) in idiopathic myelofibrosis include platelet-derived growth factor (PDGF), fibroblast growth factor (FGF)-beta, transforming growth factor (TGF)-beta, platelet factor-4, interleukin (IL)-1, calmodulin, beta-thromboglobulin
- Clonal cells affected include megakaryocytes and platelets
- PDGF has little effect on collagen synthesis while TGF-beta is pivotal as it is a potent inducer of collagen synthesis
- Monocytes-macrophages produce TGF-beta and IL-1 with their role being deduced from animal model of osteomyelosclerosis
- Radiation exposure: high incidence in survivors of atomic bombs
- Exposure to benzene compounds
- A clonal stem cell disorder due to multiple chromosomal abnormalities (13q-, 20q-, partial trisomy 1q, trisomy 8, and 12p-), most of which are associated with a poor prognosis
- Secondary myelofibrosis includes 50% of patients having polycythemia vera
- Other causes of secondary myelofibrosis include essential thrombocythemia, myeloproliferative disorders, and myelodysplastic syndrome

Contributory or predisposing factors

- History of cancer
- History of radiation exposure
- Essential thrombocythemia
- Granulomatous disease
- Autoimmune illnesses

- Hodgkin's disease
- Metastatic tumors
- Acute lymphoblastic leukemia
- Renal osteodystrophy
- Rickets

EPIDEMIOLOGY

Incidence and prevalence

INCIDENCE

- Only 0.01 cases per 1000 persons diagnosed annually
- Incidence 0.73/100,000 (males) and 0.40/100,000 (female)
- 1600 new cases/year in the US

Demographics

AGE

- Most commonly affects persons in sixth to eighth decade of life
- Median age at diagnosis: 54–62 years
- 20% of patients are younger than 55 years
- 70% of patients older than 60 years

GENDER

Females reportedly outnumber males 2:1.

GENETICS

- May be associated with mutations in ras oncogenes in stem cells
- Other abnormalities include C group chromosome duplications and deletions at loci 20q and 13q. Chromosomal abnormalities are associated with a poor prognosis

DIFFERENTIAL DIAGNOSIS

Polycythemia vera

Polycythemia vera is a primary myeloproliferative syndrome involving a pluripotent stem cell.

FEATURES

- Erthrocytosis with hypervolemia
- Varying degrees of thrombosis, leukocytosis, and splenomegaly
- Headache
- Weakness
- Itching
- Palpable liver
- Plethora

Acute myelofibrosis

Acute myelofibrosis is a much more acute severe syndrome than agnogenic myeloid metaplasia (represents a form of acute leukemia and treated as such).

FEATURES

- Fever, wasting, infection
- Absence of splenomegaly
- Cytopenias
- The red blood cell morphology characteristic of myelofibrosis is absent
- Increase in myloblasts in marrow and peripheral blood
- Marrow fibrosis

Essential thrombocythemia

Essential thrombocythemia is a persistent thrombocytosis for which no cause can be determined.

FEATURES

- Clumps of platelets with peripheral blood smear
- Transient cerebral ischemia
- Weakness
- Headache
- Parethesias
- Dizziness
- Visual disturbances
- Finger and toe thrombosis, which may require amputation
- Deep vein thrombosis
- Priapism
- Bone marrow findings of megakaryocyte hyperplasia
- Hepatomegaly and splenomegaly are not necessarily pronounced

Tuberculosis

Tuberculosis is an infection of the lungs caused by *Mycobacterium tuberculosis.*

FEATURES

- Fever
- Night sweats
- Cough
- Hemoptysis
- Scanty nonpurulent sputum
- Weight loss
- Pleuritic chest pain

Chronic myelogenous leukemia

Chronic myelogenous leukemia is a myeloproliferative disorder characterized by increased proliferation of granulocytes.

FEATURES

- Splenomegaly, hepatomegaly, left upper quadrant abdominal pain
- Leukocytosis
- Anemia
- Thrombocytosis or thrombocytopenia (later in the course of the disease)
- Tiredness, fatigue, weight loss
- Low-grade fever
- Bleeding, petechiae, ecchymoses

Splenomegaly

Splenomegaly is enlargement of the spleen.

FEATURES

Commonly occurs in blood disorders including some forms of anemia or lack of platelets.

SIGNS & SYMPTOMS

Signs

- Splenomegaly
- Hepatomegaly
- Lymphadenopathy
- Fever
- Pallor
- Weight loss
- Pathologic fractures

Symptoms

- One-third of patients are asymptomatic at time of diagnosis
- 40% have constitutional symptoms including low-grade fever, bone pain, shortness of breath, weight loss, pruritus, night sweats, and fatigue
- Easy bruising or bleeding
- Abdominal pain or fullness
- Pallor due to anemia in more than 50% of patients
- Oral thrush

ASSOCIATED DISORDERS

- Acute megakaryoblastic leukemia
- Acute myeloid leukemia
- Chronic myelogenous leukemia
- NonHodgkin's lymphoma
- Essential thrombocythemia
- Langerhans' cell histiocytosis
- Sickle cell disease
- Fanconi's anemia
- Vitamin D deficiency
- Tuberculosis
- Visceral leishmaniasis
- Histoplasmosis
- Systemic lupus erythematosus
- Gray platelet syndrome
- Osteopetrosis

- Hyperparathyroidism
- Hypoparathyroidism
- Pernicious anemia
- Gaucher's disease

INVESTIGATION OF THE PATIENT

Direct questions to patient

Q **What is your occupation?** Exposure to toxins including benzene and radiation may predispose patients to myelofibrosis

Q **How old are you?** Myelofibrosis may occur at any age, but most frequently occurs in the sixth to eighth decade of life

Q **What symptoms are you experiencing?** Patients typically present with complaints of pallor and abdominal pain. Other symptoms may include night sweats, fever, or shortness of breath

Q **Have you had any type of cancer?** Hodgkin's disease, tumor metastasis, and acute lymphoblastic leukemia are a few neoplastic diseases that may be associated with myelofibrosis

Q **Have you been exposed to high amounts of radiation either medically or occupationally?** Previous exposure to radiation may be a risk factor for myelofibrosis

Q **Do you have a history of any other hematologic abnormalities?** Essential thrombocytothemia and polycythemia vera may progress to myelofibrosis

Family history

Q **Has anyone in your family had similar symptoms?** Chromosomes are abnormal in one-third of cases: Ph1 absent, C group chromosomes may be duplicated (trisomy 9 or 21), and deletions have been detected at loci 20q and 13q. Abnormal karyotype is associated with a poor prognosis.

Examination

- **What is the patient's color like?** Pallor is often a presenting complaint. Anemia is present in over 50% of patients
- **Take the patient's temperature.** Low-grade fever is common
- **Palpate the abdomen.** Hepatomegaly or splenomegaly suggests a myeloproliferative disorder and warrants blood work
- **Palpate for lymph nodes.** Lymphadenopathy may be present
- **Examine the skin.** Bruising and scratch marks from pruritus may be present

Summary of investigative tests

- Peripheral blood smear provides evidence of cell abnormalities
- Complete blood count (CBC) with differential may reveal leukocytosis, erythrocytosis, and a variable platelet count
- Bone marrow biopsy diagnostically reveals fibrosis
- Bone X-rays may show osteopetrosis
- Blood chemistries may be abnormal
- Karyotype analysis may be performed to estimate prognosis

DIAGNOSTIC DECISION

After a physical examination revealing pallor and hepatomegaly/splenomegaly, a CBC, peripheral blood smear, and blood chemistries should be obtained. A bone marrow biopsy revealing fibrosis is diagnostic of myelofibrosis.

CLINICAL PEARLS

If myeloid/red blood cell (RBC) precursors (leukoerythroblastosis) are present in the peripheral smear and the patient has splenomegaly, then suspect myelofibrosis (and perform bone marrow aspirate/biopsy).

THE TESTS
Body fluids
PERIPHERAL BLOOD SMEAR

Description
- Blood specimen required
- Myelofibrosis reveals a normocytic anemia in over 50% of patients
- RBC mass increased in 15% cases of myelofibrosis
- Erythrocytosis is usually masked by splenomegaly-induced hemodilution
- Leukocytosis occurs in 50% of patients, which is severe in 11% of patients
- Platelet count can show thrombocytopenia in 40% of patients and thrombocytosis in 30% of cases

Advantages/Disadvantages
- Advantage: detects abnormal cells, which may be characteristic of the disease
- Disadvantage: not definitively diagnostic

Abnormal
- Moderate numbers of polychromatophilic RBCs
- Varying numbers of late-stage nucleated RBCs
- Moderate RBC anisocytosis and poikilocytosis
- Tear-drop shaped RBCs are characteristic of the disease

COMPLETE BLOOD COUNT WITH DIFFERENTIAL

Description
Blood specimen.

Advantages/Disadvantages
- Advantage: may detect abnormalities in RBC or white blood cell (WBC) levels
- Disadvantage: not definitively diagnostic

Normal
- Hematocrit: male, 40.7–50.3% (0.407–0.503); female, 36.1–44.3% (0.0361–0.433)
- Hemoglobin: male, 13.8–17.2g/dL (8.56–10.70mmol/L); female, 12.1–15.1g/dL (7.50–9.36mmol/L)
- Erythrocyte count: male, 4.5–5.7x10^6/mcL (4.5–5.7x10^{12}/L); female, 3.9–5.0x10^6/mcL (3.9–5.0x10^{12}/L)
- Mean corpuscular hemoglobin: 26.7–33.7pg/cell (1.66–2.09fmol/cell)
- Mean corpuscular hemoglobin concentration: 32.7–35.5g/dL (20.3–22.0mmol/L)
- Mean corpuscular volume: 80–97.6mcm^3 (80–97.6fL)
- Leukocytes, total: 3.8–9.8x10^3/mcL (3.8–9.8x10^9/L)
- Lymphocytes: 1.2–3.3x10^3/mcL (1.2–3.3x10^9/L)
- Mononuclear cells: 0.2–0.7x10^3/mcL (0.2–0.7x10^9/L)
- Granulocytes: 1.8–6.6x10^3/mcL (1.8–6.6x10^9/L)
- Platelets: 140–440x10^3/mcL (140–440x10^9/L)

Abnormal
- Hemoglobin of <8g/dL in 25% patients with folate deficiency and iron-deficiency anemia being rare
- The reticulocyte count is usually increased
- RBC mass increased in 15% of cases but erythrocytosis usually masked by splenomegaly induced hemodilution
- Leukocytosis is common around 12–50x10^3/mcL with a leftward shift
- Platelet counts may be high or low

Drugs, disorders and other factors that may alter results
Leukocytosis may occur during a severe chronic infection, severe hemolysis, and with malignant neoplasms.

BLOOD CHEMISTRIES
Description
Blood specimen.

Advantages/Disadvantages
- Advantage: may detect abnormalities in blood chemistries
- Disadvantage: not definitively diagnostic

Normal
- Uric acid: 3–8mg/dL (179–476mcmol/L)
- Lactate dehydrogenase (LDH): 100–250 IU/L (1.67–4.17mckat/L)
- Alkaline phosphatase: 38–126 IU/L (0.63–2.10mckat/L)

Abnormal
- Uric acid and LDH are often elevated
- Alkaline phosphatase is variable but tends to decrease with time
- Keep in mind the possibility of a false-positive result

Drugs, disorders and other factors that may alter results
Chronic inflammation tends to cause elevations in alkaline phosphatase.

KARYOTYPE
Description
Blood specimen.

Advantages/Disadvantages
Advantages:
- May give an indication of prognosis – abnormal karyotype confers poor prognosis
- May identify individuals genetically predisposed

Disadvantage: not definitively diagnostic

Abnormal
- Ph1 absent
- C group chromosome duplication
- Deletions at 20q or 13q
- Keep in mind the possibility of a false-positive result

Cause of abnormal result
Laboratory error.

Biopsy
BONE MARROW BIOPSY
Description
- Bone marrow specimen
- The grading system applicable including: grade 1 (reticulin fibrosis), 2 (collagenous fibrosis), to 3 (osteomyelosclerosis)

Advantages/Disadvantages
Advantage: diagnostic, and aids in prognosis

Disadvantages:
- Painful
- May be difficult to aspirate

Abnormal
- Aspirate is frequently hypocellular or dry
- Fibrotic marrow
- Increased blasts may be observed
- Megakaryocytes are often increased
- Colony-forming units-C in marrow are decreased (while in peripheral blood often increased)
- Increased reticular staining of biopsy
- The grading system applicable includes grade 1 (reticulin fibrosis), 2 (collagenous fibrosis), and 3 (osteomyelosclerosis)

Cause of abnormal result
Leukemia – increased blasts.

Imaging
BONE X-RAYS
Description
- Bone X-rays can be useful in myelofibrosis
- Sclerosis seen in 50% of patients; usually involving the axial skeleton
- Osteolytic lesions are rare

Advantages/Disadvantages
- Advantage: may indicate osteoporosis or more commonly osteopetrosis
- Disadvantage: radiation exposure

Abnormal
- Sclerosis seen in 50% of patients; usually in the axial skeleton
- Osteolytic lesions are rare
- Decreased bone density
- Opacity (osteopetrosis)

Drugs, disorders and other factors that may alter results
Congenital abnormalities of bone.

CONSIDER CONSULT

- Refer to oncologist if radiation, chemotherapy, or interferon will be utilized
- Refer to hematologist for consideration of bone marrow transplant (BMT)

IMMEDIATE ACTION

If patient is severely anemic, order a red blood cell (RBC) transfusion.

PATIENT AND CAREGIVER ISSUES

Impact on career, dependants, family, friends

- Affected individuals may experience unusual tiredness, or bone, joint, and abdominal pain that may interfere with quality of life
- Depending upon career, it is possible to continue working, but many patients reassess the role of work in their life and make career changes to less stressful types of work
- If a BMT is part of the treatment plan, patients will require 6–12 months of leave from employment
- The disease is associated with watchful waiting to determine trends in blood counts that will ultimately be linked to overall prognosis

Patient or caregiver request

- **What is myelofibrosis?** A disease of the bone marrow in which collagen builds up fibrous scar tissue inside the marrow cavity. The outcome is that blood is of poor quality
- **How is myelofibrosis diagnosed?** A bone marrow biopsy provides conclusive diagnosis of the disorder
- **Will a bone marrow biopsy hurt?** Opioid pain medications or local anesthesia may be utilized to assist in coping with marrow biopsies
- **How often does a bone marrow biopsy need to be repeated?** Usually once a year to determine the state of the marrow or as needed to assess progression of the disease
- **What symptoms are likely to occur with myelofibrosis?** Tiredness, diarrhea, fluid retention in the abdomen, pain in abdomen, bones, and joints, visual disturbances, and potentially skin eruptions
- **What causes the abdominal pain?** Because the blood is of poor quality, the liver and spleen try to compensate by making blood themselves
- **Why do I experience early satiety after each meal?** Due to large spleen pushing against your stomach. Eating smaller amounts of food more frequently (e.g. six times a day instead of three times a day) may help
- **What is the prognosis?** Prognosis is highly variable, ranging from less than a year to >15 years
- **What are the treatment options?** Blood transfusions if RBC counts fall too low, chemotherapy to control platelets and white blood cell (WBC) counts, interferon to modulate the immune system, and BMTs are among potential treatment options

MANAGEMENT ISSUES

Goals

- To treat or prevent anemia
- To increase quality of life (e.g. by making patient transfusion-independent)
- To cure (if a patient is a candidate for allogeneic stem cell transplant)

Management in special circumstances

- Prolonged chemotherapy may damage organs and make patient less able to withstand chemotherapy prior to a BMT
- It is unclear if prior interferon treatment has a negative impact on BMTs

SUMMARY OF THERAPEUTIC OPTIONS
Choices
- Treatment regimens have not been defined through randomized trials
- Glucocorticoids such as prednisone or methlyprednisolone may be helpful to increase RBC survival rates
- Anobolic steroids, such as nandrolone decanoate, may also be utilized to elevate hematocrit levels
- Iron and folate may be given to correct deficiencies when present
- RBC transfusion is required for severe anemia
- Painful splenomegaly may be treated with anagrelide, interferon, or irradiation treatments but sometimes requires splenectomy
- BMT, with allogeneic stem-cell transplantation, may potentially be curative
- Autologous stem cell transplantation may lead to improvement in the quality of life (e.g. having patient become transfusion-independent)

Clinical pearls
The key issue revolves around the decision of who should be offered allogeneic stem cell transplant (usually those patients younger than 45, in advanced stage of the disease).

FOLLOW UP
Plan for review
- Monthly checks of blood work in early stages of disease to determine whether patient is stable or deteriorating
- If disease is in early stages and patient is stable, checks may be performed at 2- to 3-month intervals

Information for patient or caregiver
- If abdominal pain becomes too severe, the spleen may be removed
- It may be helpful to join a support group

DRUGS AND OTHER THERAPIES: DETAILS
Drugs
PREDNISONE

Steroidal anti-inflammatory.

Dose

5–60mg/day orally. May be given as a single morning dose or divided two to four times throughout the day.

Efficacy
- Controls the rate of protein synthesis, depresses migration of fibroblasts, and stabilizes lysosomes to prevent inflammation
- Efficacy in some cases of myelofibrosis may reflect an underlying autoimmune process or suppression of a proliferating clone

Risks/Benefits

Risks:
- Use caution when administering to patients with congestive heart failure, diabetes mellitus, glaucoma, renal disease, ulcerative colitis, or peptic ulcer
- Use caution when administering to the elderly
- Prednisone taken in doses >7.5mg for 3 weeks or longer may lead to clinically relevant suppression of the pituitary-adrenal axis

Side-effects and adverse reactions

- Side-effects are minimized by short duration of therapy
- Cardiovascular system: hypertension, thromboembolism
- Central nervous system: insomnia, euphoria, depression, psychosis, seizures
- Endocrine: adrenal suppression, impaired glucose tolerance, growth suppression in children
- Eyes, ears, nose, and throat: cataract, glaucoma, blurred vision
- Gastrointestinal: dyspepsia, peptic ulceration, esophagitis, oral candidiasis
- Musculoskeletal: proximal myopathy, osteoporosis
- Skin: delayed healing, acne, striae, fragile skin

Interactions (other drugs)

■ Aminoglutethimide (increased clearance of prednisone) ■ Warfarin (alters clotting time) ■ Antidiabetics (hypoglycemic effect inhibited) ■ Salicylates (increased clearance of salicylates) ■ Antihypertensives (effects inhibited) ■ Rifampin (may inhibit hepatic clearance of prednisone) ■ Oral contraceptives (enhanced effects of corticosteroids) ■ Diuretics (effects inhibited) ■ Barbiturates (increased clearance of prednisone) ■ Nonsteroidal anti-inflammatory drugs (NSAIDs) (increased risks of bleeding) ■ Cardiac glycosides (toxicity increased) ■ Isoniazid (reduced plasma levels of isoniazid) ■ Cholestyramine, colestipol (may reduce absorption of corticosteroids) ■ Ketoconazole ■ Clarithromycin, erythromycin, troleandomycin (may enhance steroid effect) ■ Cyclosporine (may increase levels of both drugs; may cause seizures)

Contraindications

■ Systemic infection ■ Avoid live virus vaccines in those receiving immunosuppressive doses ■ History of tuberculosis ■ Cushing's syndrome ■ Recent myocardial infarction

Acceptability to patient

Side-effects may limit utility.

Follow up plan

- Potassium and blood sugar must be monitored during long-term therapy
- Patients should routinely be evaluated for edema, hypertension, cardiac symptoms, mental status changes, and weight gain

Patient and caregiver information

- Take with food to minimize gastrointestinal discomfort
- Avoid abrupt discontinuation
- Wear medical alert bracelet
- Notify clinician if you experience fatigue, anorexia, nausea, vomiting, diarrhea, weight loss, weakness, dizziness, or low blood sugar when discontinuing therapy

METHYLPREDNISOLONE

Steroidal anti-inflammatory medication.

Dose

30mg/kg for 3 days followed by 20mg/kg for 4 days, 10mg/kg for 7 days, 5mg/kg for 7 days, 1mg/kg until blood counts are adequate, then wean as tolerated. Doses should be given each morning.

Efficacy

- Controls the rate of protein synthesis, depresses migration of fibroblasts, and stabilizes lysosomes to prevent inflammation
- Efficacy in some cases of myelofibrosis may reflect an underlying autoimmune process or suppression of a proliferating clone
- Steroids are not usually used alone but rather are used in protocols with other medications

Risks/Benefits

Risks:

- Overwhelming septicemia if patient has an infection
- Loss of control of blood glucose in those with diabetes
- Use caution in elderly due to risk of diabetes and osteoporosis
- Use caution in patients with psychosis, seizure disorders, myasthenia gravis, congestive heart failure, hypertension, ulcerative colitis, peptic ulcer, or esophagitis

Side-effects and adverse reactions

- Side-effects are minimized by short duration of therapy
- Cardiovascular system: hypertension, thromboembolism
- Central nervous system: insomnia, euphoria, depression, psychosis, seizures
- Endocrine: adrenal suppression, impaired glucose tolerance, growth suppression in children
- Eyes, ears, nose, and throat: cataract, glaucoma, blurred vision
- Gastrointestinal: dyspepsia, peptic ulceration, esophagitis, oral candidiasis, nausea, vomiting
- Musculoskeletal: proximal myopathy, osteoporosis
- Skin: delayed healing, acne, striae

Interactions (other drugs)

■ Aminoglutethamide ■ Antidiabetics ■ Barbiturates ■ Cholestyramine ■ Ketoconazole ■ Colestipol ■ Clarithromycin, erythromycin ■ Cyclosporine ■ Isoniazid ■ Troleandomycin ■ NSAIDs ■ Oral contraceptives ■ Rifampin ■ Salicylates

Contraindications

■ Systemic infection ■ Avoid live virus vaccines in those receiving immunosuppressive doses

Acceptability to patient

Side-effects may limit utility.

Follow up plan

- Potassium and blood sugar must be monitored during long-term therapy
- Patients should routinely be evaluated for edema, hypertension, cardiac symptoms, mental status changes, and weight gain

Patient and caregiver information

- Take with food to minimize gastrointestinal discomfort
- Avoid abrupt discontinuation
- Wear medical alert bracelet
- Notify clinician if you experience fatigue, anorexia, nausea, vomiting, diarrhea, weight loss, weakness, dizziness, or low blood sugar when discontinuing therapy

NANDROLONE DECANOATE

Anabolic steroid medication.

Dose

By deep intramuscular injection, preferably into the gluteal muscle:

- Women – 50–100mg/week
- Men – 100–200mg/week

Efficacy

May produce a sustained increase in hematocrit.

Risks/Benefits

Risks:

- Risk of peliosis hepatis
- Edema with or without congestive heart failure may be a serious complication in patients with pre-existing cardiac, renal, or hepatic disease
- Geriatric patients treated with androgenic anabolic steroids may be at an increased risk for the development of prostatic hypertrophy and prostatic carcinoma
- Risk of virilization in women
- Insulin or oral hypoglycemic dosage may need adjustment in diabetic patients who receive anabolic steroids
- Use with caution in children

Side-effects and adverse reactions

- Central nervous system: habituation, excitation, insomnia, depression
- Gastrointestinal: nausea, vomiting, diarrhea
- Genitourinary
- Hematologic: bleeding in patients on concomitant anticoagulant therapy
- Metabolic: cholestatic jaundice with, rarely, hepatic necrosis and death, decreased glucose tolerance
- Skin: hirsutism and male pattern baldness in women, acne
- Other: deepening of the voice in women

Genitourinary (in men):

- Prepubertal – phallic enlargement and increased frequency of erections
- Postpubertal – inhibition of testicular function, testicular atrophy and oligospermia, impotence, chronic priapism, epididymitis, and bladder irritability

Genitourinary (in women):

- Clitoral enlargement
- Menstrual irregularities
- Gynecomastia

Genitourinary (in both sexes):

Increased or decreased libido.

Interactions (other drugs)

■ **Anticoagulants** ■ **Oral hypoglycemic agents**

Contraindications

■ **Known or suspected carcinoma of the prostate or the male breast** ■ **Pregnancy category X** ■ **Carcinoma of the breast in females with hypercalcemia (androgenic anabolic steroids may stimulate osteolytic bone resorption)** ■ **Nephrosis or nephrotic phase of nephritis**

Acceptability to patient

Side-effects may limit utility.

Follow up plan

- Frequent urine and serum calcium levels should be obtained (discontinue if hypercalcemia develops)
- Females should routinely be evaluated for signs of virilization
- Liver function tests, lipids, hematocrit, and hemoglobin should be periodically obtained
- Monitor growth rate in children

Patient and caregiver information

- Voice may deepen
- Do not take if pregnant
- Notify clinician if you experience abdominal pain, yellowing of the skin or eyes, darkened urine

IRON

Dose

- 100–200mg oral elemental iron divided three times daily
- Ferrous fumarate is 33% elemental iron
- Ferrous gluconate is 12% elemental iron
- Ferrous sulfate is 2% elemental iron

Efficacy

Treats iron-deficiency anemia.

Risks/Benefits

Risks:

- Use caution in patients with elevated serum ferritin levels
- The treatment of any anemic condition should be under the advice and supervision of a physician. As oral iron products interfere with absorption of oral tetracycline antibiotics, these products should not be taken within 2h of each other
- Accidental overdose of iron-containing products is a leading cause of fatal poisoning in children under 6 years

Side-effects and adverse reactions

Gastrointestinal: nausea, vomiting, bloating, abdominal discomfort, black stools, diarrhea, constipation (leading to colic), anorexia.

Interactions (other drugs)

■ Antacids ■ Quinolones ■ Penicillamine ■ Alkalinizers ■ Tetracycline ■ Doxycycline ■ Methyldopa ■ Calcium carbonate ■ Vitamin E ■ Levodopa ■ Cimetidine ■ Nizatidine ■ Ranitidine ■ Famotidine ■ Chloramphenicol ■ Pancreatic enzymes

Contraindications

■ Hypersensitivity to any iron-containing supplement ■ Hemochromatosis ■ Hemosiderosis ■ Pregnant women and nursing mothers should not use more than RDA amounts (30 and 15mg/day, respectively) ■ Ulcerative colitis ■ Regional enteritis ■ Hemolytic anemia

Acceptability to patient

Well tolerated.

Follow up plan

Periodic RBC indices should be monitored.

Patient and caregiver information

- Best absorbed on an empty stomach; may be taken with food to prevent gastrointestinal upset
- Drink liquid iron preparations diluted in water or juice, and through a straw to prevent stains of teeth
- Iron changes stool color to black or dark green

FOLATE

Dose

1mg orally daily.

Efficacy

- Treats anemia caused by folate deficiencies; folate is required for synthesis and maintenance of normal erythropoiesis
- Folate stimulates RBC, WBC, and platelet production

Risks/Benefits

Risk: use caution in patients with undiagnosed anemia

Side-effects and adverse reactions

- Respiratory: bronchospasm (rare)
- Skin: itching and rash

Interactions (other drugs)

- **Anticonvulsants** ■ **Cholestyramine** ■ **Colestipol** ■ **Colchicine** ■ **Fluoxetine** ■ **Metformin** ■ **Pyrimethamine** ■ **Phenobarbital** ■ **Lithium** ■ **Lometrexol** ■ **Methotrexate** ■ **Phenytoin** ■ **NSAIDs** ■ **Sulfasalazine**

Contraindications

Hypersensitivity to folic acid.

Acceptability to patient

Well tolerated.

Follow up plan

Periodic complete blood count (CBC) with RBC indices and serum folate should be monitored.

ANAGRELIDE

Dose

- 0.5mg four times daily or 1mg twice daily by mouth
- Dose may be adjusted after at least one week to the lowest amount required to keep platelet count <600,000 cells/mm^3
- Do not increase dose by >0.5mg/day in any one-week period
- Do not exceed 10mg/day or 2.5mg in a single dose

Efficacy

Reduces platelet counts.

Risks/Benefits

Risks:

- Anagrelide should be used with caution in patients with known or suspected heart disease, and only if the potential benefits of therapy outweigh the potential risks
- Use caution with renal and hepatic impairment

Side-effects and adverse reactions

- Cardiovascular system: palpitations
- Central nervous system: headache, dizziness
- Gastrointestinal: diarrhea, abdominal pain, flatulence
- Musculoskeletal: asthenia
- Respiratory: dyspnea

Interactions (other drugs)

None listed.

Contraindications

- **Pregnancy category C** ■ **The safety and efficacy of anagrelide in patients under the age of 16 years have not been established**

Follow up plan

Platelet count should be monitored every 2 days during the first week then weekly thereafter until maintenance dosage is attained.

Patient and caregiver information

- Weekly monitoring of platelets is essential
- Notify clinician of any bleeding

INTERFERON-ALPHA 2B

Dose

A wide variety of dosages have been used and it is probably best to consult current literature or the manufacturer. Dosages have ranged between 1 and 6 million units injected subcutaneously daily.

Efficacy

Alters the synthesis of DNA, RNA, and cellular proteins.

Risks/Benefits

Risks:

- Use caution in patients with seizure disorders, cardiac disease, pulmonary disease, diabetes mellitus, renal or hepatic disease, dental disease, thyroid disease, or psoriasis
- Use caution in the elderly
- Use caution in patients who are pregnant or breast-feeding
- Adverse effects are generally dose-related
- Flu-like symptoms are common

Side-effects and adverse reactions

- Cardiovascular system: chest pain, hypertension, edema, arrhythmias, myocardial infarction, cardiomyopathy
- Central nervous system: depression, suicidal ideation, dizziness, anxiety, confusion, paresthesias, insomnia, seizures, coma, flu-like symptoms
- Eyes, ears, nose, and throat: retinal hemorrhage, visual impairment
- Gastrointestinal: nausea, vomiting, diarrhea, weight loss, abdominal pain, taste disturbances, raised liver enzymes, gastrointestinal bleeding
- Hematologic: blood dyscrasias
- Metabolic: hyperthyroidism, hypothyroidism, hyperglycemia
- Skin: injection site reaction, rash, alopecia, pruritus, exacerbation of psoriasis, dry skin
- Respiratory: cough, dyspnea, sinusitis

Interactions (other drugs)

- **Aldesleukin** ■ **Aminophylline, theophylline** ■ **Antineoplastic agents** ■ **Zidovudine**

Contraindications

- **Benzyl alcohol hypersensitivity** ■ **History of depression or severe psychiatric disorders**
- **Visceral AIDS-related Kaposi's sarcoma associated with rapidly progressive disease**
- *E. coli* **protein hypersensitivity** ■ **Immunosuppression** ■ **Intramuscular injections**
- **Neonates, children under one year** ■ **History of hepatitis, autoimmune disease**
- **Women of child-bearing age (unless undertaking contraceptive measures)**

Acceptability to patient

- Side-effects may lead patients to be noncompliant. In some patients, the adverse effects subsided after 6 weeks; however, other patients reported feeling poorly throughout the duration of treatment
- Difficult to give self-injections

Follow up plan

Bone marrow histology and CBCs with RBC indices and platelet counts are required periodically.

Patient and caregiver information

- Drink plenty of fluids
- Influenza-like symptoms may subside with continued treatment
- Acetaminophen may alleviate fever and headache
- Use smallest gauge needle possible
- Find a spot you can tolerate injecting a needle into – the abdomen works well for many people

Surgical therapy

SPLENECTOMY

Removal of spleen.

Efficacy

May reduce pain associated with splenomegaly or infarct.

Risks/Benefits

Risks:

- Postoperative pain
- Infection, bleeding, or thrombosis in 30%
- Postoperative mortality is 10%
- Increased blast transformation
- Liver failure
- Increased extramedullary metaplasia
- Worsening of subclinical disseminated intravascular coagulation

Benefits:

- Alleviates splenic infarction
- May improve RBC indices for less need of blood transfusions
- May improve portal hypertension
- Response may be evaluated using iron studies
- May improve symptoms

Acceptability to patient

Tolerated.

Follow up plan

Blood count monitoring.

Patient and caregiver information

- Patient may be more susceptable to certain infections
- Should always let treating physician or dentist know that the spleen has been removed

Radiation therapy

SPLENIC IRRADIATION

Splenic irradiation may reduce spleen size and alleviate painful symptoms.

Efficacy

May improve the quality of life in patients with myelofibrosis refractory to usual treatments but does not induce a sustained improvement.

Risks/Benefits
Risk: radiation exposure

Benefits:
- May reduce constitutional symptoms
- May reduce spleen size
- May reduce spleen pain

Acceptability to patient
Radiation treatment is difficult to tolerate.

Follow up plan
- Monitor splenic response
- Monitor blood counts

Other therapies

RED BLOOD CELL TRANSFUSION
Injection of healthy blood into the circulation of a patient whose blood is deficient in quantity or quality.

Efficacy
To prevent RBC counts from falling too low.

Risks/Benefits
- Risk: small risk that blood may be contaminated with HIV, hepatitis, or other diseases
- Benefit: may boost energy levels

Acceptability to patient
Tolerated.

Follow up plan

Periodic blood counts are required.

BONE MARROW TRANSPLANTATION

Transplantation of the tissue contained within the internal cavities of the bones.

Efficacy

- BMT is the only curative modality known
- Investigational protocols using cord cell transplantation, nonmyeloablative allotransplantation, and myeloablation plus autologous stem cell support are currently under investigation

Risks/Benefits

Risks:

- High risk of death or disease. Mortality risk prevents this procedure in patients older than 50–55 years of age
- May require one year of sick leave from work
- Possibility of tissue rejection with BMT
- Expensive

Benefits:

- May offer a cure
- May slow progression of disease

Acceptability to patient

High risk of disease, infection, and death with BMT.

Follow up plan

Frequent blood counts are required.

OUTCOMES

EFFICACY OF THERAPIES

- The efficacy of therapies varies tremendously on individual patient responses
- Treatment of idiopathic myelofibrosis is complex as direct empirical evidence is lacking
- Treatment of idiopathic myelofibrosis should be based on inductive reasoning
- Treatment of secondary myelofibrosis includes treating the underlying cause as this has been shown to prolong survival

Review period

12 months (this is a rare disease with not many related clinical trials).

PROGNOSIS

- Prognosis is variable with mortality occurring anywhere from within one year of diagnosis to 10–15 years
- Age at time of transplant and karyotype are also important predictors of treatment response
- The leading causes of death in idiopathic myelofibrosis are infections (pneumonia – most common), cardiac failure, and thrombosis/bleeding
- The median survival time of idiopathic myelofibrosis is 5 years and ranges from one to 20 years
- The prognosis of secondary myelofibrosis is dependent on the cause and whether it is responsive to treatment, and ranges from a few months to over 15 years

Clinical pearls

Lille's scoring system (based on low hemoglobin (<10g/dL) and low (<4x10^9/L) or high (>30x10^9/L) white blood cells) is commonly used to predict the course of the disease. Those patients with none of these features have median survival of 93 months; those with two of these adverse features have median survival of 13 months. The age does not appear to be a prognostic factor.

Therapeutic failure

Splenectomy may be performed if splenomegaly is not responsive to other modalities.

Recurrence

Other therapies should be considered – treatment is based on inductive reasoning and reviewing the limited evidence available on the treatment of myelofibrosis.

Deterioration

- Bone marrow transplantation may be performed as a last resort if suitable donor source is identified
- Other therapies are still considered experimental but include thalidomide and antiangiogenesis agents

Terminal illness

- Patients with myelofibrosis may be informed that their life-expectancy should be thought of in terms of months/years rather than decades
- Patients may want to re-evaluate their occupation and other stresses to re-evaluate their priorities
- The disease involves a great deal of watchful waiting as blood cell counts are monitored and further treatments are initiated as appropriate

COMPLICATIONS

Hypoparathyroidism is sometimes seen in patients with myelofibrosis.

PREVENTION

There is really no way to prevent myelofibrosis as it is unclear what causes the disease and as it is often secondary to other myeloproliferative or neoplastic illnesses.

RISK FACTORS

- Prior history of cancer or other hemoproliferative illnesses
- Previous radiation exposure may be a risk factor

MODIFY RISK FACTORS

Lifestyle and wellness

ENVIRONMENT

Exposure to radiation and benzene compounds may be predisposing factors to myelofibrosis.

SCREENING

Routine screening is not recommended as the disease is rare.

PREVENT RECURRENCE

Patients with myelofibrosis tend to deteriorate over time, and are not likely to recover and get the disease again.

RESOURCES

ASSOCIATIONS

MPD Research Center
115 East 72nd Street
New York, NY 10021
Tel: (800) HELP-MPD
http://inform.acor.org/mpd/mffaq.html

American Cancer Society
1599 Clifton Road NE
Atlanta, GA 30329
Tel: (404) 320-3333
www.cancer.org

International Bone Marrow Transplant Registry
8701 Watertown Plank Road
PO Box 26509
Milkwaukee, WI 53226
Tel: (414) 456-8325
Fax: (414) 456-6530
E-mail: ibmtr@mcw.edu
www.ibmtr.org

National Bone Marrow Transplant Link
20411 W 12 Mile Road, Suite 108
Southfield, MI 48076
Tel: (800) 546-5268
E-mail: nbmtlink@aol.com
comnet.org/nbmtlink

KEY REFERENCES

- Pizzo PA, Poplack DG. Principles and practice of pediatric oncology, 3rd edn. Philadelphia: Lippincott-Raven Publishers, 1997
- Anderson JE, Tefferi Ayalew, Craig F, et al. Myeloablation and autologous peripheral blood stem cell rescue results in hematologic and clinical response in patients with myeloid metaplasia with myelofibrosis. Blood 2001;98:586–92. Medline
- Balduini CL, Bertolino G, Noris P, et al. Effect of anagrelide on platelet count and function in patients with thrombocytosis and myeloproliferative disorders. Haematologica 1992;77:40–3. Medline
- Bouabdallah R, Coso D, Gonzague-Casabianca L, et al. Safety and efficacy of splenic irradiation in the treatment of patients with idiopathic myelofibrosis: A report on 15 patients. Leuk Res 2000;24:491–5. Medline
- Cervantes F, Barosi G, Demory J-P, et al. Myelofibrosis with myeloid metaplasia in young individuals: disease characteristics, prognostic factors and identification of risk groups. Br J Haem 1998;102:684–90. Medline
- Cetingul N, Yener E, Oztop S, et al. Agnogenic myeloid metaplasia in childhood: a report of two cases and efficiency of intravenous high dose methylprednisolone treatment. Acta Paediatr Jpn 1994;36:697–700. Medline
- Guardiola P, Anderson JE, Bandini G, et al. Allogeneic stem cell transplantation for agnogenic myeloid metaplasia: a European group for blood and marrow transplantation. Blood 1999;93:2831–8. Medline
- Inoue Y, Matsubara A, Okuya S, et al. Myelofibrosis and systemic lupus erythematosus: reveral of fibrosis with high-dose corticosteroid therapy. Acta Haematol 1992;88:32–6. Medline
- Italian Consensus Conference on Diagnostic Criteria for Myelofibrosis with Myeloid Metaplasia. Br J Haem 1999;104:730–7. Medline
- Tefferi A, Mesa RA, Nagorney DM, et al. Splenectomy in myelofibrosis with myeloid metaplasia: a single-institution experience with 223 patients. Blood 2000;95:2226–32. Medline

- Weinfeld A, Swolin B, Westin J. Acute leukaemia after hydroxyurea therapy in polycythemia vera and allied disorders: prospective study in efficacy and leukemogenicity with therapeutic implications. Eur J Haematol 1994;52:134–9. Medline
- Yoon S-Y, Li C-Y, Mesa RA, et al. Bone marrow effects of anagrelide therapy in patients with myelofibrosis with myeloid metaplasia. Br J Haem 1999;106:682–8
- Jefferi A. Myelofibrosis with myeloid metaplasia. N Engl J Med 2000 342:1255–65
- Barosi G. Myelofibrosis with myeloid metaplasia diagnostic definition and prognostic classification for clinical studies and treatment guidelines. J Clin Oncol 1999;17:2594–970

FAQS

Question 1

What experimental approaches might be considered?

ANSWER 1

Thalidomide, autologous peripheral blood stem cell transplants, and use of STI-571 are currently actively under investigaton.

Question 2

Does course of the disease differ between young and old patients?

ANSWER 2

No. It appears that the same features adversely affect both young and older patients (i.e. levels of hemoglobin, white blood count, and abnormal karyotype).

Question 3

Is radiation to the spleen harmless?

ANSWER 3

No. Radiation can cause prolonged pancytopenia secondary to ablation of active hematopoietic tissues in extramedullary sites.

Question 4

What is a leading cause of death in idiopathic myelofibrsosis?

ANSWER 4

Infections (pneumonia, being most common), followed by cardiac failure.

Question 5

Can high-dose chemotherapy followed by autologous peripheral blood stem cell transplant prolong survival in patients with idiopathic myelofibrsosis?

ANSWER 5

This is not known. The main goal of treatment is still palliative, i.e. to have some patients become transfusion-independent.

CONTRIBUTORS

Dennis F Saver, MD
Benjamin Djulbegovic, MD, PhD
Januario E Castro, MD

OSTEOSARCOMA

SUMMARY INFORMATION

DESCRIPTION

- Osteosarcoma is a rare primary malignant tumor arising in bone, the tumor cells producing bone, or osteoid
- Occurs predominantly in adolescents and young adults, or as a complication of Paget's disease in adults (usually late middle-aged or elderly)
- Strong association with previous radiation exposure
- Most tumors arise in the distal femur or proximal tibia
- A highly malignant tumor; only 20% of patients with localized resectable primary tumors survive without relapse when treated only by surgical resection
- Management is based on chemotherapy and surgery with limb salvage if possible
- Osteosarcomas rarely arise in extraskeletal sites, including the mediastinum, retroperitoneum, lungs, breast, and uterus

URGENT ACTION

- Any child or adolescent presenting with pain, and especially swelling, in or around any bone needs urgent and thorough assessment
- Consider the diagnosis of osteosarcoma in adults with Paget's disease, especially if bone pain changes in character, nature, site, or if there is new bony swelling

KEY! DON'T MISS!

- Pain and/or swelling in a joint which the patient attributes to minor trauma when the severity of the symptoms or signs seems disproportionate to the injury sustained
- Any night-time bone pain should always be investigated (don't dismiss as 'growing pains')
- The development of seemingly mild symptoms or signs in a survivor of childhood cancer, especially Ewing's tumor or retinoblastoma
- The development of new or changing bone symptoms in middle-aged or elderly patients with Paget's disease

BACKGROUND

ICD9 CODE

- 170.9 Neoplasms, bone (periosteum), primary malignant
- M9180/3 Osteosarcoma

SYNONYMS

- Osteosarcoma
- Osteogenic sarcoma
- Primary malignant bone sarcoma

CARDINAL FEATURES

- Osteosarcoma is a rare and highly malignant primary bone tumor
- It commonly presents with persistent pain and swelling around any joint in an otherwise well patient
- About 50% of tumors arise in the femur, followed by the tibia, humerus, pelvis, jaw, fibula, and ribs in descending order of frequency
- Osteosarcoma arising in Paget's disease often develops in flat bones, is usually aggressive and metastasizes early. It may present in this group with a sudden increase in bone pain
- A substantial number of osteosarcomas occur as secondary malignancies in patients previously treated for a different primary tumor, especially childhood malignancies such as retinoblastoma or Ewing's sarcoma
- Ionizing radiation and external beam radiation have also been associated with an increased incidence of soft-tissue or bone sarcomas
- Radiographic findings are characteristic and consist of: dense (blastic) or lucent (lytic) areas in the affected bones, nearly always in the metaphyses; periosteal sunburst patterns; peripheral Codman's triangles; and poorly defined tumor margins
- Variants include parosteal (juxtacortical) osteosarcoma in which new bone formation is particularly dense (better prognosis), and periosteal osteosarcoma (intermediate prognosis)
- The most common cell type of osteosarcomas is central (medullary). It is characterized by areas of necrosis, atypical mitoses, and malignant cartilage
- The other subtypes are all less common, including: telangiectatic; intraosseous well differentiated (low grade, associated with the most favorable prognosis and can be successfully treated with radical excision of the primary tumor alone); small cell; surface (peripheral); parosteal (juxtacortical); well differentiated (low grade); periosteal (low-to-intermediate grade); high-grade surface
- Stage varies from localized to metastatic. Skip metastases in the bone of origin may occur and carrys a poorer prognosis than local disease. In metastatic disease, tumor deposit may be seen in other bones and organs. Distant metastases are found in 10–20% of patients at diagnosis. 85–90% of metastatic disease is in the lungs. Presentations with multiple bone metastases carry a very poor prognosis

CAUSES

Common causes

- Most cases of osteosarcoma are of unknown cause
- A substantial number of osteosarcomas occur as secondary malignancies in patients previously treated for a different primary tumor, especially in patients who have had a childhood malignancy
- The secondary osteosarcoma may occur many years later, and is most commonly associated with successfully treated retinoblastoma and Ewing's sarcoma
- In patients who survived childhood Ewing's sarcoma, the relative risk may be increased by 350 times, although the absolute risk is about 7%

- For patients who are cured of the familial from of retinoblastoma, there is a 500 times increased risk of subsequently developing osteosarcoma
- In other childhood cancers the relative risk of developing later osteosarcoma is about 30 times, but the absolute risk is only 0.1–0.5%
- In middle-aged and elderly patients with Paget's disease there is an association with the secondary development of osteosarcoma. It is not known why this is, and the association appears unrelated to the therapies used to manage the Paget's disease
- There is a higher incidence in identical twins, which supports the hypothesis of associated genetic alterations

Rare causes

- Ionizing radiation: workers exposed to radium (which was used in the manufacture of luminous clocks and watches) in the early 20th century led to high rates of radium poisoning and, among other effects, later development of osteosarcomas of the distal skeleton. The cumulative risk of developing osteosarcoma was as high as 70% over the ensuing 50 years
- External beam radiation can result in soft-tissue or bone sarcomas (including osteosarcoma) in 1/3000–5000 treated patients, with a latency period of 5–30 years
- About 4% of cases of osteosarcoma are associated with germline p53 mutation of chromosome 17p

Serious causes

- Previously treated malignancies
- Paget's disease
- Ionizing radiation

EPIDEMIOLOGY

Incidence and prevalence

INCIDENCE

- About 750 new cases/year in the US
- About 150 new cases/year in the UK

FREQUENCY

- Osteosarcoma accounts for 3–4% of all childhood malignancies
- The commonest malignant tumor of bone (31% of the total)

Demographics

AGE

- Peak age is 12–24 years, during and after the adolescent growth spurt
- Smaller peak at 50–80 years

GENDER

- More common in boys than girls (1.5:1)
- In older adults, males and females equally affected

RACE

There are no racial differences in the incidence of osteosarcoma.

GENETICS

- Increased incidence in identical twins
- Increased risk of osteosarcoma in patients cured of familial retinoblastoma, associated with loss of both alleles at 13q14
- Loss of heterozygosity and mutation of the p53 tumor suppressor gene on chromosome 17p can be found in sporadic osteosarcoma
- The Li-Fraumeni syndrome is known to be related to a germline mutation in p53. This is a familial cancer syndrome in which sarcomas in childhood are associated with an increased incidence of cancer in close relatives

GEOGRAPHY

More common in temperate climates.

SOCIOECONOMIC STATUS

There are no socioeconomic factors in the etiology of osteosarcoma.

DIFFERENTIAL DIAGNOSIS

The main differential diagnosis will depend on the age of the patient:

- Age 0–5 years: osteosarcoma and Ewing's sarcoma can occur
- Age 10–20 years: osteosarcoma, bone cysts, and chondroblastoma are more likely
- Age 20–40: parosteal osteosarcoma and giant cell tumors are more likely
- Age over 40 years: metastatic carcinomas are the commonest bone cancers, with myeloma relatively common in patients aged over 50 years
- Age 50–80: osteosarcoma may arise in pre-existing Paget's disease

Ewing's sarcoma

Malignant tumor of unknown histogenesis.

FEATURES

- Age of onset 10–15 years
- Painful soft-tissue mass
- Often feels warm
- Usually affects midshaft of a long bone
- Systemic symptoms are common with lethargy, weight loss, and fever

Muliple myeloma

Multiple myeloma is a hematologic plasma cell tumor localized in the bone marrow. It can generate bone deformity and fractures resembling those found in osteosarcoma.

FEATURES

- Age of onset usually over 40 years
- Male:female ratio 2:1
- Usually presents with systemic features including anorexia, weight loss, and bone pain
- Usually found in the axial bones rather than the long, extra-axial bones favored by osteosarcoma
- Can present as a solitary lesion
- The most common presentation is with severe constant back pain
- Subsequent imaging reveals a destructive skeletal lesion
- Other organs eventually become involved leading to anemia, more bone pains, renal insufficiency, bacterial infections, and dysproteinemia
- Secondary amyloidosis can occur, leading to cardiac failure and nephrotic syndrome

Chondrosarcoma

Chondrosarcoma is a malignant tumor of cartilage that may develop primarily or secondarily from transformation of a benign osteocartilaginous exostosis or enchondroma.

FEATURES

- Age of onset: 40–60 years
- Male:female = 2:1
- Presents as painful swelling
- Commonly affects the pelvis, upper femur, and shoulder girdle

Fibrosarcoma and liposarcoma

Very rare tumors arising from soft tissues. Osteosarcoma very rarely presents in the soft tissues.

FEATURES

- Very rare
- Can affect any soft-tissue type at any site

- Present in elderly or middle-aged patients
- Often painless, with no systemic features
- Diagnosis usually made from biopsied material
- Diagnosis may be serendipitous (e.g. after excision biopsy of presumed lipoma)

Metastatic bone disease

A large number of tumors can metastasize to the bones. The most common, in order, are: carcinoma of the bronchus; carcinoma of the breast; carcinoma of the prostate; carcinoma of the colon; thyroid carcinoma; carcinoma of the kidney; Ewing's tumor; neuroblastoma; carcinoid tumors.

FEATURES

- Symptoms and signs from the primary tumor will usually, but not invariably, be present
- There may be severe, unremitting pain in the affected bone
- The proximal shafts of bones are commonly affected
- Metastatic bone disease most commonly involves the ribs, pelvis, and proximal femur
- The first presentation may be with a pathologic fracture

Osteomyelitis

Osteomyelitis is an acute or chronic infection of bone, either from direct traumatic inoculation or secondary to hematologic or contagious spread.

FEATURES

- Usually affects the tibia and/or fibula in children
- Localized inflammation often secondary to trauma
- Often local cellulitis and/or hematoma
- Abrupt fever
- Lethargy, malaise, irritability
- Involved bone is painful and tender

Malignant fibrous histiocytoma of bone

A rare malignant spindle cell tumor of bone.

FEATURES

- Similar anatomical distribution to osteosarcoma
- Age of onset 30–50 years
- Most commonly affects the diaphysis of bones
- Treatment is the same as for osteosarcoma

Myositis ossificans

Myositis characterized by bony deposits or by ossification of muscles.

FEATURES

The features of this rare disorder are often the same as those observed in osteosarcoma, and occasionally the cellular components of this lesion may suggest malignancy. In fact, some individuals have undergone unnecessary amputations due to an erroneous diagnosis.

SIGNS & SYMPTOMS

Signs

- Firm swelling around the affected bone
- Tenderness and local warmth may also be present
- The neighboring joints may show limitation of movement secondary to the swelling
- The overlying skin appears normal
- There may be systemic signs such as cachexia, lymphadenopathy, or anemia if metastasis has occurred

Symptoms

- The affected area will be painful
- The pain is often mild, but may be continuous, worse at night, or intermittent
- The patient usually feels well
- Patients with pre-existing Paget's disease may complain of new bone pain of a different intensity, duration, or from a new anatomical site

ASSOCIATED DISORDERS

- Children and young adults: previous childhood tumors, especially Ewing's tumor or retinoblastoma
- Middle-aged or elderly patients: Paget's disease

KEY! DON'T MISS!

- Pain and/or swelling in a joint which the patient attributes to minor trauma when the severity of the symptoms or signs seems disproportionate to the injury sustained
- Any night-time bone pain should always be investigated (don't dismiss as 'growing pains')
- The development of seemingly mild symptoms or signs in a survivor of childhood cancer, especially Ewing's tumor or retinoblastoma
- The development of new or changing bone symptoms in middle-aged or elderly patients with Paget's disease

CONSIDER CONSULT

- Early referral of any adolescent or young adult with bone pain which persists and for which there is no obvious cause is advised for investigation and diagnosis
- Middle-aged and elderly patients with previously diagnosed Paget's disease who experience sudden changes in bone pain intensity or site should also be referred for investigation and diagnosis
- Any patient whose radiographs are consistent with or suspicious of osteosarcoma should be referred
- Referral should be to medical centers that have a multidisciplinary team of cancer specialists with experience in treating cancers that occur in childhood and adolescence
- Patients with proven or suspected osteosarcoma should be evaluated by an orthopedic oncologist familiar with the surgical management of this disease. This evaluation should take place before any initial biopsy is taken since an inappropriately performed biopsy may jeopardize a limb-sparing procedure

INVESTIGATION OF THE PATIENT

Direct questions to patient

Q **Do you feel well?** Patients often have no systemic symptoms and feel very well

Q **Where is your pain?** Most cases of osteosarcoma present with pain, usually of the distal femur or proximal tibia, especially in adolescence. Sometimes there is very little local pain. Osteosarcoma complicating Paget's disease usually affects the flat bones, especially of the face

Q **Is the pain constant or only on moving?** Typically, any pain in osteosarcoma is constant or intermittent, with no clear patterns of exacerbating or relieving factors

Q **Do you have the pain at night?** Night-time pain in a bone is always a symptom which requires full investigation and should never be ignored

Q **Have you noticed any swelling where you have the pain?** Firm, sometimes tender, swelling may appear around the site of bone pain from osteosarcoma, but swelling is not invariably present

Q **Did the pain begin before the swelling?** Usually the pain is present for many weeks before any swelling becomes apparent

- **Have you injured the part of the body where you have the pain?** Pain in a bone may only be brought to attention following minor trauma. Consider the diagnosis of osteosarcoma in adolescents whose pain or swelling following minor trauma appears to be disproportionately severe for the degree of trauma, or where the pain or swelling persist longer than expected
- **Do you have Paget's disease?** (Middle-aged and elderly patients.) There is an association between Paget's disease and an increased incidence of concomitant osteosarcoma. Any patient with Paget's disease who complains of a sudden increase in the intensity of bone pain, or a change in the site or nature of bone discomfort, needs full assessment and the possibility of a diagnosis of osteosarcoma should be borne in mind

Contributory or predisposing factors

- **Have you ever had any cancer or tumor?** There is a high relative risk of patients already treated for a childhood cancer later developing osteosarcoma. This is especially true of patients who have survived Ewing's sarcoma or retinoblastoma
- **If so, what treatment did you have?** Osteosarcoma is more common in patients who have received high-dose radiation therapy
- **Have you ever had any radiation therapy or worked with radiation or radioactive materials?** Osteosarcoma is also more common in patients who have been accidentally or occupationally exposed to radioactive materials in the past. The increased risk may last 40–50 years

Family history

- **Has anyone else in your family had any type of cancer?** There is a rare familial syndrome (the Li-Fraumeni syndrome) in which childhood sarcomas are associated with an increased incidence of cancer at an early stage in close relatives.

Examination

- **General examination:** may be entirely normal with no local signs
- **Examination of the limb or bone where pain is arising:** usually there is diffuse, firm swelling around the affected bone. The affected area may be tender or warm
- **Examination of the joints:** there may be limitation of movement of the nearest joint
- **Chest examination:** will usually be normal even if lung metastases are present

Summary of investigative tests

- Plain X-rays: plain X-rays of the affected bone should always be ordered as the initial investigation; a plain chest X-ray is needed to exclude lung metastases (present in 20% of cases at presentation)
- Biopsy of suspicious lesion: the result will confirm or refute the diagnosis (may be performed by a specialist)
- Isotope bone scan will help exclude skeletal metastases (normally performed by a specialist)
- Magnetic resonance imaging (MRI) scan of affected area and, if needed, of any areas of high isotope uptake on isotope bone scanning will delineate tumor extent and can determine the extent of the soft-tissue component and intramedullary extension (may be performed by a specialist)
- Computed tomographic (CT) scan of thorax. This is a more sensitive method of assessing the presence and extent of any lung metastasis (may be performed by a specialist)
- Serum alkaline phosphatase is frequently elevated and can be used as an approximate guide to disease activity

DIAGNOSTIC DECISION

The main recommendations for osteosarcoma management are that:

- The clinical diagnosis is based on appropriate clinical and radiologic findings
- The final diagnosis is pathologic and the biopsy should be performed by the surgeon who will subsequently perform the definitive surgery

- Surgical biopsy must be of adequate size and performed by an experienced surgeon
- The therapeutic strategy for osteosarcoma is based on surgery with neoadjuvant and adjuvant chemotherapy given in experienced centers. Inclusion of high-dose methotrexate is recommended for children, and the dose of methotrexate must be adapted for adults. Inclusion of children and adults clinical trials is recommended
- Treatment of metastatic osteosarcoma is based on chemotherapy and surgery to lung metastases which may be curative. Amputation is rarely appropriate. Inclusion of children and of adult clinical trials for metastatic osteosarcoma is recommended
- At the present time, there are no clear data on which to base guidelines for timing and duration of follow up studies in this condition

CLINICAL PEARLS

- There have been numerous identified prognostic features for patients with conventional localized high-grade osteosarcoma, including age, size of tumor, skip lesions, lactate dehydrogenase level, and alkaline phosphatase level
- MRI is the single most useful study in evaluating the intraosseous and extraosseous extent of the primary tumor and in detecting intramedullary or transarticular 'skip' metastases

THE TESTS

Body fluids

SERUM ALKALINE PHOSPHATASE

Description

Venous blood sample.

Advantages/Disadvantages

- Advantage: levels will be raised in some cases of osteosarcoma
- Disadvantage: there is weak correlation between tumor activity and serum alkaline phosphatase levels

Normal

30–120 IU/L.

Abnormal

- Keep in mind the possibility of a false-positive result
- Elevated levels are not specific for osteosarcoma

Cause of abnormal result

Increased osteocyte cell turnover.

Drugs, disorders and other factors that may alter results

- Levels may be raised due to physiologic bone growth in adolescence and puberty
- Biliary obstruction, cirrhosis, liver disease
- Paget's disease
- Osteomalacia
- Hyperthyroidism, hyperparathyroidism
- Bone metastases, other bone neoplasms
- Healing fractures
- Multiple myeloma
- Myelofibrosis
- Pregnancy
- Drugs such as estrogens, erythromycin, and phenothiazines

Biopsy

BONE BIOPSY

Description

- Bone biopsy for suspected osteosarcoma is best performed by a specialist
- Biopsy should be carried out only after an initial evaluation of the patient by an orthopedic oncologist familiar with the surgical management of the disease. An inappropriately performed biopsy may jeopardize a limb-sparing procedure
- Local, regional, or general anesthesia may be required, depending on the accessibility of the site to be biopsied and the age and wishes of the patient

Advantages/Disadvantages

Advantages:

- Allows accurate tissue diagnosis, therefore allowing planning of the most appropriate therapy
- May result in limb-sparing surgery

Disadvantages:

- Risks from anesthesia
- Bleeding
- Infection
- Inadequate or inappropriate material collected
- Contamination of superficial tissues with bone tumor

Abnormal

- Keep in mind the possibility of a falsely normal result
- The commonest histologic appearances are of anaplastic mesenchyma with foci of osteoid matrix
- Osteoblastic, chondroblastic, and fibroblastic areas can occur
- Classical osteosarcoma arises in the center of the bone
- Parosteal osteosarcoma arises in the diaphyses on the surface of the bone, and there is no medullary involvement

Imaging

PLAIN X-RAYS

Description

Plain X-rays of the bone carrying the suspected lesion, including films of the joints proximal and distal to any lesion, and a plain chest X-ray, are essential prerequisites before any other tests are contemplated in diagnosing osteosarcoma.

Advantages/Disadvantages

Advantages:

- Inexpensive
- Readily available
- False-negative results are uncommon
- The risks from radiation exposure are minimal, especially for X-rays of peripheral limbs and the chest

Abnormal

- Generally, there is a destructive lesion in the metaphyseal region of a long bone (typically the distal femur or proximal tibia)
- There is usually new bone formation, in spicules
- The lesion will stop at the unfused epiphysis, but not at the fused epiphysis
- There is destruction of the cortex, which may extend subperiosteally, lifting the periosteum (Codman's triangle)

- Parosteal osteosarcoma is associated with dense new bone formation and exostoses, with patchy calcification and involvement of the subadjacent medulla
- Chest X-ray may reveal typical appearances of secondary spread, pulmonary nodules, hilar lymphadenopathy, or malignant effusions
- Pulmonary metastases will be apparent on a plain chest X-ray in about 20–30% of cases of osteosarcoma at presentation

COMPUTED TOMOGRAPHY

Description

A CT scan of the affected region and of the chest may be essential in planning of the most appropriate management of osteosarcoma.

Advantages/Disadvantages

Advantages:

- Provides information on soft-tissue extension and can help locate calcification within the matrix of the tumor
- Can help localize tissues for biopsy or guide percutaneous biopsy
- Can help in planning tumor resection
- Can help evaluate disseminated disease
- Useful for patient follow up during and after therapy
- The most sensitive method of detecting pulmonary metastases and nodules

Disadvantage: relatively high radiation dose

MAGNETIC RESONANCE IMAGING

Advantages/Disadvantages

Advantages:

- MRI may complement the plain radiograph and CT scan
- Particularly useful for defining the intramedullary extent of the growth
- Can help assess soft-tissue spread
- Can help assess the response to chemotherapy
- Can help assess the presence of skip lesions in the medulla
- Noninvasive
- No radiation exposure

Disadvantages:

- Expensive
- Spatial resolution is better with CT scanning

CONSIDER CONSULT

- Any patient in whom the diagnosis of osteosarcoma is a possibility, whether on clinical or radiologic grounds
- Refer to an orthopedic oncologist in a center which has experience in managing such tumors, and which has a multidisciplinary team able to meet the needs of the patient
- Any patient whose symptoms and signs suggest a possibility of osteosarcoma should receive X-rays of the suspected bones and of the chest

IMMEDIATE ACTION

- If a patient is receiving chemotherapy and becomes febrile or unwell, contact the patient's specialist urgently
- If such advice is not available, arrange emergency room assessment

PATIENT AND CAREGIVER ISSUES

Impact on career, dependants, family, friends

- A diagnosis of malignancy is devastating at any age, but may be particularly so in children and young adults
- The patient will have anxieties and fears about possible amputation and the subsequent effects on self-esteem, self-confidence, and on future employment and career choice
- There may also be profound emotional and psychologic effects on the patient's family (especially parents and siblings), friends, and school or college colleagues
- If the osteosarcoma occurs in a patient previously successfully treated for another cancer, the emotional and psychologic effects may be even more profound

Patient or caregiver request

- **Can I be cured of my cancer?** Many patients, especially the young, consider the prognosis of all cancers to be worse than the reality
- **Will I need amputation or other destructive surgery?** This is often the worst fear, and may not be readily apparent
- **Will I die?** Many children and young adults are afraid of death and of voicing their fears

Health-seeking behavior

- **How much have you heard or read about your condition so far?** Many patients will have read, talked about, or looked up their condition in books, magazines, or on the Internet
- **Where did this information come from?** Make sure the patient's sources of information are reliable and sensible
- **What would you like to discuss first?** Allow the patient and their family to set the agenda for the exchanges of information

MANAGEMENT ISSUES

Goals

- To cure the patient
- To salvage the affected limb, if at all possible
- If limb salvage is not possible, to provide comprehensive and ongoing rehabilitation, both physical and psychologic, and help with reintegration and employment
- If cure is impossible, to provide the best possible quality of life for as long as possible
- To meet the physical, emotional, social, and psychologic needs of the patient and their caregivers

Management in special circumstances

- The risks and benefits of surgical and nonsurgical management options need to be fully discussed

- If there is a strong possibility of curing the tumor by amputation plus chemotherapy, the patient's informed wishes must be taken into account
- Cure at all costs may need to be altered to a slightly lower probability of cure with the avoidance of amputation or mutilating surgery

SPECIAL PATIENT GROUPS

Osteosarcoma is primarily a disorder of children and young adults, so the needs and wants of the patient and their family or carers must be taken in to account.

PATIENT SATISFACTION/LIFESTYLE PRIORITIES

- Patients and their carers must decide whether limb amputation improves the prognosis significantly enough to justify the procedure
- The positive effects of life with a prosthetic limb should not be ignored; participation in most occupations and many sports is still possible
- Meeting other patients who have undergone amputations may be helpful

SUMMARY OF THERAPEUTIC OPTIONS

Choices

- It is imperative that patients with proven or suspected osteosarcoma have an initial evaluation by an orthopedic oncologist familiar with the surgical management of this disease. This evaluation should be done prior to the initial biopsy, as an inappropriately performed biopsy may jeopardize a limb-sparing procedure
- Randomized clinical trials have established that both neoadjuvant and adjuvant chemotherapy are effective in preventing relapse in patients with nonmetastatic occult tumors
- Multidrug chemotherapy is the mainstay of therapy. The introduction of intensive and complex chemotherapy has led to a dramatic increase in the survival for patients with osteosarcoma
- Chemotherapy is employed before surgery (induction or neoadjuvant chemotherapy) using combinations of cisplatin, carboplatin, cyclophosphamide, doxorubicin, etoposide, and methotrexate, as well as postoperatively. More recently, ifosfamide has been added
- Surgery is also usually required in the treatment of osteosarcoma, but amputations are being replaced by conservative surgery. Massive internal prostheses are inserted after removal of the tumor. Functional results are better for femoral and tibial tumors than for humeral ones. Conservative limb-preserving surgery is also successfully used for pelvic tumors
- The use of preoperative chemotherapy allows systemic treatment to be started early, allows time for the production of an endoprosthesis, allows for shrinking of the tumor, making surgery easier, and allowing histologic assessment of response when the tumor is resected
- The treatment of pulmonary metastases is similar to that of the primary tumor – adjuvant chemotherapy followed by surgical excision of the metastasis then further chemotherapy. Computed tomographic (CT) scanning should always be used. Adjuvant chemotherapy after amputation or surgery may delay or prevent pulmonary metastases but may also reduce the number of metastases when they do occur
- For lesions that cannot be surgically removed, intensive chemotherapy and high-dose, localized radiation is used

Clinical pearls

- Neoadjuvant chemotherapy increases the number of patients who are able to undergo a limb-sparing operation instead of amputation. For patients who receive chemotherapy prior to surgery, the degree of tumor necrosis observed postoperatively is highly predictive of disease-free survival, local recurrence, and overall survival
- The only feature that consistently predicts outcome is the degree of histologic necrosis following induction chemotherapy. Patients with >95% necrosis in the primary tumor after induction chemotherapy have a better prognosis than those with lesser amounts of necrosis
- If limb-sparing is contemplated, the biopsy should be performed by the surgeon who will do the definitive operation, as incision placement is crucial

Never

Never assume a patient will require amputation until he or she has been fully assessed by a specialist with experience in managing osteosarcoma.

FOLLOW UP

All patients should be carefully followed up for at least 5 years. Full evaluation of the local site and of the lungs should be undertaken.

Plan for review

- There should be postoperative evaluation of the local site, including radiography, at 3, 6, and 12 months, then at 2, 3, and 5 years, and symptomatically thereafter
- CT scans of the chest should also be taken at these times
- Local recurrence should be evaluated using plain X-rays and magnetic resonance imaging (MRI) if there is no significant hardware present, and by plain X-rays alone if there is significant hardware present (unless the type and location of the hardware allow MRI scanning)

Information for patient or caregiver

- Osteosarcoma is an uncommon cancer of the bone
- Recent advances in therapy have led to considerable improvements in prognosis (expect a 70–75% 5-year survival rate)
- Amputation is avoided if at all possible

DRUGS AND OTHER THERAPIES: DETAILS

Surgical therapy

- Surgical removal of the primary tumor is the mainstay of managing osteosarcoma
- Limb-sparing surgery is carried out if at all possible, involving removal of the malignant bone tumor without amputation and replacement of bones and joints with allografts or prosthetic devices
- If limb-sparing surgery is contemplated, the biopsy should be performed by the surgeon who will do the definitive procedure
- Surgical removal of pulmonary metastases should be attempted following adjuvant chemotherapy as for primary tumors

SURGICAL REMOVAL OF THE PRIMARY TUMOR

Surgery can be by local excision, amputation, or rotationplasty.

Efficacy

- Adequate surgical excision of the primary tumor remains the best chance of cure, especially when combined with adjuvant chemotherapy
- Surgery should be undertaken only after adequate imaging to delineate the extent of the tumor
- Surgery should only be attempted by a specialist with experience in orthopedic cancer, and who is part of a specialist multidisciplinary team

Risks/Benefits

Risks:

- Anesthesia
- Bleeding
- Infection
- Poor wound healing

Benefits:

- Increased survival
- Increased chance of retaining a functional limb
- Reduced risk of malignant spread

Acceptability to patient

- As surgery offers the best chance of cure, it is generally highly acceptable
- The decision to amputate or attempt tumor removal and prosthesis insertion needs to be agreed by the specialist team and the fully informed patient and carers
- Remember that amputation and the fitting of a good prosthesis may allow quicker and better final functional outcomes than limb salvage surgery

Follow up plan

Follow up should be for at least 5 years, irrespective of the type of surgery carried out.

Patient and caregiver information

- The option of amputation or limb salvage surgery needs careful consideration
- Intensive rehabilitation will be necessary, especially if a prosthetic limb is fitted

Chemotherapy

COMBINATION CHEMOTHERAPY

The chemotherapy protocols for the management of osteosarcoma currently include combinations of the following agents:

- Cisplatin
- Carboplatin
- Cyclophosphamide
- Doxorubicin
- Ifosfamide
- Etoposide
- High-dose methotrexate

Efficacy

Overall relapse-free survival rates vary from 50–80% in trials using these agents in combination.

Risks/Benefits

Risks:

- The short-term risks of neutropenia, granulopenia, and anemia can be life-threatening
- Side-effects such as severe nausea, diarrhea, vomiting, asthenia, anorexia, hair loss, and pruritus can be very troublesome

Benefit: using these agents in combination with surgery significantly increases the overall osteosarcoma survival rate

Acceptability to patient

Overall, the dramatic increase in survival from using combinations of these agents far outweighs the negative side-effects, therefore, their acceptability is high.

Follow up plan

Follow up is recommended at 1, 3, and 6 months, and at 1, 2, 3, and 5 years postoperation.

Patient and caregiver information

Information about ongoing clinical trials is available from the National Cancer Institute.

CISPLATIN

Given under specialist instruction; dose is based on body surface area calculation.

Risks/Benefits

Risks:

- Must be administered under specialist supervision
- Should not be used in patients with hearing impairment
- Should not be used in myelosuppressed patients
- Use caution with renal impairment
- Peripheral blood counts should be monitored weekly

Benefits:

- Decreases tumor size
- Decreases risk of recurrence
- Improves survival
- Increased likelihood of limb salvage

Side-effects and adverse reactions

- Central nervous system: fatigue
- Eyes, ears, nose, and throat: ototoxicity
- Gastrointestinal: nausea, vomiting, anorexia
- Genitourinary: sexual dysfunction
- Hematologic: bone marrow suppression
- Metabolic: renal toxicity
- Skin: alopecia

Interactions (other drugs)

■ Unstable in D_5W ■ May precipitate with aluminum ■ Should not be mixed with metoclopramide, sodium bicarbonate solutions, sodium thiosulfate, 5-fluorouracil, or mesna ■ Pyridoxine plus hexmethylmelamine (may affect response duration)

Contraindications

■ Hypersensitivity to cisplatin or platinum-containing preparations ■ Renal impairment

CARBOPLATIN

Given under specialist instruction; dose is based on body surface area calculation.

Risks/Benefits

Risks:

- Must be administered under specialist supervision
- Will typically cause nausea, vomiting, tiredness, fall in white cell count, hair loss, and neuropathy
- Bone marrow suppression is dose related and may be severe, resulting in infection and/or bleeding. Anemia may be cumulative and may require transfusion support
- Should not be employed in patients with severe bone marrow depression or significant bleeding
- Bone marrow suppression is increased in patients who have received prior therapy, especially regimens including cisplatin
- Carboplatin has limited nephrotoxic potential, but concomitant treatment with aminoglycosides has resulted in increased renal and/or audiologic toxicity

Side-effects and adverse reactions

- Cardiovascular system: bradycardia, hypotension
- Central nervous system: infections, peripheral neuropathy, ototoxicty, asthenia

- Gastrointestinal: diarrhea, nausea, vomiting, mucositis
- Hematologic: neutropenia, leukopenia, thrombocytopenia, anemia
- Musculoskeletal: arthralgia, myalgia
- Skin: alopecia

Interactions (other drugs)

Nephrotoxic compounds (may potentiate renal effects of these compounds).

Contraindications

■ Safety and efficacy in pediatric patients have not been established ■ Pregnancy category D ■ Breast-feeding ■ Patients with a history of severe allergic reactions to cisplatin or other platinum-containing compounds, or mannitol

CYCLOPHOSPHAMIDE

Given under specialist instruction; dose is based on body surface area calculation.

Risks/Benefits

Risks:

- Use caution when administering with radiation therapy
- The risks of bone marrow supression and hepatotoxicity must be weighed against the limited evidence for real therapeutic benefit in established renal involvement in Henoch-Schoenlein purpura

Benefits:

- Decreased tumor size
- Increased likelihood of limb salvage
- Decreased risk of recurrence
- Improves survival

Side-effects and adverse reactions

- Cardiovascular system: cardiotoxicity (at high doses)
- Central nervous system: dizziness, headache
- Gastrointestinal: nausea, vomiting, diarrhea
- Genitourinary: amenorrhea, azoospermia, ovarian fibrosis, sterility, hematuria, hemorrhagic cystitis, neoplasms
- Hematologic: leukopenia, myelosuppression, panycytopenia, thrombocytopenia
- Metabolic: bone marrow supression
- Respiratory: fibrosis
- Skin: alopecia, dermatitis

Interactions (other drugs)

■ Phenobarbital increases the metabolism rate and leukopenic activity of cyclophosphamide ■ Cyclophosphamide causes a marked and persistent inhibition of cholinesterase activity and potentiates the effect of succinylcholine chloride ■ If a patient has been treated with cyclophosphamide within 10 days of general anesthesia, the anesthesiologist should be alerted

Contraindications

■ Serious infections, including chicken pox and herpes zoster ■ Myelosuppression ■ Hypersensitivity to cyclophosphamide

DOXORUBICIN

Given under specialist instruction; dose is based on body surface area calculation.

Risks/Benefits
Risks:
- Must be administered under specialist supervision
- Will typically cause nausea, vomiting, tiredness, fall in white cell count, hair loss, and neuropathy
- Special attention must be given to the cardiotoxicity induced by doxorubicin
- Cardiomyopathy and/or congestive heart failure may be encountered several months or years after discontinuation of doxorubicin therapy

Benefits:
- Decreased tumor size
- Increased likelihood of limb salvage
- Decreased risk of recurrence
- Improves survival

Side-effects and adverse reactions
- Cardiovascular system: cardiotoxicity, phlebosclerosis
- Central nervous system: acute nausea and vomiting, mucositis, peripheral neurotoxicity
- Eyes, ears, nose, and throat: conjunctivitis, and lacrimation
- Hematologic: secondary acute myeloid leukemia
- Hypersensitivity reactions: fever, chills, urticaria
- Genitourinary: red coloration to the urine for 1–2 days after administration
- Skin: severe cellulitis, vesication, and tissue necrosis

Interactions (other drugs)
■ Paclitaxel ■ Progesterone ■ Verapamil ■ Cyclosporine

Contraindications
■ Hypersensitivity to doxorubicin ■ Pregnancy category D ■ Breast-feeding ■ Marked myelosuppression induced by previous treatment with other antitumor agents or by radiotherapy ■ Previous treatment with complete cumulative doses of doxorubicin, daunorubicin, idarubicin, and/or other anthracyclines and anthracenes

ETOPOSIDE
Given under specialist instruction; dose is based on body surface area calculation.

Risks/Benefits
Risks:
- Specialist supervision required
- Patients being treated with etoposide must be frequently observed for myelosuppression
- Risk of anaphylactic reaction manifested by chills, fever, tachycardia, bronchospasm, dyspnea, and hypotension

Benefits:
- Decreased tumor size
- Increased likelihood of limb salvage
- Decreased risk of recurrence
- Improves survival

Side-effects and adverse reactions
- Hematologic: anemia, thrombocytopenia, leukopenia
- Gastrointestinal: nausea, vomiting, abdominal pain, anorexia, stomatitis
- Skin: alopecia

Interactions (other drugs)

None listed.

Contraindications

■ Safety and effectiveness in pediatric patients have not been established ■ Pregnancy category D ■ Hypersensitivity to etoposide

IFOSFAMIDE

Given under specialist instruction; dose is based on body surface area calculation.

Risks/Benefits

Risks:

- Must be administered under specialist supervision
- Risks of hemorrhagic cystitis, confusion, and coma
- Should not be used with severely depressed bone marrow function
- Use caution with renal impairment

Benefits:

- Decreased tumor size
- Increased likelihood of limb salvage
- Decreased risk of recurrence

Side-effects and adverse reactions

- Cardiovascular system: cardiotoxicity, hypotension, hypertension
- Central nervous system: toxicity, somnolence, confusion, hallucinations, coma, fever
- Gastrointestinal: nausea, vomiting, anorexia, constipation
- Genitourinary: urotoxic side-effects, hemorrhagic cystitis
- Hematologic: severe myelosuppression, hematuria
- Metabolic: renal impairment, liver impairment
- Skin: alopecia, dermatitis, delayed wound healing

Interactions (other drugs)

None known.

Contraindications

■ Known hypersensitivity to ifosfamide ■ Severely depressed bone marrow function ■ Pregnancy and breast-feeding ■ Safety and efficacy in children have not been established

METHOTREXATE

Given under specialist instruction; dose is based on body surface area calculation.

Efficacy

Overall relapse-free survival rates vary from 50–80% in trials using these agents in combination.

Risks/Benefits

Risks:

- Increased likelihood of limb salvage
- Many side-effects

Benefits:
- Improves survival
- Decreased tumor size
- Decreased risk of recurrence

Side-effects and adverse reactions
- Central nervous system: dizziness, headaches, malaise, undue fatigue
- Cardiovascular: hypotension, pericarditis, pericardial effusion
- Gastrointestinal: nausea, vomiting, abdominal distress, ulcerative stomatitis
- Hematologic: leukopenia, decreased resistance to infection
- Other: chills and fever

Interactions (other drugs)

■ Nonsteroidal anti-inflammatory drugs should not be administered prior to or concomitantly with the high doses of methotrexate because it has been reported to elevate and prolong serum methotrexate levels, resulting in deaths from severe hematologic and gastrointestinal toxicity ■ Toxicity may be increased by certain drugs, such as salicylates, phenylbutazone, phenytoin, and sulfonamides. Renal tubular transport is also diminished by probenecid and use of methotrexate with this drug should be carefully monitored ■ In the treatment of patients with osteosarcoma, caution must be exercised if high-dose methotrexate is administered in combination with a potentially nephrotoxic chemotherapeutic agent (e.g. cisplatin) ■ Penicillins may reduce the renal clearance of methotrexate; increasing hematologic and gastrointestinal toxicities

Contraindications

■ Pregnancy ■ Breast-feeding ■ Chronic liver disease ■ Hypersensitivity to methotrexate ■ Patients with overt or laboratory evidence of immunodeficiency syndromes ■ Patients with pre-existing blood dyscrasias, such as bone marrow hypoplasia, leukopenia, thrombocytopenia, or significant anemia

Acceptability to patient

Patients (mainly younger patients) might be reluctant in accepting chemotherapy due to side-effects such as nausea and vomiting and also alopecia which implies a change in appearance.

Follow up plan

Will vary according to chemotherapy scheme adopted.

Patient and caregiver information
- It has to be clear that it is a long course of treatment involving many visits to the hospital and innumerous blood examinations to control neutropenia and infection
- The side-effects will sometimes cause discomfort to the patient, and life-threatening infections might occur due to neutropenia
- Although difficult to go through, chemotherapy has an undeniable impact in treating osteosarcoma and this has to be clearly stated both to patient and caregiver

OUTCOMES

EFFICACY OF THERAPIES

- The most effective management of osteosarcoma is the use of preoperative combination chemotherapy, followed by surgical removal of the primary tumor (preferably by using limb-salvage procedures and avoiding amputation), and postoperative chemotherapy using the same combinations of agents
- Adjuvant chemotherapy using combinations which include high-dose methotrexate, doxorubicin, cyclophosphamide, cisplatin, etoposide, carboplatin, and ifosfamide has been shown to result in overall relapse-free survival rates from 50–80%

Treatment options for nonmetastatic, completely resectable high-grade osteosarcoma are:

- Preoperative chemotherapy followed by extirpative surgery (amputation, limb salvage, or rotationplasty)
- Postoperative pathologic evaluation of the tumor measures the degree of response to the initial chemotherapy
- If the tumor shows evidence of response to the chemotherapy combination, the combination is continued
- If the tumor did not respond, an alternative regimen is used

Review period

Patients should be reviewed at 1, 3, and 6 months after surgery and then at years 1, 2, 3, and 5.

PROGNOSIS

- Overall, about 70–80% of patients with osteosarcoma will be alive and disease-free 5 years after diagnosis
- Patients with localized disease have a better prognosis than those with overt metastatic disease
- Axial skeleton primary tumors have the greatest risk of progression and death
- Resectability of the tumor is the most important prognostic feature
- Osteosarcomas of the facial bones and other flat bones have a good prognosis if the bone is removed
- Patients with osteosarcoma as a second malignancy share the same prognosis as patients with newly diagnosed disease if they are treated with surgery and multiagent chemotherapy
- Adults who have osteosarcomas associated with Paget's disease or with previous exposure to ionizing radiation have a much poorer prognosis. Such tumors are usually not amenable to extirpation, and adjuvant chemotherapy has not yet proved effective in prolonging survival in these patients
- The most important prognostic feature is the histologic response to preoperative chemotherapy
- Patients with >95% necrosis in the primary tumor after induction of chemotherapy have a better prognosis than those with lesser amounts of necrosis

- Up to 20% of patients have radiologically detectable metastases at diagnosis
- Overall event-free survival is about 20% for patients with metastases at diagnosis, although this proportion may rise if the metastases are few or single and can be completely excised
- The prognosis after metastectomy is better if the lesions are unilateral, if there are fewer than six, if they are entirely resected, and if they appear late after chemotherapy has stopped
- Event-free survival for malignant fibrous histiocytoma and osteosarcoma are similar

Clinical pearls

- Patients requesting limb-sparing operations do not appear to be at greater risk for development of local or distant relapse than patients having transmedullary amputations
- The administration of sequential multiagent adjuvant chemotherapy has significantly improved the disease-free survival for patients without metastasis
- The risk of local recurrence appears to be no greater in patients completing limb-preserving procedures than for those having an amputation

Therapeutic failure

- If conventional therapy fails or is not possible, patients should be enrolled in a clinical trial which will usually involve high-dose chemotherapy plus radiation
- Details of these trails can be found on the National Cancer Institute's website

Recurrence

- Recurrence of osteosarcoma occurs most commonly in the lungs
- Treatment should be by surgical excision, if possible, and chemotherapy
- The prognosis is poor for patients with bony metastases, especially if they are multiple or unresectable
- Patients who relapse with a local recurrence have a worse prognosis (<10% survival at 5 years) than patients who relapse with metastases alone (25% disease-free survival at 5 years)

Deterioration

Deterioration can be from local relapse or from later metastases.

Terminal illness

- Care of the terminally ill will include the provision of adequate analgesia and antinausea management
- Emotional and psychologic help will also be needed

CONSIDER CONSULT

Any patient who has had treatment for osteosarcoma should be referred back to the specialist center which treated the patient if there are any symptoms and signs of local recurrence or metastases (usually to the lungs and bones). Symptoms and signs may include pain and swelling of or around any bone, cough, chest pain, or hemoptysis.

PREVENTION

- As the causes of osteosarcoma are not proven, there are no generally agreed preventative measures specific for this disorder
- Refinements in the management of other malignancies, such as retinoblastoma, may reduce the frequency of subsequent osteosarcoma in these patients
- Exposure to ionizing radiation, especially in the workplace, should be avoided

RISK FACTORS

- Second cancers: patients previously treated for another primary malignancy (such as Ewing's sarcoma and retinoblastoma) are at slightly greater risks of developing later osteosarcoma
- Paget's disease: there is an association with the secondary development of osteosarcoma. It is not known why this is, and the association appears unrelated to the therapies used to manage the Paget's disease
- Ionizing radiation: workers exposed to radium in the early 20th century led to high rates of radium poisoning and later development of osteosarcomas of the distal skeleton. The cumulative risk of developing osteosarcoma was as high as 70% over the ensuing 50 years
- External beam radiation: can result in soft-tissue or bone sarcomas (including osteosarcoma) in 1/3000–5000 treated patients, with a latency period of 5–30 years
- Li-Fraumeni syndrome: relatives of patients with this syndrome are at higher risk of developing osteosarcomas and other tumors

MODIFY RISK FACTORS

Reduce or eliminate exposure to ionizing radiation.

SCREENING

- Screening for osteosarcoma is not recommended at present as the screening method would need to use X-rays, and the risk:benefit ratio is not proven
- It is not known whether screening patients who have survived a primary cancer such as Ewing's sarcoma or retinoblastoma, or who have Paget's disease, or who have relatives with Li-Fraumeni syndrome is worthwhile
- Currently, screening is not recommended

PREVENT RECURRENCE

Complete surgical excision of the primary tumor, and of any pulmonary metastases, with intensive chemotherapy, will reduce recurrence rates.

ASSOCIATIONS

National Cancer Information Service
Public Information Office
Building 31, Room 10A03
32 Center Road, MSC 2580
Bethesda, MD 20892–2580
Tel: (800) 4-CANCER (800) 422-6237)
www.cancer.gov

American Cancer Society
1599 Clifton Road NE
Atlanta, GA 30329–4257
Tel: (404) 320-3333
Toll-free: (800) ACS-2345
www.cancer.org

National Comprehensive Cancer Network
50 Huntingdon Drive, Suite 200
Rockledge, PA 19046
Tel: (215) 728-4788
Fax: (215) 728-3877
E-mail: information@nccn.org
www.nccn.org

American Society of Clinical Oncology
1900 Duke Street, Suite 200
Alexandria, VA 22314
Tel: (703) 299-0150
Fax: (703) 299-1044
E-mail: asco@asco.org
www.asco.org

KEY REFERENCES

- Agarwal S, Agarwal T. Fine needle aspiration of bone tumors. Cancer Detect Prev 2000;24:602–9
- Berquist TH, Dalinka MK. Bone tumors. American College of Radiology. ACR Appropriateness Criteria. Radiology 2000;215:261–4
- Shin KH, Moon SH. Tumor volume change as a predictor of chemotherapeutic response in osteosarcoma. Clin Orthop 2000;376:200–8
- Philip T, Blay JY. Osteosarcoma. Br J Cancer 2001;84:78–80
- Weeden S, Grimer RJ. The effect of local recurrence on survival in resected osteosarcoma. Eur J Cancer 2001;37:39–46
- Davis AM, Bell RS, Goodwin PJ. Prognostic factors in osteosarcoma: a critical review. J Clin Oncol 1994;12:423–31. Review
- Smith MA, Ungerleider RS. Influence of doxorubicin dose intensity on response and outcome for patients with osteogenic sarcoma and Ewing's sarcoma. J Natl Cancer Inst 1991;83:1460–70
- Philip T, Blay JY. Standards, options and recommendations (SOR) for diagnosis, treatment and follow-up of osteosarcoma. Groupe de travail SOR [in French]. Bull Cancer 1999;86:159–76. Review
- Chuman H. Evidence-based chemotherapy for patients with bone and soft part sarcoma [in Japanese]. Gan To Kagaku Ryoho 2000;27:192–202. Review
- Link MP. The multi-institutional osteosarcoma study: an update. Cancer Treat Res 1993;62:261–7

FAQS

Question 1

Why can't I or the general surgeon in my service perform the biopsy?

ANSWER 1

Because it might change the patient's prognosis concerning the definitive surgery. If limb-sparing (removal of the malignant bone tumor without amputation and replacement of bones or joints with allografts or prosthetic devices) is contemplated, the biopsy should be performed by the surgeon who will do the definitive operation, as incision placement is crucial.

Question 2

Is there any difference in survival depending upon the kind of surgery performed?

ANSWER 2

There is no difference in overall survival between patients treated by amputation and those treated with a limb-sparing procedure. Limb-sparing procedures should be planned only when the preoperative staging indicates that it is possible to achieve wide surgical margins. If the pathologic examination of the surgical specimen shows inadequate margins, an immediate amputation should be considered, especially if the histologic response to preoperative chemotherapy was poor.

Question 3

What is the role of chemotherapy in the treatment of osteosarcoma?

ANSWER 3

Neoadjuvant chemotherapy increases the number of patients who are able to undergo a limb-sparing operation instead of amputation. For patients who receive preoperative chemotherapy, the degree of tumor necrosis observed postoperatively is highly predictive of overall survival. Adjuvant chemotherapy is effective in preventing relapse or recurrence in patients with localized resectable primary tumors and both neoadjuvant and adjuvant chemotherapy are effective in preventing relapse in patients with nonmetastatic occult tumors.

Question 4

What are the prognostic factors for osteosarcoma?

ANSWER 4

- Patients with localized disease have a much better prognosis than those with metastatic disease
- The site of the primary tumor is important. Axial skeleton primary tumors have the greatest risk of progression and death
- Resectability of the tumor is the most important prognostic feature because this tumor is very resistant to radiation therapy
- Other factors include age of patient, size of tumor, skip lesions, lactate dehydrogenase level, and alkaline phosphatase level
- The only feature that consistently predicts outcome is the degree of histologic necrosis following induction chemotherapy. Patients with >95% necrosis in the primary tumor after induction chemotherapy have a better prognosis than those with lesser amounts of necrosis

CONTRIBUTORS

Gordon H Baustian, MD
Luciana G O Clark, MD
Januario E Castro, MD

PANCREATIC CANCER

SUMMARY INFORMATION

DESCRIPTION

- Pancreatic cancer is the fourth leading cause of cancer death in men and the fifth in women
- Often presents late with advanced disease
- 5-year survival for all patients with pancreatic cancer is only 3%
- Histologically, 95% are adenocarcinomas arising from duct cells
- Surgical resection offers prospect for cure in small tumors (<2cm) limited to the pancreas

URGENT ACTION

- Evidence of life-threatening gastrointestinal hemorrhage mandates immediate surgical or endoscopic intervention
- Evidence of deep vein thrombosis secondary to malignancy requires anticoagulation

KEY! DON'T MISS!

- Rapidly progressive abdominal pain with raised amylase indicative of acute pancreatitis
- Biliary colic and jaundice accompanied by fever and chills (Charcot's triad) with or without evidence of sepsis indicative of acute cholangitis
- Deep vein thrombosis secondary to malignancy

ICD9 CODE

- 157.9 Neoplasm, pancreas
- 157.0 Neoplasm, pancreas: head
- 157.1 Neoplasm, pancreas: body
- 157.8 Neoplasm, pancreas: neck
- 157.2 Neoplasm, pancreas: tail

SYNONYMS

Pancreatic adenocarcinoma.

CARDINAL FEATURES

- Most commonly diagnosed in sixth and seventh decades of life
- Most arise in the ductal epithelium of pancreatic head as adenocarcinoma
- Four-fifths of patients present with advanced disease
- Frequently characterized by jaundice, epigastric or back pain, and cachexia
- May result in biliary or pancreatic duct obstruction and cause ascending cholangitis or pancreatitis
- Poor prognosis regardless of treatment

CAUSES

Common causes

Unknown.

Rare causes

Familial pancreatic cancer may be present in 3–5% of cases.

Contributory or predisposing factors

- Cigarette smoking increases risk 2- to 3-fold
- Diabetes mellitus type 1, especially juvenile onset, and long-standing diabetes mellitus type 2 increase risk 2- to 3-fold
- New onset diabetes is probably an independent marker for pancreatic cancer as well
- History of gastric resection increases risk 2- to 3-fold
- Pernicious anemia increases risk 2- to 3-fold
- Chronic pancreatitis
- Alcohol use
- Cholelithiasis
- High-fat, animal protein diet
- N-nitroso compounds found in processed meat products are known carcinogens for laboratory animals but have not been directly linked to pancreatic cancers in humans
- The contribution of caffeine to pancreatic cancer is controversial

EPIDEMIOLOGY

Incidence and prevalence

INCIDENCE

- 0.1/1000 for men
- 0.072/1000 for women
- 0.12/1000 for African-Americans

FREQUENCY

- 29,000 new cases per year in US
- 28,900 deaths ascribed to this cancer

Demographics

AGE

- Rare before age 50
- Peak incidence seen in the sixth and seventh decades of life

GENDER

- Pancreatic cancer is slightly more common in males than in females. This difference is most prominent in younger patients
- Recent trends indicate that the incidence is approaching 1:1 as pancreatic cancer becomes more common in women

RACE

- More common in African-Americans who carry an excess risk of 30–40% compared with Caucasians
- Less common in Asians and Hispanics

GENETICS

- Rare familial clusters of pancreatic cancer have been described
- 7% of patients with pancreatic cancer have a family history of pancreatic cancer
- Ki-ras mutations found in 85–90% of pancreatic cancers
- Mutations in p16INK4 result in 13-fold increase in pancreatic cancer
- C-erb B12 oncogene seen in 20% of pancreatic cancers
- Inactivated p53 seen in 50–70% of pancreatic cancers

DIFFERENTIAL DIAGNOSIS

Chronic pancreatitis

The key features of chronic pancreatitis are as follows:

FEATURES

- Like pancreatic cancer, may present with epigastric/back pain; weight loss; pancreatic mass; and elevated serum CA 19-9, bilirubin, and alkaline phosphatase level
- Patients with chronic pancreatitis usually have history of recurrent pancreatitis
- Definite differential diagnosis needs biopsy of the pancreatic mass

Cholangiocarcinoma

A bile duct cancer that can involve extrahepatic or intrahepatic bile ducts.

FEATURES

- Like pancreatic cancer, can present with jaundice, abdominal pain, pruritus, weight loss, elevated transaminase/bilirubin
- Endoscopic retrograde cholangiopancreatography (ERCP) with cholangiogram can identify the site of tumor involvement
- May be associated with primary sclerosing cholangitis, *Clonorchis sinensis*, and ulcerative colitis

Ampulla of Vater adenocarcinoma

The key features of this type of adenocarcinoma are as follows:

FEATURES

- Like pancreatic cancer, can present with pancreatitis; jaundice; abdominal tenderness; palpable gallbladder; and elevated alkaline phosphatase, bilirubin, transaminase, and amylase
- May be associated with familial polyposis and Gardner's syndrome

Endocrine tumors of pancreas

Rare tumors, representing 5% of pancreatic cancers and include insulinoma, glucagonoma, VIPoma, somatostatinoma, GRFoma, PPoma, and nonfunctioning pancreatic endocrine tumors.

FEATURES

Symptoms often depend on hormones secreted by the tumor and can include symptoms related to hypoglycemia or hyperglycemia, muscle spasm, skin flushing, and diarrhea.

Rare pancreatic tumors

Uncommon forms of pancreatic tumors include acinar carcinoma, cystadenocarcinomas, epidermoid carcinomas, unclassified large cell or small cell carcinoma, lymphomas, and sarcomas.

FEATURES

- Prognosis may be significantly better in the case of lymphoma compared with pancreatic adenocarcinoma
- Rare pancreatic tumors may be associated with multiple endocrine neoplasia syndrome

SIGNS & SYMPTOMS

Signs

- Cachexia
- Jaundice
- Excoriations from pruritus

- Glucose intolerance
- Palpable gallbladder (Courvoisier's law states that a palpable, nontender gallbladder is unlikely to be due to stones in a patient with obstructive jaundice)
- Palpable pancreatic mass
- Ascites
- Supraclavicular lymph node enlargement
- Venous thrombosis
- Migratory superficial phlebitis (Trousseau's syndrome)
- Pancreatitis
- Gastric outlet obstruction
- Hepatomegaly
- Splenomegaly
- Hemorrhage from duodenum erosion by cancer
- Blood-positive stool

Symptoms

Symptoms are usually vague and nonspecific and thus contribute to delayed diagnosis:

- Jaundice with or without dark urine, pale claylike stool, pruritus
- Abdominal/epigastric pain that is gnawing, often radiating to back, indicative of advanced disease (70–90%)
- Weight loss (70–100%)
- Anorexia
- Weakness
- Leg/back pain
- Psychiatric complaints (e.g. depression), sense of dread or of impending doom
- Melena
- Steatorrhea from pancreatic exocrine insufficiency

KEY! DON'T MISS!

- Rapidly progressive abdominal pain with raised amylase indicative of acute pancreatitis
- Biliary colic and jaundice accompanied by fever and chills (Charcot's triad) with or without evidence of sepsis indicative of acute cholangitis
- Deep vein thrombosis secondary to malignancy

CONSIDER CONSULT

- Refer to surgeon for possible laparoscopy if imaging studies fail to locate tumor but clinical suspicion remains high
- Refer to gastroenterologist for endoscopy if imaging studies fail to locate tumor but clinical suspicion remains high

INVESTIGATION OF THE PATIENT

Direct questions to patient

- Q **When did your symptoms begin?** Early pancreatic cancer is often asymptomatic, with symptoms appearing late in the disease
- Q **How is your appetite?** Many patients with pancreatic cancer are anorexic
- Q **Have you been losing weight?** Weight loss is a common finding in pancreatic cancer, resulting from anorexia
- Q **Have you noticed any dark urine or pale stools?** Jaundice secondary to biliary obstruction is an early manifestation of pancreatic cancer
- Q **Do you have any pain?** Patients with pancreatic cancer often complain of gnawing epigastric pain that may radiate to the back
- Q **Does your pain improve when leaning forward?** Abdominal pain that improves when flexing the trunk forward is frequently pancreatic in origin

Q **Have you noticed any black stools or blood from your rectum?** Periampullary tumors may cause heme-positive stool. Gastric varices result from portal hypertension

Q **Have you ever vomited blood or ground coffee-like material?** Bleeding from duodenal erosion can cause heme-positive stool, bright red blood per rectum, melena, and hematemesis

Q **Have you been experiencing excessive thirst, urination, or eating?** Patients with pancreatic cancer can develop glucose intolerance with diabetic symptomatology

Q **Have you had leg pain or noticed that one leg is bigger than the other?** Many cancers induce hypercoagulable states that can lead to deep vein thrombosis

Contributory or predisposing factors

Q **Do you smoke?** Tobacco abuse is a risk factor for pancreatic cancer

Q **Do you have diabetes?** Long-standing type I or II diabetes is a risk factor for pancreatic cancer

Q **Do you have a history of chronic pancreatitis?** Chronic inflammatory conditions of the pancreas have been suggested as a predisposing factor for pancreatic cancer

Family history

Q **Is there a family history of pancreatic cancer?** Rare forms of familial pancreatic cancer are described.

Examination

- **Perform a general examination,** looking for evidence of weight loss or wasting. Patients may be cachectic from anorexia with severe and at times rapid weight loss
- **Examine the skin and sclera.** One of the most common symptoms of pancreatic cancer is jaundice; look for yellow skin with possible excoriations from scratching and scleral icterus
- **Perform an abdominal examination.** Examine for evidence of ascites, palpable masses in the gallbladder, gallbladder enlargement, hepatomegaly, and splenomegaly. 70% of pancreatic cancers form in the head of the pancreas and may be a significant size before becoming symptomatic
- **Palpate the supraclavicular area.** Examine for possible lymph node enlargement
- **Examine the legs.** Venous thrombosis is a recognized complication of neoplastic disease classically presenting as a unilateral edematous lower extremity
- **Perform a urine dipstick examination** to confirm that there is bilirubin or urobilinogen in the urine

Summary of investigative tests

- CA 19-9 is of use to primary care physicians as a nonspecific tumor marker for follow up of pancreatic cancer after treatment, but it is not useful for screening of asymptomatic patients. Very high levels are considered highly suggestive of pancreatic cancer
- Percutaneous needle aspiration biopsy provides tissue for definitive diagnosis of pancreatic malignancy vs other pancreatic processes
- Abdominal ultrasound and abdominal computed tomography (CT) scan can identify a pancreatic mass and are ordered by primary care physicians and specialists
- Staging to determine resectability and to rule out locally advanced and metastatic disease usually consists of abdominal CT, pelvic CT, and chest X-ray
- ERCP, endoscopic ultrasonography, and CT/ultrasound-guided fine-needle aspiration are normally ordered by specialists to obtain definite diagnosis and to confirm staging

DIAGNOSTIC DECISION

- Clinical presentation of weight loss, obstructive jaundice, and abdominal pain suggests diagnosis
- Definitive diagnosis requires biopsy for histologic confirmation
- CT can localize mass and is the principal diagnostic modality

- If CT fails to identify mass but clinical suspicion remains high, ERCP or endoscopic ultrasound may be indicated
- Laparoscopy/laparotomy may be needed to confirm diagnosis but should be avoided as first-line measure if possible
- Consider laparoscopy and laparoscopic ultrasonography before explorative laparotomy
- Endoscopic ultrasound can evaluate nodal disease, vascular invasion, and extent of local disease
- Laboratory testing cannot confirm or exclude a diagnosis
- Elevated amylase, lipase, alkaline phosphatase, gamma-glutamyl transpeptidase (GGT), hepatic aminotransferases (alanine aminotransferase (ALT) and aspartate aminotransferase (AST)), and bilirubin are indicative of a biliary/pancreatic process but are not diagnostic
- Serologic markers such as CA 19-9 and carcinoembryonic antigen are available
- An abnormal CA 19-9 is found in up to 80% of all patients with pancreatic cancer
- Tissue inhibitor of metalloproteinase-1 (TIMP-1) is under investigation as a serum marker

Guidelines

Guidelines have been developed by the Society for Surgery of the Alimentary Tract [1].

THE TESTS

Body fluids

CANCER ANTIGEN 19-9 TUMOR MARKER (CA 19-9, CARBOHYDRATE ANTIGEN 19-9)

Description

Venous blood, 7–10mL in a red-top tube.

Advantages/Disadvantages

Advantages:

- Elevated in 74% of pancreatic cancer patients when using a cut-off value of >40U/mL
- Safe, simple, and inexpensive
- Can be used to follow treatment response and recurrence in pancreatic cancer

Disadvantage: not adequately sensitive or specific for screening because of the low incidence of pancreatic cancer in the general population; sensitivity 79–91%, specificity 93%

Normal

Less than 37U/mL.

Abnormal

- Elevated CA 19-9 may indicate pancreatic cancer
- Keep in mind the possibility of a false-positive result

Cause of abnormal result

Elevated level is due to release of CA 19 from damaged pancreatic cells.

Drugs, disorders and other factors that may alter results

Mild CA 19-9 elevation seen with cholelithiasis, cystic fibrosis, inflammatory bowel disease, and pancreatitis.

Biopsy

PERCUTANEOUS NEEDLE ASPIRATION BIOPSY

Description

Pancreatic tissue obtained using CT or ultrasound-guided fine-needle aspiration (FNA).

Advantages/Disadvantages

Advantages:

- Invasive diagnostic procedure of choice
- Provides tissue for definitive diagnosis of pancreatic malignancy vs other pancreatic processes
- Sensitivity 90%, specificity approaches 100%

Disadvantages:

- FNA must be avoided in patients with tumors suitable to resection because FNA may seed the peritoneum with malignant cells
- Complications include bleeding and bowel perforation
- Biopsy needle must penetrate pancreatic mass significantly because neoplasm is often surrounded by fibrosis, inflammation, and edema
- Superficial biopsy of pancreatic neoplasm may yield false negative, showing only pancreatitis

Normal

Normal pancreatic tissue.

Abnormal

- Abnormal histology consistent with pancreatic carcinoma
- Keep in mind the possibility of a false-positive result

Cause of abnormal result

- Pancreatic adenocarcinoma
- Pancreatitis
- Other pancreatic tumors

Imaging

ULTRASOUND

Description

Ultrasonic examination of the pancreas and surrounding structures.

Advantages/Disadvantages

Advantages:

Endoscopic ultrasound the test of choice if available:

- Sensitivity 99%
- Specificity 100%
- Can visualize small intrapancreatic islet cell tumors
- Detected 99% of tumors found at surgery in one study
- Can visualize pancreatic mass and rule out gallbladder disease
- Pancreatic masses may be identified, even if the pancreatic contour is not distorted (an advantage over CT scan)
- Common bile duct obstruction may be visualized

Disadvantages:

Transabdominal ultrasound:

- Sensitivity 60–67%
- Specificity 40%
- Safe, no radiation exposure
- Not specific

Normal

Do not exclude the diagnosis of pancreatic cancer.

Abnormal

- A mass may be seen within the pancreas
- Dilated intrahepatic ducts may be seen
- Keep in mind the possibility of a false-positive result

Cause of abnormal result

- Pancreatic adenocarcinoma
- Pancreatitis
- Pancreatic cyst or pseudocyst
- Other pancreatic tumors

COMPUTED TOMOGRAPHY SCAN WITH CONTRAST

Description

- CT scan of the abdomen and pelvis
- Accuracy can be enhanced by using contrast
- Sensitivity only 53% for tumors <3cm

Dual-phase spiral CT scan much more accurate:

- Sensitivity 85–95% overall
- Sensitivity 67% for tumors <15mm
- Sensitivity 100% for tumors >15mm

Advantages/Disadvantages

Advantages:

- Noninvasive diagnostic and staging procedure of choice
- Superior to ultrasound with better reproducibility and ability to accurately define the head, body, and tail of pancreas
- Sensitivity 90% for pancreatic cancer
- Metastases may be visualized

Disadvantages:

- Contraindicated in those with contrast/iodine allergy
- False-positive 5–10%

Normal

Makes less likely the diagnosis of pancreatic cancer, but do not exclude it.

Abnormal

- Evidence of pancreatic tumor (and metastases)
- Keep in mind the possibility of a false-positive result

Cause of abnormal result

- Pancreatic adenocarcinoma
- Pancreatitis
- Pancreatic cyst or pseudocyst
- Other pancreatic tumors

CHEST X-RAY

Advantages/Disadvantages

Advantage: evaluates presence of metastatic disease.

Normal

No pulmonary lesion identified.

Abnormal

- Pulmonary lesion identified
- Keep in mind the possibility of a false-positive result

Cause of abnormal result

Metastatic disease.

Special tests

ENDOSCOPIC RETROGRADE CHOLANGIOPANCREATOGRAPHY

Description

Performed only by specialists for diagnosis or palliation.

Advantages/Disadvantages

Advantages:

- Sensitivity 90% for pancreatic cancer
- Brush cytology frequently performed concurrently
- May be used to relieve obstruction of biliary/pancreatic duct

Normal

No masses or strictures identified.

Abnormal

- Pancreatic or biliary duct stricture
- Keep in mind the possibility of a false-positive result

Cause of abnormal result

- Pancreatic cancer
- Chronic pancreatitis
- Pancreatic duct stricture
- Biliary duct stricture
- Ampulla of Vater adenocarcinoma

TREATMENT

CONSIDER CONSULT

- Urgent surgical referral mandated for evidence of acute pancreatitis/cholangitis or major hemorrhage
- Multidiscipline team approach offers best patient satisfaction and enhanced survival
- Refer to oncologist for co-ordination of treatment and chemotherapy
- Refer to experienced upper gastrointestinal surgeon for possible surgical resection
- Refer to radiation-oncologist for palliation or combination therapy
- Refer to gastroenterologist or surgeon for biliary or small bowel obstruction
- Refer to a dietitian for nutritional support
- Referral to a clinical trial may be appropriate given poor prognosis

IMMEDIATE ACTION

- Acute gastrointestinal bleed requires surgical, gastroenterologic, or interventional radiologist referral
- Deep vein thrombosis requires anticoagulation
- Hospital admission is required for acute pancreatitis or cholangitis

PATIENT AND CAREGIVER ISSUES

Patient or caregiver request

- **Is there a possibility of cure?** Patients may be aware of certain cancers having a worse prognosis than others
- **Will my family members get a similar cancer?** Patients are often aware that some cancers are inherited and may worry that other family members will develop the disease

MANAGEMENT ISSUES

Goals

- Initiate evaluation for endoscopic, surgical, radiation, or chemotherapeutic therapy
- Pain control and patient comfort should be a priority
- Anticipate and manage anxiety and depression
- Evaluate social support
- Determine desire for resuscitative measures and attitudes toward hospice care if palliative care is the only treatment option

SUMMARY OF THERAPEUTIC OPTIONS

Choices

- For some patients there will be few treatment options and emphasis of care will be on quality of life and pain control
- Nearly 80% of patients presenting with pancreatic cancer have locally advanced or metastatic disease
- Only 10–20% of patients are candidates for resection
- First treatment choice and only chance for cure is surgical resection with pancreatectomy or pancreaticoduodenectomy followed by adjuvant (postoperative) chemoradiotherapy. Preoperative chemotherapy and/or radiotherapy is under evaluation
- Vascular invasion, metastatic disease, and extensive local disease usually preclude resection
- Second treatment choice is chemoradiotherapy with or without surgical palliation
- Chemoradiotherapy may make a formerly unresectable tumor resectable
- Chemoradiotherapy without surgery is used only for palliation
- 5-fluorouracil (5-FU) and gemcitabine are the mainstays of chemotherapy, with gemcitabine emerging as the preferred chemotherapeutic agent. Gemcitabine was found to improve the quality of life of these patients. Gemcitabine use is linked to a modest improvement in survival
- Metastatic and locally advanced disease usually treated with chemotherapy or chemoradiotherapy

- Supportive care only can be an option for some patients with advanced disease
- Endoscopic retrograde cholangiopancreatography (ERCP) is used to treat biliary obstruction
- Immunotherapy, gene therapy, and mucin-directed monoclonal antibodies/vaccines are under investigation
- Address lifestyle issues in all patients

Guidelines

- Guidelines have been developed by the Society for Surgery of the Alimentary Tract. Surgical treatment of pancreatic cancer [1].
- The Cancer Care Ontario Practice Guidelines Initiative has produced the following guidelines. Use of gemcitabine in the treatment of advanced pancreatic adenocarincoma [2].

Clinical pearls

- Only 10–20% of patients are candidates for resection
- Treatment with chemotherapy or chemoradiation is effective in palliation
- The use of morphine is not precluded in pancreatic cancer

FOLLOW UP

Plan for review

- Following treatment, relief of symptoms, and recurrence/spread of disease should be evaluated
- Bilirubin, alkaline phosphatase, aspartate aminotransferase (AST), alanine aminotransferase (ALT), and gamma-glutamyl transpeptidase (GGT) can be checked to evaluate persistent or recurrent biliary obstruction
- Ultrasound, endoscopy, or CT may be helpful to evaluate resolution or persistent biliary obstruction
- Decreased CA 19-9 level may indicate therapeutic efficacy
- Rising CA 19-9 level may indicate disease progression or recurrence
- Chest X-ray may be indicated to rule out metastasis
- Abdominal/pelvic CT may be indicated to evaluate efficacy of treatment and rule out metastasis

Information for patient or caregiver

- Patients should understand that surgery is an option for only 20–25% of patients, with the postoperative 5-year survival rate being 20% for patients submitted to complete resection. Patients with unresectable disease live an average of 6–10 months with current treatment
- Most patients will ultimately have to make decisions about end-of-life care and be educated regarding options
- Appropriate hospice, home health care referral can be made depending upon the patient's social and financial support and personal preference

DRUGS AND OTHER THERAPIES: DETAILS

Surgical therapy

- Complete tumor resection offers only hope for cure
- Surgical eligibility is usually confined to those patients with disease limited to pancreatic head
- Vascular invasion, metastatic disease, and extensive local disease usually preclude resection
- Postoperative prognosis still grave, with an 86% recurrence rate and a 5-year survival rate of 20% for those with completely resected tumors
- Positive lymph nodes and locally advanced disease confer a worse prognosis
- Chest X-ray and abdominal/pelvic CT scan with contrast must be performed prior to surgery to rule out metastatic/locally advanced disease
- Percutaneous transhepatic biliary drainage (PTBD) may be used for palliative relief of biliary obstruction
- PTBD has a 33% early and an 86% late complication rate with an 81% 'technical success rate'

- Surgery is an option for biliary decompression, diversion, and gastric outlet obstruction; mean survival postsurgical bypass is less than 6 months
- Morbidity rate for biliary enteric bypass: 15%
- Perioperative mortality rate for biliary bypass: 15–30%
- Surgical bypass may be superior to PTBD with less morbidity and mortality

PANCREATECTOMY

Usually involves resection of pancreas, spleen, greater omentum, duodenum, lymph nodes, and subtotal gastrectomy.

Efficacy

- May affect long-term survival in about 20% of patients
- Surgically suitable candidates who undergo pancreatectomy and experience recurrence survive three to four times longer than those patients who do not undergo surgery

Risks/Benefits

Risk: total pancreatectomy can result in loss of pancreatic exocrine/endocrine function, leading to brittle diabetes and malabsorption

Benefits:

- Chemical splanchnicectomy for pain control can be performed concurrently
- Mortality rate less than 15%

Evidence

- Surgical resection represents the only chance for cure [1] *Level C*
- The procedure of choice for tumors of the pancreatic body/tail is distal pancreatectomy with splenectomy [1] *Level C*

Acceptability to patient

Pancreatectomy associated with significant morbidity that may be unacceptable to some patients given dismal prognosis.

Follow up plan

- Educate patient about the signs and symptoms of malabsorption and treat with pancreatic enzymes should pancreatic insufficiency occur
- Monitor serum blood sugar level and treat diabetes
- Ensure adequate postoperative pain control
- Observe for wound infection

PANCREATICODUODENECTOMY (WHIPPLE'S RESECTION)

- Usually involves resection of the pancreatic head, distal stomach, duodenum, common bile duct, gallbladder, and truncal vagotomy followed by pancreaticojejunostomy, choledochojejunostomy, and gastrojejunostomy
- Limited to patients whose cancer is confined to the pancreatic head

Efficacy

- Rarely effects cure
- Procedure of choice for small lesions confined to pancreatic head
- May also be used for palliation, especially in young otherwise healthy patients
- The highest surgical mortality rates and long-term survival are achieved at hospitals with the most experience with the procedure

Risks/Benefits
Risk: complication rate 5–10% and includes delayed gastric emptying, gastrointestinal hemorrhage, intra-abdominal abscess, and pancreatic fistula

Benefits:
- Only opportunity for cure
- Less risk of brittle diabetes and malabsorption
- Chemical splanchnicectomy for pain control can be performed concurrently
- Mortality rate less than 5%

Evidence
- Surgical resection represents only chance for cure [1] *Level C*
- Tumors confined to pancreatic head should be treated with pancreaticoduodenectomy (with or without preservation of the pylorus) [1] *Level C*

Acceptability to patient
- Pancreaticoduodenectomy may be associated with significant morbidity that may be unacceptable to some patients given poor prognosis
- Hospital stay usually less than 2 weeks

Follow up plan
- Educate patient about the signs and symptoms of malabsorption and treat with pancreatic enzymes should pancreatic insufficiency occur
- Monitor serum blood sugar level and treat diabetes
- Ensure adequate postoperative pain control
- Observe for wound infection or evidence of anastomotic leak or bleed

Radiation therapy

EXTERNAL BEAM RADIATION THERAPY
- Usually used in combination with surgery and chemotherapy
- May be combined with brachytherapy
- May be used preoperatively to reduce tumor burden
- Used as single-agent therapy for palliation in patients with back/abdominal pain from retroperitoneal invasion/liver metastases
- Patients with pain recalcitrant to conventional analgesia and radiation therapy may benefit from neurolytic celiac plexus block
- Survival may be improved by combined adjuvant chemoradiotherapy with 5-FU (median survival 20 months vs 11 months)

Efficacy
- Improves survival when combined with surgery and chemotherapy (20 months vs 11 months)
- No significant impact on survival when used as monotherapy
- Efficacious when used for palliation of abdominal/back pain

Risks/Benefits
- Risk: radiation exposure with potential for radiation damage to surrounding structures (e.g. biliary tree, bowel, pancreas)
- Benefit: may offer palliation, reduce tumor size and pain

Evidence
Radiotherapy may improve survival when used as adjuvant therapy:
- Radiation therapy and 5-FU may be beneficial in patients without evidence of distant metastases [1] *Level C*

- Standard treatment for unresectable locoregional disease is radiation therapy plus 5-FU or gemcitabine alone [3] *Level C*
- A randomized controlled trial (RCT) compared high-dose radiation therapy alone, high-dose radiotherapy with 5-FU, and moderate-dose radiation plus 5-FU in patients with locally unresectable pancreatic cancer. The combination therapy groups showed a significant improvement in survival when compared with radiation therapy alone. There was no significant difference noted between the two combination groups [4] *Level P*
- Pancreatic cancer patients were treated with either surgery alone or in combination with radiotherapy (external beam radiation therapy (EBRT) or intraoperative radiation therapy (IORT)) in a prospective trial. A survival advantage was noted with the combination therapy for patients with T3 tumors and positive nodes [5] *Level P*
- A retrospective analysis compared surgery alone with surgery and adjuvant radiation therapy (either EBRT or IORT). A significant survival benefit was noted for EBRT and surgery compared with surgery alone. IORT and surgery was found to have a borderline significant increase in survival. Patients managed with all three therapies had the best median survival rate [6] *Level S*

Acceptability to patient

- Aggressively manage nausea, vomiting, and diarrhea, which can limit patient compliance
- Profound fatigue is common during radiation therapy; instruct patient to get adequate rest
- Warn patient about potential skin irritation over radiated site

Follow up plan

- Evaluate patient for symptomatic improvement
- Evaluate patient for recurrence of disease or reduction in tumor burden
- Follow bilirubin, amylase, lipase, and transaminase for evidence of radiation-induced organ damage

Patient and caregiver information

- Advise patient to receive adequate rest to limit profound fatigue
- Advise patient that radiation therapy may cause nausea, vomiting, and diarrhea, all of which can be managed

Chemotherapy

- Combination chemotherapy is used in conjunction with surgery with or without radiotherapy if the aim is to cure
- Single-agent chemotherapy is used for palliation
- Gemcitabine is the mainstay of pancreatic cancer chemotherapy in palliative setting
- Neoadjuvant (chemotherapy before surgery) chemotherapy is under investigation
- Survival after complete resection may be improved by combined adjuvant chemoradiotherapy with 5-FU (median survival 20 months vs 11 months)
- Specific chemotherapy is usually prescribed by an oncologist and administered in an outpatient or hospital setting

5-FLUOROURACIL

- Used in combination chemotherapy and radiation therapy before or after surgery when the aim is to cure
- Used with radiation therapy and other chemotherapeutic agents for palliation
- Acts as radiosensitizing agent
- Multiple clinical trials combining 5-FU with other chemotherapeutic agents are being performed with variable results

Efficacy

May improve survival when used in combination therapy (20 months vs 11 months).

Risks/Benefits

Risks:

- Specialist advice must be followed
- Bone marrow suppression
- Impaired hepatic or renal function
- High-dose pelvic irradiation
- Previous use of alkylating agents
- Discontinue as soon as signs of toxicity appear (diarrhea, watery stools, frequent bowel movements, gastrointestinal ulceration and bleeding, hemorrhage, leukopenia, stomatitis or esophagopharyngitis, thrombocytopenia, vomiting)

Side-effects and adverse reactions

- Cardiovascular system: Angina, myocardial ischemia
- Central nervous system: Headache, nystagmus, acute cerebellar syndrome
- Gastrointestinal: Stomatitis, esophagopharyngitis, diarrhea, emesis, nausea, vomiting
- Hematological: Bone marrow suppression, leukopenia, thrombocytopenia, agranulosis, pancytopenia, anemia
- Ophthalmic: Photophobia
- Skin: Alopecia, dermatitis, photosensitivity

Interactions (other drugs)

- Leucovorin calcium ■ Cimetidine ■ Filgrastim ■ Metronidazole

Contraindications

- Hypersensitivity to fluorouracil ■ Severe hematological toxicity ■ Depressed bone marrow ■ Gastrointestinal hemorrhage ■ Poor nutritional state ■ Serious infections

Evidence

5-FU when used in combination with radiation therapy may improve survival for patients with pancreatic carcinoma:

- A RCT compared radiation therapy alone and in combination with 5-FU for locally unresectable pancreatic carcinoma. Patient survival rate was improved in the combination treatment group [7] *Level P*
- Standard treatment for unresectable locoregional disease is radiation therapy plus 5-FU or gemcitabine alone [3] *Level C*
- A RCT compared high-dose radiation therapy alone, high-dose radiotherapy with 5-FU, and moderate-dose radiation plus 5-FU in patients with locally unresectable pancreatic cancer. The combination therapy groups showed a significant improvement in survival when compared with radiation therapy alone. There was no significant difference noted between the two combination groups [4] *Level P*

Acceptability to patient

- Nausea, vomiting, diarrhea, gastrointestinal ulceration, and neurologic toxicity manifesting as ataxia and somnolence may limit compliance
- Warn patient about the possibility of skin rash and hand-foot syndrome

Follow up plan

- Follow complete blood count because myelosuppression is a major complication
- Aggressively manage nausea, vomiting, and diarrhea to prevent dehydration
- Monitor skin reaction, including hand-foot syndrome
- Monitor and treat oral mucositis

Patient and caregiver information

Warn patient of high side-effect profile while reassuring that side-effects can be managed.

GEMCITABINE

- First drug to demonstrate an improvement in the quality of life for the palliative treatment of advanced pancreatic cancer
- Linked to a modest but significant improvement in survival
- Potent radiosensitizing agent
- Nucleoside antimetabolite

Efficacy

- Causes a modest improvement in the median survival of patients with advanced/metastatic disease when compared with 5-FU alone
- Improves the quality of life in patients with advanced and unresectable pancreatic cancer

Risks/Benefits

Risks:

- Use caution with renal or hepatic impairment
- Safety and efficacy have not established in children
- Should not be used during pregnancy and breast-feeding
- Patients should be monitored for myelosuppression

Side-effects and adverse reactions

- Cardiovascular system: myocardial infarction, cerebrovascular accident, arrhythmia, hypertension
- Central nervous system: fever
- Gastrointestinal: nausea, vomiting
- Hematolgical: myelosuppression,
- Metabolism: proteinuria, hematuria
- Respiratory: dyspnea, bronchospasm
- Skin: alopecia, rash, pruritus

Interactions (other drugs)

None listed.

Contraindications

- Hypersensitivity to gemcitabine
- Should not be used during pregnancy and breast-feeding
- Safety and efficacy have not established in children

Evidence

There is evidence for the use of gemcitabine in the treatment of advanced symptomatic pancreatic carcinoma:

- Gemcitabine is a treatment option for patients with advanced or unresectable pancreatic cancer [2] *Level C*
- An RCT compared gemcitabine with 5-FU for the management of pain in patients with advanced symptomatic carcinoma of the pancreas. A modest improvement in survival was noted in the gemcitabine group. Gemcitabine was more effective than 5-FU for symptomatic relief [8] *Level P*

Acceptability to patient

- Myelosuppression is a dose-limiting toxicity
- May cause influenza-like symptoms that some patients may find unacceptable
- Gastrointestinal complaints include nausea, vomiting, diarrhea, and constipation but are usually mild
- Warn patient about the possibility of alopecia (rare), pruritus, edema, and skin rash

Follow up plan

- Follow complete blood count because myelosuppression is a dose-limiting toxicity
- Monitor liver function tests for hepatotoxicity and urinalysis for nephrotoxicity (hematuria and proteinuria)
- Aggressively manage nausea, vomiting, and diarrhea

Patient and caregiver information

Warn patient of high side-effect profile while reassuring that side-effects can be managed.

Endoscopic therapy

ENDOSCOPIC RETROGRADE CHOLANGIOPANCREATOGRAPHY

- Primarily used to relieve biliary or gastric obstruction through insertion of stent
- Large-caliber metal stents favored over smaller plastic stents
- If ERCP not successful, urgent transhepatic cholangiography with stent placement may be indicated
- Studies have documented no significant difference in complications, length of stay, and survival rate between operative and nonoperative biliary decompression; however, nonoperative palliation associated with less cost
- If ERCP-guided stenting is not possible, then stenting through radiologic catheter placement should be considered

Efficacy

Endoscopic endoprosthesis insertion success rate: 90%.

Risks/Benefits

Risks:

- Complications include perforation, bleeding, duodenal obstruction, and stent occlusion/migration
- Stent occlusion rate varies from 8 to 30%
- Intraoperative mortality rate for endoscopic endoprosthesis: 0–2%
- Perioperative mortality rate for endoscopic endoprosthesis: 10–18%

Benefit: ERCP-guided stent insertion may have less morbidity and mortality when compared with percutaneous stent placement

Evidence

Endoscopic management of obstructive jaundice is recommended for patients who are not candidates for surgical cure:

- Endoscopic placement of a stent is a recommended treatment option for patients with biliary obstruction secondary to pancreatic carcinoma, who are not candidates for curative resection [3] *Level C*
- An endoscopically placed stent is effective for the palliation of obstructive jaundice with less morbidity than surgical bypass [1] *Level C*

Acceptability to patient

- Sedation needed for ERCP
- Up to 10% of 'survival time' may be spent hospitalized
- Can effectively relieve jaundice and pruritus and decrease risk of cholangitis

Follow up plan

Evaluate patient for recurrent biliary obstruction, and repeat stenting/debridement may be indicated.

OUTCOMES

EFFICACY OF THERAPIES

- Prognosis is poor for the majority of patients, regardless of what therapy is employed
- Combined surgery and chemoradiotherapy offer the best survival advantage but can be prohibited by the patient's clinical condition

Evidence

- PDxMD are unable to cite evidence that meets our criteria for evidence for surgical management of pancreatic carcinoma
- Combination therapy with external beam radiation therapy and 5-fluorouracil (5-FU) may improve survival in patients with locally unresectable pancreatic cancer [4,7] *Level P*
- Gemcitabine may be more effective than 5-FU for symptomatic relief in patients with advanced pancreatic carcinoma. Gemcitabine may also confer a survival advantage [8] *Level P*

PROGNOSIS

- Extremely poor, with overall 5-year survival rate less than 5%
- Long-term survival rate is 0.4%
- For locally advanced disease, the median survival is 6–10 months
- For metastatic disease, the median survival is 3–6 months
- 5-year survival rate for patients with advanced disease is less than 1%; most die within one year
- For patients undergoing surgical resection, median survival is 10–18 months
- For surgical candidates, 5-year postoperative survival rate is about 20–25%
- Survival may be improved by combined adjuvant chemoradiotherapy with 5-FU (20 months vs 11 months)
- Tumor grade, stage, and resection margin status are the best predictors of survival following surgery
- Severe abdominal pain is often indicative of splanchnic nerve involvement and advanced nonresectable disease

Therapeutic failure

- Consider entry into clinical trial
- Pain control and quality of life should be a priority

Recurrence

- Recurrence tends to be local, occurring 1–2 years postresection
- Hepatic metastases may occur early in disease
- Chemotherapy alone with gemcitabine confers better quality of life but rarely produces significant clinical response
- Immunotherapy with and without chemotherapy is under investigation
- Entry into clinical trial should be strongly considered
- Radiation therapy can reduce tumor burden
- Pain control and quality of life should be a priority

Deterioration

- Consider entry into a clinical trial
- Pain control and quality of life should be a priority

Terminal illness

- Pain control and patient comfort are a priority
- Assist patient and family in dealing with end-of-life issues
- Cachexia usually develops

COMPLICATIONS

- Tumor may cause biliary or pancreatic duct obstruction; refer to gastroenterologist or surgeon for stenting or bypass
- Pain is a frequent complaint and should be managed aggressively
- Gastrointestinal bleeding and small bowel obstruction may occur
- Deep vein thrombosis is a recognized complication of malignancy
- Monitor blood sugar level and treat diabetes
- Malabsorption may occur, especially after pancreatectomy

CONSIDER CONSULT

- Consider referral to an academic-university center for clinical trial entry
- Referral to hospice for treatment failure or clinical deterioration
- Referral to pain specialist for intractable pain

PREVENTION

There are no known interventions that have been shown to prevent pancreatic cancer.

RISK FACTORS

- Alcohol: there is an association between chronic pancreatitis and pancreatic cancer, and patients who have a history of pancreatitis should abstain from alcohol
- Tobacco: there is an association between smoking and pancreatic cancer, and patients who wish to reduce their risk of pancreatic cancer should stop smoking

MODIFY RISK FACTORS

With the exception of rare hereditary forms of pancreatic cancer, there are no known definite risk factors for pancreatic carcinoma.

Lifestyle and wellness

TOBACCO

Tobacco use should be discouraged.

ALCOHOL AND DRUGS

Alcohol use should be discouraged, especially in patients with a history of pancreatitis.

FAMILY HISTORY

Familial clusters of pancreatic cancer have rarely been described.

SCREENING

- Use of serologic markers or ultrasound are not recommended for screening in asymptomatic individuals, according to the American Academy of Family Physicians. Periodic Health Examinations, Summary of AAFP Policy Recommendations and Age Charts
- Use of serologic markers, ultrasound, and abdominal palpation in asymptomatic individuals is not recommended for screening for pancreatic cancer [9]

PREVENT RECURRENCE

- Complete surgical resection is the only intervention that can prevent recurrence
- Chemoradiotherapy may prolong disease-free survival

ASSOCIATIONS

American Cancer Society
Tel: (800) ACS-2345
www.cancer.org/

American Association for Cancer Research
Public Ledger Building, Suite 826
150 South Independence Mall West
Philadelphia, PA 19106–3483
Tel: (215) 440-9300
Fax: (215) 440-9313
www.aacr.org/

American Society of Clinical Oncology
1900 Duke Street
Suite 200
Alexandria, VA 22314
Tel: (703) 299-0150
Fax: (703) 299-1044
E-mail: asco@asco.org
www.asco.org/

M.D. Anderson Cancer Center
1515 Holcombe Blvd
Houston, TX 77030
Tel: (800) 392-1611
www.mdanderson.org/

National Coalition for Cancer Survivorship
1010 Wayne Avenue, Suite 505
Silver Springs, MD 20910–5600
Tel: (800) 622-7937
E-mail: info@cansearch.org
www.cansearch.org

National Hospice and Palliative Care Organization
1700 Diagonal Road, Suite 300
Alexandria, VA 22314
Tel: (800) 658-8898
E-mail: helpline@nhpco.org
www.nhpco.org

Pancreatic Cancer Action Network
P.O. Box 4809
Palos Verdes, CA 90272
Tel: (877) 272-6226
E-mail: information@pancan.org
www.pancan.org

National Cancer Institute
NCI Public Inquiries Office
Building, 31, Room 10A31
31 Center Drive, MSC 2580
Bethesda, MD 20892–2580
Tel: (301) 435-3848
E-mail: cancermail@icicc.nci.nih.gov
www.nci.nih.gov/

KEY REFERENCES

- DeVita VT, Hellman S, Rosenberg SA, eds. Cancer: principles & practices of oncology, 5th edn. New York: Lippincott-Raven, 1997
- Sleisenger MH, Fordtran JS, Weisiger RA, Billhartz LE, eds. Sleisenger & Fordtran's gastrointestinal and liver disease, 6th edn. New York: WB Saunders, 1998
- Cotran RS, Kumar V, Collins T, eds. Robbins pathological basis of disease, 5th edn. Philadelphia: WB Saunders, 1994
- Abeloff MD. Clinical oncology, 2nd edn. New York: Churchill Livingstone, 2000
- Gullo L, Pezzilli R, Morselli Labate AM. Diabetes and the risk of pancreatic cancer. N Engl J Med 1994;331(2):81–4
- American Gastroenterological Association Technical Review on the epidemiology, diagnosis and treatment of pancreatic ductal adenocarcinoma. Gastroenterology 1999;117:1464–84

Evidence references and guidlines

1 Society for Surgery of the Alimentary Tract. Surgical treatment of pancreatic cancer. Patient Care Committee, 2000. Available at the National Guideline Clearinghouse

2 The Cancer Care Ontario Practice Guidelines Initiative have produced the following guidelines. Use of gemcitabine in the treatment of advanced pancreatic adenocarcincoma. Provincial Gastrointestinal Cancer Disease Site Group 1998. Available at the National Guidelines Clearinghouse

3 American Gastroenterological Association Medical Position Statement: Epidemiology, diagnosis, and treatment of pancreatic ductal adenocarcinoma. Gastroenterology 1999;117:1463–4

4 Moertel CG, Frytak S, Hahn RG, et al. Therapy of locally unresectable pancreatic carcinoma: a randomized comparison of high dose (6000 rads) radiation alone, moderate dose radiation (4000 rads plus 5-flurouracil), and high dose radiation plus 5-fluorouracil: The Gastrointestinal Tumor Study Group. Cancer 1981;48:1705–10

5 Hosotani R, Kogire M, Arii S, et al. Results of pancreatectomy with radiation therapy for pancreatic cancer. Hepatogastroenterology 1997;44:1528–35
6 Dobelbower RR, Merrick HW, Khuder S, et al. Adjuvant radiation therapy for pancreatic cancer: a 15-year experience. Int J Radiat Oncol Biol Phys 1997;39:31–7
7 The Gastrointestinal Tumor Study Group. A multi-institutional comparative trial of radiation therapy alone and in combination with 5-fluorouracil for locally unresectable pancreatic carcinoma. Ann Surg 1979;189:205–8
8 Burris HA, Moore MJ, Anderson J, et al. Improvements in survival and clinical benefit with gemcitabine as first-line therapy for patients with advanced pancreas cancer: a randomized trial. J Clin Oncol 1997;15:2403–13
9 United States Preventative Services Task Force. Guide to Preventative Services, 2nd edn. Baltimore: Williams & Wilkins, 1996, p167-73. Available from the National Guidelines Clearinghouse

FAQS

Question 1

Can we treat pain related to pancreatic cancer with morphine?

ANSWER 1

Yes. There is no contraindication of morphine use in such patients.

Question 2

Is the pancreatic biopsy linked to a very high index of complication?

ANSWER 2

No. The index of complication of this procedure is not so high that it can preclude its realization.

Question 3

Can the biopsy be precluded in patients with pancreatic mass not suitable for surgery if the CA 19-9 is very high?

ANSWER 3

No. The histopathologic diagnosis is required before any specific treatment can be conducted.

CONTRIBUTORS

Russell C Jones, MD, MPH
Otavio A Clark, MD
Naixi N Chen, MD

PITUITARY ADENOMA

SUMMARY INFORMATION

DESCRIPTION

- Pituitary adenomas are benign neoplasms of the anterior pituitary
- Symptoms result from either excess secretion of a pituitary hormone, mass effect of the tumor on local structures, or from destruction of the normal gland producing hypopituitarism
- They are classified in two ways: as secretory or nonfunctional and by size (tumors <10mm are called microadenomas and those >10mm are called macroadenomas)

URGENT ACTION

- Patients with sudden change in sensorium, headache, stiff neck, fever, ophthalmoplegia, or visual loss need an immediate magnetic resonance imaging or a thin section noncontrast computed tomography scan of the pituitary and the orbits
- Patient should be presumed to have anterior pituitary insufficiency, in which case they are at risk for vascular collapse with sudden deficiencies in adrenococorticotropic hormone and cortisol
- Blood tests should be obtained for cortisol and T4 levels
- A glucocorticoid dose adequate for stress and cerebral edema should be started (dexamethasone 2mg every 6h)
- Urgent endocrinologic, ophthalmologic, and neurosurgical evaluation should be considered and obtained when clinically warranted

KEY! DON'T MISS!

- Pituitary apoplexy may result from hemorrhagic infarction of a pituitary adenoma
- Loss of adrenocorticotropic hormone and thyroid-stimulating hormone due to a tumor can lead to severe and life-threatening adrenal insufficiency and hypothyroidism
- Galactorrhea has been reported in 14–33% of men with marked hyperprolactinemia but in practice is less common

ICD9 CODE

- 253 Pituitary adenoma
- 253.0 Acromegaly
- 253.1 Prolactinoma

SYNONYMS

- Pituitary tumor or adenoma
- Prolactin-secreting tumor or prolactinoma
- Growth hormone-secreting tumor or somatotrophin-secreting – the clinical syndrome is acromegaly
- Cushing's disease or ACTH secreting tumor
- Thyrotropin or TSH-secreting tumor
- Nonfunctional or gonadotroph and nonsecreting tumors

CARDINAL FEATURES

- Pituitary adenomas are benign neoplasms of the anterior pituitary
- Symptoms result from excess secretion of pituitary hormones, dysfunction in the compressed areas of the pituitary, or from mass effect of the tumor impinging on local structures
- Large tumors are >10mm and are referred to as macroadenomas
- Small tumors are <10mm and are referred to as microadenomas
- Pituitary adenomas are also classified as secretory or nonfunctional
- Secretory tumors include prolactin-secreting adenomas, growth hormone (GH)-secreting adenomas, corticotrophin-secreting adenomas, and thyrotropin-secreting adenomas
- Nonfunctional adenomas – sometimes called nonsecreting adenomas – may be gonadotropin-secreting or may not secrete any detectable hormone
- Adenomas that secrete gonadotropins or the subunits are called nonfunctional as gonadotropin hypersecretion has little clinical effect
- Gonadotropin and nonsecreting adenomas generally present as macroadenomas with headache, visual disturbances, or hypopituitarism
- Some adenomas are capable of secreting both prolactin and GH
- Therapy for pituitary adenomas includes transphenoidal surgery, pituitary radiation, and pharmacotherapy, depending on the cell type and size of the adenoma

CAUSES

Common causes

Pituitary adenomas are monoclonal benign neoplasms of epithelial origin.

EPIDEMIOLOGY

Incidence and prevalence

INCIDENCE

- Pituitary adenomas are common
- Asymptomatic microadenomas (1cm diameter or less) are found in 6–24% of unselected autopsies
- Symptomatic adenomas account for 10–15% of all intracranial tumors treated by neurosurgeons
- In 35% of cases, pituitary adenomas are invasive without demonstrating histologic malignancy

PREVALENCE

In autopsy studies, 6–24% of adults have small pituitary tumors.

FREQUENCY

- Pituitary adenomas are 10–15% of all intracranial neoplasms, and the most common cause of hormone hyper- and hyposecretion in adults
- Prolactinomas make up 35% of all pituitary adenomas and are responsible for up to 20% of unexplained cases of primary or secondary amenorrhea
- Gonadotroph and nonsecreting adenomas are about 30% of all pituitary adenomas or about 10 persons/million/year
- GH-secreting pituitary adenomas account for 20% of all adenomas
- Adenomas secreting both prolactin and GH account for about 7% of all adenomas
- Corticotrophin (ACTH)-secreting adenomas account for about 7% of all adenomas
- Thyrotropin-secreting tumors are about 1% of pituitary adenomas

Demographics

GENDER

- Thyrotropin-secreting adenomas: there is a slight female:male predominance of 1.7:1
- Corticotropin-secreting pituitary adenomas: there is a female:male predominance of 8:1

GENETICS

- Pituitary adenomas may be part of the multiple endocrine neoplasia type 1 (MEN-1) syndrome, which consists of parathyroid neoplasia, pituitary neoplasia, pancreatic islet cell neoplasia, carcinoid, or lipomas
- It can also be part of rare genetic syndromes, such as McCune-Albright syndrome and Carney's syndrome
- Transmission is autosomal dominant

DIFFERENTIAL DIAGNOSIS

The differential diagnosis of a pituitary adenoma is based on the types of hormone the adenoma secretes.

Prolactin-secreting pituitary adenoma

Other causes of hyperprolactinemia include:

- Pregnancy, breast-feeding, and breast stimulation
- Hypothyroidism
- Drug ingestion (phenothiazines, haloperidol, antidepressants, metoclopramide, estrogen, calcium channel blockers, H_2 receptor antagonists, antihypertensives (methyldopa, reserpine, verapamil))
- Chronic renal failure
- Nonsecretory pituitary adenomas
- Hypothalamic lesion
- Head, chest, or spinal cord trauma

Growth hormone-secreting pituitary adenoma

Other causes of acromegaly include: ectopic production of growth hormone (GH)-releasing hormone from carcinoid, pancreatic, hypothalamic, or other types of tumors.

Corticotropin-secreting pituitary adenoma

This is the most common cause of endogenous Cushing's syndrome. Other causes of Cushing's syndrome include:

- Ectopic sources of overproduction of corticotrophin (adrenocorticotropic hormone (ACTH)) (small-cell carcinoma of the lung, bronchial carcinoid, intestinal carcinoid, pancreatic islet cell tumors, medullary carcinoma of the thyroid, pheochromocytoma, ovarian tumors)
- Sources of excess glucocorticoids (adrenal adenomas, adrenal carcinoma)
- Iatrogenic causes are the most common cause of Cushing's syndrome

Thyrotropin-secreting pituitary adenomas

Other causes of thyroid-stimulating hormone (TSH) elevation include:

- Primary hypothyroidism
- Syndrome of pituitary resistance to thyroid hormone

Gonadotroph and nonsecreting adenomas

The most common differential diagnosis for nonsecreting adenomas include:

- Craniopharyngioma
- The 'empty sella' syndrome
- Chordomas
- Colloid cysts and lipomas
- Dermoids, teratomas and ectopic pinealomas
- Gliomas (especially the chiasmatic type)
- Meningiomas, metastatic tumors, aneurysms
- Granulomas (e.g. tuberculosis and sarcoid)

Pituitary incidentalomas

- Autopsy studies suggest 10–20% of people have pituitary microadenomas
- Microadenomas are sometimes identified by magnetic resonance imaging (MRI) when the scan was obtained for other reasons, and up to 10% of otherwise normal individuals have evidence of a mass on imaging
- These microadenomas are referred to as incidentalomas and require evaluation for biochemical activity and propensity for growth

SIGNS & SYMPTOMS

Signs

Nonfunctioning pituitary adenomas are usually large macroadenomas at diagnosis:

- Bitemporal hemianopia can occur due to compression of optic chiasm
- There may be hypopituitarism and hypogonadism due to destruction of pituitary gland
- Pathologic fractures may occur from osteoporosis

Prolactin-secreting adenomas (represents about 40% of pituitary adenomas):

- May present during pregnancy (or be worsened by it)
- Men and postmenopausal women generally have larger tumors at time of diagnosis
- There may be decreased visual acuity and visual field deficits, especially bitemporal hemianopia. Ophthalmoplegia may also be present
- Females of reproductive age may present with galactorrhea, amenorrhea, or vaginal dryness
- Osteoporosis may lead to pathologic fractures

GH-secreting pituitary adenomas frequently are macroadenomas at diagnosis:

- May present with visual field deficits
- There may be gigantism in children, acromegaly in adults
- The patient may have coarse facial features, oily skin, hyperhydrosis, and prognathism
- Hypertension, hyperglycemia
- Osteoarthritis and carpal tunnel syndrome
- May present with signs of hypopituitarism

Corticotropin-secreting pituitary adenoma produces a classical appearance:

- The patient may have a round face, truncal obesity, and a dorsocervical fat pad (buffalo hump)
- Hirsutism, acne, stria, thin skin, and bruising may be present
- Menstrual disorders can occur as well as hypertension and hyperglycemia

Thyrotropin-secreting pituitary adenoma produces thyrotoxicosis:

- Goiter may be present
- Visual impairment can occur

Symptoms

- Symptoms from macroadenomas are usually due to mass effect
- Patient may report headache and visual field deficits
- Symptoms from microadenomas are usually due to effects of aberrant hormone levels
- Patient may report infertility, impotence or dyspareunia

ASSOCIATED DISORDERS

Central hypogonadism is caused by inadequate amounts of gonadotropins, which usually present as amenorrhea or infertility.

KEY! DON'T MISS!

- Pituitary apoplexy may result from hemorrhagic infarction of a pituitary adenoma
- Loss of ACTH and TSH due to a tumor can lead to severe and life-threatening adrenal insufficiency and hypothyroidism
- Galactorrhea has been reported in 14–33% of men with marked hyperprolactinemia but in practice is less common

CONSIDER CONSULT

- In general, macroadenomas (adenomas >10mm) are referred to endocrinologists for definitive diagnosis and treatment. These patients need assessment of their present pituitary functional status regardless of whether the therapy chosen will be surgical or pharmacologic

- Larger adenomas should also be referred to an ophthalmologist for assessment of visual fields
- Patients suspected of having Cushing's disease need to be managed by an endocrinologist. MRI findings are not sufficient to make a diagnosis of Cushing's disease nor can the MRI be used to exclude the diagnosis
- Primary care physicians (PCPs) who choose to treat prolactin-secreting microadenomas need to eliminate other causes of hyperprolactinemia prior to initiating therapy. A microadenoma identified on MRI of the pituitary may not be the source of the hyperprolactinemia. Causes such as drug use, sexual practices, and hypothyroidism need to be eliminated. If the PCP is not comfortable making this determination, the patient should be referred to an endocrinologist

INVESTIGATION OF THE PATIENT

Direct questions to patient

- Q **Do you have any problems with driving your car or with your peripheral vision?** Patients with macroadenomas may develop compression at the optic chiasm and temporal visual field losses
- Q **Are menstrual cycles regular? Any history of infertility, diminished libido, vaginal dryness or impotence, and decreased beard growth?** These questions help elicit symptoms of hypogonadism with low levels of circulating sex hormones that can accompany pituitary adenomas. In general, any woman with regular menstrual cycles (off oral contraceptives) does not have significant pituitary disease
- Q **Do you have headaches?** Patients with macroadenoma more commonly present with a headache. However, even patients with a microadenoma can have this presentation
- Q **Is there a history of galactorrhea?** This may be a presenting complaint in prolactinoma; a pregnancy history is necessary to determine whether galactorrhea may be physiologic. Check for a history of drug use as several kinds of illegal drugs (as well as prescription drugs) may cause galactorrhea. Breast stimulation from sexual activity may also cause hyperprolactinemia
- Q **Have you noticed a change in your appearance?** Increases in glove, shoe, hat, or ring size may be noticed by patients with elevated levels of GH. Ask if anyone has commented about their change in appearance. Cushing's disease and acromegaly are insidious in presentation. Sometimes a patient seeks medical attention after a family member or friend that hasn't seen the patient in a while comments about a marked change in appearance
- Q **Have you noticed recent weight loss, increased appetite, heat intolerance, or tremor?** Hyperthyroidism symptoms suggest thyrotropin-secreting adenoma

Family history

- Q **Is there a family history of pituitary or glandular diseases?** Pituitary adenomas are a part of the syndrome multiple endocrine neoplasia type 1 (MEN-1), as well as Carney's syndrome and McCune-Albright syndrome.

Examination

Macroadenomas (examine for signs of hypopituitarism):

- Pallor
- Hypotension
- Visual field defects

Prolactin-secreting tumors:

- Galactorrhea
- Hypogonadism
- Osteoporosis

GH-secreting tumors:

- Coarse facial features
- Oily skin
- Prognathism

- Carpal tunnel syndrome
- Osteoarthritis
- Hypertension
- Hyperhydrosis

Corticotropin-secreting pituitary adenoma:
- Truncal obesity
- Round face
- Dorsocervical fat pad (buffalo hump)
- Hirsutism
- Acne
- Menstrual disorders
- Hypertension
- Stria
- Bruising
- Thin skin

Thyrotropin-secreting pituitary adenoma:
- Thyrotoxicosis
- Goiter
- Visual impairment

Summary of investigative tests

- Serum prolactin is a blood test that evaluates prolactin secretion. This hormone is secreted physiologically in pregnancy for milk production. Hypersecretion of this hormone can occur if a prolactin-secreting adenoma develops in the pituitary. Additionally, any pituitary adenoma that causes stalk compression interferes with inhibition of prolactin secretion by the hypothalmus. Patients with elevated prolactin levels present with symptoms such as galactorrhea, amenorrhea, or infertility
- High-sensitivity TSH and thyroid function tests are used to evaluate the integrity of the pituitary thyroid axis when a pituitary adenoma is present. A large macroadenoma of any cell type may compromise the pituitary's ability to secrete TSH and result in central hypothyroidism. Alternatively, a patient presenting with hyperthyroidism may be found to have a nonsuppressible TSH level and need to be further evaluated for TSH-secreting pituitary adenoma
- Urinary or serum beta human gonadotropin hormone is used to exclude pregnancy in female patients. This is important in interpreting normal hormone levels, especially prolactin levels, which vary with pregnancy
- Insulin-like growth factor-1 (IGF-1) is the most useful screening test for acromegaly
- GH secretion is pulsatile, even with adenomas, and does not correlate as well as IGF-1 to the clinical manifestations of acromegaly. Patients in whom acromegaly is suspected should be screened with IGF-1
- A 50–100g oral glucose tolerance test is still considered the gold standard in the diagnosis of acromegaly. When patients with acromegaly are given a glucose load, their GH will not suppress to <2mcg/L as it will in normal subjects (this test is usually obtained by specialist)
- An ACTH level can be obtained in patients suspected of having Cushing's disease. Demonstrating inappropriately elevated ACTH with elevated cortisol levels is not simple. As with other pituitary hormones, ACTH secretion is pulsatile and unless it is exceedingly elevated, it may be difficult to obtain a diagnostic value. Additionally, very elevated ACTH values do not suggest a pituitary source of the ACTH but rather an ectopic ACTH-producing neoplasm (small cell lung carcinoma, bronchial carcinoid, medullary carcinoma of the thyroid, pheochromocytoma, paraganglioma). Further evaluation of Cushing's disease is best left to an endocrinologist, and is discussed in Cushing's syndrome

- Dexamethasone suppression test and the corticotrophin-releasing hormone (CRH) test are dynamic tests of function to determine if excess secretion of adrenal hormones is due to pituitary dysfunction. These tests require administration and interpretation by an endocrinologist
- Alpha subunit is a blood test that can be obtained when considering the diagnosis of thyrotropin-secreting, gonadotroph-secreting, or nonsecreting pituitary adenomas. Any of these adenomas may secrete alpha subunits and this will assist diagnosis
- MRI of the pituitary is the best imaging procedure for defining the anatomy of the pituitary. However, not every adenoma is clinically significant, so it is important to perform MRIs only on patients in whom clinical indications exist. Additionally, MRI is not as useful in Cushing's disease – not identifying an adenoma by MRI in patients clinically suspected of having Cushing's disease should not deter further workup. Many neurosurgeons believe MRI of the pituitary is inadequate even when an adenoma is identified, as clinically significant ACTH-secreting pituitary adenomas may be very small; what seems to be an adenoma on MRI may be an incidentaloma. Computed tomographic (CT) scan of the pituitary is only appropriate if MRI is unavailable or contraindicated
- Assessment of visual fields: helps determine the extension of the tumor. A larger tumor that extends beyond the confines of the sella turcica can cause headache and visual abnormalities. The classic presentation is bitemporal hemianopia from compression of the optic chiasm by a tumor that extends superiorly. If the chiasm is prefixed or if the tumor extends posteriorly, compression of a single optic tract produces a homonymous visual field defect. Lateral extension into the cavernous sinus can cause impaired oculomotor function involving cranial nerves III, IV, and VI, and the V_1 and V_2 divisions of cranial nerve V, either singly or in combination

DIAGNOSTIC DECISION

- When considering the diagnosis of pituitary adenoma, there are many issues to consider. The clinical presentation must be consistent with a syndrome caused by a pituitary tumor. Blood tests and MRI are then employed to identify the hormonal abnormalities and the pituitary adenoma
- Initial laboratory tests for evaluating a small prolactinoma should include prolactin, high-sensitivity TSH, and thyroid function tests to rule out hypothyroidism and as well as a pregnancy test. MRI of the pituitary should be obtained in patients with hyperprolactinemia not due to pregnancy, drug use, or hypothyroidism
- For patients in whom acromegaly is suspected the initial evaluation should include a random GH level (results of <1.0mcg/L exclude active acromegaly) and IGF-1 level (if elevated above age-related normal range, acromegaly is suggested)
- Patients with acromegaly will require a prolactin level to exclude co-secretion of prolactin and GH, as well as functional testing of the other pituitary hormonal functions. Patients will also need MRI of the pituitary and a visual field assessment as these tumors tend to be large at the time of diagnosis. Functional testing is usually performed by an endocrinologist
- Patients in whom Cushing's disease is suspected are initially evaluated for Cushing's syndrome. Cushing's disease is difficult to diagnose and treat, so these patients are best handled by physicians and centers that specialize in this disease
- In patients with hyperthyroidism and nonsuppressible TSH, a diagnosis of TSH-secreting adenoma should be considered. An MRI of the pituitary and alpha subunit blood test will help distinguish between a pituitary adenoma and pituitary resistance to thyroid hormone. Because these adenomas tend to be large at the time of diagnosis, visual field assessment and functional testing of the other pituitary hormonal functions is advised. These cases are rare and best managed by an endocrinologist
- Patients with gonadotroph or nonsecreting pituitary adenomas generally have large tumors at the time of presentation. These patients need an MRI of the pituitary to delineate the lesion, as well as an assessment of visual fields

- Prolactin levels are essential and may be elevated by stalk compression, but it is vital to exclude the possibility of a prolactinoma since initial therapy for a prolactinoma is likely medical rather than surgical. This is a determination that may be best left to an endocrinologist
- High-sensitivity TSH, thyroid function tests, IGF-1 levels, and 24h urine for free cortisol are also useful for excluding other pituitary hypersecretory states

CLINICAL PEARLS

- Patients with large tumors are at risk for compromise of other anterior pituitary functions due to compression of normal pituitary tissue, causing GH, corticotropin, luteinizing hormone (LH), follicle-stimulating hormone (FSH), or thyrotropin deficiency, singly or in combination
- Patients that come to medical attention should be screened with prolactin, high-sensitivity TSH, thyroid function tests, IGF-1, FSH, LH, alpha subunit, and cortisol after overnight dexamethasone suppression which will exclude pituitary hypersecretion syndromes
- If tests are positive, further testing is needed. If tests are negative, serial MRIs of the pituitary are needed every 6–12 months initially and then less frequently to evaluate the propensity for growth. A growing lesion will need resection or other appropriate therapy
- In men, suppression of hyperprolactinemia and restoration of gonadal function can cause an increase in radial shaft bone density but little change in vertebral bone density; suppression of hyperprolactinemia without restoration of gonadal function does not increase bone density
- In a patient with acromegaly, joint pain from accelerated osteoarthrosis may be misdiagnosed as degenerative arthritis. Arthralgias occur in 62–75% of acromegalic patients, and arthropathy is present in 16–62%
- The diagnosis of Cushing's syndrome may be made incidentally by X-ray findings of healed fractures (e.g. rib) with no known history of fracture. Because of the severe pain normally associated with a rib fracture, a painless rib fracture should always raise the possibility of this syndrome
- Gonadotropin adenomas are most commonly diagnosed in middle-aged or older men (mean age 45) who seek medical attention because of visual abnormality or headaches. The distinction between a nonsecretory adenoma and a gonadotrop adenoma may not be possible clinically or biochemically and may require electron microscopic or immunocytochemical study of the excised tumor

THE TESTS

Body fluids

SERUM PROLACTIN

Description

- Venous blood sample
- Useful in diagnosing pituitary adenoma if >100ng/mL (>100mcg/L)
- If prolactin is <100ng/mL (<100mcg/L), consider another source of hyperprolactinemia

Advantages/Disadvantages

Advantage: useful in diagnosing pituitary adenoma if >100ng/mL (>100mcg/L)

Diasadvantages:

- Prolactin levels of twice normal value can be found in normal subjects
- Prolactin is secreted in a pulsatile fashion and may require serial samples to detect abnormality if small adenoma if present

Normal

Normal prolactin levels are <20ng/mL (<20mcg/L) unless patient is pregnant or breast-feeding.

Abnormal

- Level of prolactin elevation correlates with tumor size
- Prolactin levels between 20–100ng/mL (20–100mcg/L) suggest microadenoma or another cause of hyperprolactinemia
- Prolactin levels above 200ng/mL (200mcg/L) suggest macroadenoma
- Prolactin levels between 100–200ng/mL (100–200mcg/L) may be due to adenoma or from compression of pituitary stalk by adenoma of any cell type
- Keep in mind the possibility of a false-positive result

Cause of abnormal result

- Prolactinomas secrete prolactin in excessive amounts
- Stalk compression prevents delivery of dopamine to the anterior pituitary – dopamine inhibits prolactin secretion

Drugs, disorders and other factors that may alter results

Other medical conditions may elevate prolactin:

- Pregnancy and breast-feeding
- Hypothyroidism
- Drug ingestion
- Other pituitary diseases causing stalk compression
- Chronic renal failure

HIGH-SENSITIVITY THYROID-STIMULATING HORMONE AND THYROID FUNCTION TESTS

Description

Venous blood specimen.

Advantages/Disadvantages

Advantages:

- Evaluation of pituitary thyroid axis
- Useful in differentiating primary from central hypothyroidism and hyperthyroidism

Normal

- High sensitivity TSH assay: 0.6–4.6mcU/mL (0.6–4.6mU/L)
- Thyroxine: 4–11mcg/dL (51–142nmol/L)
- Tri-iodothyronine resin uptake: 25–35% (0.25–0.35)

Abnormal

- The diagnosis of TSH-secreting adenoma should be considered when a TSH value is normal or elevated and the other thyroid function tests suggest hyperthyroidism
- Keep in mind the possibility of a false-positive test

Cause of abnormal result

TSH secretion by an adenoma is autonomous of normal feedback mechanisms.

Drugs, disorders and other factors that may alter results

- Estrogen, pregnancy, familial syndromes, and liver disease can increase serum protein binding of T4 and result in elevated levels of total T4
- When this occurs in the presence of a nonsuppressed TSH, the possibility of a TSH-secreting adenoma arises
- Obtaining a free T4 level to exclude hyperthyroidism is helpful in this scenario

URINARY OR SERUM HUMAN GONADOTROPIN HORMONE

Description

- An immunoassay that measures free beta subunits plus intact beta-human chorionic gonadotropin (hCG)
- Simple blood test or urine test
- Urine test is done by collecting the first-morning urine (usually contains the highest concentration of beta-hCG); however, any sample is suitable for testing. Sample should be collected in a plastic container

Advantages/Disadvantages

Advantages:

- Useful in diagnosing pregnancy
- Simple test with rapid result
- Especially important in hyperprolactinemia

Normal

- Plasma level: <3mIU/mL (3IU/L)
- Urine: negative

Abnormal

- Plasma level >3mIU/mL
- Beta-hCG present in the urine

Cause of abnormal result

- Pregnancy
- Ectopic pregnancy
- Abortion
- Trophoblastic and other germ cell tumors including extra-gonadal tumors
- Keep in mind the possibility of a false-positive result

GROWTH HORMONE

Description

- After a glucose tolerance test, GH should suppress to <2ng/mL, but fails to do so in patients with acromegaly
- Random GH levels are not generally useful for diagnosing acromegaly, but the diagnosis can be excluded if the GH level in a random blood sample is very low

Advantages/Disadvantages

Advantages:

- Simple blood test
- The demonstration of elevated and unsuppressible serum GH levels following glucose administration helps to confirm the diagnosis in adults with signs and symptoms of acromegaly, and more rarely in children or adolescents with gigantism

Normal

Normal GH levels vary with metabolic conditions.

Abnormal

- Levels outside of the normal ranges
- >2ng/mL after glucose tolerance test
- Keep in mind the possibility of a false-positive result

Cause of abnormal result
GH-secreting adenoma.

INSULIN-LIKE GROWTH FACTOR-1
Description
- IGF-1, also referred to as somatomedin-C (or Sm-C), is one of a class of peptides whose serum concentrations are regulated principally by human GH and nutritional intake
- In general, to diagnose acromegaly it is necessary to document elevated basal GH levels and failure to suppress GH levels with an oral glucose challenge to <2ng/mL

Advantages/Disadvantages
Advantages:
- A good screening test for GH excess is IGF-1, which has age-adjusted normal values and correlates well with the level of activity of GH
- Serum IGF-1 concentrations are reliably and predictably elevated in patients with acromegaly and in children with gigantism due to excess of pituitary GH

Disadvantages:
- Care should be taken with interpretation of elevated IGF-1 serum values in pubertal patients; however, because levels are normally increased at this time and may be as much as four to five times adult concentration.
- Pregnancy is also associated with high serum levels

Normal
- Women: 0.45–2.2U/mL (0.45–2.2kU/L)
- Men: 0.34–1.9U/mL (0.34–1.9kU/L)

Abnormal
Levels that are elevated when compared with age-adjusted normal values suggest acromegaly.

Cause of abnormal result
IGF-1 is a GH-mediated growth factor produced largely by the liver. Its levels are more constant in the blood than GH, which is pulsatile in nature.

Drugs, disorders and other factors that may alter results
- Systemic illnesses
- Poor nutrition

CORTICOTROPIN
Description
- Cushing's disease is diagnosed by elevated ACTH in the presence of elevated cortisol levels
- Abnormal changes in cortisol levels may be due to hypothalamic, pituitary, or adrenal malfunction. If undiagnosed and untreated, these disorders can lead to severe metabolic imbalance, which may be life-threatening

Advantages/Disadvantages
- Advantage: ACTH levels are useful in distinguishing corticotropin-dependent from corticotropin-independent hypercortisolism
- Disadvantage: sample collection and processing are complicated and delicate and failure to process correctly leads to erroneous results

Normal
20–100pg/mL (4–22pmol/L).

Abnormal

- ACTH levels are suppressed in patients with adrenal adenomas or adrenal carcinomas
- ACTH levels are detectable in patients with ectopic corticotropin syndromes, Cushing's disease, or ectopic CRH production
- Levels >200pg/mL suggest ectopic ACTH-producing neoplasm
- Levels <10pg/mL suggest adrenal neoplasm

CORTISOL (URINARY)

Description

- All causes of Cushing's syndrome (except glucocorticoid medication) are associated with increased 24h urinary cortisol
- The most common causes of Cushing's syndrome are bilateral adrenal hyperplasia (due to pituitary ACTH hypersecretion, Cushing's disease), pituitary adenoma, or corticotroph hyperplasia

Advantages/Disadvantages

- Advantage: urinary free cortisol is an excellent test for diagnosis of endogenous Cushing's syndrome and for assessing responses to dexamethasone suppression tests
- Disadvantage: patient has to collect 24h urine

Normal

Urinary free cortisol: 55–275nmol/24h (20–100mcg/day).

Abnormal

Values outside of the normal range.

ALPHA SUBUNIT

Description

Alpha subunit of TSH can be secreted in measurable amounts by thyrotropin-secreting adenomas, gonadotropin-secreting adenomas, and nonsecreting adenomas.

Advantages/Disadvantages

Advantage: useful in differentiating TSH-secreting pituitary adenoma from central resistance to thyroid hormone

Abnormal

- Central resistance of thyroid hormone: the ratio of alpha subunit to TSH is <1
- Thyrotropin-secreting adenoma: the ratio of alpha subunit to TSH is >1

Imaging

MAGNETIC RESONANCE IMAGING OF THE PITUITARY

Advantages/Disadvantages

Advantages:

- Imaging study of choice for the pituitary; it can identify adenomas as small as 2mm
- High-resolution MRI is about 90% sensitive in detecting adenomas

Disadvantages:

- Some adenomas, particularly ACTH-secreting adenomas, may be too small to detect by MRI
- MRI studies alone cannot be used to define the existence of an adenoma and must be interpreted in conjunction with the clinical picture and biochemical findings
- MRI is contraindicated in patients with severe claustrophobia, cardiac pacemakers, ferromagnetic aneurysm clips, or movable metal prostheses

Other tests

ASSESSMENT OF VISUAL FIELDS

Description

- Basic assessment of visual fields can be done by confrontation testing by the PCP
- If macroadenoma is found on MRI of the pituitary, more refined automated method of assessing visual fields should be obtained by an ophthalmologist
- Large pituitary tumors may result in impingement of the optic chiasm and cause bitemporal visual field defects

Advantages/Disadvantages

Advantage: this test is important in monitoring the success of therapy and in following growth of the tumor

TREATMENT

CONSIDER CONSULT

- Initial therapy for all macroadenomas except prolactinomas is trans-sphenoidal hypophysectomy. These patients will need referral to a neurosurgeon
- An endocrinologist should be involved to assess functional capacity of the pituitary both pre- and postoperatively and then to evaluate the need for permanent hormone replacement

IMMEDIATE ACTION

Patient needs immediate referral to neurosurgery for all macroadenomas when visual field is compromised.

PATIENT AND CAREGIVER ISSUES

Patient or caregiver request

- There has been controversy in the medical literature in the past about the association between estrogen-containing products (such as oral contraceptives or hormone replacement therapy) and the growth of prolactinomas
- While these tumors may grow in pregnancy, administering estrogen for contraception or hormone replacement is not contraindicated. These patients should be monitored closely
- Pituitary adenomas and/or surgery can affect fertility, but with the help of pituitary replacement therapies, patients can conceive

MANAGEMENT ISSUES

Goals

- Eliminate effects due to the mass of the tumor
- Reduce elevated pituitary hormone levels to normal
- Ameliorate end-organ effects of elevated pituitary hormone levels
- Avoid damage to remaining normal hypothalamic or pituitary function
- Minimize other potential adverse effects of therapy

Management in special circumstances

- Hemorrhage into a pituitary adenoma is not an uncommon event
- Unselected autopsy studies reveal 1–3% of persons with adenomas have hemorrhage involving more than 25% of the gland
- If the patient has MEN-1 syndrome, careful follow up with an endocrinologist is essential

COEXISTING DISEASE

Patients with diabetes mellitus, bleeding disorders, pituitary radiation, pneumoenphalography, carotid angiography, mechanical ventilation, trauma, and upper respiratory infection are at increased risk of hemorrhage into a pituitary adenoma.

COEXISTING MEDICATION

- Patients on systemic anticoagulants are at increased risk for hemorrhagic infarction into the pituitary
- Possible pituitary hemorrhage/apoplexy needs to be considered if patient has a pituitary adenoma and develops another medical condition necessitating systemic anticoagulation

SPECIAL PATIENT GROUPS

- In general, physicians should try to limit fetal exposure to bromocriptine to as short a period as possible
- Patients with microprolactinomas should be advised to stop bromocriptine after missed menses and have pregnancy confirmed

- Bromocriptine has not been shown to cause spontaneous abortions, ectopic pregnancies, trophoblastic disease, multiple pregnancies, or congenital malformations
- Long-term follow up of women who took bromocriptine throughout pregnancy shows no excess ill effect but the numbers are very limited
- Women with microadenomas who become pregnant are at 2% risk for significant symptomatic enlargement
- Women with macroadenomas are at 16% risk of significant symptomatic enlargement
- Women with previous surgery, radiation, or both are at 4% risk of significant symptomatic enlargement
- Bromocriptine has been used during pregnancy to reduce symptomatic tumor enlargement
- Prolactin levels are not useful in pregnancy. Prolactin levels may not always rise with tumor growth and may not always rise during pregnancy. Periodic magnetic resonance imaging (MRI) and visual field testing is advisable in patients with macroprolactinomas

PATIENT SATISFACTION/LIFESTYLE PRIORITIES

- Postpartum lactation is not contraindicated and has not been shown to encourage tumor growth
- Bromocriptine resumption must be delayed to permit postpartum lactation

SUMMARY OF THERAPEUTIC OPTIONS

Choices

- In general, there are three therapeutic choices for pituitary adenomas: surgery, radiation, or pharmacologic therapy. The best choice depends on the overall health status of the patient, the cell type of the adenoma, and the size of the adenoma
- Microprolactinoma: the first choice in patients with symptomatic microprolactinoma are dopamine agonists such as bromocriptine
- Macroadenoma: dopamine agonists are also the first choice in patients with macroadenomas, but if there is compromise of vision and no immediate response (within one week) to the bromocriptine, then trans-sphenoidal surgery is necessary. Cabergoline, a newer dopamine agonist, may be more potent than bromocriptine and may be useful in patients who fail therapy with bromocriptine. Radiation has limited effect on prolactinomas
- Growth hormone (GH)-secreting tumor: the first-choice therapy is trans-sphenoidal surgery and the second choice is bromocriptine or somatostatin analogs such as octreotide, or radiation
- Corticotrophin (ACTH)-secreting tumor: the first choice is trans-sphenoidal surgery and the second choice is radiation plus cortisol decreasing medications
- Thyroid-stimulating hormone (TSH)-secreting tumor: the first choice is trans-sphenoidal surgery; most of these patients also require radiation to control the adenoma. The next option is somatostatin analogues such as octreotide
- Gonadotroph-secreting tumor: the first choice for gonadotroph or nonsecreting tumors is trans-sphenoidal surgery. The second choice is radiation, which may be used if surgery fails to ablate the tumor
- Following surgical removal of the pituitary adenoma, the patient may have reduced or absent secretion of pituitary hormones. This hypopituitarism needs to be evaluated by an endocrinologist, and management of hormone replacement therapies is a priority

Clinical pearls

- Successful treatment of prolactinoma involves administration of a dopamine agonist. Some patients require more than one type of treatment to correct prolactin levels and decrease tumor size. In addition to medical and surgical therapy, pituitary radiation may be employed, usually as adjunctive therapy
- The results of dopamine agonist treatment is the same in macro- and microprolactinomas. Reduction in tumor size, improvement in visual abnormalities, and partial suppression of serum prolactin are usually evident before the serum prolactin level reaches the normal range

- In patients with acromegaly, even if all tests of GH secretion are normal postoperatively, late recurrence can occur. The incidence of recurrence is not known, but after an average follow up of 2–3.5 years, rates can be as high as 13%
- In patients with Cushing's syndrome, if the effects of excessive cortisol production are marked and if there is concern about operative morbidity, medical therapy to inhibit cortisol synthesis (ketoconazole or metyrapone) should be initiated before surgery

Never

A patient should never have trans-sphenoidal surgery for a pituitary adenoma without first obtaining a prolactin level.

FOLLOW UP

Follow up depends on the type of adenoma and the chosen therapy.

Plan for review

- Assess remaining tumor mass and the effects of remaining tumor mass by MRI and visual fields
- Check that pituitary hormone levels have normalized
- Assess symptomatic improvement that may occur from end-organ effects of normalizing pituitary hormones
- Assess damage to residual pituitary
- Review side-effects patient may be experiencing from chosen therapies

Information for patient or caregiver

- Many of the complications of untreated or poorly treated pituitary adenomas are not immediately apparent to the patient
- Some women prefer not dealing with monthly menstrual cycles, but they need to understand that not menstruating is a sign of inadequate sex hormone levels and puts them at risk for osteoporosis later in life

DRUGS AND OTHER THERAPIES: DETAILS

Drugs

BROMOCRIPTINE

The most widely used dopamine agonist is bromocriptine. Other dopamine agonists include cabergoline, which may be useful when patients cannot tolerate bromocriptine.

Dose

The initial adult dose of bromocriptine mesylate for hyperprolactinemic indications:

- 1.25–2.5mg/day
- An additional 2.5mg may be added to the treatment regimen as tolerated every 3–7 days, until an optimal therapeutic response is achieved
- The therapeutic dosage usually is 5–7.5mg and ranges from 2.5–15mg/day
- Medication should be taken with food

The initial adult dose of bromocriptine mesylate for acromegaly:

- 1.25–2.5mg at bedtime with food for 3 days
- An additional 1.25–2.5mg should be added to the treatment regimen as tolerated every 3–7 days until the patient obtains optimal therapeutic benefit
- The usual optimal therapeutic dosage range of bromocriptine mesylate varies from 20 to 30mg/day in most patients
- The maximal dosage should not exceed 100mg/day

Efficacy

- Microprolactinomas: 80–90% of patients respond with normoprolactinemia and return of ovulatory cycle
- Macroprolactinomas: 60–70% of patients respond with substantial shrinkage in tumor size and have improvement in visual fields if affected
- Acromegaly: 20% response if used after surgery

Risks/Benefits

Risks:

- Use caution in hepatic or renal disease
- Use caution in hypotension and concurrent hypertensive medications
- Use caution in children and in pregnancy

Benefits:

- Highly effective in treatment of prolactin-secreting tumors
- Decreases serum prolactin levels
- Decreases tumor size
- Restores gonadal function
- Decreases long-term risk of osteoporosis

Side-effects and adverse reactions

- Side-effects are lessened if the drug is started at a low dose
- Transvaginal administration of bromocriptine has been reported to cause fewer gastrointestinal side-effects
- Cardiovascular system: postural hypotension, vasospasm of fingers and toes
- Central nervous system: headache, dizziness, drowsiness, confusion, hallucinations, dyskinesia
- Eyes, ears, nose, and throat: visual disturbances
- Gastrointestinal: nausea, vomiting, diarrhea, anorexia, bleeding, dry mouth

Interactions (other drugs)

■ Erythromycin (increased bromocriptine levels) ■ Isometheptene (hypertension) ■ Neuroleptics (in patients with pituitary adenomas, may inhibit bromocriptine's ability to lower prolactin levels) ■ Drugs which have dopamine antagonist activity, e.g. phenothiazines, butyrophenones (may decrease efficacy of bromocriptine)

Contraindications

■ Severe ischemic and peripheral vascular disease ■ Uncontrolled hypertension ■ Lactation ■ Sensitivity to ergot preparations

Acceptability to patient

- Side-effects such as nausea, vomiting, and postural hypotension are generally seen early in therapy; this usually improves with continued therapy
- May help to start therapy at night

Follow up plan

- Microprolactinomas: follow up with repeat prolactin measurement at 3 and 12 months, and then annually. Consider withdrawal of medication every 2–3 years to check for remission. Consider neurosurgery if patient is intolerant of medication, has no response or no return of menses, or patient prefers surgery
- Macroprolactinomas: follow up with repeat prolactin levels at 3, 6, 9, and 12 months. Repeat MRI at 3–6 months and then annually until prolactin normalizes or maximum tumor shrinkage is obtained

- Smallest effective dose of bromocriptine should be used to maintain tumor shrinkage
- Treat hypogonadism, hypoadrenalism, and hypothyroidism but check need for long-term replacement when prolactin normalizes or maximum tumor shrinkage occurs
- Consider cabergoline, surgery, and/or radiotherapy if patient is intolerant of bromocriptine or if prolactin levels or tumor size continue to increase despite maximal therapy
- Cabergoline may be especially useful when compliance is questionable
- Consider surgery in patients presenting with visual or cranial nerve problems, if no improvement occurs within 7 days of initiating therapy

Patient and caregiver information

- Use measures to prevent orthostatic hypotension
- Importance of medication compliance needs to be stressed
- If the patient cannot tolerate the side-effects, alternate therapies exist; the patient needs to communicate any difficulty tolerating medications as poor compliance is the major hindrance to this therapy

CABERGOLINE

Long-acting dopamine agonist.

Dose

- Starting adult dose is 0.25mg twice weekly
- The dose can be increased by 0.25mg twice weekly up to a dose of 1mg twice weekly according to the patient's serum prolactin level
- Dosage increases should not occur more rapidly than every 4 weeks, so that the patient's response to each dosage level may be assessed

Efficacy

Appears to be as effective as bromocriptine in the treatment of hyperprolactinemia and may be better tolerated.

Risks/Benefits

Risks:

- Regional enteritis (past or present)
- Ulcerative colitis (past or present)
- History of antibiotic-induced colitis
- Risk of serious pleuro-pulmonary inflammatory-fibrotic reaction
- Risk of vasoconstriction in patients with unstable coronary angina and Raynaud's syndrome
- Dopamine agonists in general should not be used in patients with pregnancy-induced hypertension, e.g. preclampsia and eclampsia, unless the potential benefit is judged to outweigh the possible risk

Benefits:

- May be easier to tolerate
- May be useful in patients who fail to respond to bromocriptine

Side-effects and adverse reactions

- Cardiovascular system: hypotension
- Central nervous system: somolence, confusion, hallucinations
- Gastrointestinal: nausea, vomiting, constipation

Interactions (other drugs)

- Phenothiazines
- Butyrophenones
- Thioxanthines
- Metoclopramide

Contraindications

- **Safety and effectiveness of cabergoline in pediatric patients have not been established**
- **Hypersensitivity to cabergoline** ■ **Pregnancy category B**

Acceptability to patient

- Teratogenic effects have not been reported
- Gastrointestinal symptoms, headache, and dizziness are less severe with cabergoline than bromocriptine

Follow up plan

Guidelines for use of cabergoline are not yet established but it is likely that they will be similar to those for bromocriptine.

OCTREOTIDE

Somatostatin analog.

Dose

- The initial adult dose of octreotide acetate for the treatment of acromegaly is 50mcg subcutaneously or intravenously three times daily
- The dose most commonly found to be effective is 100mcg three times daily, but some patients require up to 500mcg three times daily for maximum effectiveness

Efficacy

- Effective treatment for acromegaly; if surgery is contraindicated, if surgery is unsuccessful, or while awaiting the effects of radiation therapy
- Effective in 40–60% of cases
- Many endocrinologists feel octreotide is indicated in bromocriptine nonresponders: efficacy of bromocriptine can be determined in 3 months; if ineffective, octeotide should be used
- Symptom improvement is greater than biochemical remission
- Can also be used after surgical debulking in patients with TSH-secreting tumors

Risks/Benefits

Risks:

- Single doses of octreotide acetate have been shown to inhibit gallbladder contractility and decrease bile secretion
- Octreotide acetate alters the balance between the counter-regulatory hormones, insulin, glucagon, and GH, which may result in hypoglycemia or hyperglycemia
- Octreotide acetate may alter absorption of dietary fats in some patients
- In patients with severe renal failure requiring dialysis, the half-life of octreotide acetate may be increased, necessitating adjustment of the maintenance dosage

Benefit: improves most symptoms of acromegaly, including diabetes, hypertension, sleep apnea

Side-effects and adverse reactions

- Cardiovascular system: sinus bradycardia, conduction abnormalities, and dysrhythmias
- Central nervous system: fatigue, dizziness, headache, and weakness
- Gastrointestinal: nausea, vomiting, diarrhea, distension, flatulence, and pancreatitis
- Metabolic: hyperglycemia, hypoglycemia, hypothyroidism, and goiter
- Musculoskeletal: myalgia and Bell's palsy
- Skin: alopecia and local pain on injection

Interactions (other drugs)

Patients taking insulin, oral hypoglycemic agents, beta-blockers, calcium channel blockers, or agents to control fluid and electrolyte balance will require dose adjustments of these treatments.

Contraindications

■ **Pregnancy** ■ **Breast-feeding** ■ **Gall bladder disease** ■ **Diabetes mellitus**

Acceptability to patient

- Generally well tolerated
- May sustain gastrointestinal side-effects due to effects on bowel motility

Follow up plan

- Monitor thyroid function tests, serum glucose, vitamin B12 levels
- Monitor heart rate in patients on beta-blockers or calcium channel blockers
- In patient having had surgery and on octreotide, measure GH and insulin-like growth factor-1 (IGF-1) at least every 6 months until levels stabilize
- Monitor for gallstones, consider biliary ultrasound
- Consider colonoscopy
- Monitor for osteoporosis

Patient and caregiver information

- Gallstones are a serious concern when using this medication
- Symptoms of biliary colic should be discussed with the patient

Surgical therapy

TRANS-SPHENOIDAL ADENOMECTOMY

Efficacy

- Response is defined as normalization of hormone secretion or ablation of tumor mass and is generally only required for tumors resistant to dopamine agonists
- Prolactin-secreting tumors: microadenomas 55% response; macroadenomas 20% response
- GH-secreting tumors: microadenomas 70% response; macroadenomas 50% response
- Adrenocorticotropic hormone (ACTH)-secreting tumors: microadenomas 80–90% response; macroadenomas 50% response
- TSH-secreting tumors: surgery with irradiation 67% response
- Gonadotroph or nonsecreting tumors (with endpoint of improved vision): 70% response

Risks/Benefits

Risks:

- Surgical mortality rate for all types of secreting and nonsecreting tumors is 1%
- Surgical major morbidity is 7%, rates are lower for microadenomas
- Transient diabetes insipidus is the most common complication but is permanent only about 1% of the time

Acceptability to patient

Patients are more accepting of trans-sphenoidal surgery than the alternative, craniotomy, which is used only for very large tumors.

Follow up plan

- Prolactin-secreting adenomas: different series report various cure rates. If the preoperative prolactin level is <10,000ng/mL (<10,000mcg/L), recurrence rates are 40–90% with preservation of pituitary function. If the postoperative prolactin level is normal, recurrence rates are 10–40% over 5 years, so serum prolactin levels should be followed intermittently even if prolactin returns to normal initially

- Acromegaly: assess 6–12 weeks postsurgery. If surgery leaves residual tumor, options include repeat surgery, pituitary radiotherapy, medical therapy, or any combination. If basal GH is <2mcg/L, review annually or less frequently with GH and IGF-1. Inquire about headaches and check visual field if GH is >2mcg/L. Repeat MRI scan if GH rises consistently during follow up
- Cushing's disease: a biochemical assessment can be performed within 7 days of surgery; these patients benefit from long-term follow up with an endocrinologist so that recovery of the hypothalamic-pituitary adrenal axis can be assessed, reoccurrences detected, and steroid replacement monitored
- TSH-secreting tumors: only about one-third of tumors are cured surgically; MRI monitoring is needed and most patients will require irradiation and/or octreotide
- Gonadotroph and nonsecreting tumors: early imaging to detect tumor at 2–3 months postoperatively; an MRI should be done at 6–12 months and then at 1–5 year intervals to determine if the tumor has returned. Cortisol requirement can be assessed prior to discharge and again at 6–12 weeks after surgery. If hormonal deficits persist past 12 weeks, they are likely to be permanent

Patient and caregiver information

While initial results of surgery may be encouraging, the patient needs to be made aware of the possibility of reoccurrence. The need for long-term follow up needs to be stressed.

Radiation therapy

PITUITARY RADIATION

Efficacy

- Not recommended as primary therapy for any pituitary adenomas; however, it is a useful adjunct therapy in GH-secreting, TSH-secreting, corticotropin-secreting, gonadotroph, or nonsecreting adenomas
- May be primary therapy for patients who are unable to have surgery

Risks/Benefits

Risks:

- There is a significant risk of hypopituitarism – ranging from 25 to 50%
- Radiation therapy may result in damage to the optic chiasm and oculomotor nerves
- Potential risk of second extrapituitary brain tumor
- A newer procedure using a gamma knife may have better safety profile but this has yet to be established

Acceptability to patient

Generally used in patients who are not surgical candidates or have failed surgery.

Follow up plan

Given high rate of subsequent hypopituitarism, in addition to monitoring active disease, patients need to be followed for hypopituitarism at least annually.

Patient and caregiver information

Patients need to be familiarized with symptoms of hypopituitarism and the importance of regular screening for hypopituitarism.

OUTCOMES

EFFICACY OF THERAPIES

- Great advances in the management of pituitary tumors have resulted from the better visualization available with magnetic resonance imaging (MRI)
- In general, microadenomas respond better to the primary therapeutic approach of choice – dopamine agonists for prolactinomas and surgery for other types of adenomas
- Macroadenomas frequently require more than a single therapeutic modality for cure or control
- Macroprolactinomas that fail to respond to dopamine agonists require surgery
- Other types of macroadenomas that fail to respond adequately to surgery alone should be referred for pharmacologic and/or radiation therapy

PROGNOSIS

Prognosis depends on the size of the adenoma, the cell type, and the propensity for growth.

Clinical pearls

- The medical conditions associated with acromegaly (hypertension, coronary heart disease, diabetes) contribute to a shorter life span, making early diagnosis crucial
- In retrospective reviews, acromegalic patients have a risk of premature mortality, usually from cardiovascular and pulmonary causes. However, lowering the serum growth hormone concentrations appears to reduce the risk of premature mortality
- Pituitary apoplexy occurs when the tumor undergoes infarction, hemorrhage, or both. The sudden occurrence of severe headache followed by visual disturbances usually leads to a consideration of subarachnoid hemorrhage, but a computed tomographic or MRI scan readily makes the diagnosis
- Octreotide infusion can improve visual defects caused by nonfunctioning and gonadotropin-secreting adenomas in approximately half the patients treated. Patients who respond usually demonstrate improvement within 4 days

Therapeutic failure

- The initial therapy for prolactinomas is dopamine agonists; if this therapy fails the next option to consider is surgery
- The initial therapy for other types of pituitary tumors is surgery; if surgery is not successful, options to consider include further surgery, radiation therapy, or appropriate pharmacologic agents

Recurrence

- Recurrences can occur in patients who were treated for microprolactinomas with dopamine agonist therapy, which was discontinued when the prolactin normalized and normal pituitary hormonal function returned
- These patients should receive another trial of dopamine agonists unless the patient's preference is for surgery

Deterioration

- In general, patients with poorly responsive pituitary tumors are also under the care of an endocrinologist
- Octreotide should be considered in any patient with acromegaly or thyroid-stimulating hormone-secreting pituitary adenomas who has had radiation therapy or is awaiting its effects
- Patients with Cushing's disease awaiting the effects of radiation therapy need to be started on steroidogenic inhibitors

Terminal illness

Terminal illness from pituitary adenomas is rare but aggressive adenomas can be locally invasive and destroy structures surrounding the pituitary such as the optic chiasm and cerebral blood vessels.

COMPLICATIONS

- Hypopituitarism may result from the aggressive growth of a pituitary tumor, or secondary to radiation therapy or surgery for macroadenomas. It develops insidiously and may have catastrophic implications if not diagnosed. Patients may present when stressed by an intercurrent illness and vascular collapse has developed
- Osteoporosis is a complication of any pituitary adenoma that causes hypogonadism
- Infertility may result from macroadenomas, but replacement therapies exist so fertility may be restored
- Pituitary hemorrhages are a relatively common occurrence. Pituitary apoplexy is an extreme case
- Cranial nerve deficits may occur and are due to extension into the cavernous sinus
- Hydrocephalus may occur and is due to extension in the third ventricle compressing the foramen of Monro
- Diabetes insipidus may occur and is due to compression of hypothalmus or pituitary stalk

CONSIDER CONSULT

- Patients who have failed therapy for prolactinomas with dopamine agonists will require referral to an experienced neurosurgeon. This is a decision which will be made in concert with the endocrinologist
- Patients who have failed to improve significantly with trans-sphenoidal surgery for nonprolactin-secreting adenoma may benefit from radiation therapy as well as pharmacotherapy. In general, this decision involves the endocrinologist, the neurosurgeon, and the primary care physician

PREVENTION

Pituitary adenomas are not preventable.

RESOURCES

ASSOCIATIONS

American Association of Clinical Endocrinologists
1000 Riverside Avenue, Suite 205
Jacksonville, FL 32204
Tel: (904) 353-7878
Fax: (904) 353-8185
www.aace.com

KEY REFERENCES

- Clayton RN, Wass J. Pituitary tumors: recommendations for service provision and guidelines for management of patients. Summary of a consensus statement of a working party from the endocrinology and diabetes committee of the Royal College of Physicians and the Society for Endocrinology in conjunction with the research unit of the Royal College of Physicians. J R Coll Physicians Lond 1997;31:628–36
- Shimon I, Melmed S. Management of pituitary tumors. Ann Intern Med 1998;129:472–83
- Molitch M, ed. Medical knowledge self assessment program in the subspecialty of endocrinology and metabolism. American College of Physicians, 1995: p12–22
- Thorner M, et al. Anterior pituitary. In: Wilson JD. Williams book of endocrinology, 9th edn. Philadelphia: WB Saunders, 1998
- Pellegrini I, Rasolonjanahary R, Gunz G, et al. Resistance to bromocriptine in prolactinomas. J Clin Endocrinol Metab 1989;69:500–9
- Nelson PB, Goodman M, Maroon JC, et al. Factors in predicting outcome from operation in patients with prolactin-secreting pituitary adenomas. Neurosurgery 1983;13:634–41
- Bengtsson BA, Eden S, Ernest I, et al. Epidemiology and long-term survival in acromegaly. A study of 166 cases diagnosed between 1955 and 1984. Acta Med Scand 1988;223:327–35
- Bates AS, Van't Hoff W, Jones JM, et al. An audit of outcome of treatment in acromegaly. Q J Med 1993; 86:293–9
- Sonino N, Boscaro M, Paoletta A, et al. Ketoconazole treatment in Cushing's syndrome: experience in 34 patients. Clin Endocrinol (Oxf) 1991;35:347–52

FAQS

Question 1

Why do some patients with prolactinoma respond to the treatment with dopamine agonists and others don't?

ANSWER 1

The clinical response to medical therapy and the number and affinity of tumor dopamine receptors are correlated. Surgically resected adenomas from bromocriptine-responsive patients have twice as many dopamine receptors and higher binding affinity for dopamine than do adenomas from bromocriptine-resistant patients. These observations probably explain occasional tumor growth during bromocriptine therapy, loss of responsiveness, and occasional metastasis of tumors.

Question 2

How can one predict the results of trans-sphenoidal surgery in a patient with prolactinoma?

ANSWER 2

The most important factors predictive of successful surgery are the preoperative serum prolactin concentration and the tumor size and stage (degree of invasion of parasellar structures). Of 266 women with prolactinoma, a normal postoperative serum prolactin level was achieved in 86% when the preoperative prolactin concentration was 20–250 ng/mL (20–250mcg/L), in 48% when the preoperative concentration was 250–500ng/mL (250–500mcg/L), and in 6% when the preoperative concentration was >1000ng/mL (>1000mcg/L); similar results have been reported in hyperprolactinemic men.

Question 3
What is the main cause of death in an acromegalic patient?

ANSWER 3
Cardiovascular disease is the most common cause of death in acromegalic patients. In approximately 80% of acromegalic patients, cardiac enlargement, usually an increase of left ventricular mass, can be detected by echocardiography and is independent of hypertension or ischemic heart disease.

Question 4
What is the prognosis in acromegaly?

ANSWER 4
Acromegalic patients have a risk of premature mortality, usually from cardiovascular and pulmonary causes. Survival may be reduced by an average of 10 years compared with the general population. However, lowering the serum growth hormone concentrations appears to reduce the risk of premature mortality. Increased awareness of the early symptoms and signs of acromegaly, ease of diagnosis, ability to determine the correct cause, results of modern trans-sphenoidal pituitary microsurgery (which demonstrate that the smaller the tumor at the time of operation, the better the outcome), and results of radiotherapy and medical therapy all suggest that patients with acromegaly are more likely to be cured today than in the past.

Question 5
What is the role of medical therapy for Cushing's disease?

ANSWER 5
Medical therapy for Cushing's disease is adjunctive only. It is used to reduce cortisol production in preparing an extremely ill patient for surgery and to maintain normal plasma cortisol levels while awaiting the full effects of radiation. Other medical therapies, such as the use of cyproheptadine and bromocriptine to reduce pituitary corticotropin secretion, are effective in few patients. Those who respond to bromocriptine may have intermediate lobe tumors, but this concept is unconfirmed.

CONTRIBUTORS
Gordon H Baustian, MD
Otavio A Clark, MD
Dinesh S Rao, MD

PLEURAL MALIGNANT MESOTHELIOMA

SUMMARY INFORMATION

DESCRIPTION

- Pleural malignant mesothelioma is a malignant neoplasm of the pleura
- It is uncommon and occurs mainly in men aged 40–60 years
- There is a very strong causal link with asbestos exposure, first described as recently as 1960
- The risk of pleural malignant mesothelioma increases with the time from exposure and with the total cumulative dose of exposure. The risk is not related to cigarette smoking
- The prognosis is poor, and if inoperable there is no generally effective treatment

ICD9 CODE

163. Malignant neoplasm of pleura.

SYNONYMS

- Pleural mesothelioma
- Malignant mesothelioma
- Pleuroperitoneal malignant mesothelioma
- Malignant pleural mesothelioma

CARDINAL FEATURES

- A history of asbestos exposure. The longer and stronger the exposure, the more the risk. A history of exposure to crocidolite fibers is usual
- There is a latent period between the exposure to asbestos and the development of pleural malignant mesothelioma of at least 20 years
- Insidious onset of symptoms with good general health
- Breathlessness of insidious but fairly rapid onset
- Chest pains, nonpleuritic, often continuous and severe
- Characteristic chest X-ray changes that include pleural effusion and irregular protuberant opacities of the inner chest wall
- Poor prognosis, with little effective treatment
- Incurable disease; few patients can have a long-term survival if treated in early stages
- Distant metastases occur frequently but may not be clinically apparent

CAUSES

Common causes

Asbestos exposure:

- Asbestos occurs as amphiboles (straight, rod-like fibers) or chrysotile (silky, serpentine fibers). Amphibole fibers can be categorized by fiber size into amosite, anthophyllite, or crocidolite. Crocidolite fibers are cleared from the lungs more slowly than any other asbestos fibers, which may account for its greater pathogenicity
- Mesothelioma is more likely after exposure to amphibole (especially crocidolite) than chrysotile fibers of asbestos
- The risk of mesothelioma is related to the total cumulative dose of exposure
- Exposure is highest in asbestos miners and workers exposed to cutting or grinding asbestos
- Naturally occurring minerals cause high rates of mesothelioma in a few communities in Cyprus, Greece, and Turkey
- The mean latent period between first exposure to asbestos and mesothelioma is around 35–40 years and is rare under 20 years
- More rarely, mesothelioma may occur in patients with a history of indirect exposure to asbestos. Examples include via the clothes of relatives who had direct asbestos exposure, or through environmental contamination from a nearby asbestos factory
- The risks of developing mesothelioma from, for example, a deteriorating asbestos ceiling in an office or school are very small

The risk of mesothelioma is not affected by smoking.

Rare causes

- A possible link with simian virus 40, which contaminated polio vaccine in the 1950–60s has been postulated

- Such a link may explain the rapid rise in the condition since the 1960s, and partly explains why only a relatively small proportion of people who are exposed to asbestos will develop mesotheliomas
- The proof of the link, however, fails to stand up to vigorous epidemiologic scrutiny

Serious causes

Asbestos exposure: there is a history of significant asbestos exposure in >90% of proven cases of pleural malignant mesothelioma.

EPIDEMIOLOGY

Incidence and prevalence

- The incidence and prevalence of asbestosis will peak in the early 21st century before rapidly declining
- Better protection for asbestos miners and workers, and stricter environmental protection laws were introduced in the 1960s and 1970s, resulting in less asbestos-related diseases, especially mesotheliomas, 35–40 years later

INCIDENCE

- 3–7 cases/million population per year in the US
- 3–10 cases/million population per year in the UK
- One case/million population per year with no history of asbestos exposure
- 50,000–90,000 cases/million population who have had significant exposure to asbestos
- Thus, most (70–80%) cases are secondary to asbestos exposure

FREQUENCY

- About 5–9% of occupationally exposed individuals will develop pleural malignant mesothelioma
- It is not known why only a small number are so affected
- There are about 2200 new cases per year in the US

Demographics

AGE

40–60 years.

GENDER

Male:female = 3:1.

GEOGRAPHY

Cases of pleural malignant mesothelioma are clustered in population centers that have/had high concentrations of industries in which asbestos is/was used, e.g. ports, dockyards, shipbuilding, railway works, automobile parts manufacturing, and heavy engineering plants.

SOCIOECONOMIC STATUS

Pleural malignant mesothelioma is more common in blue-collar workers, as they will have been more likely to have had significant exposure to asbestos.

DIFFERENTIAL DIAGNOSIS

Carcinoma of the lung

Carcinoma of the lung usually occurs in smokers or ex-smokers, in late middle-age. Asbestos exposure increases the risk of lung cancer, especially in smokers.

FEATURES

- Chest X-ray may reveal a suspicious unilateral mass in lung cancer
- However, both mesothelioma and lung cancer may produce a unilateral pleural effusion
- Bronchial carcinoma may be the most difficult to differentiate as it is common while mesothelioma is not, and bronchial carcinoma may present with unusual features
- Even pleural fluid microscopy and pleural biopsy results may not easily distinguish the two conditions, and a definitive diagnosis may not be made until necroscopy

Metastatic cancers

Cancers of the breast, stomach, uterus, and pancreas commonly metastasize to the lung and may produce some initial diagnostic confusion. Lymphomas, especially Hodgkin's and lymphosarcomas, can cause pleural effusions.

FEATURES

Metastatic cancers usually result in bilateral pleural effusions, and there are no other apparent pleural abnormalities.

Other causes of pleural effusions

Pleural effusions can result from a variety of inflammatory or infective causes, including pneumonias, sarcoidosis, and rheumatoid arthritis.

FEATURES

- There are usually specific or systemic symptoms and signs or chest X-ray changes to help differentiate these disorders from pleural malignant mesothelioma
- Pleural effusions without any other radiologic clues are usually associated with pulmonary tuberculosis, small deposits of other intrathoracic malignancies, or Meigs's syndrome (ovarian fibromyoma with hydrothorax and/or hydroperitoneum)

Asbestos exposure and benign pleural effusion

Benign pleural effusions are uncommon in patients who have been exposed to asbestos; 2–3% of such patients will develop benign pleural effusions. Benign effusions are less common following chrysotile exposure.

FEATURES

- Benign effusions are often unilateral and usually small (<500mL)
- They do not usually cause dyspnea, or produce only mild dyspnea if the effusion is large
- Pleuritic chest pain occurs in two-thirds of cases
- They usually spontaneously resolve within a few months, leaving persistent costophrenic blunting on the chest X-ray
- Occasionally they recur repeatedly

SIGNS & SYMPTOMS

Signs

- Initially the patient will be in good general health
- As the disease progresses there will be emaciation and dyspnea at rest

- Signs are those of pleural effusion or thickening: dull percussion note and decreased breath sounds, the extent of which are not limited by anatomical boundaries; sometimes there are bronchial breath sounds, especially above the effusion; and the affected side moves poorly
- Signs of pleural effusion are usually unilateral
- Clubbing is unusual (about 10% of cases of pleural malignant mesothelioma)
- Pulmonary osteoarthropathy arthritis pain (distal extremities with periosteal new bone formation) is unusual, but may be severe
- Tumor masses may track through biopsy or drain sites and appear as visible or palpable masses
- Vocal cord paralysis and Horner's syndrome on the same side as the tumor can occasionally occur as late complications
- Profuse sweating may occur

Symptoms

- Symptoms are usually of insidious onset
- Breathlessness: usually of fairly gradual, insidious onset, worse on exertion, but with no accompanying wheeze
- As the tumor progresses, breathlessness becomes more severe and occurs at rest
- Rapidly escalating breathlessness can occur if fluid accumulates rapidly in the pleural space or in the tumor itself
- Cough, which may be intractable, and which is nonproductive, is common
- Chest pain is nearly universal, may be nonspecific, dull, constant, and severe. It is not usually pleuritic in nature
- The pain may radiate to the ipsilateral shoulder or abdomen
- Local invasion of the brachial plexus may cause pain, paresthesia, and weakness on the ulnar side of the ipsilateral arm
- Tiredness, weight loss, and nonspecific malaise may develop in the later stages
- Hemoptysis is rare

ASSOCIATED DISORDERS

- Calcified pleural plaques, a marker of asbestos exposure, are very often seen on chest X-ray
- Peritoneal malignant mesothelioma: associated with heavier asbestos exposure and for longer periods than that for pleural mesotheliomas. About 20% of all malignant mesothelioma are peritoneal
- Pleural malignant mesothelioma overall occurs twice as commonly as peritoneal mesothelioma
- For patients who were first exposed to asbestos in the 1920s, the ratio of new pleural to peritoneal mesothelioma was 1:5, by the 1950s this had altered to 3:1
- Malignant mesothelioma can rarely arise in the pericardium and tunica vaginalis testis

CONSIDER CONSULT

Referral of all cases of suspected pleural malignant mesothelioma is mandatory:

- To confirm or refute the diagnosis (even if histologic proof is never achieved), staging, and prognosis
- For medico-legal reasons, as most patients will be eligible for compensation from their former employers or from their state

INVESTIGATION OF THE PATIENT

Direct questions to patient

Q **Is there any history of asbestos exposure?** Usually the exposure is occupational, first occurred at least 20 years ago, and was recurrent or persistent. A history of appreciable exposure is usual, and failure to elicit such a history should cast doubt on a diagnosis of pleural malignant mesothelioma without confirmatory tests

Q **How quickly did the symptoms start?** An abrupt and sudden onset or a very prolonged, insidious onset over many years would not be usual

- **Are you, or were you, a heavy smoker?** Although pleural malignant mesothelioma can and does occur in smokers, smoking is not a risk factor for the development of pleural malignant mesothelioma; smoking is a strong risk factor for lung cancer
- **Do your symptoms include coughing up blood?** Hemoptysis is unusual in pleural malignant mesothelioma
- **Are there any nonchest symptoms, such as arthritis or abdominal pains?** Such features may indicate other diagnoses, such as rheumatoid arthritis or nonpleural malignancies
- **Have you noticed any changes in your hands?** Clubbing is rare with pleural malignant mesothelioma, but pulmonary osteoarthropathy is more common

Contributory or predisposing factors

- **Did you ever work with asbestos, or in a building with asbestos lagging, or do any close relatives work with or have a history of working with asbestos?** Pleural malignant mesothelioma is much more common after prolonged or high-dose asbestos exposure, but can occur after seemingly more trivial or secondary exposure.

Examination

- **Check for signs of a pleural effusion.** Pleural malignant effusions nearly always present with signs of a pleural effusion
- **Check if the patient's fingers are clubbed.** If they are, this suggests lung cancer rather than mesothelioma
- **Check for evidence of pulmonary osteoarthropathy arthritis** (distal extremities with periosteal new bone formation). This can occur in lung cancer as well as with mesothelioma

Summary of investigative tests

- Chest X-ray: this is essential in all cases for the diagnosis of pleural malignant mesothelioma
- Computed tomograhy (CT) scans of the chest: will help to accurately differentiate the cause of an abnormal chest X-ray
- Pleural fluid cytology: usually performed by a specialist, but the results may be available for the primary care physician (PCP) to discuss with the patient. It is performed on fluid aspirated from the pleural space and is often hard to interpret because normal mesothelial cells can appear malignant. Sensitivity varies from 25% to >60%, depending on the experience of the laboratory and cytologist. It can be especially difficult to differentiate accurately between mesothelioma cells and cells from a secondary pleural malignancy. Counts and distribution of asbestos fiber types are also helpful but are diagnostic of previous asbestos exposure, not of pleural malignant mesothelioma. Typically, counts are less than in asbestosis, but higher than in controls. Ultrasound and CT-guided biopsy should be used to increase the likelihood of accurate diagnosis
- Pleural fluid chemistry: usually performed by a specialist, but the results may be available for the PCP to discuss with the patient. This test will show a high protein content characteristic of an exudate, often be bloodstained, and have a high hyaluronic acid content although this has low sensitivity and specificity
- Sputum examination under the microscope may reveal asbestos bodies
- Closed pleural biopsy: usually performed by a specialist, but the results may be available for the PCP to discuss with the patient. It is invasive and requires a local or even general anesthetic. Tumor cells may infiltrate the needle track or incision site. Trephine biopsy minimizes this risk, and may allow larger samples to be obtained
- Biopsy analysis may not be diagnostic; definite diagnoses may be possible in only 40–60% of biopsy specimens. Histologic diagnosis can be difficult because of the pleomorphic nature of mesothelioma. It can be especially difficult to differentiate mesothelioma from secondary adenocarcinoma of the pleura, usually from the lung, and it is also difficult to accurately distinguish malignant from benign pleural disease. Electron microscopy or immunohistochemical techniques using carcinoembryonic antigen, or stains for human milk fat globule 1 and 2, and alpha-1 antichymotrypsin may help
- Care should always be taken before performing pleural aspiration as the tumor often grows along any needle track or surgical incision

DIAGNOSTIC DECISION

There are no specific diagnostic guidelines but the British Thoracic Society Standards of Care Committee recommends the following strategy [1].

Diagnosis is suspected on the basis of:

- A history of significant asbestos exposure in the past
- Symptoms and signs, especially chest pain
- Chest X-ray changes showing pleural effusion or thickening

Diagnosis is confirmed by:

- CT scanning of the chest
- Pleural aspiration of fluid for cytology and culture
- Pleural biopsy, guided by CT if possible, if not surgical or thoracoscopic biopsy

Consider bronchoscopy and mediastinoscopy on any patient fit enough for the procedure, to allow accurate staging and assessment of the prognosis.

In practice, although a noninvasive expectant course seems logical in suspected cases, many patients will not tolerate the uncertainty and will prefer that definitive diagnostic procedures are undertaken. Pathologic confirmation of the diagnosis is, therefore, recommended unless the patient is frail or has extremely advanced disease.

CLINICAL PEARLS

- Pleural malignant mesothelioma may occasionally present with unexplained chest pain and a normal chest radiograph
- Symptomatic metastatic disease is unusual at presentation
- Negative pleural biopsy and cytology results do not exclude mesothelioma and should lead to further investigations
- Bilateral disease rarely occurs at presentation but is more common in the terminal phases

THE TESTS

Body fluids

SPUTUM EXAMINATION

Description

- Sputum can be collected by spontaneous expectoration or after inhalation of an irritating aerosol (e.g. hypertonic saline)
- Examination of the sputum under the microscope may reveal asbestos bodies

Advantages/Disadvantages

Advantage: noninvasive.

Cause of abnormal result

Past exposure to asbestos.

Imaging

CHEST X-RAY

Description

Plain posteroanterior and lateral views of the chest.

Advantages/Disadvantages

Advantages:

- Usually diagnostic (a normal chest X-ray is very unusual with mesothelioma)
- Inexpensive, safe, and easy to perform
- Can be repeated

Abnormal

- Calcified pleural plaques indicate previous asbestos exposure and are not diagnostic of mesothelioma, merely providing evidence of asbestos exposure
- Pleural plaques may be absent in proven cases of mesothelioma attributable to asbestos exposure
- The appearances of the pleural tumor vary according to the stage at which the disease is first seen, its distribution, and whether or not it is associated with an effusion
- Pulmonary fibrosis is seen in 20% of cases of pleural malignant mesothelioma (50% of abdominal types)
- Pleural effusions are nearly always seen
- Pleural thickening may be seen above the fluid or after aspiration
- Later, an irregular lobulated opacity that lines part or all of one inner chest wall is characteristic. Such opacities may extend into the lung field
- Occasionally, a hilar mass is seen if the greater part of the tumor lies within the mediastinum
- In advanced disease, there is contraction of the affected hemithorax

COMPUTED TOMOGRAPHY SCAN OF CHEST

Description

CT of the structures of the thorax.

Advantages/Disadvantages

- Advantage: CT scan of the chest will demonstrate all the features described for the chest X-ray, but more clearly
- Disadvantage: more costly and not universally available

Abnormal

- Calcified pleural plaques indicate previous asbestos exposure and are not diagnostic of mesothelioma, merely providing evidence of asbestos exposure
- Pulmonary fibrosis is seen in 20% of cases of pleural malignant mesothelioma (50% of abdominal types)
- Pleural effusions are nearly always seen
- Pleural thickening may be seen above the fluid or after aspiration
- Later, a lobulated outline to the thickening is characteristic
- In advanced disease, there is contraction of the affected hemithorax
- Demonstration of chest wall invasion by CT scanning is highly suggestive of malignant rather than benign pleural disease

TREATMENT

CONSIDER CONSULT

If referral is logistically difficult:

- Any patient with known or suspected asbestos exposure presenting with symptoms or signs of possible mesothelioma or pleural effusion should have a chest X-ray as soon as possible
- If this is abnormal, arrange a computed tomography (CT) scan if the changes are equivocal
- Otherwise, consider pleural aspiration and possible pleural biopsy (bearing in mind neither is completely diagnostic), referral at this stage, or watchful waiting

PATIENT AND CAREGIVER ISSUES

Patient or caregiver request

- Many patients equate any exposure to asbestos, however inert and transient, with high risks to their health
- There is a great deal of public anxiety and misinformation about the risks of asbestos exposure
- Many people will be at no or low risk of developing pleural malignant mesothelioma because of their trivial or low-grade asbestos exposure, but perceive themselves to be at high risk. Education and reassurance are needed
- Many people who have had significant exposure to asbestos may not realize the implications, especially if the exposure was some time ago

Health-seeking behavior

Are you still at risk of asbestos exposure? This is now unlikely in North America, Australasia, or western Europe due to strict health and safety laws, but may be more likely elsewhere.

MANAGEMENT ISSUES

Goals

- To relieve the symptoms of breathlessness, chest pain, and cough
- To diagnose accurately, so that a realistic prognosis can be formulated
- To provide comprehensive, holistic palliative care

Management in special circumstances

PATIENT SATISFACTION/LIFESTYLE PRIORITIES

Patients are seeking relief of their symptoms, a diagnosis, and thus a prognosis.

SUMMARY OF THERAPEUTIC OPTIONS

Choices

There are no specific published treatment guidelines, but the British Thoracic Society Standards of Care Committee recommend the following strategy [1]:

- There is no established effective therapeutic option for the management of pleural malignant mesothelioma
- There is certainly no curative treatment
- Treatment will depend on the stage of the tumor, and the wishes and general health of the patient
- Staging is important for the correct selection of patients for surgery, and for entry into any clinical trials

There is no first-line therapy or established hierarchy of management options. The following have been used:

- Radical surgery is worth considering in cases of localized disease in otherwise healthy patients
- Pleural aspiration and pleurodesis are useful for recurrent pleural effusions
- Many cytotoxic agents have been tried, but none are very successful

- Radiotherapy may provide pain relief, and fast neutron therapy may prevent growth of tumor through biopsy sites
- Opiate analgesics remain the mainstay of treatment in the later stages of the disease; other conventional analgesics, e.g. nonsteroidal anti-inflammatory drugs (NSAIDs) and analgesic patches, can be used
- A number of newer agents, including gene therapy and lovastatin, are under trial

Never

Never fail to take seriously any respiratory or chest symptoms in a patient known to have had significant asbestos exposure in the past. Examine carefully and have a low threshold for ordering a chest X-ray.

FOLLOW UP

- During and immediately after any active therapy of any sort
- As needed after active therapy, but monthly when well, increasingly frequently thereafter, to provide support and symptomatic relief when needed

Plan for review

- There is no generally effective therapy and the prognosis is poor
- Regular follow up, of increasing frequency, will provide support and succor to the patient, and attention to symptom relief, even if the course of the disease cannot be altered
- If the diagnosis has not been definitely established, regular reviews are needed (at least monthly) and any changes in symptoms or signs that suggest alternative diagnoses must be investigated and in turn followed up

Information for patient or caregiver

- Most patients will need to know their diagnosis and subsequent prognosis
- The patient may wish to include family and friends in making any decisions regarding investigations and therapies

DRUGS AND OTHER THERAPIES: DETAILS

Surgical therapy

- Surgical intervention can be by aspiration of a pleural effusion (often repeatedly), pleurodesis, pleurectomy, or radical pleuropneumonectomy
- These therapies are usually carried out by specialists who are part of a multidisciplinary team

PLEURAL ASPIRATION AND PLEURODESIS, PLEURECTOMY

- Recurrent aspiration of pleural effusions and chemical pleurodesis are useful for control of symptomatic effusions
- Pleural aspiration may also help in the diagnosis of pleural malignant mesothelioma
- If an effusion repeatedly reforms despite several aspirations, and especially if the effusion reforms rapidly, chemical pleurodesis may be attempted using intrapleural talc, bleomycin, tetracycline, doxycycline, or minocycline
- Open pleurectomy and decortication can be used for controlling pleural effusions
- A more recent and safer alternative is video-assisted thoracic surgery, which allows for partial pleurectomy or cytoreductive surgery
- Of the agents used in pleurodesis, talc is the most effective and cheapest but produces the most pain and usually requires a general anesthetic; bleomycin is the least effective and most expensive. The tetracyclines are therefore most commonly used

Efficacy

- Good for symptomatic relief of problems caused by pleural effusions
- Overall efficacy awaits evaluation and trials

Risks/Benefits

Risks:

- Aspiration may need to be repeated quite frequently (often daily)
- There is a significant risk of tumor cells infiltrating the needle tracks
- Pleurodesis is a discomforting procedure and may require systemic analgesia and instillation of local anesthetic with the sclerosing agent

Benefits:

- Aspiration is relatively safe, pleurodesis marginally less so
- Both provide good short-term symptomatic relief of breathlessness and dyspnea
- Video-assisted thoracic surgical pleurectomy is an effective treatment to control pleural fluid in mesothelioma and is safer than open pleurectomy and decortication, with a low morbidity and mortality

Acceptability to patient

High if symptomatic.

Follow up plan

Follow-up chest X-rays are always needed to exclude pneumothorax or pneumomediastinum in the early stages, and recurrence if symptoms recur.

Patient and caregiver information

- The therapy is for symptomatic relief and will not alter the course of the disease
- Aspiration may need to be repeated, often frequently
- There is a risk of tumor cells infiltrating the needle tracks

RADICAL PLEUROPNEUMONECTOMY

- This involves surgical excision of the affected pleura and any lobes of the lungs showing evidence of infiltration or spread
- Surgery is likely to be fairly extensive
- There are no randomized controlled trials to establish the role of radical surgery
- Surgery should only be performed in centers where there is an interest and experience in performing extrapleuropneumonectomies

Efficacy

- The overall effectiveness is low
- Results from surgery are better in patients with relatively localized disease, of the epithelial-type histologically, who are otherwise well, and when surgery is undertaken soon after diagnosis

Risks/Benefits

- Risk: there is an appreciable peri- and postoperative mortality and morbidity from the surgery
- Benefit: a very small proportion of patients treated by radical surgery may have an improved prognosis, but it is difficult to accurately predict individual benefits from the surgery

Patient and caregiver information

- Patients must be made aware that results from surgery in this condition are disappointing and that such surgery carries risks of morbidity and mortality
- Given the limited life expectancy for patients following diagnosis of pleural malignant mesothelioma, patients need to balance the prospect of increased life expectancy against the poorer quality of a limited life while recuperating from major, invasive surgery

Radiation therapy

Palliative radiotherapy may reduce symptoms arising from chest wall tumor masses.

PALLIATIVE RADIOTHERAPY

- This can be given for pain relief or to shrink tumor bulk if there are problems arising from that bulk
- Radiotherapy has also been used to attempt to reduce the risk of tumor growth through biopsy sites

Efficacy

- Effective palliation of pain and pressure symptoms arising from chest wall tumor masses, especially if there is pain arising from invasion of a nerve root, rib, or vertebra
- Results are not as good for more diffuse or nonspecific pain
- Fast neutron therapy via a cyclotron may provide better results

Risks/Benefits

Risks:

- Side-effects are temporary and include nausea, vomiting, diarrhea, local skin burns, and alopecia (rare)
- Local radiotherapy may increase the incidence of local spread, probably because it disturbs the immunologic defenses
- Breathlessness is rarely improved by radiotherapy

Benefits:

- Benefits are also temporary, but allow partial or complete relief of local pain and pressure symptoms
- Best results occur following the early use of radiotherapy after any invasive procedures, and when it is given in three daily fractions
- When given for chest wall pains or masses, the best results occur after the early use of radiotherapy for 2 weeks' duration

Acceptability to patient

High if the tumor mass is causing troublesome symptoms.

Follow up plan

Follow-up chest X-rays are needed periodically, especially if local symptoms recur.

Patient and caregiver information

The treatment will provide symptom relief, but is of no long-term benefit and is not curative.

Chemotherapy

- Various chemotherapeutic agents have been tried either in combination or singly
- The treatments are discussed together as none are significantly more effective
- All patients should have the opportunity to discuss the advantages and disadvantages of chemotherapy with an oncologist or respiratory specialist
- If chemotherapy is used, it should be part of a clinical trial

CYTOTOXIC THERAPY

- All the usual cytotoxic agents used in cancer chemotherapy have been tried singly or in combination
- None has been found to give very encouraging results

Efficacy

- Doxorubicin is the best-documented chemotherapeutic agent to show activity but only produces small objective responses in <20% of cases
- Evidence for cisplatin is no better
- Combinations of doxorubicin and cisplatin has been reported to show some activity in up to 25% of cases

Risks/Benefits

Risks:

- Systemic cytotoxic agents may cause more extensive dissemination of the mesothelioma, probably because they disturb the immunologic defenses
- Side-effects of doxorubicin include cardiotoxicity and bone marrow suppression. These effects are more marked after radiation therapy
- Cisplatin causes severe nausea and vomiting

Evidence

A prospective trial (no control group) assessed the efficacy of cisplatin and gemcitabine for 21 patients with advanced pleural mesothelioma. 10 patients had a partial response to treatment, nine patients had no change, and two patients were noted to have progressive disease. 90% of the responding patients had significant symptomatic improvement [2] *This study does not meet the criteria for level P*

Acceptability to patient

The small expected benefit in terms of life expectancy must be weighed against the side-effects and decline in quality of life for each patient.

Follow up plan

Regularly and frequent (daily) follow up while on treatment, and at intervals thereafter (weekly initially).

Patient and caregiver information

The likely side-effects and risks of treatment must be explained as well as the small possibility of benefit.

Other therapies

NEWER THERAPEUTIC APPROACHES

New therapeutic approaches include:

- Gene therapy: e.g. introduction of 'suicide' genes that make the tumor cells susceptible to antiviral agents, and genes to stimulate natural defense mechanisms against tumors. Examples of the latter include cytokine genes to stimulate natural killer cell activity and the heat shock protein gene to increase presentation of tumor antigens
- Photodynamic therapy: this employs a red laser light to activate drugs that have a cytotoxic effect
- Immunotherapy: various types of immunotherapy have been tried, including intrapleural and systemic interleukin-2 and interferon. It is not proven that they are more effective therapies than chemotherapy
- Lovastatin, a well-tolerated drug commonly used to treat high cholesterol, has shown positive results as an adjunctive, or secondary, drug treatment to inhibit mesothelial cell growth. This drug is not, however, in clinical trials
- Vinorelbine: mesothelioma is generally unresponsive to most chemotherapy treatment, but vinorelbine has been shown to have a response rate of nearly 25% in patients with mesothelioma and low toxicity

Efficacy

The efficacy of these treatments is still unproven.

Evidence

- A randomized controlled trial (RCT) compared surgery and chemotherapy with and without intraoperative photodynamic therapy. Survival and local control were not significantly improved in the group receiving photodynamic therapy [3] *Level P*

- A prospective trial (no control group) assessed the efficacy of vinorelbine in 29 patients with malignant pleural mesothelioma. A response in 24% of patients was noted, 55% had stable disease, and 21% had disease progression while receiving treatment. A benefit for vinorelbine was noted in a quality-of-life analysis [4] *This study does not meet the criteria for level P*
- A physiologic study found that lovastatin induced apoptosis in human malignant mesothelioma cells. Mesothelioma cell viability was decreased in a dose-dependent manner [5] *Level S*

Acceptability to patient

Many patients prefer to be entered into trials of unproven treatments given the overall poor prognosis with any of the established therapeutic options.

Patient and caregiver information

Patients must be made aware that such treatments may or may not be of use.

PALLIATIVE CARE

- Good pain relief often difficult to achieve
- The pain from invasive tumor can be severe and intractable, especially if there is nerve root involvement
- Most patients need symptom palliation from the time of diagnosis onward
- Conventional analgesia using opiates and nonsteroidal anti-inflammatory drugs (NSAIDs) will usually be needed
- Opiates may need titrating up to high doses, which should be given regularly
- Oral tablets, capsules, or liquids may be preferred
- Many patients will benefit from analgesic patches (e.g. fentanyl), or slow-release preparations of oral morphine or its derivatives
- In more terminal disease, a constant subcutaneous dose of opiate may be administered using a syringe driver and continuous infusion
- Analgesia may need supplementation by tricyclic antidepressants, benzodiazepines, local radiotherapy, local or regional nerve blocks, transcutaneous electrical stimulation of nerves, or acupuncture

Efficacy

Varies. Referral to a palliative care specialist or pain clinic may be needed if adequate and sustained pain relief is proving difficult.

Risks/Benefits

- Risk: common side-effects are constipation (treated with laxatives, fluids, and dietary manipulation), and nausea and vomiting (regular oral or parenteral antiemetics may be needed)
- Benefit: pain is debilitating and very unpleasant so all attempts at providing analgesia usually provide more benefit than risk

Acceptability to patient

High.

Follow up plan

Once adequate analgesia has been achieved, the frequency and amount of analgesic drug doses need reviewing and reducing to the minimum effective levels.

Patient and caregiver information

- Potential problems with addiction and habituation need addressing
- The benefits of adequate analgesia on quality of life need to be discussed
- Palliative care should aim to provide relief from pain and other physical symptoms, and to respond the emotional, psychological, social, and spiritual needs

OUTCOMES

EFFICACY OF THERAPIES

- In general the outcome is poor
- Median survival is 12–18 months from initial presentation
- There is no evidence that current therapy affects survival
- Standard therapy for all but localized mesothelioma is generally not curative. Although some patients will survive long-term with aggressive treatment regimens, it remains unclear if overall survival has been altered by the various treatment modalities and combinations
- Extrapleural pneumonectomy in selected patients with early-stage disease may improve recurrence-free survival, but its impact on overall survival is unknown
- Decortication and pleurectomy can provide symptomatic relief from recurrent effusions and tumor bulk
- The addition of radiation therapy and/or chemotherapy following surgical intervention has not led to increased survival

Evidence

PDxMD are unable to cite evidence that meets our criteria for evidence.

Review period

Review at least monthly, but more frequently as the disease progresses.

PROGNOSIS

- Prognosis is poor
- There is a rapid demise in the 12 months after diagnosis
- Many patients die within 4 months of diagnosis
- Most patients die from primary lesions rather than metastatic effects
- Death is usually from respiratory failure or bronchopneumonia

Therapeutic failure

- The prognosis for pleural malignant mesothelioma is poor, and there is usually no effective treatment
- Symptom relief is most important at all stages
- Initially, analgesia and relief of dyspnea are the priorities
- In the later stages, adequate analgesia may require escalating treatments

Deterioration

- Palliative therapy will need to be instigated whenever the patient deteriorates
- Early involvement of a pain relief service is desirable
- Breathlessness is often multifactorial and a variety of approaches may be necessary for palliation

Terminal illness

- Palliation of all symptoms, if possible
- Analgesia is paramount, but often difficult to achieve
- Drug therapy may need augmentation by nerve blocks or transcutaneous electrical nerve stimulation
- Acupuncture may also help
- Attention should be paid to adopting an holistic approach to the patient, and addressing their psychological and social needs and fears as well as their physical symptoms

COMPLICATIONS

- Pleural malignant mesothelioma may spread into the pericardium or through the diaphragm into the peritoneum (most common)
- It also commonly metastasized. Postmortem studies show that about 50–70% of pleural malignant mesothelioma have metastasized, but the metastases are not usually clinically apparent
- Common sites of metastases are regional lymph nodes, lungs, adrenals, central nervous system, liver, and pericardium
- Death occurs from cachexia, asthenia, pleural and pulmonary infiltration, and eventual respiratory failure, or from bronchopneumonia

CONSIDER CONSULT

Early in the course of the disease:
For consideration of any of the therapeutic options: chemotherapy, radiotherapy, pleural aspiration or pleurodesis, radical surgery.

As the disease progresses:

- For help with the control of symptoms
- For therapeutic pleural aspiration if the primary care physician is unable to do this
- For help from other medical specialists or from professions allied to medicine: psychologists, acupuncturists, relaxation therapists, as well as palliative care specialists

PREVENTION

- The greatest risk factor by far is asbestos exposure
- Over the next 20–30 years, the incidence of pleural malignant mesothelioma should fall drastically as the effects of health and safety laws governing the use of asbestos take effect

RISK FACTORS

Asbestos exposure: the longer and more concentrated the exposure, the greater the risk.

MODIFY RISK FACTORS

- Reduction of asbestos exposure: since the 1960s and 1970s, there have been great changes in the health and safety laws regarding the permissible levels of asbestos exposure
- There is also a system of no-fault compensation available in many countries and states
- Together, these measures have led to a prediction that cases of mesothelioma will peak in the early 21st century and then rapidly decline
- The lag between implementing the public health regulations and laws and clinical effect reflects the lag between asbestos exposure and the manifestation of clinical disease

SCREENING

- Screening of patients who have been exposed to significant amounts of asbestos is not undertaken because there is no effective early intervention that alters the outcome
- If such a therapy did became available, screening of those at risk (i.e. patients who have had an appreciable exposure to asbestos) would seem sensible
- Mesothelioma probably starts to grow about 10 years, on average, before clinical manifestations appear

CHEST X-RAY

This would be the screening method of choice should an effective early intervention ever become available.

ASSOCIATIONS

American Lung Association
1740 Broadway
New York, NY 10019
Tel: (212) 315-8700
Toll-free: (800) 586-4872
www.lungusa.org

National Cancer Institute
NCI Publications and Information Office
Building 31, Room 10A03
31 Center Drive
MSC 2580
Bethesda, MD 20892–2580
Tel: (301) 405-3848
Toll-free: (800) A-4-CANCER
www.nci.nih.gov

American Cancer Society
1599 Clifton Road NE
Atlanta, GA 30329–4257
Tel: (404) 320-3333
Toll-free: (800) ACS-2345
www.cancer.org

KEY REFERENCES

- Bowne K. Asbestos-related diseases. In: Parkes WR. Occupational lung disorders. MA: Butterworth,1994, p411–514
- Rudd RM. Asbestos-related disease. In: Brewis RAL, Corrin B, Geddes DM, Gibson GJ, eds. Respiratory medicine. Philadelphia: WB Saunders, 1998, p557–63
- www.mesotheliomaweb.org
- Aisner J, Sigman LM. The role of chemotherapy in the treatment of malignant mesothelioma. In: Antman K, Aisner J, eds. Asbestos-related malignancy. Orlando (FL): Grune and Stratton, 1987, p385–99
- Ardizzoni A, Rosso R, Salvatia F. Activity of doxorubicin and cisplatin combination chemotherapy in patients with diffuse pleural malignant mesothelioma. Cancer 1991;67:2984–90
- Baris YI. The clinical and radiological aspects of 185 cases of pleural malignant mesothelioma. In: Wagner JC, Davis W, eds. Biological effects of mineral fibres. Lyon: International Agency for Research on Cancer Scientific Publications No.30, 1980:937–41
- Blake PR, Catterall M, Emerson PA. Pleural mesothelioma treated by fast neutron therapy. Thorax 1985;40:72–5
- Boron M, Couston A, Livornese L, Schalet N. Mesothelioma following exposure to asbestos: a review of 72 cases. Chest 1973;64:641–6
- Browne K, Smither WJ. Asbestos-related mesothelioma: factors discriminating between pleural and peritoneal sites. Br J Ind Med 1983;40:145–52
- Edge JR, Choudary SR. Malignant mesothelioma of the pleura in Barrow-in-Furness. Thorax 1978;33:26–30
- Elmes PC, Simpson MJC. The clinical aspects of mesothelioma. Q J Med 1976;179:427–33
- Enterline PE. Mortality among asbestos products workers in the United States. Ann N Y Acad Sci 1965;132:156–65
- Epler GR, McCloud TC, Gaensler EA. Prevalence and evidence of benign asbestos pleural effusion in a working population. J Am Med Assoc 1982;247:617–22
- Greenberg M, Davies TA. Mesothelioma register, 1967–68. Br J Ind Med 1974;31:91–104
- Hillerdal G. Malignant mesothelioma 1982: review of 4710 published cases. Br J Did Chest 1983;77:321–30
- Hinds MW. Mesothelioma in the United States. Incidence in the 1970s. J Occup Med 1978;20:469–71
- Kinnear WJM, Johnston IDA, Hall IP. Key topics in respiratory medicine. Oxford: Bios, 1999, p6–9

- Mårtensson G, Hagberg S, Petterson P, Thiringer G. Asbestos pleural effusion: a clinical entity. Thorax 1987;42:646–51
- McDonald JC, Armstrong B, Case B. Mesothelioma and asbestos fiber type. Cancer 1989;63:1544–9
- McDonald AD, Mc Donald JC. Malignant mesothelioma in North America. Cancer 1980;46:1650–6
- McDonald AD, Magner D, Eyssen G. Primary malignant mesothelioma in Canada, 1960–1968. Cancer 1973;31:869–76
- Mbidde EK, Harland SJ, Calvert AH, Smith IE. Phase II trial of carboplatin (JM8) in treatment of patients with malignant mesothelioma. Cancer Chemother Pharmacol 1986;18:288–93
- Newhouse MI, Berry G, Wagner JC. Mortality of factory workers in east London 1933–1980. Br J Ind Med 1985;42:4–10
- Peto J, Seidman H, Selikoff IJ. Mesothelioma mortality in asbestos workers: implications for models of carcinogenesis and risk assessment. Br J Cancer 1982;45:124–6
- Pooley FD. Mesothelioma in relation to exposure. In: Bogovski P, ed. Biological effects of asbestos. Lyon: International Agency for Research on Cancer, 1973, p222–5
- Ribak J, Lilis R, Suzuki Y, et al. Malignant mesothelioma in a cohort of asbestos insulation workers. Br J Ind Med 1988;45:182–7
- Robinson BWS, Musk AW. Benign asbestos pleural effusion. Thorax 1981;36:895–900
- Williams CJ. Respiratory system. In: Williams CJ, ed. Cancer biology and management: an introduction. New York: John Wiley and Sons, 1990, p235–9
- Zidar BL, Pugh RP, Schiffer LM. Treatment of six cases of mesothelioma with doxorubicin and cisplatin. Cancer 1983;52:1788–91

Evidence references and guidelines

1. British Thoracic Society Standards of Care Committee. Statement on malignant mesothelioma in the United Kingdom. Thorax 2001;56:250–65
2. Byrne MJ, Davidson JA, Musk AW, et al. Cisplatin and gemcitabine treatment for malignant mesothelioma: a phase II study. J Clin Oncol 1999;17:25–30. Medline
3. Pass HI, Temeck BK, Kranda K, et al. Phase III randomized trial of surgery with and without intraoperative photodynamic therapy and postoperative immunochemotherapy for malignant pleural mesothelioma. Ann Surg Oncol 1997;4:628–33
4. Steele JP, Shamash J, Evans MT, et al. Phase II study of vinorelbine in patients with malignant pleural mesothelioma. J Clin Oncol 2000;18:3912–7. Medline
5. Rubins JB, Greatans T, Kratzke RA, et al. Lovastatin induces apoptosis in malignant mesothelioma cells. Am J Respir Crit Care Med 1998;157:1616–22. Medline

Clinical trials and review articles

For details of ongoing clinical trials see: http://www.cancer.gov/ search/clinical_trials (85 closed trials listed under the search heading 'Mesothelioma,' 15 open trials)

- Sugarbaker DJ, Flores RM, Jaklitsch MT, et al. Resection margins, extrapleural nodal status and cell type determine post-operative long-term survival in trimodality therapy of malignant pleural mesothelioma: results in 183 patients. J Thorac Cardiovasc Surg 1999;117:54–65. Medline
- Ball DL, Cruikshank DG. The treatment of malignant mesothelioma of the pleura: review of a 5-year experience, with special reference to radiotherapy. Am J Clin Oncol 1990;13:4–9. Medline
- Butchart G. Contemporary management of malignant pleural mesothelioma. Oncol 1999;4:488–500. Medline
- Byrne MJ, Davidson JA, Musk AW, et al. Cisplatin and gemcitabine treatment for malignant mesothelioma. J Clin Oncol 1999;17:25–30. Medline
- Ryan CW, Herndon J, Vogelzang NJ. A review of chemotherapy trials for malignant mesothelioma. Chest 1998;113:66–73S. Medline
- Pass HI, Temeck BK, Kranda K, et al. Phase III randomized trial of surgery with and without intraoperative photodynamic therapy and postoperative immunochemotherapy for malignant pleural mesothelioma. Ann Surg Oncol 1997;4:628–33. Medline

- Upham JW, Garlepp MJ, Musk AW, Robinson BW. Malignant mesothelioma: new insights into tumor biology and immunotherapy as a basis for new treatment approaches. Thorax 1995;50:887–93. Medline
- Steele JP, Shamash J, Evans MT, et al. Phase II study of vinorelbine in patients with malignant pleural mesothelioma. J Clin Oncol 2000;18:3912–7. Medline
- Rusch VW, Piantadosi SP, Holmes EC. The role of extrapleural pneumonectomy in malignant pleural mesothelioma. A Lung Cancer Study Group trial. J Thorac Cardiovasc Surg 1991;102:1–9. Medline
- Rusch VW, Saltz L,Venkatraman E, et al. A phase II trial of pleurectomy/decortication followed by intrapleural and systemic chemotherapy for malignant pleural mesothelioma. J Clin Oncol 1994;12:1156–63. Medline
- Ong ST, Vogelzang NJ. Chemotherapy in malignant pleural mesothelioma: a review. J Clin Oncol 1996;14:1007–17. Medline
- Nakano T, Chahinian AP, Shinjo M, et al. Cisplatin in combination with irinotecan in the treatment of patients with malignant pleural mesothelioma: a pilot phase II clinical trial and pharmacokinetic profile. Cancer 1999;85:2375–84. Medline
- Kasseyet S, Astoul P, Boutin C. Results of a phase II trial of combined chemotherapy for patients with diffuse malignant mesothelioma of the pleura. Cancer 1999;85:1740–9. Medline
- Fizazi K, Caliandro R, Soulié P, et al. Combination raltitrexed (Tomudex(R))-oxaliplatin: a step forward in the struggle against mesothelioma? The Institut Gustave Roussy experience with chemotherapy and chemo-immunotherapy in mesothelioma. Eur J Cancer 2000;36:1514–21. Medline
- Halme M, Knuuttila A, Vehmas T, et al. High-dose methotrexate in combination with interferons in the treatment of malignant pleural mesothelioma. Br J Cancer 1999 Aug 80:1781–5. Medline
- Sugarbaker DJ, Jaklitsch MT, Liptay MJ. Mesothelioma and radical multimodality therapy: who benefits? Chest 1995;107:345S–50S. Medline

FAQS

Question 1

Are there patients still at risk by exposure to asbestos?

ANSWER 1

Yes. Asbestos was banned some years ago, but there are still some people alive who were exposed to it.

Question 2

Will all patients need chemotherapy and/or radiotherapy?

ANSWER 2

No. There is no specific treatment available. Supportive care alone can be an option.

Question 3

Should patients exposed to asbestos have any special screening program?

ANSWER 3

There is no specific program of screening for asbestos exposure. Some agencies have recommended that patients with previous exposure be submitted to routine check-up and counseling to stop smoking.

CONTRIBUTORS

Fred F Ferri, MD, FACP
Otavio A Clark, MD
Januario E Castro, MD

PORPHYRIA

SUMMARY INFORMATION

DESCRIPTION

- Group of seven predominantly inherited metabolic disorders, caused by deficiencies of enzymes of the heme biosynthetic pathway
- Clinically characterized by cutaneous or acute neuropsychiatric symptoms; often present with severe abdominal pain
- Acute neuropsychiatric porphyrias can be life-threatening, but attacks can be aborted by early administration of hematin
- Latency is common, and some carriers only become symptomatic after exposure to precipitating factors such as alcohol or certain drugs
- When a patient is diagnosed with porphyria, the whole family must be screened so that precipitating factors can be avoided in anyone found to be a carrier

URGENT ACTION

Acute symptoms may need immediate hospitalization.

ICD9 CODE

277.1 Disorders of porphyrin metabolism.

SYNONYMS

- Delta-aminolevulinic aciduria, ALAD porphyria
- Swedish porphyria, pyrroloporphyria, intermittent acute porphyria
- Gunther disease
- Porphyria variegata, South African porphyria, protocoproporphyria, Royal malady
- Protoporphyria, erythrohepatic protoporphyria
- Toxic porphyria

CARDINAL FEATURES

- Group of metabolic disorders that are predominantly inherited although they may be acquired
- Caused by a partial or nearly complete deficiency of enzymes of heme biosynthetic pathway
- Seven different kinds of porphyria have been distinguished, representing discrete deficiencies of each of the seven enzymes beyond the first and rate-limiting step of the pathway
- Dysfunction of each specific enzyme causes a unique pattern of abnormally elevated levels of porphyrins and/or their precursors to accumulate in tissues, and to be excreted in urine and stool
- Clinical presentation depends on associated enzyme and mode of inheritance and is often influenced by metabolic and environmental factors
- Clinically characterized by cutaneous or acute neuropsychiatric symptoms and syndromes, or both
- Cutaneous manifestation is typically cutaneous photosensitivity which can be severe
- Acute neuropsychiatric manifestations are most typically abdominal pain, constipation, dysesthesia, muscular paralysis, and respiratory failure which can be fatal; attacks can be aborted by early administration of hematin
- Latency is common and there can be asymptomatic or minimally symptomatic carriers
- Some carriers only become symptomatic after exposure to an additional agent or factor capable of inducing disease expression

Classification (from most to least common):

- Porphyria cutanea tarda (includes hepatoerythropoietic porphyria)
- Acute intermittent porphyria
- Erythropoietic protoporphyria
- Variegate porphyria
- Hereditary coproporphyria
- Congenital erythropoietic porphyria

Also occur as:

- Hepatic porphyrias (delta-aminolevulinic acid dehydratase deficiency porphyria, acute intermittent porphyria, variegate porphyria, hereditary coproporphyria, porphyria cutanea tarda), in which the excess porphyrin production occurs in the liver
- Erythropoietic porphyrias (erythropoietic protoporphyria, congenital erythropoietic porphyria), in which excess porphyrin production occurs in the bone marrow

Also occur as:

- Acute porphyrias (delta-aminolevulinic acid dehydratase deficiency porphyria, acute intermittent porphyria, variegate porphyria, hereditary coproporphyria), which typically cause neuropsychiatric problems, often manifested as a severe abdominal pain and are associated with excess production and excretion in urine of porphobilinogen and delta-aminolevulinic acid

- Nonacute porphyrias (porphyria cutanea tarda, congenital erythropoietic porphyria, erythropoietic protoporphyria), in which porphobilinogen and delta-aminolevulinic acid are not produced in excess

Also according to their mode of inheritance:
- Autosomal dominant (acute intermittent porphyria, variegate porphyria, hereditary coproporphyria, porphyria cutanea tarda, erythropoietic protoporphyria)
- Autosomal recessive (delta-aminolevulinic acid dehydratase deficiency porphyria, congenital erythropoietic porphyria)

CAUSES

Common causes

Porphyrias are predominantly inherited; inherited mutant gene encodes the specific enzyme deficiency (in order of sequence of enzymes in heme biosynthetic pathway):
- Delta-aminolevulinic acid dehydratase deficiency causes delta-aminolevulinic acid dehydratase deficiency porphyria
- Porphobilinogen deaminase deficiency causes acute intermittent porphyria
- Uroporphyrinogen III synthase deficiency causes congenital erythropoietic porphyria
- Uroporphyrinogen decarboxylase deficiency causes porphyria cutanea tarda
- Coproporphyrinogen oxidase deficiency causes hereditary coproporphyria
- Protoporphyrinogen deficiency causes variegate porphyria
- Ferrochelatase deficiency causes erythropoietic protoporphyria

Porphyria cutanea tarda may also be acquired:
- Hepatitis C virus
- Specific exposure to polyhalogenated hydrocarbons (e.g. hexachlorobenzene)
- Alcohol
- Estrogens

Contributory or predisposing factors

All porphyrias:
- Liver disease
- Hepatitis C
- Infection
- Heavy alcohol use
- Major surgery

Acute intermittent porphyria, variegate porphyria, hereditary coproporphyria, delta-aminolevulinic acid dehydratase deficiency porphyria:
- Drugs: estrogen and progesterone from contraception and hormone replacement therapies (although may be beneficial in some patients in prevention of cyclic menstrual attacks); danazol; griseofulvin; rifampin, sulfonamides, chloramphenicol and primidone; diclofenac; phenobarbital, carbamazepine, valproic acid, clonazepam, chlordiazepoxide and meprobamate; imipramine; chlorpropamide and metoclopramide; methyldopa and glutethimide; ergotamine; pyrazinamide; carisoprodol; ethchlorvynol; and pentazocine, mephenytoin, succinimides, and pyrazolones
- Steroids: endogenous steroid hormones, sex steroid preparations
- Menstrual cycle: in presence of high levels of progesterone
- Pregnancy

- Fasting
- Emotional and physical stress
- Substance misuse: particularly marijuana, ecstasy, amphetamines, and cocaine
- Smoking

Porphyria cutanea tarda:
- Drugs: nonsteroidal anti-inflammatory drugs, sulfonylureas, busulfan
- Estrogens, especially from oral contraceptives
- Iron supplements

EPIDEMIOLOGY

Incidence and prevalence

PREVALENCE
- Porphyria cutanea tarda: 0.1/1000
- Acute intermittent porphyria, erythropoietic protoporphyria, variegate porphyria: 0.01–0.1/1000
- Hereditary porphyria: <0.01/1000
- Delta-aminolevulinic acid dehydratase deficiency porphyria, congenital erythropoietic porphyria: very rare

Demographics

AGE
- Congenital erythropoietic porphyria: early childhood
- Erythropoietic protoporphyria: older childhood
- Acute intermittent porphyria, variegate porphyria, hereditary coproporphyria, delta-aminolevulinic acid dehydratase deficiency porphyria: young adult
- Porphyria cutanea tarda: middle age

GENDER
- Erythropoietic protoporphyria, congenital erythropoietic porphyria: males and females equally affected
- Porphyria cutanea tarda: generally more common in males; however, female incidence is increasing in association with oral contraceptive and alcohol use
- Acute intermittent porphyria, variegate porphyria, hereditary coproporphyria, delta-aminolevulinic acid dehydratase deficiency porphyria: more common in females

RACE

More common in Caucasians than African-Americans or Asians.

GENETICS
- Autosomal dominant: acute intermittent porphyria, variegate porphyria, hereditary coproporphyria, porphyria cutanea tarda, erythropoietic protoporphyria
- Autosomal recessive: delta-aminolevulinic acid dehydratase deficiency porphyria, congenital erythropoietic porphyria

GEOGRAPHY

Variegate porphyria has a substantially higher incidence in South Africa of 3/1000; most cases have been traced to a single union between two Dutch settlers in 1680.

DIAGNOSIS

DIFFERENTIAL DIAGNOSIS

Acute, intermittent porphyria, variegate porphyria, hereditary coproporphyria, delta-aminolevulinic acid dehydratase deficiency porphyria:

- Lead poisoning
- Hereditary tyrosinemia
- Guillain-Barré syndrome

Porphyria cutanea tarda:

- Systemic lupus erythematosus (SLE)
- Scleroderma

Systemic lupus erythematosus

SLE is a multisystem, autoimmune, inflammatory condition that is markedly more common in women than men.

FEATURES

- Skin lesions, especially an erythematosus rash in a 'butterfly' distribution across bridge of the nose and on cheeks; also vasculitis on the fingertips, urticaria, and purpura on the nailfolds (in porphyria cutanea tarda rash is usually bullous, frequently occurs on exposure to sunlight, and often heals with scarring)
- Arthritis
- Fever
- Anorexia
- Oral ulcers
- Eye pain and redness
- Chest pain and shortness of breath
- Nausea, vomiting, diarrhea
- Psychosis/delirium
- Alcohol is not generally a precipitating factor (unlike in acute intermittent porphyria)
- Urinary excretion of uroporphyrin is not increased (unlike in porphyria cutanea tarda)

Scleroderma

Scleroderma is a chronic disease of unknown etiology, ranging from a mild disease affecting the skin to a systemic disease that can cause death.

FEATURES

- Cutaneous manifestations include digital ulcerations, thickening of digits, hyper- and hypopigmentation, scaling skin, narrowed oral aperture (in porphyria cutanea tarda rash is usually bullous, frequently occurs on exposure to sunlight, and often heals with scarring)
- Hand swelling and joint stiffness
- Proximal muscle weakness
- Gastrointestinal manifestations, including dysphagia, diarrhea, nausea, and vomiting
- Hypertension
- Peripheral and trigeminal neuropathy
- Urinary excretion of uroporphyrin is not increased (unlike in porphyria cutanea tarda)

Lead poisoning

Lead poisoning is a consequence of a high body burden of lead.

FEATURES

- Abdominal cramps
- Constipation

- Weight loss
- Metallic taste
- Tremor
- Peripheral neuritis usually painless and limited to extensor muscles
- Serious neurologic-development consequences in children
- Seizures
- Coma
- Renal failure

Hereditary tyrosinemia

FEATURES

- Onset between the ages of 2 weeks and one year
- Recurrent, acute, hepatic crises: fever, irritability, vomiting, hepatomegaly, jaundice, hypoglycemia, melena, hematemesis, hematuria. Progression to liver failure and death may occur
- Recurrent, acute, peripheral neuropathy: severe pain in legs, vomiting, paralytic ileus, weakness, and paralysis
- Renal involvement

Guillian-Barré syndrome

Guillain-Barré syndrome is a group of demyelinating diseases, causing acute progressive weakness.

FEATURES

- Acute, progressive weakness of all four limbs
- Areflexia associated with the muscle weakness
- Pain common, especially back, legs, and extremities
- Gait disorder common
- Dysesthesias, paresthesias (often perioral)
- Respiratory muscle paralysis may occur
- Usually no abdominal symptoms that are prominent in porphyria-related neuropathy

SIGNS & SYMPTOMS

Signs

Porphyrias with cutaneous signs

Porphyria cutanea tarda:

- Cutaneous photosensitivity
- Vesicles and bullae on face, dorsum of hands and feet, forearms, and legs
- Vesicles superseded by crusting, superficial scar, or milia formation (small white plaques)
- Pink to red-brown urine may be present on standing

Erythropoietic protoporphyria:

- Childhood onset of cutaneous photosensitivity in light-exposed areas
- Exacerbation of symptoms in spring and summer
- Artificial lights may also cause photosensitivity, especially surgical room lights
- Gallstones, sometimes at a very early age, are common
- Hepatic disease is unusual but may be severe and life-threatening
- Labial grooving and onycholysis may occur after excessive exposure

Congenital erythropoietic porphyria:

- Presents in early childhood except in very mild cases
- May be expressed in utero as brownish amniotic fluid
- Pink to red-brown staining of diapers or urine
- Severe cutaneous photosensitivity, resembling that of porphyria cutanea tarda but more severe

- Subepidural bullous lesions contain a porphyrin-rich fluorescent fluid
- Lesions heal slowly, progressing to crusted erosions and leaving pigmented scars
- Lesions are prone to rupture and become infected
- Erythrodontia, with red fluorescence under ultraviolet light
- Hemolytic anemia with enlarged spleen and porphyrin-rich gallstones
- Pathologic fractures or vertebral compression-collapse and shortness of stature as a result of erythroid hyperplasia of bone marrow
- Mutilating deformities, developing over a period of years or if there is extreme injury by light exposure (e.g. with phototherapy for neonatal jaundice); epidermal atrophy, sclerodermoid plaques with calcification, scarring alopecia, destruction of nasal and auricular cartilage, and microstomia; osteolysis of terminal phalanges produces shortened and contracted digits
- Ocular abnormalities may be present – ectropion, blepharitis, keratoconjunctivitis, scleromalacia, and corneal scarring leading to mutilation of eyelids and blindness

Porphyrias with neuropsychiatric signs

Acute intermittent porphyria:

- Rarely occurs before puberty
- Acute onset of symptoms lasting from a few days to several months
- Recurrent attacks tend to be similar in a given individual
- Pink to red-brown urine may be present on standing
- Abdominal pain, which is steady and generalized more often than localized, possibly cramping
- Abdomen is soft with no rebound tenderness or other signs of peritoneal irritation. Dilated bowel loops may be palpable
- Ileus with distention and decreased bowel sounds is common; sometimes increased bowel sounds with diarrhea
- Urinary retention
- Tachycardia, hypertension, restlessness, fine tremors, and excess sweating may be due to sympathetic overactivity
- Peripheral motor neuropathy which rarely develops apart from abdominal symptoms, and does not develop in all patients
- Weakness most commonly begins proximally in legs but may involve arms and distal extremities. May be difficult to detect. It can be asymmetrical and focal
- Tendon reflexes initially little affected or hyperactive, but decreased or absent with advanced neuropathy
- Cranial and sensory nerves can be affected
- Progression to respiratory and bulbar paralysis and death
- Sudden death may occur, presumably from cardiac arrhythmia
- Hyponatremia resulting in seizures
- If attack resolves, paresis will usually disappear within a few days of abdominal pain
- Poor eye contact, miserable demeanor, lack of spontaneous speech associated with depression
- Hyperventilation and tremor associated with anxiety
- Persecutory ideation and hallucinations

Delta-aminolevulinic acid dehydratase deficiency porphyria:

- May present in childhood
- Otherwise neuropsychiatric signs identical to acute intermittent porphyria

Porphyrias with cutaneous and neurovisceral signs

Variegate porphyria:

- Neuropsychiatric signs identical to acute intermittent porphyria
- Photosensitivity and cutaneous lesions clinically and histologically indistinguishable from porphyria cutanea tarda

- Cutaneous manifestations may occur apart from the neuropsychiatric symptoms
- Pink to red-brown urine may be present on standing

Hereditary coproporphyria:
- Neurovisceral signs identical to acute intermittent porphyria
- Photosensitivity and cutaneous lesions similar to porphyria cutanea tarda and variegate porphyria occur in 30% of cases (less commonly than in variegate porphyria)
- Cutaneous manifestations may occur apart from the neurovisceral symptoms
- Pink to red-brown urine may be present on standing

Symptoms

Porphyrias with cutaneous symptoms

Porphyria cutanea tarda:
- Sun-evoked blistering and skin fragility
- Facial hypertrichosis (conspicuous in women)
- Hyper- or hypo-pigmentation of affected skin
- Thickening and scarring of affected skin may occur if exposure is intense and repeated
- Pink to red-brown urine may be present
- Photo-onycholysis is occasionally present

Erythropoietic protoporphyria:
- Stinging or painful burning sensations in skin (particularly hands and face) after exposure to sun, usually, but not always followed by erythema and edema
- Petechiae or more rarely purpura, vesicles, and crusting may develop and persist for several days after sun exposure
- Thickening of affected skin and mild scarring may occur if sun exposure is intense and repeated

Congenital erythropoietic porphyria:
- Pink to dark-brown staining of diapers/urine
- Severe cutaneous photosensitivity, resembling that of porphyria cutanea tarda but more severe
- Alopecia and hypertrichosis
- Photo-onycholysis
- Blindness may occur

Porphyrias with neurovisceral symptoms

Acute intermittent porphyria:
- Abdominal pain
- Nausea and vomiting
- Constipation
- Dysuria, urinary retention, and incontinence may occur
- Pink to red-brown urine may be present
- Occasionally mild fever, sweating, restlessness, and tremor occur
- Pain in the limbs, head, neck, or chest
- Muscle weakness
- Sensory loss
- Seizures
- Anxiety, depression, insomnia, disorientation
- Hallucinations and paranoia

Delta-aminolevulinic acid dehydratase deficiency porphyria:
Neurovisceral symptoms identical to acute intermittent porphyria.

Porphyrias with cutaneous and neurovisceral symptoms

Variegate porphyria:
- Neurovisceral symptoms identical to acute intermittent porphyria
- Photosensitivity and cutaneous lesions identical to porphyria cutanea tarda
- Pink to red-brown urine may be present

Hereditary coproporphyria:
- Neurovisceral symptoms identical to acute intermittent porphyria
- Photosensitivity and cutaneous lesions similar to porphyria cutanea tarda
- Pink to red-brown urine may be present

ASSOCIATED DISORDERS

Porphyria cutanea tarda:
- HIV
- Hepatitis C
- Hepatocellular carcinoma
- Excess tissue iron storage associated with inheritance of hemochromatosis genes

Acute intermittent porphyria:
- Chronic hypertension
- Impaired renal function
- Hepatocellular carcinoma
- Chronic depression

CONSIDER CONSULT

Refer to specialist if a diagnosis of porphyria is highly suspected or confirmed by laboratory findings.

INVESTIGATION OF THE PATIENT

Direct questions to patient

- Q **How long have you had your (neuropsychiatric) symptoms/abdominal pain? Have you had them before?** Acute porphyric attacks are usually self-limiting and recurrent
- Q **Are you having any difficulties urinating?** Acute porphyric attacks often present with dysuria, retention, and incontinence
- Q **Are you sleeping well?** Insomnia may present with neurologic signs and symptoms in acute porphyric attacks
- Q **Do your (cutaneous) symptoms worsen after exposure to sun?** Cutaneous symptoms in porphyria are photosensitive
- Q **Have you emigrated to the US from South Africa?** There is a high prevalence of variegate porphyria in South Africa
- Q **Are you pregnant?** Porphyria has variable course in pregnancy

Contributory or predisposing factors

- Q **Does the patient have hepatitis C?** Up to 80% of patients with porphyria cutanea tarda have hepatitis C
- Q **What is your drinking pattern?** Alcohol use is associated with porphyria
- Q **Are you taking any medications?** There are a number of drugs that may precipitate porphyria
- Q **Are you taking steroids?** Use of sex steroid preparations may precipitate porphyria
- Q **Are you taking oral contraceptive or replacement estrogen?** Porphyria may develop in women taking estrogen
- Q **Have you recently been treated for prostrate cancer?** Porphyria may develop in men taking estrogen for prostrate cancer

- Q **Are your symptoms related to your menstrual cycle?** Porphyria may develop in the presence of high levels of progesterone during luteal phase and resolve at menses. Such attacks are likely to be cyclic
- Q **Have you recently had major surgery?** Acute porphyric attacks have been known following surgery, possibly triggered by stress or barbiturate anesthesia; cutaneous manifestations of congenital erythropoietic porphyria can be seriously exacerbated by lights in operating rooms
- Q **Have you had any recent infections?** Porphyria may develop postinfection
- Q **Have you recently been dieting or fasting?** Acute porphyria attack may develop in individuals with low carbohydrate intake
- Q **Are you HIV-positive?** HIV-positive individuals are at an increased risk of developing porphyria
- Q **Are there any signs of liver disease?** Liver disease is associated with porphyria

Family history

- Q **Is there any other member of your family who has a similar illness?** Except in a few acquired forms, porphyria is an inherited disorder.

Examination

- **Examine urine**. Pink to red-brown staining on standing may suggest porphyrin excretion in urine indicative of porphyria cutanea tarda, acute intermittent porphyria, variegate porphyria, hereditary coproporphyria, congenital erythropoietic porphyria
- **Examine skin on hands and face**, and other sun-exposed areas for signs of cutaneous photosensitivity. Look for vesicles, crusting, superficial scar, milia formation, friability, facial hypertrichosis, hyper- or hypopigmentation
- **Examine teeth** with and without Wood's Light. Congenital erythropoietic porphyria shows erythrodontia with red fluorescence under ultraviolet light. Labial grooving occurs after excessive sun exposure in erythropoietic protoporphyria
- **Examine nails**. Onycholysis may present with other cutaneous photosensitivities after excessive sun exposure
- **Examine abdomen**. Ileus with distention and decreased bowel sounds is common in acute porphyric attack. Sometimes increased bowel sounds with diarrhea
- **Perform a full neurologic examination**. Check motor strength in all limbs
- **Measure blood pressure**. Hypertension may occur in acute porphyric attack and can be chronic
- **Listen for tachycardia**. Tachycardia may occur in acute porphyric attack
- **Consider patient's affect**. Depression may occur with other neurovisceral symptoms in acute porphyric attack and may be chronic and suicidal
- **Perform mental state examination**. Anxiety, disorientation, hallucinations, and paranoia can all occur with other neurovisceral symptoms in acute porphyric attack

Summary of investigative tests

- Fresh urine sample should be sent, protected from light, to the laboratory for delta-aminolevulinic acid (ALA), porphobilinogen (PBG), and total porphyrin testing when an acute porphyric attack is suspected (as in acute intermittent porphyria, variegate porphyria, hereditary coproporphyria, and delta-aminolevulinic acid dehydratase deficiency porphyria). Normal levels of ALA, PBG, and total porphyrins excludes all acute porphyrias as potential causes of symptoms
- Venous blood sample should be sent to laboratory for total plasma porphyrin test when it is suspected that skin photosensitivity might be due to porphyria. Normal plasma porphyrin levels exclude porphyria as a cause of cutaneous symptoms; however, to definitively rule out variegate porphyria the measurement must be carried out by a simple and direct fluorometric test since plasma porphyrins in variegate porphyria are mostly covalently bound to plasma porphyrins
- Measurement of plasma or erythrocyte porphyrin can be carried out if congenital erythropoietic porphyria or erythropoietic protoporphyria are suspected. Normally performed by a specialist

Other tests:

- Quantitative analysis of porphyrins (uroporphyrin, coproporphyrin, protoporphyrin, and PBG) in urine and feces can be carried out (normally by a specialist) to differentiate types of porphyria:
- Urinary uroporphyrin is increased in congenital erythropoietic porphyria and porphyria cutanea tarda
- Urinary ALA is increased in delta-aminolevulinic acid dehydrase-deficiency porphyria
- Urinary ALA and PBG are elevated in acute intermittent porphyria
- Urinary ALA, PBG and coproporphyrin are elevated in hereditary coproporphyria and variegate porphyria
- Fecal uroporphyrin and coproporphyrin are increased in congenital erythropoietic porphyria
- Fecal protoporphyrin is increased in erythropoietic protoporphyria and variegate porphyria
- Fecal coproporphyrin is increased in hereditary coproporphyria
- Fecal isocoproporphyrin is increased in porphyria cutanea tarda

DIAGNOSTIC DECISION

- Strong clinical suspicion of acute porphyric attack demands immediate action. Testing must be carried out before treatment is instigated to gain a definitive diagnosis
- Diagnosis is by testing

CLINICAL PEARLS

Porphyria cutanea tarda is not associated with abdominal pain and acute intermittent porphyria is not associated with skin lesions.

THE TESTS

Body fluids

DELTA-AMINOLEVULINIC ACID, PORPHOBILINOGEN, AND TOTAL PORPHYRIN TEST

Description

Urine sample for color reaction with Ehrlich's reagent.

Advantages/Disadvantages

Advantage: sample easy to collect.

Normal

Negative test result (no ALA, PBG, or porphyrin present in urine).

Abnormal

- Positive test result (ALA, PBG, or porphyrin present in urine)
- Keep in mind the possibility of a false-positive test

Cause of abnormal result

Strong likelihood of symptomatic acute porphyria (acute intermittent porphyria, hereditary coproporphyria, variegate porphyria, delta-aminolevulinic acid dehydratase-deficiency porphyria).

TOTAL PLASMA PORPHYRINS TEST

Description

Venous blood sample.

Advantages/Disadvantages

Advantages:

- Sample easy to collect
- Can help to exclude photosensitivity

Normal

Negative test (no porphyrins present in plasma).

Abnormal

Positive test (porphyrins present in plasma).

Cause of abnormal result

Strong likelihood of cutaneous photosensitivity due to porphyria (porphyria cutanea tarda, erythropoietic protoporphyria, congenital erythropoietic porphyria, variegate porphyria, or hereditary coproporphyria).

TREATMENT

CONSIDER CONSULT

- Refer to specialist if chronic symptoms progress
- Refer to specialist if acute symptoms reoccur

IMMEDIATE ACTION

Recurrent acute symptoms may need immediate hospitalization.

PATIENT AND CAREGIVER ISSUES

Impact on career, dependants, family, friends

- Recurrent porphyria attacks can significantly affect patient's ability to work
- All family members must be screened for the porphyria and, if carriers, should avoid precipitating factors

Health-seeking behavior

- **Have you tried any treatments or alternative therapies yourself?** As porphyria may be cyclic or recurrent, patients may report miraculous cures with self-treatment if this coincides with recovery
- **Have you been taking any pain relief?** Some over-the-counter medications exacerbate porphyria
- **Have you presented at ER?** Frequent visits to ER or another medical facility may indicate that the disorder has a recurrent nature

MANAGEMENT ISSUES

Goals

- To resolve acute porphyric attack
- To reduce cutaneous manifestations
- To reduce chronic symptoms
- To prevent reoccurrence of acute and chronic symptoms
- To prevent occurrence of signs and symptoms in family members

Management in special circumstances

There is a risk of permanent neurologic damage, including respiratory paralysis and death if a severe acute porphyric attack is not treated promptly

COEXISTING DISEASE

- Epilepsy can be difficult to treat in patients with a neuropsychiatric porphyria because standard epileptic drugs can precipitate an acute attack. Gabapentin is now the drug of choice
- Impaired renal function may result in anemia; in this instance phlebotomy would be contraindicated in the treatment of porphyria, and low-dose chloroquine should be used

COEXISTING MEDICATION

Certain drugs must be avoided in porphyria.

In an acute porphyric attack:

- Hormonal contraception and hormone replacement therapy (including estrogen and progesterone – although they may be beneficial in some patients in prevention of cyclic menstrual attacks)
- Hormonal treatment: danazol
- Fungicide: griseofulvin
- Antibiotics: sulfonamides, rifampin, chloramphenicol, primidone
- Nonsteroidal anti-inflammatory drugs (NSAID): diclofenac
- Anticonvulsants: phenobarbital, carbamazepine, valproic acid, clonazepam

- Anxiolytics: chlordiazepoxide, meprobamate
- Antidepressant: imipramine
- Chlorpropamide
- Antiemetic: metoclopramide
- Centrally acting beta-blockers: methyldopa and glutethimide
- Ergot alkaloid: ergotamine
- Antitubercular agent: pyrazinamide
- Muscle relaxant: carisoprodol
- Sedative: ethchlorvynol
- Pentazocine
- Mephenytoin
- Succinimides
- Pyrazolones

In porphyria cutanea tarda:
- NSAIDs
- Sulfonylureas
- Busulfan
- Estrogens, especially in oral contraceptives

SPECIAL PATIENT GROUPS

Pregnant women:
- Acute porphyric attacks may occur during pregnancy, when estrogen concentrations are high
- Patient should be advised to avoid pregnancy until she has been in remission for at least 2 years. Aminolevulinic acid can cross the placenta and possibly cause toxicity to develop in the fetal brain
- If acute attacks do occur during pregnancy they should be treated in the normal way

Menstruating women:

Cyclic attacks of acute intermittent porphyria can be treated with long-acting agonists of luteinizing hormone-releasing hormone to induce a chemical menopause.

PATIENT SATISFACTION/LIFESTYLE PRIORITIES

Sun-seeking behavior should be discontinued in all patients with cutaneous manifestations.

SUMMARY OF THERAPEUTIC OPTIONS
Choices
Porphyrias with cutaneous manifestations

Porphyria cutanea tarda:
- Avoidance of precipitating factors: alcohol, estrogen supplements, certain drugs (NSAIDs, sulfonylureas, busulfan), and iron supplements
- Removal of iron stores by phlebotomy, 500mL of blood every 2 weeks, to achieve mild anemia
- Low-dose chloroquine, or if possible phlebotomy and chloroquine combined, for those in whom phlebotomy is contraindicated
- Avoidance of sun through protective clothing and use of topical sunscreens effective in the 400–410nm portion of the spectrum (Soret band)
- In hepatoerythropoietic porphyria, phlebotomy is not effective

Erythropoietic protoporphyria:
- Avoidance of sun through protective clothing and use of topical sunscreens effective in the 400–410nm portion of the spectrum (Soret band)
- Oral administration of beta-carotene 120–180mg daily to afford some systemic photoprotection
- Phlebotomy and chloroquine are not effective

Congenital erythropoietic porphyria:

- Avoidance of exposure to sunlight including special protective clothing, wide brimmed hats, gloves, and use of topical sunscreens effective in the 400–410nm portion of the spectrum (Soret band)
- Oral administration of beta-carotene 120–180mg daily to afford some systemic photoprotection
- Splenectomy may partially or completely relieve the hemolytic anemia and reduce photosensitivity, but it is not always beneficial and not always warranted by the degree of anemia
- Transfusion of sufficient blood to suppress erythropoiesis is effective but results in iron overload

Porphyrias with neuropsychiatric manifestations

Acute porphyric attack in acute intermittent porphyria, delta-aminolevulinic acid dehydratase-deficiency porphyria, variegate porphyria, and hereditary coproporphyria:

- Remove precipitating factors when possible
- Intravenous glucose 10%, 300–500g daily
- Heme therapy (hematin) infused intravenously if symptoms are severe or if carbohydrate loading is not effective within 12–24h
- Gabapentin to control seizures; correction of hypomagnesemia may also reduce seizure activity
- Correction of fluid and electrolyte imbalance
- Safe analgesics and narcotics for pain as required
- Beta-adrenergic blocking agents for tachycardia and hypertension, but cautiously or not at all in patients with hypovolemia
- Phenothiazines such as chlorpromazine to control nausea, vomiting, anxiety, agitation, and psychosis
- Selective serotonin reuptake inhibitors for depression
- Bladder distention may require catheterization
- Maintain patient's morale and alleviate fear

Acute intermittent porphyria:

- Prevention of acute porphyric attack is the cornerstone of treating these patients: lifestyle changes, restricted use of medications, and stress management. A commonsense assessment must be made of benefit vs risk of restricting medications; an acute attack is less likely to be precipitated if disease is latent, if patient has previously only had a single attack, and if concentration of urinary porphobilinogen and aminolevulinic acid are normal at time of prescribing drug
- Gabapentin can be used for long-term seizure control
- Selective serotonin reuptake inhibitors for depression

Delta-aminolevulinic acid dehydratase deficiency porphyria:

Similarities in symptoms between delta-aminolevulinic acid dehydratase deficiency porphyria and acute intermittent porphyria suggest that management of former should probably be the same as that for acute intermittent porphyria.

Porphyrias with cutaneous and neuropsychiatric manifestations

Variegate porphyria:

- Prevention of acute porphyric attack is the cornerstone of treating these patients: lifestyle changes, restricted use of medications, and stress management
- Gabapentin can be used for long-term seizure control
- Avoidance of sun through protective clothing and use of topical sunscreens effective in the 400–410nm portion of the spectrum (Soret band)

- Selective serotonin reuptake inhibitors for depression
- Phlebotomy and chloroquine are not effective

Hereditary coproporphyria:
As for variegate porphyria.

Never

Never commence hematin treatment until diagnosis is confirmed by laboratory testing, as hematin treatment will negate the results. Glucose 10% should be commenced immediately pending laboratory results.

FOLLOW UP

- Follow up lifestyle changes and avoidance of other precipitating factors in neuropsychiatric porphyrias to prevent acute porphyric attack
- Follow up use of topical sunscreens and appropriate clothing, and avoidance of precipitating factors in cutaneous porphyrias to prevent permanent scarring and, in congenital erythropoietic porphyria, deformities

Plan for review

- Treatment review should be carried out by specialist
- Follow up of preventive measures should be individualized depending on ability of the patient to comply

Information for patient or caregiver

Patients with neuropsychiatric porphyrias:

- Must avoid precipitating factors
- Need to carry a drugs list with them with details of drugs thought to be unsafe

Patients with cutaneous porphyrias:

- Must avoid precipitating factors
- Need to wear adequate sun protection

DRUGS AND OTHER THERAPIES: DETAILS

Drugs

CHLOROQUINE

Dose

125mg chloroquine phosphate twice weekly for photosensitivity in porphyria cutanea tarda when phlebotomy is contraindicated.

Efficacy

Effective, but relapse may occur when therapy is discontinued.

Risks/Benefits

Risks:

- Use caution in hepatic disease or alcoholism, psoriasis or eczema, blood dyscrasias or G6PD deficiency, neurologic disease
- Use caution in children

Side-effects and adverse reactions

- Gastrointestinal: nausea, vomiting, diarrhea, anorexia
- Hematologic: blood cell disorders
- Central nervous system: seizures, headache, stimulation, fatigue
- Ears, eyes, nose, and throat: visual disturbances, tinnitus, vertigo
- Skin: eruptions, rashes, exfoliative dermatitis

Interactions (other drugs)

- Chlorpromazine
- Cimetidine
- Cyclosporine
- Digoxin
- Mefloquine
- Methotrexate
- Magnesium trisilicate, kaolin products
- Penicillamine
- Praziquantel

Contraindications

- Retinal changes, ocular disease
- Psoriasis

Acceptability to patient
Usually very acceptable to patients with few side-effects.

Follow up plan
Monitor response to treatment and check liver function every 3–6 months.

Patient and caregiver information
Report any visual changes (e.g. blurred vision, difficulty with focusing) to physician.

BETA-CAROTENE BEADLETS

Dose

- Adult: 30–300 mg (1–10 capsules) per day
- Child under 14 years: 30–150 mg (1–5 capsules) per day. Capsules may be opened and the contents mixed in orange or tomato juice to aid administration

Efficacy
Increased tolerance to sunlight occurs in many but not all patients after 3–4 weeks of treatment, and protective effect may last up to 8 weeks after cessation of the drug.

Risks/Benefits
Risks:

- Use caution in patients with impaired renal or hepatic function
- Use caution in nursing mothers

Benefit: can lessen effects of photosensitivity especially when used in conjunction with topical sunscreens and protective clothing

Side-effects and adverse reactions
Gastrointestinal: some patients may have occasional loose stools while taking beta-carotene.

Acceptability to patient
Usually acceptable, with few side-effects.

Follow up plan
Monitor serum carotene level (therapeutic range of 10–15mcmol/L) and adjust drug dosage accordingly if needed.

GLUCOSE 10%

Dose
Intravenous 300–500g daily for mild symptoms of acute porphyric attack, especially when carbohydrates cannot be tolerated orally.

Efficacy
Historically has been effective for milder symptoms of acute porphyric attack.

Risks/Benefits
Benefit: no side-effects and easily administered

Contraindications
No significant contraindications recorded.

Acceptability to patient
Usually very acceptable to patients.

Follow up plan
Every 3 months or when patient suffers acute porphyric attacks.

Patient and caregiver information
Early administration of intravenous glucose during an acute porphyric attack may be most effective.

HEMATIN
Dose
For severe acute porphyric attack, or acute porphyric attack not responding to carbohydrate treatment:
- Intravenous infusion of 1–4mg/kg/day
- In more severe cases this dose may be repeated no earlier than every 12h
- No more than 6mg/kg of hematin should be given in any 24-h period

Efficacy
Effective if administered early in acute porphyric attack.

Risks/Benefits
Risk: transient, mild anticoagulant effects have been observed during clinical studies

Benefits:
- Can prevent irreversible sequelae and death in severe, acute porphyric attack
- Can be used prophylactically in patients with severe, recurrent attacks

Side-effects and adverse reactions
- Metabolism: reversible renal shutdown has occurred with administration of excessive doses
- Other: may cause phlebitis after administration through small arm veins

Interactions (other drugs)
Drugs which increase the activity of delta-aminolevulinic acid synthetase (such as estrogens, barbituric acid derivatives, and steroid metabolites) should be avoided.

Contraindications
No significant contraindications recorded.

Acceptability to patient
Usually very acceptable to patients.

Follow up plan
Every 3 months or when patient suffers acute porphyric attacks .

Patient and caregiver information
Early administration of intravenous hematin during an acute porphyric attack may be most effective.

GABAPENTIN

Dose

- The effective dose of gabapentin is 900–1800mg/day given in divided doses (three times a day)
- The starting dose is 300mg three times a day

Efficacy

Effective in patients of all ages with partial crises.

Risks/Benefits

Risks:

- Use caution in pregnancy and breast-feeding
- Use caution in renal impairment and in the elderly
- Gabapentin may be associated with teratogenesis, the significance in humans is unknown
- Do not withdraw abruptly

Benefit: can be used safely in combination with other antiepileptic drugs

Side-effects and adverse reactions

- Cardiovascular system: hypertension
- Central nervous system: drowsiness, dizziness, paresthesias, depression, amnesia, nystagmus, ataxia, tremor, irritability, dysarthria
- Eyes, ears, nose, and throat: rhinitis, pharyngitis, visual disturbances
- Hematologic: leukopenia
- Gastrointestinal: nausea, vomiting, weight gain, dyspepsia, dry mouth, constipation, flatulence, anorexia, glossitis
- Genitourinary: impotence
- Musculoskeletal: fatigue, back pain, asthenia, malaise, myalgia
- Skin: purpura, abrasion, pruritus

Interactions (other drugs)

- **Antacids**
- **Cimetidine**

Acceptability to patient

Some patients will not tolerate dose above 300mg three times a day due to increased fatigue, somnolence, and dizziness.

Follow up plan

Initially at 4 weeks and then every 3–6 months as needed.

Surgical therapy

SPLENECTOMY

Should be considered for hemolytic anemia in congenital erythropoietic porphyria if anemia is fairly severe.

Efficacy

May partially or completely relieve the hemolytic anemia and may also lead to reduced porphyrinuria and photosensitivity, but is not always beneficial.

Risks/Benefits

- Risk: of major surgery
- Benefit: in severe and deforming condition

Acceptability to patient
Usually acceptable when potential benefits and limited risks are considered.

Follow up plan
Follow up by hematology specialist.

Patient and caregiver information
Postsplenectomy patient may be more susceptible to certain infections such as pneumococcal pneumonia and be vaccinated against these before surgery.

Other therapies

PHLEBOTOMY

For the treatment of porphyria cutanea tarda:
- 450mL of blood at intervals of 1–2 weeks, to achieve mild anemia
- Initial values of ferritin and transferrin iron saturation in serum should be obtained

Efficacy
Leads to clinical and biochemical remission in virtually every case.

Risks/Benefits
- Risk: may cause iron-deficiency anemia
- Benefit: relatively easy to perform

Acceptability to patient
Formation of new skin lesions ceases gradually and full recovery often extends over several months to a year or more.

Follow up plan
Regular follow up values of ferritin and transferrin iron saturation in serum, and should be obtained. The optimal approach is to achieve:
- Normal levels of transferrin iron saturation in serum
- Near 2mcg/dL (20mcg/L) of serum ferritin

TOPICAL SUNSCREENS

Topical sunscreens must be effective in the 400–410nm portion of the spectrum (Soret band) to be useful. The only readily available preparations are opaque formulations containing oxidates of zinc or titanium.

Efficacy
Effectively reduce consequences of sun exposure if applied correctly.

Risks/Benefits
Benefit: protection against sun exposure

Acceptability to patient
Patient may find topical sunscreens unpleasant to apply and wear.

Patient and caregiver information
- Topical sunscreens must be effective in the 400–410nm portion of the spectrum (Soret band) to be useful
- Instructions on the packaging must be adhered to
- Can help prevent scarring

STRESS MANAGEMENT

Patients with high levels of stress and poor coping responses may be referred to a psychologist or occupational therapist for stress management.

Risks/Benefits

Benefit: beneficial to general health

Acceptability to patient

Stress management techniques may be difficult for some patients to adhere to.

Patient and caregiver information

Patients should be made aware that stress can be a precipitating factor in acute porphyric attack.

LIFESTYLE

All porphyrias:

Alcohol consumption increases risk of disease expression and patients should be encouraged to abstain.

Acute porphyric attack:

- Illicit drug use, crash dieting or fasting, and smoking all increase risk of acute porphyric attack and patients should be encouraged to completely avoid these triggers
- A diet high in carbohydrate may help to prevent an acute porphyric attack

Porphyria cutanea tarda:

Use of iron supplements may trigger symptoms of porphyria cutanea tarda and patients should be told not to use them.

RISKS/BENEFITS

- Risk: alcoholics and drug users are at risk of withdrawal symptoms
- Benefit: abstinence from alcohol, illicit drugs and smoking, as well as avoidance of crash diets and fasting, benefit general health

ACCEPTABILITY TO PATIENT

- Majority of problem drinkers/alcoholics and drug users have great difficulty in reducing their intake
- Majority of smokers have at least some difficulty stopping
- Fasting may be associated with religious practice

FOLLOW UP PLAN

Monitor adherence to lifestyle changes at follow up.

PATIENT AND CAREGIVER INFORMATION

Inform patients of importance of adhering to treatment even if symptoms have improved.

EFFICACY OF THERAPIES

- Most porphyria symptoms can be controlled successfully once diagnosis is confirmed and patient knows how to avoid the known precipitating factors
- Acute attacks can usually be controlled with intravenous heme therapy if initiated early

Review period

- Must be individualized for each patient
- A review is warranted if patient starts to experience more frequent acute attacks or develops new symptoms
- Any new medication should also be reviewed by physician to ensure safety with porphyria

PROGNOSIS

- Patients who are asymptomatic or minimally symptomatic have unaffected longevity
- Patients who are more symptomatic are treatable and if so, do well
- Neurologic manifestations (e.g. peripheral neuropathy, neurosis, depression, hemiplegia), can be permanent or the patient may take years to recover
- Depression can be associated with suicide
- Acute porphyric attacks have a 1% mortality rate

Clinical pearls

One negative workup does not exclude porphyria(s) as an explanation of a patient's symptoms. Maintain high index of suspicion, particularly after 'negative' (unnecessary) surgery.

Therapeutic failure

In patients unresponsive to beta-carotene:

- PUVA treatment can be given three times a week until a total UVA dose of 120–200J/cm^2 is reached. In younger children, UVB phototherapy can be given four times a week until a total dose of 1–1.5J/cm^2 is received
- Pyridoxine has been associated with a reduction in photosensitivity without evidence of adverse effects

COMPLICATIONS

Renal failure:

- Can occur as a complication in porphyria cutanea tarda; these patients lack the renal excretory pathway for porphyrins, leading to higher levels in plasma and tissues
- If patient has anemia, phlebotomy will not be tolerated
- Chloroquine-porphyrin complexes are not filtered out by standard hemodialysis, but high-flux hemodialysis may be of some benefit
- Administration of recombinant erythropoietin mobilizes stored iron and relieves the anemia so that phlebotomies can be carried out to induce remission
- In the event of therapeutic failure, porphyria cutanea tarda is fully resolved after renal transplantation

Liver failure:

- Liver failure can occur as a complication in erythropoietic protoporphyria
- Treatment to minimize the hepatotoxic effects of protoporphyrin in erythropoietic protoporphyria are nonconclusive
- Liver transplantation as a life-saving measure is the only treatment available once severe liver damage has occurred

CONSIDER CONSULT

- Patients should be referred to specialists when they develop renal or liver failure from porphyria.

PREVENTION

Prevention should focus on screening family members of patients diagnosed with porphyria, and educating those known to be carriers in avoidance of precipitating factors.

RISK FACTORS

All porphyrias:
Family history: the porphyrias are a group of predominantly inherited disorders.

In acquired porphyria cutanea tarda, it appears that uroporphyrinogen decarboxylase can be deactivated by any of the following, giving rise to acquired porphyria cutanea tarda, although exact mechanisms involved are unknown:

- Hepatitis C virus: in some parts of the world as many as 80% of patients with porphyria cutanea tarda are chronically infected with hepatitis C
- Specific exposure to polyhalogenated hydrocarbons (e.g. hexachlorobenzene): there have been several reported outbreaks of porphyria cutanea tarda associated with toxic exposure, most notably >3000 people in Turkey (1956–61) as a result of exposure to a seed wheat fungicide
- Alcohol: heavy alcohol intake has been reported in 25–100% of patients
- Estrogens: association of estrogen ingestion and expression of porphyria cutanea tarda has been reported frequently but only in a very small percentage of patients who ingest estrogen, suggesting an underlying predisposition

MODIFY RISK FACTORS

Lifestyle and wellness

ALCOHOL AND DRUGS

- Excessive alcohol consumption is associated with many diseases as well as porphyria, and all individuals should be advised to limit alcohol consumption to the equivalent of 30mL (men) or 15mL (women) of ethanol per day
- Alcoholics giving up will require a special program

ENVIRONMENT

Exposure to polyhalogenated hydrocarbons should be avoided.

FAMILY HISTORY

If a family member suffers from porphyria, all relatives should be screened.

DRUG HISTORY

Benefits outweigh risks of estrogen use.

SCREENING

- Dominant mode of inheritance of acute porphyrias, occurrence of asymptomatic gene carriers, and risk of developing potentially fatal attacks of neuropsychiatric origin on exposure to a wide range of common precipitating factors, make it essential to exclude or confirm diagnosis of neuropsychiatric porphyrias in all relatives of individuals with diagnosed porphyria
- Relatives with latent porphyria can be educated on avoided precipitating factors
- Exclusion of carrier status avoids the need for screening future generations of that particular family branch

MEASUREMENT OF HEME BIOSYNTHETIC ENZYMES

Measurement of heme biosynthetic enzymes in red blood cells or lymphocytes can detect the presence of delta-aminolevulinic acid dehydratase, porphobilinogen deaminase, uroporphyrinogen III cosynthase, and uroporphyrinogen decarboxylase.

Cost/efficacy

- Test is inexpensive
- Test results are difficult to interpret and should be performed by a laboratory that has expertise in porphyria

MOLECULAR GENETIC ANALYSIS

Molecular analysis of specific porphyria-causing gene defect in any one family. Porphyria-causing gene is sequenced from a small blood sample.

Cost/efficacy

- Expensive and time-consuming
- Definitive identification of carriers of gene defect and thus those at risk of developing porphyria

PREVENT RECURRENCE

- Recurrence should be prevented as much as possible by avoiding precipitating factors
- In severe, recurrent, acute porphyric attack, hematin can be used prophylactically
- Recurrence of cutaneous symptoms can be avoided by maintaining mild anemia by phlebotomy as required

RESOURCES

ASSOCIATIONS

American Porphyria Foundation
PO Box 22712
Houston, TX 77227
Tel: (713) 266-9617
www.enterprise.net/apf/

KEY REFERENCES

- Thadani H, Deacon A, Peters T. Diagnosis and management of porphyria. BMJ 2000;320:1647–51
- Chapters on porphyria: Diagnosis and management. In: Djulbegovic B, ed. Reasoning and decision making in hematology. New York: Churchill Livingstone, 1992, p67–71
- Anderson KE. The porphyrias. In: Goldman: Cecil textbook of medicine, 21st edn. Philadelphia: WB Saunders, 2000
- Bottomley SS, Lee, GR. Porphyria. In: Lee: Wintrobe's clinical hematology, 10th edn. Philadelphia: Lippincott Williams &Wilkins, 1999
- Sassa S. The Porphyrias. In: Behrman: Nelson textbook of pediatrics, 16th edn. Philadelphia: WB Saunders, 2000

FAQS

Question 1

Can porphyria present both with acute abdominal symptoms and skin disorders?

ANSWER 1

Yes. Hereditary coproporphyria and variegate porphyria may present with acute abdominal symptomatology and skin sensitivity. However, the most common type – acute intermittent porphyria – presents with abdominal pain (and other neuropsychiatric and gastrointestinal symptoms) but not skin sensitivity. On the other hand, porphyria cutanea tarda and protoporphyria are not associated with gastrointestinal symptoms.

Question 2

Why is that so?

ANSWER 2

It is because porphyrin precursors, which accumulate in acute intermittent porphyria, are associated with gastrointestinal and neuropsychiatric symptoms, while accumulation of porphyrins alone leads to skin lesions.

Question 3

Can a quick urine screening test rule out acute intermittent porphyria?

ANSWER 3

No. A qualitative test using the Watson-Schwartz or Hoesch test are too insensitive to rule out porphyria. 24-h urine collection for quantitative determination of porphobilinogen and delta-aminolevulinic acid are necessary to diagnose/rule out acute intermittent porphyria. A normal result in a symptomatic patient rules out acute intermittent porphyria, hereditary coproporphyria, and variegate porphyria with high likelihood.

CONTRIBUTORS

Fred F Ferri, MD, FACP
Benjamin Djulbegovic, MD, PhD
Naixi N Chen, MD

PROLACTINOMA

SUMMARY INFORMATION

DESCRIPTION

- Typically an intrasellar tumor of the anterior part of the pituitary gland, which secretes prolactin
- Subclassified into microadenoma (<10mm diameter) and macroadenoma (>10mm)
- Treatment depends on size and encroachment on optic chiasm
- Treatment may be medical, surgical, or radiotherapeutic – medical treatment with dopamine agonists is the preferred option
- Recurrence rates are high with surgery

URGENT ACTION

Refer urgently to neurosurgical unit patients with:

- Clinically apparent visual field defects
- Symptoms of raised intracranial pressure

Prolactinoma can uncommonly present acutely with severe headache or prostration secondary to hemorrhage in previously undiagnosed pituitary tumor – requires urgent admission, may cause hypopituitarism requiring immediate evaluation and treatment.

BACKGROUND

ICD9 CODE

253.1 Forbes-Albright syndrome.

SYNONYMS

- Forbes-Albright syndrome
- Pituitary microadenoma
- Pituitary macroadenoma

CARDINAL FEATURES

- Monoclonal tumor of anterior pituitary gland
- Most common pituitary tumor
- Results in hyperprolactinemia
- Features in women include: infertility, oligomenorrhea/amenorrhea, galactorrhea, rarely hypopituitarism, usually microadenomas
- Features in men include: decreased libido, usually macroadenomas, hypogonadism, impotence, galactorrhea (one-third of the cases), neurologic effects, headaches in nearly 50% of the cases due to raised intracranial pressure, visual loss from optic nerve compression
- Established indications for treatment of a prolactinoma are restoration of fertility and the presence of a macroadenoma
- Trans-sphenoidal resection is the preferred surgical treatment
- Clinical treatment of choice is a dopamine agonist
- Goals of therapy are to normalize prolactin, restore gonadal function, and decrease tumor size
- Long-term follow up is necessary because recurrence rates are high: up to 50% of microadenomas and nearly 90% of macroadenomas can recur
- Only rare cases of prolactin cell carcinoma have been reported

CAUSES

Common causes

- Monoclonal expansion of prolactin-secreting cell line in anterior pituitary
- Adenomas arise de novo with no known cause or predisposition

Rare causes

Prolactin cell carcinoma (extremely rare).

Serious causes

- Monoclonal expansion of prolactin-secreting cell line in anterior pituitary: if tumor is large or rapidly expanding, pressure on the optic chiasm may result in permanent loss of visual field, and damage to other nearby structures may also result. Bleeding into tumor may cause sudden collapse with pituitary insufficiency
- Prolactin cell carcinoma: extremely rarely prolactinoma may behave in a malignant manner

EPIDEMIOLOGY

Incidence and prevalence

- Most common pituitary tumor – nearly 30% of all pituitary adenomas secrete enough prolactin to cause hyperprolactinemia
- 23–27% of individuals have microadenomas at autopsy and 40% of these stain positive for prolactin
- Most of these have no evidence of endocrine dysfunction

Demographics

GENDER

- Microadenomas are more common in women
- Macroadenomas are more common in men
- No gender difference in the incidence of prolactinomas in unselected adult autopsy material

DIAGNOSIS

DIFFERENTIAL DIAGNOSIS

A serum prolactin concentration of >200ng/mL is virtually diagnostic for prolactinoma. Other causes of hyperprolactinemia (usually <200ng/mL) are as follows.

Idiopathic

- Often no cause is found for mildly elevated prolactin levels
- Normal mean levels: 8ng/mL in women and 5ng/mL in men, normal range up to 20ng/mL
- Levels >200ng/mL highly suggestive of adenoma
- Prolactin levels can vary with time of day, stress, sleep cycle, and meals
- More accurate measures can be obtained 2–3h postwaking, preprandially when patient is not distressed
- Serial measurements are recommended in patients with mild elevations

FEATURES

- No cause found
- Mildly elevated prolactin level

Physiologic – pregnancy

Levels may rise physiologically to 20 times normal by full term, with a gradual fall postpartum.

FEATURES

- Normal pregnancy
- Presence of severe headache or visual field loss in pregnancy merits referral for further investigation to exclude intracranial cause, including prolactinoma

Stress – physiologic or pathologic

Stress causes elevation of serum prolactin; levels are usually <200ng/mL.

FEATURES

- Elevated serum prolactin
- No signs or symptoms of intracranial pathology
- Signs and symptoms of hyperprolactinemia may occur
- Features of psychologic stress may be evident
- Physical stress may include intensive athletic training

Iatrogenic – drugs

- Dopamine inhibits prolactin release so drugs that block dopamine increase prolactin level, e.g. chlorpromazine, fluphenazine, haloperidol, perphenazine, promazine, domperidone, metoclopramide, sulpiride
- Neuroleptic agents and other dopamine receptor antagonists cause rapid elevation of prolactin to levels that may reach 200ng/mL
- Estrogens stimulate lactotroph growth, increasing prolactin levels
- Metoclopramide may be associated with a 15-fold increase in prolactin concentration
- Histamine type-2 receptor blockers produce hyperprolactinemia by a central mechanism
- In patients with primary hypothyroidism, hyperprolactinemia develops because of increased hypothalamic thyrotropin-releasing hormone (TRH) activity

FEATURES

- Elevated serum prolactin – can be >200ng/mL
- History of ingestion of dopamine receptor antagonists (e.g. chlorpromazine, fluphenazine, haloperidol, perphenazine, promazine, domperidone, metoclopramide, sulpiride), antihypertensives (e.g. methyldopa, reserpine, verapamil), estrogens, opiates, cimetidine

Nipple stimulation

Usually sexual, therefore patients are likely not to admit to it. Can cause galactorrhea.

FEATURES

- Elevated serum prolactin (not always – galactorrhea may be euprolactinemic)
- Galactorrhea
- Absence of intracranial localizing signs

Breast manipulation, chest wall lesions, spinal cord lesions, head trauma

Chest wall disease or manipulation may elevate serum prolactin and cause symptoms of hyperprolactinemia. Causes include chest wall surgery, skin disease, and breast cancer.

FEATURES

- Elevated serum prolactin
- Chest wall disease

Polycystic ovarian syndrome

Hyperinsulinemia is a contributory factor to ovarian hyperandrogenism.

FEATURES

- Multiple ovarian cysts in arrested development
- Hirsutism
- Obesity
- Oligomenorrhea
- Infertility
- Acne
- Insulin resistance
- Dysfunctional uterine bleeding
- Mildly elevated prolactin levels may be found, probably relating to increased hypothalamic secretion of gonadotrophin-releasing hormone (GnRH)
- Raised luteinizing hormone:follicle-stimulating hormone (LH:FSH) ratio (>3.0)
- Hirsutism, multiple ovarian cysts, and oligomenorrhea causing infertility with elevated LH:FSH ratio

Chronic liver disease

Cirrhosis may cause some of the physical signs of prolactinoma, but serum prolactin is not usually elevated.

FEATURES

- History compatible with chronic liver disease
- Skin signs: spider nevi, bruising, palmar erythema, caput medusae
- Jaundice
- Ascites
- Gynecomastia
- Hypogonadism
- Loss of body hair
- Edema
- Ataxia
- Choreoathetosis

Chronic renal failure

Chronic renal failure may cause elevated serum prolactin.

FEATURES
- Fatigue
- Edema
- Hypertension
- Skin pallor
- Bruising
- Nausea, malaise
- Pruritus
- Insomnia
- Taste disturbance
- Depression
- Altered renal function tests

Primary hypothyroidism

Primary failure of thyroid gland resulting in secondary elevation of thyroid-stimulating hormone (TSH).

FEATURES
- Elevated serum prolactin may result from suppression of hypothalamic dopamine secretion
- Coarse skin, hair, facies
- Myxedema
- Carotenemia
- Goiter
- Pericardial effusion
- Feels the cold
- Bradycardia
- Tiredness
- Peripheral neuropathy
- Carpal tunnel syndrome
- Muscular weakness
- Cerebellar ataxia

Hypothalmic disease

- Hypothalamic tumor, e.g. metastases, craniopharyngioma, germinoma, cyst, glioma, hamartoma, infiltration (sarcoid, tuberculosis, histiocytosis X, granuloma, cranial irradiation)
- Any damage to the hypothalamus may result in decreased secretion of dopamine, which inhibits prolactin release from the anterior pituitary
- Serum prolactin concentrations are usually <100ng/mL

FEATURES
- Elevated serum prolactin
- Symptoms of pituitary insufficiency – loss of gonadotropins, corticosteroids
- Signs of raised intracranial pressure
- Other symptoms and signs of relevant causative disease
- Hypothalamic abnormality found on computed tomography (CT)/magnetic resonance imaging (MRI)

Pituitary disease

- Pituitary infiltration – sarcoid, histiocytosis, granuloma, tuberculosis, other anterior pituitary tumor
- Serum prolactin is elevated in acromegaly (growth hormone-secreting anterior pituitary tumor), gonadotrope adenoma, meningioma, Cushing's disease

FEATURES

- Seen on CT/MRI
- Features of optic chiasm pressure may be seen
- Features of raised intracranial pressure may be seen
- Prolactin levels usually <200ng/mL
- Features of other hormonal excess

Ectopic prolactin-secreting tumor

Rare feature of hypernephroma, bronchogenic carcinoma.

FEATURES

- Elevated serum prolactin – may be very high
- Signs and symptoms indistinguishable from prolactinoma of anterior pituitary except no tumor found on radiologic investigation

SIGNS & SYMPTOMS

Signs

- Signs vary with age, sex, duration of hyperprolactinemia, and tumor size
- Often chance radiologic discovery with no signs
- Signs can be due to mass effects of the tumor or to hyperprolactinemia itself

All patients may show:

- Bitemporal hemianopsia secondary to optic chiasm compression
- Decreased visual acuity
- Visual field deficits (only in macroadenoma as microadenoma is intrasellar)
- Ophthalmoplegia
- Impairment of cranial nerves III, IV, VI, and first and second divisions of trigeminal nerve
- Collapse due to hemorrhage into tumor
- Hypopituitarism
- Osteopenia on X-ray

Women of reproductive age commonly show:

- Galactorrhea
- Signs of prolonged estrogen deficiency – atrophic vaginitis, thinning of pubic hair, loss of labial fat pads, reduction in breast size

Men may also present with:

- Decreased beard and body hair (long-standing hypogonadism)
- Testes usually soft but of normal size (>12mL volume)
- Galactorrhea – less common in men; demonstration may require vigorous breast manipulation
- Gynecomastia is uncommon
- Breasts may appear enlarged due to fatty tissue

Symptoms

- Presentation varies with age and sex, duration of hyperprolactinemia, and tumor size
- Often asymptomatic and chance discovery: may be incidentally imaged when a CT or MRI scan is obtained because of head trauma or for evaluation of headaches

All patients may present with:

- Headache (63% – but 27% of individuals without prolactinoma have headache)
- Apathy 63%, making this an important differential diagnosis of depressive illness in men as well as women
- Bitemporal hemianopsia secondary to optic chiasm compression

- Altered vision – blurring, needing new spectacle prescription
- Microadenomas are intrasellar, so visual abnormalities do not occur, but headache occurs more often than in normal individuals
- Ophthalmoplegia
- Squint
- Double vision
- Uncommonly severe headache with prostration secondary to hemorrhage into tumor
- Hemorrhage into tumor may rarely cause hypopituitarism requiring immediate evaluation and treatment
- Rarely, seizures as large tumors extend into temporal lobe

Women of reproductive age commonly present with:
- Primary amenorrhea
- Amenorrhea
- Oligomenorrhea
- Menorrhagia
- Infertility
- Galactorrhea in 30–80%
- Symptoms of prolonged hypoestrogenism
- Decreased libido
- Vaginal dryness
- Dyspareunia
- Microadenoma (most premenopausal, hyperprolactinemic women)

Men may present with:
- Decreased libido (83%)
- Weight gain (69%)
- Complete or partial impotence – many realize that there is a problem only after successful treatment
- Infertility
- Decreased or softer beard and body hair
- Galactorrhea (less common in men)
- Gynecomastia (uncommon)
- Fatty breast enlargement

CONSIDER CONSULT

- Always urgently admit patients with severe headache and collapse or where there is clinical suspicion of intracranial bleeding – all require urgent radiologic evaluation by MRI
- Always refer pregnant women with known pituitary adenoma for specialist team management including ophthalmologist, obstetrician, and endocrinologist
- Always refer patients with markedly raised prolactin for radiologic evaluation

INVESTIGATION OF THE PATIENT

Direct questions to patient

Questions depend very much on age, sex, and presentation, but might include the following.

Galactorrhea:

Q **For how long have you noticed it?** Women may have had galactorrhea for many years – this is usually due to nipple stimulation and may date back to when they last breast-fed

Q **Is it spontaneous/staining your clothes or does it only appear when you express it?** Spontaneous galactorrhea is of much greater significance than expressed galactorrhea – continuing expression will encourage production

- **Could you be pregnant?** Pregnancy increases serum prolactin, and spontaneous galactorrhea is common from the midsecond trimester
- **Have you breast-fed recently? Did the milk production stop afterwards or has it continued?** Galactorrhea may continue for many months after breast-feeding and indefinitely if the woman continues to express it. Postbreast-feeding galactorrhea may last longer if breast-feeding has been prolonged
- **Has anything like this ever happened before/have you ever had blood tests because of milk production or abnormal hormones before?** Women occasionally reveal a previous history of prolactinoma

Fertility:

- **What are your periods like? Are they regular? Are they heavy?** Dysfunctional uterine bleeding and oligomenorrhea are both suggestive of elevated prolactin levels
- **Are you trying for a baby? For how long have you been trying? Have you had any tests for this?** Hyperprolactinemia causes anovulation – ovulation induction is usually needed to conceive
- **Are you using any contraception?** Estrogens may cause elevation in serum prolactin
- **Have you gained or lost weight recently?** Dramatic weight change may signify underlying illness, including psychiatric illness, or may be the cause of cause anovulation

Intracranial features:

- **Do you suffer from headaches? What are they like?** Frequent headache is common – 27% of people without prolactinoma suffer from regular headaches while 63% of patients with prolactinoma do so. Headache due to raised intracranial pressure is likely to be present on sitting up in the morning, exacerbated by coughing and straining, and is often occipital – it may also lead to other headaches, e.g. tension headache, migraine
- **Have they been any worse recently?** Change in headache type or pattern may indicate new disease
- **Are they worse when you cough or sneeze? Are they there when you wake or when you sit up in bed, or do they worsen towards the end of the day?** Tension headaches worsen through the day; headache of intracranial cause is present on first sitting up in the morning

General questions:

- **Do you feel basically well or unwell?**
- **Are you on any medication?** Remember to ask about herbal remedies and drugs of abuse – opiates may cause hyperprolactinemia, alcohol may cause liver disease, and an extensive list of medication may cause hyperprolactinemia
- **Are you seeing another doctor about any problems?** This may give clues to the presence of other underlying disease or drug use
- **Have you noticed any problems with your vision?** A positive response should generate further questions on precise symptoms, looking for diplopia, visual field loss, altered acuity, eye pain
- **Has anything else changed?** It is always useful to ask some open questions in case patients have noticed other symptoms such as gynecomastia
- **Is your mood good or do you feel that you could be low?** Stress and depression cause moderate elevation of prolactin levels and are a very common cause
- **Do you feel more tired than usual?** Tiredness and malaise are common in prolactinoma (and in stress, depression, and other chronic illness)
- **Do you feel your sex drive has altered recently?** There are many other causes of female and male sexual dysfunction, but if a pattern suggestive of raised prolactin is emerging then this is another positive finding
- **Do you (women) have any pain or discomfort during intercourse?** Dyspareunia may be suggestive of vaginitis secondary to low estrogen levels due to hyperprolactinemia but may also have other causes

Examination

- **Does the patient look well?** In rare instances where hypopituitarism has resulted from tumor extension or bleeding, patient may look and feel unwell. In chronic renal or liver disease, patients may be pale or jaundiced and have lost weight
- **Has a male patient lost body hair?** Beard hair may be unusually sparse and soft in hyperprolactinemia
- **Does the patient look hypothyroid?** Hypothyroidism causes coarsening of skin, hair, and facies, sometimes with obvious goiter
- **Is the patient's acuity altered?** Check with a Snellen chart using pinhole vision if necessary
- **Are the patient's visual fields affected?** Test visual fields to confrontation, which is likely to reveal only large visual field defects
- **Are the fundi normal?** Look for papilledema
- **Are the patient's cranial nerves affected?** Test nerves of eye movement and facial sensation, all of which may rarely be affected by tumor extension to cavernous sinus
- **Are the patient's breasts altered?** Look for signs of galactorrhea, and for real or apparent gynecomastia in men
- **Is the patient's blood pressure normal?** Hypotension may be a sign of pituitary failure
- **Is the patient's chest wall normal in appearance?** Chest wall disease (including skin disease) may cause hyperprolactinemia and galactorrhea
- **Does the patient's abdomen feel normal?** Liver disease may cause a palpable liver and ascites. Concealed pregnancy of advanced stage may be revealed only on examination of the abdomen

Summary of investigative tests

- Serum prolactin level: if the cause of the hyperprolactinemia is not apparent after history and physical examination, medication review, and measurement of thyroid hormone, radiographic evaluation of the pituitary should be undertaken
- MRI: usually performed by a specialist, MRI is superior to CT in delineating tumor size and determining whether there is lateral or suprasellar tumor extension
- Stimulation and suppression tests of prolactin secretion with TRH, chlorpromazine, levodopa, or insulin-induced hypoglycemia are sometimes described, but are not valuable in the differential diagnosis of hyperprolactinemia

DIAGNOSTIC DECISION

- Prolactin-secreting macroadenomas (>1cm) cause marked elevations of prolactin (about 1000ng/mL) and a macroadenoma that is accompanied by a prolactin level of <200ng/mL is unlikely to be a prolactinoma
- Some patients with sustained hyperprolactinemia have no radiographic evidence of a tumor (idiopathic hyperprolactinemia)

CLINICAL PEARLS

- The likelihood for blindness is great because, in the absence of endocrine symptoms, visual loss is the usual initial manifestation
- The most common visual abnormality is bitemporal hemianopsia secondary to compression of the optic chiasm
- Lateral extension of the tumor into the cavernous sinus can cause impaired oculomotor function involving cranial nerves III, IV, and VI, and the V1 and V2 divisions of cranial nerve V, either singly or in combination
- Occasionally large tumors may extend into the temporal lobe and cause seizures

THE TESTS

Body fluids

SERUM PROLACTIN LEVEL

Description

- Blood test
- Because prolactin secretion is episodic and stress may raise prolactin concentrations, a low or borderline level should be confirmed by obtaining several samples
- The diagnosis of hyperprolactinemia is confirmed by demonstration of sustained elevation of serum levels

Advantages/Disadvantages

Advantages:

- Easy to perform
- Serum prolactin concentration of 200ng/mL or greater in the presence of a macroadenoma (>1cm) is most likely a prolactinoma
- Serum prolactin levels of <200mcg/L in the setting of a large pituitary tumor are usually elevated because of the mechanical effects of nonprolactin-secreting tumors that cause pituitary stalk compression or interfere with dopamine transport from the hypothalamus to the anterior pituitary
- This distinction is particularly important in selecting appropriate therapy; dopamine agonist drugs reduce serum prolactin levels in both instances, but shrinkage of the tumor is unlikely with secondary hyperprolactinemia
- Patients with a prolactin-secreting microadenoma usually have serum prolactin levels <200mcg/L

Disadvantages:

- Not diagnostic of prolactinoma without radiologic evidence
- An increased serum prolactin level must be interpreted in conjunction with the anatomic findings (MRI) to determine whether the hyperprolactinemia is due to a prolactinoma or is secondary to some other process

Normal

<20mcg/L.

Abnormal

- A single prolactin measurement may be sufficient to diagnose a prolactinoma if the value is >200mcg/L
- Because prolactin is secreted in a pulsatile fashion and in response to breast manipulation, a mildly increased concentration of 20–60mcg/L may be difficult to interpret; in this situation several measurements should be made before diagnosing hyperprolactinemia

Drugs, disorders and other factors that may alter results

- Dopamine antagonists increase prolactin levels
- Estrogens stimulate lactotroph growth, increasing prolactin levels
- Neuroleptic agents and other dopamine receptor antagonists cause rapid elevation of prolactin to levels that may reach 200ng/mL
- Metoclopramide may be associated with a 15-fold increase in prolactin concentration
- Histamine type-2 receptor blockers produce hyperprolactinemia by a central mechanism
- Estrogen stimulates prolactin secretion
- In patients with primary hypothyroidism, hyperprolactinemia develops because of increased hypothalamic TRH activity

Imaging

MRI SCAN

Description

Radiologic scan.

Advantages/Disadvantages

Disadvantages:

- Expensive
- Not usually readily accessible by primary care physicians
- Needs specialist to interpret results
- Small exposure to electromagnetic radiation

Abnormal

Pituitary mass.

Cause of abnormal result

- Microadenoma
- Macroadenoma
- Other pituitary or hypothalamic mass

TREATMENT

CONSIDER CONSULT

Always refer a patient diagnosed with prolactinoma to a specialist, preferably an endocrinologist – the treatment, however, will most likely be handled by a multidisciplinary team.

IMMEDIATE ACTION

Urgent admission if patient seriously unwell with collapse or severe headache.

MANAGEMENT ISSUES

Goals

- Return hormonal hypersecretion to normal
- Reduce tumor size
- Restore gonadal function and fertility, if desired
- Correct visual or cranial nerve abnormalities
- Restore any abnormal pituitary function
- Preclude the need for chronic hormone replacement therapy
- Monitor for recurrence
- In the case of large tumors, these goals may be only partially achieved
- The established indications for treatment of a prolactinoma are restoration of fertility and the presence of a macroadenoma
- The treatment of choice is a dopamine agonist; treatment is necessarily medical if fertility is required

Management in special circumstances

COEXISTING MEDICATION

- Oral contraceptive pill – there is no human evidence that estrogen increases tumor size although trials in mice suggest that it may. It is, therefore, considered prudent to discontinue treatments containing estrogens in patients with prolactinoma
- Dopamine antagonists or other medication likely to increase prolactin levels should be discontinued

SPECIAL PATIENT GROUPS

Infertility/trying to conceive:

- Spontaneous ovulation is uncommon when a pituitary tumor is present
- Most patients with this disorder will present with galactorrhea or anovulatory cycles and infertility
- Most women with prolactin-secreting adenomas require ovulation induction to conceive
- Resumption of ovulatory menses occurs in 80–90% of hyperprolactinemic women during bromocriptine therapy – the fertility rate of these patients should be the same as that of other women of the same age
- A standard recommendation for women attempting to become pregnant is that barrier contraception should be used until there has been two or three regular cycles so that cycle length can be determined
- After discontinuation of mechanical contraception, a serum human chorionic gonadotropin (hCG)-beta measurement is made to confirm pregnancy as soon as there is a delay in expected menses
- This makes early diagnosis of pregnancy and early discontinuation of dopamine agonist therapy possible
- Nonpregnant patients who present with amenorrhea-galactorrhea and prolactin >20ng/mL should be radiologically investigated for pituitary adenoma

- Computerized axial tomography and magnetic resonance imaging (MRI) are used to evaluate the size of the pituitary gland
- If pituitary tumor is diagnosed, some specialists advise re-evaluation for growth after several months before ovulation induction
- Macroadenomas are usually treated surgically, as over one-third may develop symptoms during pregnancy
- Radiotherapy is reserved for patients who do not respond to medical or surgical treatment
- Because of the risk of tumor expansion in women with macroadenomas, a thorough ophthalmologic examination, including visual field testing, is recommended before conception is attempted so that baseline values can be documented

Pregnancy:

- Pregnancy has become increasingly common in patients with prolactinomas due to successful ovulation induction
- Most patients with a microadenoma have an uneventful pregnancy
- In those patients who become symptomatic, regression usually follows delivery
- Pituitary gland normally increases in size during pregnancy and prolactin rises to up to 20 times normal at term
- Prolactin levels do not always rise during pregnancy in women with prolactinomas
- Evaluation for prolactinoma is difficult during pregnancy due to physiologic rise in serum prolactin
- Pregnancy-induced lactotroph hyperplasia due to estrogen may cause enlargement of adenomas
- Prolactin levels do not always rise with pregnancy-induced tumor enlargement
- Radiologic diagnosis is necessary for pregnant patients with severe headaches or visual field defects

Management of the pregnant patient with a previously diagnosed prolactinoma:

- Fluctuations in serum prolactin do not correlate well with tumor growth in pregnancy
- Enlargement of the pituitary also occurs during pregnancy, but tumor expansion is rarely clinically significant
- The risk of tumor growth with a microadenoma is very small but there is a higher risk with macroadenomas (theses patients should be followed closely with formal visual field testing and/or MRI)
- Fewer than 2% of women with microadenomas develop headaches or visual deficits, and <5% have radiographic evidence of tumor expansion during pregnancy
- All dopamine agonists cross the placenta but are not associated with an increased risk of spontaneous abortion or congenital defects
- Even so, women taking a dopamine agonist should stop the drug when pregnancy is documented
- Surveillance of >2000 pregnancies indicates that bromocriptine use is not associated with an increased risk of multiple pregnancies, spontaneous abortions, ectopic pregnancy, trophoblastic disease, or congenital malformations; even so, its use during pregnancy is only indicated if symptomatic tumor enlargement occurs
- Marked elevations of serum prolactin outside the pregnant range for given gestational age may signal rapid tumor enlargement in macroadenoma
- It is not necessary to monitor serum levels throughout pregnancy in microadenoma
- Symptoms occur in 5–20% of pregnancies with previously untreated microadenoma, with most resolving after delivery
- Tumor expansion may occur during pregnancy, particularly in women with macroadenomas. The incidence of significant tumor enlargement during pregnancy is about 1.4% in women with microadenomas and 16% in women with macroadenomas
- Therapies in the event of significant tumor enlargement include surgical resection, high-dose glucocorticoid therapy, and reinstitution of bromocriptine

- Patients with macroadenomas treated with bromocriptine continuously during pregnancy do not have tumor-related complications
- Similarly, those given bromocriptine because of tumor expansion had improvement or resolution of headaches and visual field defects

Management of patient with complications during pregnancy:

- Therapy for complications in pregnancy is affected by gestational age and severity of symptoms
- If fetal maturity is present, induction of labor or cesarean delivery
- Earlier in gestation, if radiologic evidence suggests tumor enlargement, therapy should not be delayed
- Bromocriptine is the preferred therapy during pregnancy and appears to be safe in early pregnancy
- Other treatments during pregnancy include trans-sphenoidal surgery and hydrocortisone therapy
- Complications of surgery are infection, hypopituitarism, hemorrhage, and transient diabetes insipidus. Risk of these is probably not increased during pregnancy
- Following delivery, radiologic assessment of tumor size and a serum prolactin assay should be performed at the first postpartum visit

Breast-feeding with known pituitary adenoma:

- Breast-feeding is not contraindicated in the presence of a prolactin-secreting microadenoma
- Bromocriptine appears safe in breast-feeding
- Serum prolactin levels may remain elevated while nursing; caution must be used in interpreting these results

Future pregnancy planning with known pituitary adenoma:
Counseling patients regarding future pregnancies requires establishing that progression of tumor growth has not occurred.

Contraception with known pituitary adenoma:

- Oral contraceptives use has not been associated with growth of pre-existing microadenomas or their development
- Repeated pregnancies do not appear to have greater complication rate than first pregnancies

Children:

- Prolactinoma may cause primary amenorrhea but is responsible for <1% of cases
- Most are microadenomas
- Excess prolactin secretion can cause galactorrhea and suppress the reproductive system in males and females manifested as delayed or arrested puberty
- Prolactinomas may be seen in children with the McCune-Albright syndrome (i.e. precocious puberty, cutaneous café au lait spots, and polyostotic fibrous dysplasia) and in young adults with multiple endocrine neoplasia type I (MEN-I)
- Treatment is the same as for adults

PATIENT SATISFACTION/LIFESTYLE PRIORITIES
Patient will generally prefer the idea of medical therapy to surgery or radiotherapy.

SUMMARY OF THERAPEUTIC OPTIONS

Choices

- Treatment is not required in certain cases: when fertility is not an issue, treatment is controversial; microprolactinomas have a benign natural history and treatment is not necessary to prevent tumor growth; and if the hyperprolactinemia is associated with regular menses, no therapy is necessary

- Medical treatment with dopamine agonists is the first-choice approach. Available dopamine agonists include bromocriptine, pergolide, and cabergoline
- Surgical treatment via trans-sphenoidal approach is indicated for failure of medical treatment. Surgical resection of a microadenoma offers the greatest potential for cure, but the usual outcome for patients with large tumors is persistent hyperprolactinemia requiring additional therapy
- Primary treatment of prolactinoma by pituitary radiation prevents further growth of the tumor but is less effective in promoting a prompt reduction of the serum prolactin concentration, although a progressive reduction in serum prolactin concentration may occur over time. Radiotherapy is not effective as primary therapy but may be useful as adjunctive therapy with large tumors or after surgery

Clinical pearls

- The goals of treatment are to: return hormonal secretion to normal, reduce tumor size, correct visual or cranial nerve abnormalities, restore any abnormal pituitary function, and preclude the need for chronic hormone replacement therapy
- Evidence shows that preoperative treatment with bromocriptine may reduce the size of macroprolactinomas and aid in subsequent removal
- Microneurosurgical techniques make it possible to remove the tumor and leave normal pituitary intact, which reduces the requirement for replacement hormonal therapy

Never

In all patients, avoidance of estrogen is standard practice:

- Evidence suggests that estrogen may be administered without stimulating tumor growth although estrogen increases prolactin and has been associated with tumor formation in animals
- Nevertheless, estrogen should be administered with caution to women with macroadenomas, with radiographic follow up to ensure that tumor growth is not enhanced

FOLLOW UP

- Frequent follow up with prolactin measurement is necessary for all patients due to the high rates of recurrence in this disorder
- Exact frequency of visits will vary with tumor size
- Microadenoma may be followed up with serial prolactin measurements alone
- Macroadenoma is associated with a greater risk of complications, and needs radiologic and possible optic field monitoring in addition to serum prolactin measurements
- The rate of recurrence if treatment is discontinued is very high and patients should be carefully monitored
- Follow up of pregnant patients with microadenoma is to monitor for signs of complications only
- Pregnant patients with macroadenoma should be monitored by a specialist team including ophthalmologist, endocrinologist, and obstetrician

Plan for review

- Review period varies with tumor size
- Patients stable on treatment require regular review of serum prolactin measurements
- Patients with macroadenoma require radiologic follow up in addition to serum prolactin measurements
- Serum prolactin measurements are unhelpful in pregnant women with known microadenoma
- Time interval for review depends on each individual case. Many patients have a slow progression, with recurrence even 10–15 years after initial treatment

Information for patient or caregiver

Patients should be aware that:

- While the tumor is benign it is a recurrent condition and they are likely to need monitoring for years

- If they develop severe headaches or loss of vision they should consult a doctor or visit an emergency room immediately and make staff aware they have a prolactinoma
- They should avoid medications containing estrogen

DRUGS AND OTHER THERAPIES: DETAILS

Drugs

BROMOCRIPTINE

- All dopamine agonists inhibit prolactin secretion by stimulating pituitary and neuronal dopamine receptors
- Most patients will respond within 3 months
- After treatment with bromocriptine, 80–90% of women with a microprolactinoma will have normal serum prolactin levels, regular menstrual periods, and restoration of fertility
- Normalization of serum prolactin may occur within 24h, and gonadal function may normalize as early as 3 months after treatment
- Normalization of prolactin is less likely to occur in a patient with a macroadenoma, but a dopamine agonist is still first-line therapy
- Patients who fail to respond to bromocriptine or who cannot tolerate that drug may respond to another dopamine agonist
- With the exception of one report of pulmonary fibrosis in patients with Parkinson's disease, long-term therapy with bromocriptine has not been associated with complications

Dose

- Initial dosage of bromocriptine mesylate is 0.5–2mg tablet daily. An additional 2.5mg tablet may be added to the treatment regimen as tolerated every 3–7 days until an optimal therapeutic response is achieved. The therapeutic dosage usually is 5–7.5mg and ranges from 2.5 to 15mg/day
- It is uncommon for a patient to require a higher dose; size of tumor and the serum prolactin level have no bearing on the dose required
- In patients who achieve a normal serum prolactin level, dose may be reduced to 2.5mg twice daily; suppression may continue with the reduced dose
- Some patients have been given larger doses (20–30mg/day) but there is no evidence that this is more effective

Efficacy

- Most patients have a good response to dopamine agonists but some respond partially or not at all
- Most patients will respond within 3 months
- After treatment with bromocriptine 5–7.5mg daily, 80–90% of women with a microprolactinoma will have normal serum prolactin levels, regular menstrual periods, and restoration of fertility
- Normalization of serum prolactin may occur within 24h, and gonadal function may normalize as early as 3 months after treatment
- Normalization of prolactin is less likely to occur in a patient with a macroadenoma, but a dopamine agonist is still first-line therapy
- Higher dosages (10–30mg) may be necessary to obtain reduction in serum prolactin and decrease in tumor size in men and in women with macroadenomas
- Reduction in tumor size usually occurs within 4–6 weeks
- About 60% of women with macroadenomas will have more than a 50% reduction in tumor size
- Bromocriptine must be given continuously to be effective
- Discontinuation of the drug leads to a rapid return to pretreatment prolactin levels and tumor re-expansion
- Response to medical therapy and the number and affinity of tumor dopamine receptors are correlated

- Resistance to bromocriptine is uncommon, but all patients should be closely monitored during medical therapy, and surgical resection should be considered if a patient fails to respond to medical treatment
- The treatment of men with a dopamine agonist enhances libido and potency as the serum testosterone level increases
- Semen analysis (sperm count and semen volume) improves with lowering of the prolactin level to normal and restoration of pulsatile secretion of luteinizing hormone (LH) and follicle-stimulating hormone (FSH)

Risks/Benefits

Risks (disease-specific):
- Protracted medical treatment of prolactinomas may lead to marked calcification, deposition of endocrine amyloid, and perivascular and interstitial fibrosis
- This may decrease the chance for successful surgery
- Use caution in hepatic or renal disease
- Use caution in hypotension and concurrent hypertensive medications
- Use caution in children

Benefit: safe drug with few complications

Side-effects and adverse reactions
- Side-effects are lessened if the drug is started at a low dose
- Transvaginal administration of bromocriptine has been reported to cause fewer gastrointestinal side-effects
- Cardiovascular system: postural hypotension, vasospasm of fingers and toes
- Central nervous system: headache, dizziness, drowsiness, confusion, hallucinations, dyskinesia
- Eyes, ears, nose, and throat: visual disturbances
- Gastrointestinal: nausea, vomiting, diarrhea, anorexia, bleeding, dry mouth

Interactions (other drugs)

■ Alcohol ■ Antipsychotics ■ Domperidone ■ Erythromycin ■ Macrolides ■ Octreotide ■ Metoclopramide ■ Isometheptene ■ Phenylpropanolamine

Contraindications

■ Pregnancy category B ■ Severe ischemic and peripheral vascular disease ■ Lactation

Acceptability to patient

Usually well tolerated and acceptable.

Follow up plan
- Prolactin level should be checked about one month after starting the bromocriptine
- If the level has not normalized, the dose should be increased slowly

Patient and caregiver information
- Patients should be aware that if treatment is for microadenoma they should discontinue the medication if they become pregnant
- Patients should be aware they need to be followed up and treatment should not be abruptly discontinued without medical advice
- Patients should be aware of the high risk of recurrence when therapy is stopped

OTHER DOPAMINE AGONISTS

Other dopamine agonists include quinagolide, cabergoline, pergolide, and lisuride.

Cabergoline:

- Long-acting ergot derivative
- Administered once or twice weekly and is also better tolerated than bromocriptine by some patients
- Lowers prolactin concentrations, restores gonadal function, and reduces tumor size
- A more potent dopamine agonist with a very high specificity for the dopamine D_2 receptor and a long half-life

Pergolide:

- Longer duration of action
- Dosages of 50–150mcg once daily are as effective as bromocriptine in normalizing prolactin
- Approved by the US Food and Drug Administration (FDA) only for treatment of Parkinson's disease
- Lowers serum prolactin levels and has also been used to treat patients with acromegaly

Dose

Cabergoline:

- Recommended dosage of cabergoline tablets for initiation of therapy is 0.25mg twice a week. Dosage may be increased by 0.25mg twice weekly up to a dosage of 1mg twice a week according to the patient's serum prolactin level. Dosage increases should not occur more rapidly than every 4 weeks
- After a normal serum prolactin level has been maintained for 6 months, cabergoline may be discontinued, with periodic monitoring of the serum prolactin level to determine whether or when treatment with cabergoline should be reinstituted. The durability of efficacy beyond 24 months of therapy with cabergoline has not been established

Pergolide (off-label indication):
Starting dose of 0.05mg at bedtime for first 2 days; gradually increase dosage by 0.1 or 0.15mg/day every 3 days over next 12 days, then increase dose by 0.25mg/day every 3 days until optimal therapeutic dose is achieved, up to 5mg/day maximum; usual dosage range: 2–3mg/day in three divided doses.

Efficacy

- Most patients have a good response to dopamine agonists but some respond partially or not at all
- Most patients will respond within 3 months
- Normalization of serum prolactin may occur within 24h, and gonadal function may normalize as early as 3 months after treatment
- Normalization of prolactin is less likely to occur in a patient with a macroadenoma, but a dopamine agonist is still first-line therapy
- Reduction in tumor size usually occurs within 4–6 weeks
- Discontinuation of the drug leads to a rapid return to pretreatment prolactin levels and tumor re-expansion

Risks/Benefits

Risks: (Bromocriptine)

- Use caution in hepatic or renal disease
- Use caution in hypotension and concurrent hypertensive medications
- Use caution in children

Risks: (Pergolide)

- Risk of symptomatic orthostatic and/or sustained hypotension
- Risk of hallucinosis
- In the placebo-controlled trial, 2 of 187 patients treated with placebo died as compared with one of 189 patients treated with pergolide mesylate

- There have been rare reports of pleuritis, pleural effusion, pleural fibrosis, pericarditis, pericardial effusion, or retroperitoneal fibrosis in patients taking pergolide
- Use with caution when administering pergolide mesylate to patients prone to cardiac dysrhythmias
- Use with caution when administering to patients with preexisting dyskinesia

Benefit: well tolerated, very effective in most patients

Side-effects and adverse reactions

(Bromocriptine)

- Side-effects are lessened if the drug is started at a low dose
- Transvaginal administration of bromocriptine has been reported to cause fewer gastrointestinal side-effects
- Cardiovascular system: postural hypotension, vasospasm of fingers and toes
- Central nervous system: headache, dizziness, drowsiness, confusion, hallucinations, dyskinesia
- Eyes, ears, nose, and throat: visual disturbances
- Gastrointestinal: nausea, vomiting, diarrhea, anorexia, bleeding, dry mouth

(Pergolide)

- Cardiovascular system: hypotension, vasoconstriction for patients with unstable coronary angina and Raynaud's syndrome
- Central nervous system: somolence, confusion, hallucinations

Interactions (other drugs)

(Bromocriptine)

■ Erythromycin (increased bromocriptine levels) ■ Isometheptene (hypertension) ■ Neuroleptics (in patients with pituitary adenomas, may inhibit bromocriptine's ability to lower prolactin levels) ■ Drugs which have dopamine antagonist activity, e.g. phenothiazines, butyrophenones (may decrease efficacy of bromocriptine)

(Pergolide)

■ Dopamine antagonists, such as the neuroleptics (phenothiazines, butyrophenones, thioxanthenes) or metoclopramide (may diminish the effectiveness of pergolide mesylate) ■ Other drugs known to affect protein binding dopamine antagonists, such as the neuroleptics (phenothiazines, butyrophenones, thioxanthenes) or metoclopramide (may diminish the effectiveness of pergolide mesylate)

Contraindications

(Bromocriptine)

■ Pregnancy categoy B ■ Severe ischemic and peripheral vascular disease ■ Lactation

(Pergolide)

■ Hypersensitivity to pergolide and other ergot derivatives ■ Pregnancy category B ■ Safety and efficacy in pediatric patients have not been established

Acceptability to patient

Usually very acceptable: side-effects not usually severe.

Follow up plan

- Prolactin level should be checked about one month after starting the medication
- If the level has not normalized, the dose should be increased slowly

- Resistance to dopamine agonists is uncommon, but all patients should be closely monitored during medical therapy, and surgical resection should be considered if a patient fails to respond to medical treatment

Patient and caregiver information

- Patients should be aware that if treatment is for microadenoma they should discontinue the medication if they become pregnant
- Patients should be aware they need to be followed up and treatment should not be abruptly discontinued without medical advice
- Patients should be aware of the high risk of recurrence when therapy is stopped

Surgical therapy

TRANS-SPHENOIDAL MICROSURGICAL RESECTION

- Before the development of medical therapy, surgery was the most effective treatment for a prolactinoma
- If a dopamine agonist is ineffective or poorly tolerated, trans-sphenoidal surgery may be considered for treatment of a prolactinoma
- Surgery performed by an experienced neurosurgeon will normalize prolactin in 60–70% of patients with microadenomas and in about one-third of patients with macroadenomas
- Recurrence rate of hyperprolactinemia is high and the procedure should be used only in selected cases
- Surgical resection of a microadenoma offers the greatest potential for cure, but the usual outcome for patients with large tumors is persistent hyperprolactinemia requiring additional therapy

Efficacy

- Cure is effected in a minority of patients with large tumors and is associated with a risk of recurrence in all patients
- Results depend on the skill and experience of the surgeon
- Resection of microadenomas (<10mm) at centers where the procedure is performed frequently result in a return of serum prolactin levels to normal 60–87% of the time, whereas serum prolactin levels become normal in only 0–40% of patients with macroadenomas (>10mm)
- Most important factors predictive of successful surgery are the preoperative serum prolactin concentration and the tumor size and stage (degree of invasion of parasellar structures)

Risks/Benefits

Risks:

- Risk of mortality with trans-sphenoidal surgery is <1%
- Complications include CSF rhinorrhea, diabetes insipidus, infection, damage to the visual system (less common with trans-sphenoidal surgery than with craniotomy), and anterior pituitary insufficiency
- Cumulative risk for these complications is on the order of 2% for patients with microadenomas and 14% for patients with macroadenomas
- Risk of morbidity is increased with a second surgical procedure

Acceptability to patient

Little choice available if surgery is required.

Follow up plan

Intensive follow up is necessary with radiologic and serum monitoring due to the high recurrence rate.

Radiation therapy

RADIOTHERAPY

- Primary treatment of prolactinoma by pituitary radiation prevents further growth of the tumor but is less effective in promoting a prompt reduction of the serum prolactin concentration, although a progressive reduction in serum prolactin concentration may occur over time
- Stereotactic radiosurgery with the gamma knife or focused linear accelerator may produce less hypopituitarism because of the sparing of the hypothalamus with these methods but further evidence is required
- The recommended radiation dose is a total of 45Gy administered as 1.8Gy/day over 25 days. A high-energy linear accelerator, rather than a cobalt 60 teletherapy apparatus, combined with a rotational arc technique provides maximal limitation of the high-dose region and usually produces little or no hair loss
- A total radiation dose of <40Gy results in poor tumor control, and total doses >50Gy or daily doses >2Gy are associated with higher complication rates and no demonstrable improvement in the overall results

Efficacy

Primary treatment of prolactinoma by pituitary radiation prevents further growth of the tumor but is less effective in promoting a prompt reduction of the serum prolactin concentration, although a progressive reduction in serum prolactin concentration may occur over time.

Risks/Benefits

Risks:

- Complications of pituitary radiation include: hypothalamic insufficiency, hypopituitarism; optic chiasm or optic nerve injury, or both; vascular damage with stroke; brain necrosis; and development of malignant tumors (fibrosarcoma, osteosarcoma)
- Radiation-induced hypopituitarism has been best documented in acromegalic patients treated with radiotherapy, and the incidence increases with time
- Gonadotropin deficiency is most common, occurring in 47–70% of patients treated with either radiation alone or surgery and radiation
- Second most common is corticotropin deficiency (15–67%), followed by thyrotropin deficiency (15–55%)
- There have been no adequate studies of growth hormone secretion after radiotherapy, but plasma growth hormone is frequently undetectable in random measurements in these patients

Acceptability to patient

Likely to be poor – hair loss may result from cranial irradiation, possible side-effects/consequences are severe.

Follow up plan

Intensive radiologic and serum follow up due to high recurrence risk.

Patient and caregiver information

Patients need a broad idea of possible complications so as to be alert for symptoms and signs.

EFFICACY OF THERAPIES

- If left untreated the natural history of prolactinoma is not known precisely, but most grow slowly over years
- Successful treatment is most often medical with administration of a dopamine agonist
- Recurrence rates are high if treatment is stopped
- Surgery is indicated when medical therapy fails
- In addition to medical and surgical therapy, pituitary radiation may be employed, usually as adjunctive therapy
- Some patients require more than one type of treatment to correct prolactin levels and decrease tumor size
- Overall recurrence rates are high – up to 50% of microadenomas and nearly 90% of macroadenomas can recur

Review period

- A dopamine agonist is usually taken chronically and, thus, functions as a hormone 'replacement'
- Withdrawal of treatment usually results in an increase in serum prolactin concentrations and re-expansion of the tumor
- Thus, long-term follow up is always necessary whether on or off treatment
- Occasionally a patient with a microadenoma or no demonstrable tumor has no increase in prolactin concentration after discontinuing dopamine agonist therapy
- Whether spontaneous infarction of the tumor occurred is not known
- If medication is discontinued, the patient should be followed closely with frequent measurement of the serum prolactin concentration
- If the level increases, medical therapy should be restarted
- After initiating treatment a prolactin level should be checked about one month after starting the bromocriptine
- If the level has not normalized, the dose should be increased slowly
- Because of the risk of tumor expansion in women with macroadenomas, a thorough ophthalmologic examination, including visual field testing, is recommended before conception is attempted so that baseline values can be documented

PROGNOSIS

- Microadenomas are benign tumors that rarely cause serious complications but are associated with a high rate of infertility
- Macroadenomas are more likely to lead to extrasellar space-occupying effects
- Serious complications are unusual
- Dopamine agonists are highly successful in reducing tumor size and clinical manifestations including fertility in women and men
- Recurrence rates are extremely high, especially if medication is discontinued
- Recurrence rates are also high after surgery

Clinical pearls

- Although most patients have a good response to dopamine agonists, some respond partially or not at all
- The clinical response to drug therapy and the number of dopamine receptors are correlated, which explains occasional tumor growth during bromocriptine therapy, loss of responsiveness, and even metastasis of tumors
- Resistance to bromocriptine is uncommon, but all patients should be closely monitored during medical therapy; if this fails, surgical resection should be considered

- Recurrence rates with surgery over 5 years of follow up range from 10 to 50% in patients with microadenomas and from 0 to 91% in those with macroadenomas
- The usual outcome in surgery for patients with large tumors is persistent hyperprolactinemia requiring additional therapy

Therapeutic failure

If medical treatment fails then surgical treatment, with or without radiotherapy, is indicated.

Recurrence

- In recurrence where medication has been stopped, medication should be restarted
- In recurrence where medication has been continuous, surgical treatment is indicated

COMPLICATIONS

- Hyperprolactinemia is associated with impaired pulsatile gonadotropin – luteinizing hormone (LH), follicle-stimulating hormone (FSH) – release, most likely via alteration in hypothalamic luteinizing hormone-releasing hormone (LHRH) secretion
- Gonadal insufficiency is reversed with reduction of prolactin levels
- Chronic hyperprolactinemia causes decreased bone density in both men and women
- Prolactin-induced estrogen deficiency may lead to bone loss, and women with hyperprolactinemia have 25% lower spinal bone mineral than women with regular menses
- Use of dual energy X-ray absorptiometry (DEXA) to measure spinal bone density may help with treatment decisions in individual patients
- A large tumor that extends beyond the confines of the sella turcica can cause headache and visual abnormalities – classically, bitemporal hemianopsia from compression of the optic chiasm by a tumor that extends superiorly
- If the tumor extends posteriorly, compression of a single optic tract produces a homonymous visual field defect
- Lateral extension into the cavernous sinus can cause impaired oculomotor function involving cranial nerves III, IV, and VI, and the V1 and V2 divisions of cranial nerve V, either singly or in combination
- Occasionally, large tumors may extend into the temporal lobe and cause seizures
- Patients with large tumors are at risk for compromise of other anterior pituitary function due to compression of normal pituitary tissue, causing growth hormone, corticotropin, LH, FSH, or thyrotropin deficiency, singly or in combination
- Complications of surgery and radiotherapy

PREVENTION

Not specifically preventable in a general population.

PREVENT RECURRENCE

Continued dopaminergic medication is highly successful at preventing recurrence.

Reassess coexisting disease

PATIENT SATISFACTION/LIFESTYLE PRIORITIES

Patients concerned about fertility will have many questions about medication during pregnancy and the risks of tumor growth.

RESOURCES

ASSOCIATIONS

Pituitary Network Association
223 E. Thousand Oaks Blvd, #320
Thousand Oaks, CA 91360
Mailing address:
PO Box 1958
Thousand Oaks, CA 91358
Tel: (805) 496-4932
Fax: (805) 557-1161
www.pituitary.org

KEY REFERENCES

- Crosignani PG. Long-term effects of time, medical treatment and pregnancy in 176 hyperprolactinemic women. Eur J Obstet Gynecol Reprod Biol1992;44:175–80
- Piketty ML. High prolactin level. J Neurosurg 2000;92:368–9
- Dullaart RP. Evaluation of adrenal function in patients with hypothalamic and pituitary disorders: comparison of serum cortisol, urinary free cortisol and the human-corticotrophin releasing hormone test with the insulin tolerance test. Clin Endocrinol 1999;50:465–71
- Gsponer J. Diagnosis, treatment, and outcome of pituitary tumors and other abnormal intrasellar masses. Retrospective analysis of 353 patients. Medicine 1999;78:236–69
- Nishioka H. Growth potential of female prolactinomas. Surg Neurol 2001;55:213–7
- Visot A. Neurosurgery and pituitary tumors: surgical indications and outcome. Presse Med. 2001;30:401–4. French
- De Luis DA. A randomized cross-over study comparing cabergoline and quinagolide in the treatment of hyperprolactinemic patients. J Endocrinol Invest 2000;23:428–34

FAQS

Question 1

What is the best approach in treating prolactinoma when pregnancy is not an issue?

ANSWER 1

When the tumor is small, there is no clear consensus on whether to treat or to monitor the patient without therapy. Microadenomas have a benign natural history and do not progressively increase in size over time. Elevated prolactin levels do, however, suppress production of estradiol and testosterone and may place these patients at risk for premature bone loss. Women with hyperprolactinemic amenorrhea have been shown to have 25% lower spinal bone mass than women with regular menses but do not have an increased fracture rate. A close control of bone mass in hyperprolactinemic women may help with treatment decisions in individual patients. An amenorrheic patient who is not desirous of pregnancy or a postmenopausal woman with hyperprolactinemia may be treated with estrogen. Although this may induce pituitary enlargement, these women should be monitored closely for clinical signs of tumor growth. Another option is to treat them with a combination of estrogen and bromocriptine.

Question 2

What is the expected response in terms of tumor size with clinical treatment?

ANSWER 2

Dopamine agonists provoke shrinkage on pituitary adenomas which is most dramatic for macroprolactinomas and is due to cell size reduction. In one meta-analysis, 79% of 271 definite macroprolactinomas were reduced in size by at least 25%, and 89% shrank to some degree. Most shrinkage will occur during the first 3 months of treatment. About 10% of true macroadenomas do not shrink with dopamine agonists.

Question 3

What should be expected after drug withdrawal?

ANSWER 3

Drug withdrawal nearly always leads to a return of hyperprolactinemia, even after several years of treatment, although early tumor re-expansion is unusual.

CONTRIBUTORS

Gordon H Baustian, MD
Luciana G O Clark, MD
Januario E Castro, MD

RENAL CELL ADENOCARCINOMA

SUMMARY INFORMATION

DESCRIPTION

- Most cases of kidney cancer are renal cell adenocarcinoma (RCC)
- RCC can mimic many diseases, making diagnosis very challenging
- RCC spreads intravascularly and 25–30% of patients have distant metastases or locally advanced disease at presentation
- Surgery is the primary treatment for RCC
- Survival is related to disease stage and ranges from 66% for stage I to 11% for stage IV
- Patients with early-stage RCC are curable with surgery
- The stage is based on the extra-renal extension of the tumor

URGENT ACTION

- Urgent action is required for some of the complications associated with RCC, not the disease itself
- Specifically, kidney failure with acute worsening of blood urea nitrogen and creatinine levels requires admission to the hospital and possibly intensive care
- Adrenal insufficiency can occur because of proximity of the adrenal gland to the kidney tumor

KEY! DON'T MISS!

- A common manifestation of RCC is hematuria
- The first examination for patients with persistent hematuria is the urography, followed by ultrasonography
- If the results are not clear, a computerized axial tomography scan should be ordered

ICD9 CODE

- 189.0 Renal cell carcinoma
- 189.1 (renal pelvis)

SYNONYMS

- Hypernephroma
- Alveolar adenocarcinoma
- Internist's tumor (due to the different types of presentation and to the diagnostic challenge)

CARDINAL FEATURES

- Approx. 90% of all kidney cancers are renal cell adenocarcinoma (RCC)
- There are five main types of RCC: clear cell, papillary, chromophobe, collecting duct, and unclassified
- RCC is symptomatically similar to many diseases; only 5–10% of patients present with the classic triad (abdominal mass, flank pain, and hematuria)
- The main sign is hematuria (40%), followed by back/flank pain (35%) and a palpable mass (30%)
- Because the kidney is an organ in the endocrine system, RCC tumors can express many different hormones resulting in various paraneoplastic syndromes and metabolic disturbances
- Between 25 and 30% of patients have distant metastases, and 25% have locally advanced disease at presentation
- Weight loss and malaise may be indicative of metastatic disease
- RCC is a tumor that spreads via the vascular system and by direct invasion into other organ structures and lymph nodes
- Surgery is the primary treatment for RCC
- Systemic chemotherapy, immunotherapy, radiation therapy, and bone marrow transplantation are considered experimental and currently are tested in clinical trials
- Survival is related to stage and ranges from 66% for stage I to 11% for stage IV

CAUSES

Common causes

The following factors will increase the risk of RCC:

- Cigarette smoking (20–30% of all cases)
- Occupational exposure to asbestos, gasoline, petroleum products, lead, cadmium, or organic solvents
- Use of any phenacetin-containing product (banned by the US Food and Drug Administration (FDA) in 1983)
- Exposure to Thorotrast (a contrast medium)
- Obesity (especially among women, and particularly those postmenopause)
- Diabetes
- Hypertension
- High intake of well-cooked meat

Rare causes

- Hereditary conditions including familial renal carcinoma, von Hippel-Lindau (VHL) disease, papillary renal cell carcinoma, tuberous sclerosis, and autosomal dominant adult polycystic kidney disease
- Kidney disease requiring regular hemodialysis

Serious causes

- Cigarette smoking increases the risk significantly
- Chemical carcinogenicity appears to be associated with an increased risk of developing RCC
- Obesity among women increases the risk significantly

Contributory or predisposing factors

- Cigarette smoking
- Carcinogenic chemical exposure
- Obesity
- Kidney disease

EPIDEMIOLOGY

Incidence and prevalence

0.4–1/1000/year.

INCIDENCE

- 30,000 cases/year. The incidence rate of RCC is increasing and has almost doubled from the 18,000 cases reported during the 1980s to the current rate of 30,000/year
- 12,000 deaths/year

PREVALENCE

RCC accounts for 2–3% of all new cancers diagnosed per year in the US.

FREQUENCY

Increased frequency in patients with VHL disease; 35% of patients with VHL develop RCC.

Demographics

AGE

Diagnosis of RCC usually occurs in people older than 40 years, with a peak between 50 and 80 years of age. It is important to note that RCC has a long latency period, therefore patients may have been exposed to the carcinogenic agent when they were in their 20s, but the tumor is not detected until they are in their 50s or 60s.

GENDER

Males are 2–3 times more likely than females to develop RCC.

RACE

- RCC is similarly distributed among African-Americans and Caucasians
- Incidence rate among American-Hispanics is >33% more than Caucasians

GENETICS

Most cases of RCC are of sporadic origin, but people with VHL disease or other hereditary diseases associated with RCC are more likely to develop the disease.

GEOGRAPHY

- RCC is more common in urban areas than rural areas, possibly due to the increase in occupational exposure to chemical carcinogens involved in dye, leather, petroleum, plastics, and rubber production
- The US and Scandinavia have the highest incidence rates of RCC

SOCIOECONOMIC STATUS

There is no known difference in the incidence of RCC based on socioeconomic status.

DIFFERENTIAL DIAGNOSIS

- Renal cell adenocarcinoma (RCC) is symptomatically similar to many diseases, including endocrine, paraneoplastic, and metabolic diseases, making differential diagnosis difficult
- This tumor is called 'internist tumor' due to the diagnostic challenges

Transitional cell carcinoma of the renal pelvis

93% of all bladder cancers are transitional cell carcinoma of the pelvis.

FEATURES

- Hematuria
- Urinary frequency and urgency
- Dysuria
- Abdominal pain
- Flank pain
- Lymphedema
- Renal failure
- Anorexia
- Bone pain

Renal cyst

Classified according to location – cortex and medulla, or medulla.

FEATURES

- Some forms are inherited (polycystic disease)
- Abnormal kidney size, hematuria, and hypertension occur from rare to frequently

Metastatic disease

A radiologic lesion can be caused not only by kidney disease itself, but also by metastatic disease from a distant site. When a renal lesion is detected, refer for prompt diagnostic services to determine the source of the tumor, including risk factor assessments and computed tomography (CT) scans of the chest and abdomen.

FEATURES

- Metastases to the kidney occur via hematogenous spread
- In addition, a renal lesion may be caused by direct extension of a tumor from adjacent structures, including the colon

Pyelonephritis

Pyelonephritis is an infection in the upper urinary tract.

FEATURES

- Fever and rigors
- Chills
- Flank pain (very intense)
- Dysuria, polyuria, and hematuria
- Nausea and vomiting
- Headache
- Diarrhea

Angiomyolipoma

Angiomyolipoma is a rare benign kidney tumor that usually affects people with tuberous sclerosis.

FEATURES
Distinctive fat density on CT scan.

Oncocytoma

Oncocytoma is a rare benign kidney tumor that does not metastasize and is cured by surgical kidney removal. It has virtually 100% survival, despite the size of the tumor.

FEATURES
The distinction between oncocytoma and RCC usually is made only by anatomopathologic study.

Renal infarct

Renal infarct is a necrotic area in one or both kidneys, resulting from occlusion of a renal blood vessel.

FEATURES
- Upper abdominal pain (very intense, sharp in nature)
- Flank pain and tenderness
- Fever
- Anorexia
- Nausea and vomiting
- Bruit
- Enlarged kidney
- Increased urinary output

SIGNS & SYMPTOMS

Signs

- Flank or abdominal mass
- Anemia
- Polycythemia
- Hypertension
- Hepatic dysfunction
- Hypercalcemia (rare)
- Renal colic
- Left varicocele or right varicocele, which might include a caval tumor thrombus
- Supraclavicular lymphadenopathy

Symptoms

- Hematuria
- Flank pain
- Weight loss
- Fever
- Flank mass
- Classic triad: hematuria, flank pain, and flank mass

ASSOCIATED DISORDERS

- Hemorrhage
- Respiratory problems due to lung metastases
- Neurologic problems due to brain metastases
- Gastrointestinal problems due to liver metastases
- Because the kidney is an organ in the endocrine system, RCC tumors can express many different hormones resulting in various paraneoplastic syndromes and metabolic disturbances, including abnormal liver function, amenorrhea, amyloidosis, anemia, balding, cachexia, Cushing's syndrome, decreased libido, erythrocytosis, fever, galactorrhea, gynecomastia, hirsutism, hypercalcemia, hypertension, hypoglycemia, neuromyopathy, protein-wasting enteropathy, Stauffer's syndrome, and weight loss

KEY! DON'T MISS!

- A common manifestation of RCC is hematuria
- The first examination for patients with persistent hematuria is the urography, followed by ultrasonography
- If the results are not clear, a computerized axial tomography (CAT) scan should be ordered

CONSIDER CONSULT

- Refer to urologist in all cases of a kidney lesion
- Refer for intravenous pyelography or renal ultrasonography in cases of hematuria
- Refer for CT scan and ultrasonography when a renal mass is suspected or detected by an ultrasound examination
- Refer for regularly-scheduled CT scan or magnetic resonance imaging (MRI) in cases of von Hippel-Lindau (VHL) patients, hereditary papillary renal cell carcinoma, or patients on long-term dialysis treatment
- Refer for MRI with gadolinium in cases of invasion into the inferior vena cava
- Refer for renal arteriography when vasculature mapping is required
- Refer for a chest X-ray if lung metastases are suspected
- Refer for CT scan of the chest if chest X-rays indicate metastatic disease
- Refer for a bone scan if bone metastases are suspected and in patients presenting with bone pain and increased alkaline phosphatase levels

INVESTIGATION OF THE PATIENT

Direct questions to patient

Q **What symptoms do you have? How long have you had these symptoms?** Because the symptoms of RCC may mimic other diseases it is important to get a complete history. Additionally, 25–30% of patients with RCC present with metastatic or locally advanced disease, therefore duration of symptoms is important

Q **Are you experiencing blood loss in the urine? For how long?**

Patients with persistent hematuria should be investigated for RCC:

Q **Are you experiencing short breath? Do you think you are pale?** Hematuria and/or hemolysis can lead to hypochromic/microcytic anemia, sometimes with symptoms

Q **Have you experienced abdominal pain, especially in the flanks?** Up to 30% of the patients will experience some degree of pain, more commonly in the flanks. This pain may or may not be accompanied by other symptoms

Q **Do you have kidney disease? Do you undergo dialysis regularly?** Kidney disease, especially kidney disease that requires dialysis, increases the risk for RCC

Contributory or predisposing factors

Q **Do you smoke? If so, for how long have you smoked, and how much do you smoke?** Cigarette smoking increases the risk significantly for RCC

Q **Are you overweight?** Obesity increases the risk significantly for RCC, especially in women

Q **Do you have hypertension?** Hypertension is linked to RCC

Q **Are you diabetic?** Diabetes is linked to an increased risk of RCC

Q **What type of work do you do? Are you exposed to any type of chemicals during your work?** Exposure to chemical carcinogens or Thorotrast (a contrast medium) increases the risk for RCC

Q **Have you ever taken phenacetin-containing analgesics?** These medicines increase the risk for RCC and have been banned by the FDA

Q **Are you a frequent user of analgesics?** Heavy use of analgesics is linked to a high risk of RCC

Family history

Q **Has anyone in your family had kidney cancer? If so, what type and at what age?** A family history is significant in certain cases of RCC

- **Does anyone in your family have von Hippel-Lindau disease, hereditary papillary renal cell carcinoma, or hereditary renal oncocytoma?** All of these diseases increase the risk for tumor development

Examination

- **What is the patient's overall physical condition? Does the patient complain of hematuria, flank pain, fever, tiredness, edema, or other symptoms?** Many patients do not experience any symptoms during the early stage of the disease; therefore, positive symptoms may indicate advanced disease. Furthermore, patients may present with symptoms indicative of endocrine-based syndromes
- **Does the patient have a palpable mass in the abdomen or kidney regions? Are there bruits over the abdominal mass?** RCC tumors can grow large before becoming palpable, therefore a palpable mass may indicate advanced disease. A mass in the flank can be indicative of RCC
- **Does the patient have left or right varicocele?** These are associated symptoms of RCC
- **Is lymphadenopathy present?** These are associated symptoms of RCC
- **Does the patient complain of malaise or weight loss?** These two symptoms are indicative of metastatic disease
- **Are the patient's laboratory test results normal?** Anemia, erythrocytosis, polycythemia, and hypercalcemia are associated with RCC
- **Is the patient's liver, renal, and endocrine function test normal?** Abnormal results are associated with RCC
- **Do imaging studies show signs of tumor invasion or metastases?** These help diagnose RCC

Summary of investigative tests

- Laboratory tests including urinalysis, complete blood count with red blood cell indices, erythrocyte sedimentation rate (ESR), liver function tests, serum chemistry (especially blood urea nitrogen (BUN) and creatinine), alpha-fetoprotein, plasma fibrinogen, and coagulation studies can show hematuria, anemia, erythrocytosis, and abnormal function in the liver, kidney, and endocrine systems
- Imaging studies including intravenous pyelogram, renal ultrasound, abdominal CT scan or MRI of the abdomen and pelvis, and a renal arteriogram can show if a tumor is present, how large it is, how far advanced it is, and how it affects the blood flow of the kidney
- Chest X-rays and a bone scan can reveal metastatic disease

DIAGNOSTIC DECISION

- The gold standard is pathologic diagnosis
- However, the presence of a mass detected on an imaging test that is consistent with a solid tissue mass (not a cyst), positive urine cytology, and signs and symptoms consistent with RCC are suggestive of a diagnosis of RCC
- The diagnosis of RCC is strongly suggested by the combination of an imaging study with solid tissue mass present in the kidney, positive urine cytology, and signs and symptoms consistent with RCC
- The gold standard remains pathologic diagnosis after resection of the mass
- The major issue is to determine if a curative surgery can be performed
- Even for metastatic disease a nephrectomy can be recommended
- Some data have shown a survival advantage for patients with metastatic disease treated with nephrectomy

CLINICAL PEARLS

- Alterations on the hepatic enzymes are not always linked to liver metastasis
- RCC can produce these enzymes
- These changes normalize after the extraction of the kidney

THE TESTS

Body fluids

URINALYSIS

Description

Urine sample.

Advantages/Disadvantages

Advantages:

- Useful as a screening test for renal diseases
- Detects blood in the urine
- Urine cytology tests can detect cancer cells
- Detects metabolic or systemic diseases unrelated to renal disorders

Normal

All test values are within normal ranges; specifically looking for red blood cell (RBC) count within normal reference range.

- Color: light straw
- Appearance: clear
- pH: 4.5–8 (average, 6)
- Specific gravity: 1.005–1.030
- Protein: absent
- Ketones: absent
- Glucose: absent
- Occult blood: absent

Microscopic examination:

- RBCs: 0–5 (high-power field)
- White blood cells (WBCs): 0–5 (high-power field)
- Bacteria (spun speciment): absent
- Casts: 0–4 hyaline (low-power field)

Abnormal

Abnormal test results may indicate metabolic or endocrinologic disorders.

Cause of abnormal result

Hematuria secondary to carcinoma of the renal tract.

Drugs, disorders and other factors that may alter results

- High intake of vitamin C
- Some foods, such as beets or rhubarb
- Phenytoin
- Phenazopyridine
- Oral anticoagulants

COMPLETE BLOOD COUNT WITH RED CELL INDICES

Description

Blood sample.

Advantages/Disadvantages

Advantage: blood test results can determine if any abnormalities exist: anemia (29–88% of patients), polycythemia, and erythrocytosis

Normal

- Hemoglobin: males, 14–17.4g/dL (140–174g/L); females, 12–16g/dL (120–160g/L)
- RBCs: males, 4.5–5.5x10^6/mm^3 (4.5–5.5x10^{12}/L); females, 4–5x10^6/mm^3 (4–5x10^{12}/L)
- Mean corpuscular volume: 80–100mcm^3 (80–100fl)
- Mean corpuscular hemoglobin: 27–33pg
- Mean corpuscular hemoglobin concentration: 33–37g/dL (330–370g/L)
- Reticulocyte count: 0–1%
- RBC distribution width: 11.5–14.5

Abnormal

High or low hematocrit and hemoglobin.

Cause of abnormal result

- The kidney secretes erythropoietin, which is required for the maturation of bone marrow progenitor cells into mature RBCs
- This function of the kidney can be disrupted by tumor invasion; alternatively, the tumor could consist of cells that secrete erythropoietin, leading to a high hematocrit

Drugs, disorders and other factors that may alter results

- Metabolic disorders
- Endocrine disorders
- Improper laboratory testing techniques

SERUM CHEMISTRY

Description

Blood sample.

Advantages/Disadvantages

Advantages:

- Approx. 15% of patients have hypercalcemia, and a smaller number may display abnormalities in their BUN/creatinine levels
- Inexpensive, widely available test

Disadvantage: neither sensitive nor specific for RCC

Normal

- BUN: 8–20mg/dL (2.8–7.1mmol/L) (slightly higher in elderly patients)
- Creatinine: 0.6–1.3mg/dL (53.0–114.9mcmol/L)
- Calcium: males over 22 years and females over 19 years – 8.9–10.1mg/dL (2.2–2.5mmol/L)

Abnormal

- Increased calcium
- Increased BUN/creatinine

Cause of abnormal result

- Renal clearance of calcium may be affected in RCC
- Alternatively, abnormalities in vitamin D metabolism may occur
- Azotemia and renal failure can occur with RCC

Drugs, disorders and other factors that may alter results

- Metabolic disorders
- Endocrine disorders
- Improper laboratory testing techniques

LIVER FUNCTION TESTS

Description

Blood sample.

Advantages/Disadvantages

Advantage: 7% of patients with RCC have elevated liver function tests

Normal

- Alanine aminotransferase: 7–56U/L
- Aspartate aminotransferase: 5–40U/L

Abnormal

Increased liver function enzymes.

Cause of abnormal result

Hepatic dysfunction occurs without the presence of metastases from the kidney lesion; known as Stauffer's syndrome.

Drugs, disorders and other factors that may alter results

- Hepatitis, cirrhosis
- Metabolic disorders
- Endocrine disorders
- Improper laboratory testing techniques

ERYTHROCYTE SEDIMENTATION RATE

Description

Blood sample.

Advantages/Disadvantages

- Advantage: simple test, easily available
- Disadvantage: nonspecific, can be elevated in a large number of disorders

Normal

Males 0–15mm/h; females 0–10mm/h (rates increase with age).

Abnormal

Elevated in a variety of disorders.

Cause of abnormal result

- ESRs are elevated in disorders that cause inflammation, due to the increased 'stickiness' of erythrocytes when there is inflammation
- Can be elevated in RCC

Drugs, disorders and other factors that may alter results

- Infection
- Rheumatoid arthritis, systemic lupus erythematosus
- Other chronic inflammatory diseases

COAGULATION STUDIES

Description

Blood sample.

Advantages/Disadvantages

Advantages:

- Hypercoagulable states often accompany renal cell carcinoma
- Can be suggestive of RCC
- Can catch an important treatable complication of disease

Disadvantage: nonspecific test

Normal

- Activated partial thromboplastin time (APTT): 25–35s
- Prothrombin time (PT): 11–13s

Abnormal

In a state of hypercoagulability the APTT or PTT can be normal or slightly decreased.

Cause of abnormal result

- Renal failure has long been associated with a hypercoagulable state, although the mechanism is poorly understood
- RCC can be associated with renal failure

Drugs, disorders and other factors that may alter results

- Aspirin
- Other nonsteroidal anti-inflammatory drugs
- Vitamin K deficiency

PLASMA FIBRINOGEN

Description

Blood sample.

Advantages/Disadvantages

- Advantage: fibrinogen can be elevated in RCC
- Disadvantage: while the detection of elevated fibrinogen in a patient with symptoms suggestive of RCC can be helpful in diagnosis, many other conditions can also cause dysfibrinogenemia

Normal

Plasma fibrinogen: 175–350mg/dL (1.75–3.5g/L).

Abnormal

Increased plasma fibrinogen.

Cause of abnormal result

A decrease in kidney function can lead to elevated plasma fibrinogen.

Drugs, disorders and other factors that may alter results

- Metabolic disorders
- Endocrine disorders
- Improper laboratory testing techniques

Imaging

COMPUTED TOMOGRAPHY SCAN OF THE ABDOMEN AND PELVIS

Description

- Patient must be in a fasted state if an oral contrast agent is used. Fasting is not necessary if a contrast agent is not used
- Standard for diagnosis

Advantages/Disadvantages

Advantage: CT scans are generally noninvasive, but contrast agents may be used and are administered orally or intravenously

Disadvantages:

- Intravenous contrast agents may cause transient discomfort and some patients may be allergic to the agent
- Intravenous contrast agents should not be used in patients with severe hepatic or renal disease or those who are allergic to iodine
- Patients are exposed to radiation with this test
- CT scans are more expensive that ultrasonography

Normal

No dense areas on the scan; a normal CT can rule out a diagnosis of RCC in most cases.

Abnormal

Dense areas on the scan.

Cause of abnormal result

- Tumors
- Obstructions
- Calculi
- Polycystic kidney disease
- Congenital anomalies
- Fluid buildup

RENAL ULTRASONOGRAPHY

Description

- Standard for diagnosis
- Usually takes 30min

Advantages/Disadvantages

Advantages:

- Noninvasive
- Can show organ size, shape, and position
- Can detect suspicious regions in the kidney that were not detected by radionuclide tests and can determine if these regions are abscesses, cysts, or tumors
- Superior to CT scans when differentiating between cysts and tumors

Disadvantage: in some cases, the ultrasonograph is not enough to distinguish between a benign and malignant mass, and a CT should be ordered

Normal
One normal ultrasonograph is usually enough to rule out the diagnosis of RCC.

Abnormal
Abnormal structure of renal anatomy seen on ultrasonography, which can include a mass.

Cause of abnormal result
- Tumors
- Cysts
- Abscesses
- Hydronephrosis
- Renal hypertrophy
- Fluid buildup

RENAL MAGNETIC RESONANCE IMAGING OF THE ABDOMEN AND PELVIS
Description
- Contrast enhancement may be used
- Contrast with gadolinium increases the chances for finding early-stage tumors

Advantages/Disadvantages
Advantages:
- MRI and CT are equally efficient in the distinction of malignant and benign mass and in the staging of RCC
- Useful when ultrasonography/CT is contraindicated due to allergies or insufficient renal function

Disadvantages:
- MRI can detect tumors, but RCC tumors are not usually well defined
- MRI studies are more expensive than CT scans
- In the evaluation of RCC, MRI should be reserved for those patients with allergic reactions to the contrast

Normal
Normal renal structure.

Abnormal
Abnormal renal structure.

Cause of abnormal result
- Tumors
- Obstructions
- Calculi
- Polycystic disease
- Congenital anomalies
- Abnormal fluid buildup

INTRAVENOUS PYELOGRAM
Description
- Also known as excretory urography
- Patient must fast for 8h before the test, but must be well hydrated
- Rarely used

Advantages/Disadvantages

Advantages:

- Provides immediate visualization of the kidneys
- Able to show cancerous tumors and kidney damage
- Useful to evaluate hematuria

Disadvantages:

- Usually used only in specific cases which require vasculature mapping
- Not as useful as CT scans or MRI

Normal

Normal renal structure.

Abnormal

Abnormal renal structure.

Cause of abnormal result

- Tumors
- Calculi
- Polycystic disease
- Renal hypertrophy
- Pyelonephritis
- Renal tuberculosis
- Hydronephrosis
- Renovascular hypertension

Drugs, disorders and other factors that may alter results

- End-stage renal disease
- Technical complications

ANGIOGRAPHY

Description

- Patient must fast for 8h before test
- Test takes about one hour
- Rarely used

Advantages/Disadvantages

Advantages:

- Can identify the blood vessels that feed the tumor
- Simple test
- Can be useful during the surgical planning
- If a partial nephrectomy is the aim, this examination can be very helpful to the surgeon

Disadvantage: contraindicated during pregnancy, bleeding problems, allergies to the contrast agent, and end-stage renal disease

Normal

Normal vascular anatomy.

Abnormal

Abnormal vascular anatomy.

Cause of abnormal result
- Renal tumors
- Cysts
- Other renal abnormalities

Drugs, disorders and other factors that may alter results
- Recent contrast studies
- Stool or gas in the gastrointestinal tract

CHEST X-RAY
Description
Chest X-ray is useful to diagnose pulmonary metastases.

Advantages/Disadvantages
Advantages:
- Can show if the cancer has metastasized to the lungs
- Can help assess the patient's general health and the potential tolerance level for immunotherapy or surgery

Disadvantage: X-rays are usually contraindicated during the first trimester of pregnancy, but a lead apron can be used to protect the fetus

Normal
A normal X-ray should be considered enough to rule out pulmonary metastasis of RCC if there are no major reasons to believe the contrary.

Abnormal
Because normal pulmonary tissue is radiolucent, a dense area on the X-ray may indicate a tumor.

Cause of abnormal result
- Infiltrates, foreign bodies, fluid buildup, or tumors will show up as a dense area
- The type of chest X-ray can interfere with the results, e.g. portable chest X-rays may decrease the quality

BONE SCAN

Description

- Scan of the skeleton after a radioactive trace has been administered intravenously
- Rarely used, and if there are no suspicious of bone metastasis there is no reason to order a bone scan

Advantages/Disadvantages

Advantages:

- Radiation level used is low and not harmful
- A bone scan can detect abnormalities and diseases in the bones

Disadvantages:

- The patient may have an allergic reaction to the radionuclide
- Bone scans are contraindicated in pregnant or lactating women
- Bone scans cannot distinguish normal from abnormal bone formation

Normal

Hot spots will show in areas of new bone formation.

Abnormal

Hot spots will show any bone malignancy, infection, fracture, or bone abnormality.

Cause of abnormal result

- Cancer
- Infection
- Fractures

Drugs, disorders and other factors that may alter results

- Distended bladder
- Improper technique may allow the radionuclide to seep into the muscle tissue and create false hot-spots
- Antihypertensive agents

TREATMENT

CONSIDER CONSULT

- Refer patient for treatment when diagnosis of renal cell adenocarcinoma (RCC) is made or when a renal mass is suspicious
- Surgery is the standard treatment for locally contained RCC
- Management of metastatic disease is dependent upon the stage of the disease, general health of the patient, and location of the metastases

IMMEDIATE ACTION

Treat the patient for any metabolic or endocrinologic emergency.

PATIENT AND CAREGIVER ISSUES

Patient or caregiver request

- **What options do I have?** Surgery is the major treatment modality and, unless contraindicated, will always be performed, even in the presence of metastatic disease. If the tumor is restricted to the kidney, a chance of cure with the surgery is real. If there are distant metastasis, a clinical trial should be preferred. For metastatic disease, nonablative bone marrow transplant is an option. Immunotherapy with interferon prolongs life. Interleukin is another immunotherapy also in use
- **Are there any investigative treatments that I can take?** Usually the process of staging and diagnosis will require some tests. If there are suspects of genetic alterations, a genetic evaluation can be done
- **How long do I have to live?** This is impossible to predict. Low stages are often curable. For advanced disease, it has an unpredictable course. There are cases of spontaneous remission, long-term survival, and also dramatic cases with a fast advance. No marks for this have been identified
- **Will I be cured if my kidney is removed?** In stage I or II disease, the chance for a cure is about 40–50%. For other stages the chances are lower, but there are data that shown that nephrectomy is able to prolong life even in patients with metastatic disease

Health-seeking behavior

Avoidance of smoking, obesity, and exposure to carcinogens are the main behaviors that can help in preventing RCC.

MANAGEMENT ISSUES

Goals

- Accurately diagnose the patient's disease and stage
- Provide treatment that could save or prolong the patient's life
- Reduce the level of pain
- If treatment is successful, prevent recurrence

Management in special circumstances

- RCC is usually not detected until the very late stages
- 25–30% of patients present with metastatic or locally advanced disease

COEXISTING DISEASE

Renal failure: if a patient has a baseline renal failure and is already in dialysis when a RCC is diagnosed, the procedures available are limited. Surgical restrictions and drug restriction can prevent an optimal management. Each case should be evaluated and the risks and benefits from each intervention weighted.

PATIENT SATISFACTION/LIFESTYLE PRIORITIES

- If the treatment is made with curative intent and in the absence of baseline renal disease, most patients will be able to have an almost normal life, receiving the standard of care for patients with only one kidney
- If the treatment is palliative, the survival course is unpredictable, but most patients will die within 5 years, so end-of-life care can be required

SUMMARY OF THERAPEUTIC OPTIONS

Choices

- The choice of treatment depends on the stage of the disease and the general health of the patient
- Surgery is the main treatment for RCC at stages I, II, and III
- A radical nephrectomy removes the kidney, adrenal gland, and fatty tissue around the kidney
- Sometimes a regional lymphadenectomy, which removes the lymph nodes nearby, is performed with the radical nephrectomy
- A partial nephrectomy or nephron-sparing surgery removes only the part of the kidney invaded by the tumor. This type of surgery is usually performed in patients with tumors in both kidneys, tumor in only one kidney, or very small tumors (<4cm; <1.6 inches)
- Management of metastatic disease (stage IV) may include nephrectomy and surgical removal of the metastatic tumor
- There are no benefits and an increased rate of complication with adjunctive therapy on RCC. Chemotherapy, radiation therapy, and immunotherapy all failed to show a benefit in randomized studies. These treatments may be performed only in the context of a clinical trial
- Treatment with hormonal therapy has been associated with symptom relief, but very low response rates
- Arterial embolization, a surgical procedure that blocks the renal artery of the affected kidney, has been used to control bleeding in stage III
- Overall, other than surgical removal of the affected kidney, investigative treatments offered in clinical trials are the treatment options
- Overall, drug therapy for RCC is disappointing
- Interferon (IFN) and interleukin (IL) are the only drugs with effect on this disease
- Smoking cessation and weight loss should be encouraged

Clinical pearls

- The clinical course of an advanced RCC is unpredictable
- A few patients will experience long-term survival even with metastatic disease
- The RCC is one of the few tumors with documented cases of spontaneous remission, although rare

FOLLOW UP

- Follow up evaluations may consist of X-rays and imaging studies of the chest and abdomen to detect any recurrent disease
- Blood tests are used to monitor kidney and liver function
- There are no standard follow up procedures

DRUGS AND OTHER THERAPIES: DETAILS

Drugs

INTERFERON

Dose

Varies from as low as 3–20MU three times weekly.

Efficacy

An estimated survival benefit of 2.6 months, on average, is expected for patients treated with IFN.

Risks/Benefits

Risks:

- The side-effects of IFNs can preclude their use
- Use caution with children under 18 years
- Use caution with chronic progressive multiple sclerosis
- Use caution with depression and mental disorders
- Use caution with seizure disorders and heart disease
- Use caution in pregnancy
- Use caution in photosensitivity and psoriasis

Side-effects and adverse reactions

- Gastrointestinal: abdominal pain, constipation, diarrhea, vomiting
- Central nervous system: dizziness, neuropathy, behavioral changes
- Eyes, ears, nose, and throat: conjunctivitis
- Cardiovascular system: hypertension, palpitations, peripheral vascular disorders
- Genitourinary: breast pain, cystitis, dysmenorrhea
- Hematologic: lymphadenopathy, leukopenia, lymphopenia
- Respiratory: dyspnea, sinusitis
- Skin: sweating, injection site reaction
- Other: flu-like syndrome, fever, myalgia, hepatic toxicity

Interactions (other drugs)

- Aminophylline ■ Theophylline ■ Zidovudine

Contraindications

- Hypersensitivity to human albumin ■ Nursing mothers

Acceptability to patient

- Patients will accept IFN, due to possible extension of survival
- Any side-effects that occur may change the acceptability

INTERLEUKIN

Aldesleukin.

Dose

- Aldesleukin, recommended for injection treatment regimen, is administered by a 15-min intravenous infusion every 8h
- 600,000 IU/kg (0.037mg/kg) dose administered every 8h by a 15-min intravenous infusion for a maximum of 14 doses. Following 9 days of rest, the schedule is repeated for another 14 doses, for a maximum of 28 doses/course, as tolerated, although may vary from as low as 72,000–720,000 IU/kg every 8h

Efficacy

ILs are known to induce response in RCC patients, but their impact on survival is unknown.

Risks/Benefits

Risks:

- The side-effects of ILs can preclude their use
- Use caution with children under 18 years
- Use caution with chronic progressive multiple sclerosis
- Use caution with depression and mental disorders
- Use caution with seizure disorders and heart disease

Side-effects and adverse reactions

- Cardiovascular system: hypotension, tachycardia, vasodilation, myocardial infarction
- Central nervous system: chills, fever, malaise, asthenia, pain
- Gastrointestinal: abdominal pain, enlarged abdomen, diarrhea, vomiting, nausea, stomatitis, anorexia
- Hematologic: thrombocytopenia, anemia, leukopenia
- Other: sepsis, infection

Interactions (other drugs)

■ Psychotropic drugs (possible interactions) ■ Drugs with nephrotoxic (e.g. aminoglycosides, indomethacin), myelotoxic (e.g. cytotoxic chemotherapy), cardiotoxic (e.g. doxorubicin) or hepatotoxic (e.g. methotrexate, asparaginase) effects (may increase toxicity)

Contraindications

■ Sustained ventricular tachycardia (=5 beats) ■ Gastrointestinal bleeding requiring surgery ■ Cardiac tamponade ■ Intubation required >72h ■ Renal failure requiring dialysis >72h ■ Coma or toxic psychosis lasting >48h ■ Repetitive or difficult to control seizures ■ Bowel ischemia/perforation ■ Cardiac arrhythmias not controlled or unresponsive to management ■ Chest pain with ECG changes, consistent with angina or myocardial infarction ■ Hypersensitivity to human albumin ■ Pregancy category C ■ Nursing mothers ■ Safety and effectiveness in children under 18 years of age have not been established

Acceptability to patient

Any side-effects that occur may affect the acceptability.

Surgical therapy

Surgical removal of the kidney(s) is the standard treatment for RCC at stages I, II, and III. The type of surgery is dependent upon the stage.

NEPHRECTOMY

- A radical nephrectomy, which removes the entire kidney(s), adrenal gland, and surrounding fatty tissue, is usually performed for some stage I and II tumors and large stage II tumors
- A partial nephrectomy, which removes only the affected part of the kidney, is usually performed for stage I tumors that are small, or in patients with tumors in both kidneys
- A radical nephrectomy with regional lymphadenopathy, which removes the surrounding lymph nodes, is usually performed for stage III tumors
- Stage IV RCC can be treated with surgery, but with palliative objectives

Efficacy

- Radical nephrectomies are more curative than partial nephrectomies in stage I and II disease
- 5-year survival rate for stage I disease after surgery is 90–100%
- 5-year survival rate for stage II disease after surgery is 65–75%
- 5-year survival rate for stage III disease after surgery is 40–70%
- Palliative for stage IV disease

Risks/Benefits

Benefits:

- Without surgery, prognosis for survival is very poor, regardless of stage of disease
- The cure rates are >50% if the disease is diagnosed in the early stages and surgery is performed

Acceptability to patient

Although surgery is inherently invasive, the potential for a complete cure makes this type of treatment acceptable.

Follow up plan

Imaging studies and blood tests are usually used to evaluate and monitor disease recurrence.

Radiation therapy

Radiation therapy is usually used for the metastatic disease rather than the primary tumor site.

ADJUNCTIVE RADIATION THERAPY

- Radiation therapy may be used to treat patients with stage I or II disease who cannot undergo surgery due to overall poor health
- Radiation therapy to the metastatic site offers some pain relief and symptomatic control, but is not a cure
- Radiation is not beneficial in the adjuvant setting

Efficacy

Radiation therapy will not cure RCC, but may offer some pain and symptom relief at the metastatic sites.

Risks/Benefits

- Risk: radiation therapy is associated with toxicities
- Benefit: symptom relief, including decreased pain, hemoptysis control, decreased airway obstruction, cord compression prevention, and fracture prevention, have been reported with radiation therapy to the metastatic site

Acceptability to patient

Radiation therapy is associated with toxicities and may not be acceptable to patients.

Chemotherapy

SYSTEMIC CHEMOTHERAPY

Systemic chemotherapy is usually investigative in nature and reserved for recurrent disease.

Efficacy

RCC appears to be resistant to chemotherapy.

Risks/Benefits

Risk: chemotherapy is associated with varying degrees of toxicity

Acceptability to patient

The toxicities associated with chemotherapy and the lack of response may make this type of treatment unacceptable to patients.

Patient and caregiver information

Information regarding clinical trials with chemotherapy agents can be found on the website of the National Cancer Institute.

Other therapies

HORMONAL THERAPY

Treatment with systemic hormonal therapies is investigative in nature.

Efficacy

- Treatment with hormonal therapy has been associated with symptom relief but very low response rates
- No definitive benefit was found for this therapy

Risks/Benefits

Risk: hormonal therapy is not associated with significant toxicity, but patients may experience fluid retention and weight gain

Acceptability to patient

Although hormonal therapy is not associated with significant toxicity, the low response rates may make this therapy unacceptable to patients.

IMMUNOTHERAPY

Immunotherapy is usually performed with IL or cytokines, and is investigative in nature.

Efficacy

Immunotherapy is associated with tumor shrinkage and long-term responses when response occurs.

Risks/Benefits

Risk: toxicities associated with immunotherapy tend to be severe and even fatal

Acceptability to patient

The potential for a response may make this form of therapy acceptable to patient; however, the acceptability may be offset by the toxicities associated with immunotherapy.

LIFESTYLE

The risk of RCC is increased significantly in patients who smoke or who are obese (especially women). Therefore, encourage patients to quit smoking and lose weight.

RISKS/BENEFITS

Although the effects of smoking cessation and weight loss may not affect the prognosis of RCC, the overall health benefits will make the patient stronger to battle the disease.

ACCEPTABILITY TO PATIENT

Smoking cessation and weight loss are difficult for patients.

OUTCOMES

EFFICACY OF THERAPIES

- An estimated survival benefit of 2.6 months, on average, is expected for patients treated with interferon
- Interleukin is known to induce a response in renal cell adenocarcinoma (RCC) patients, but impact on survival is unknown
- Radical nephrectomies are more curative than partial nephrectomies in stage I and II disease, with 5-year survival rates of 90–100% for stage I and 65–75% for stage II disease
- Radiation therapy will not cure RCC, but may offer some pain and symptom relief at the metastatic sites
- RCC appears to be resistant to chemotherapy
- Treatment with hormonal therapy has been associated with symptom relief but very low response rates; however, no definitive benefit was found for this therapy
- Immunotherapy is associated with tumor shrinkage and long-term responses when response occurs

Review period

One year.

PROGNOSIS

- The prognosis for survival is very poor without surgery
- The prognosis for 5-year survival after surgery is dependent on the stage of the disease: stage I – 90–100%; stage II – 65–75%; and stage III – 40–70%
- Patients should consider participating in a clinical trial with systemic chemotherapy, immunotherapy, or radiation therapy if they cannot undergo surgery or if the disease recurs

Clinical pearls

The clinical course of patients with metastatic disease is unpredictable and rare spontaneous remissions and long-term survival in a few can be achieved. There is no known way to predict those who will achieve these results.

Therapeutic failure

For patients that fail first-line treatment of RCC, the choice may be a phase I or II study.

COMPLICATIONS

- Hypercalcemia
- Amyloidosis
- Hemorrhage
- Respiratory problems due to lung metastases
- Neurologic problems due to brain metastases
- Gastrointestinal problems due to liver metastases
- Bone pain due to bone metastases
- Paraneoplastic syndromes
- Metabolic syndromes
- Endocrine syndromes
- Increased sedimentation rate
- Hypertension
- Anemia
- Cachexia
- Fever
- Abnormal liver function
- Erythrocytosis
- Neuromyopathy

CONSIDER CONSULT

- Patients who have failed treatment may be eligible for participation in a clinical trial
- Refer all patients who have failed treatment to an oncologist for further management
- Depending on the patient's attitude towards treatment, consider referral to a cancer center where clinical trials are active

PREVENTION

RISK FACTORS

- Smoking: people who smoke are at a significantly increased risk for renal cell adenocarcinoma (RCC) (20–30% of all cases of RCC)
- Obesity: obese people, especially women, are at a significantly increased risk for RCC
- Chemical carcinogen exposure: exposure to chemical carcinogens significantly increases the risk for RCC

MODIFY RISK FACTORS

Lifestyle and wellness

TOBACCO

Patients should stop smoking.

DIET

High fat and well-cooked meat intake should be decreased.

PHYSICAL ACTIVITY

Patients should be physically active.

ENVIRONMENT

Exposure to any chemical carcinogens, particularly chemicals used in dye, gas, and leather production, should be avoided.

FAMILY HISTORY

Be aware of familial history of kidney cancer and hereditary kidney diseases and syndromes.

SCREENING

IMAGING STUDIES

Perform computed tomography or magnetic resonance imaging scans in patients at high risk for RCC, such as patients with a familial history of von Hippel-Lindau, hereditary papillary renal cell carcinoma, patients on long-term dialysis, or patients who present with symptoms indicative of RCC.

Cost/efficacy

- Expensive, but helpful in monitoring at-risk patients
- These imaging studies are the standard tests for detecting RCC

LABORATORY TESTS

Laboratory tests including urinalysis, complete blood count with red blood cell indices, erythrocyte sedimentation rate, liver and kidney function tests, serum chemistry (especially blood urea nitrogen and creatinine), alpha-fetoprotein and coagulation tests can show hematuria, anemia, erythrocytosis, and abnormal function in the liver, kidney, and endocrine systems.

Cost/efficacy

These studies are inexpensive, standard tests that can be ordered by the primary care physician, and are useful tools for detecting RCC and other renal disorders.

PREVENT RECURRENCE

Patients should participate in regular screening programs, including imaging and laboratory studies to monitor for tumor recurrence.

RESOURCES

ASSOCIATIONS

American Cancer Society
1599 Clifton Road, NE
Atlanta, GA 30329
Tel: (800) 227-2345
www.cancer.org

National Kidney Cancer Association
1234 Sherman Avenue, Suite 203
Evanston, IL 60202–1375
Tel: (800) 850-9132 or (847) 332-1051
Fax: (847) 332-2978
www.kidneycancerassociation.org

National Cancer Institute Cancer Information Service
NCI Public Inquiries Office
Building 31, Room 10A31
31 Center Drive, MSC 2580
Bethesda, MD 20892–2580
Tel: (800) 4-CANCER
www.nci.nih.gov

VHL (Von Hippel-Landau Disease) Family Alliance
171 Clinton Road
Brookline, MA 02445–5815
Tel: (800) 767-4845 or (627) 277-5667
Fax: (617) 734-8233
E-mail: info@vhl.org
www.vhl.org

KEY REFERENCES

- Flanigan RC, Salmon SE, Blumenstein BA, et al. Nephrectomy followed by interferon alfa-2b compared with interferon alfa-2b alone for metastatic renal-cell cancer. N Engl J Med 2001;345:1655–9
- Simons JW, Marshall FF. Kidney and ureter. In: Abeloff MD, Armitage JO, Lichter AS, Niederhuber JE, eds. Clinical oncology, 2nd edn. New York: Churchill Livingstone, Inc., 2000, p1784–94
- Renal cell carcinoma. In: Brenner BM, ed. Brenner & Rector's the kidney, 6th edn. Philadelphia (PA): W.B. Saunders, 2000, p1844–60
- What is kidney cancer (renal cell carcinoma)? Cancer Reference Information. Available on the American Cancer Society website

FAQS

Question 1

How should a patient with a renal mass detected by excretory urography be assessed?

ANSWER 1

The American Society of Radiology recommends that an ultrasound examination may be performed first. If the ultrasound does not distinguish between cystic and malignant lesions, a computed tomography scan should be ordered. The magnetic resonance imaging scan is reserved for patients with allergic reactions to the contrast.

Question 2
Is a bone scan essential to the staging of renal cell adenocarcinoma (RCC)?

ANSWER 2
No. Bone scan examination may be reserved for patients with suspicious bone metastasis.

Question 3
How should a patient with persistent hematuria be evaluated?

ANSWER 3
First, an urinary cytology may be performed (keep in mind that a negative finding is not sufficient to rule out a malignant tumor of the urinary tract). For images, an excretory urography may be the first examination, followed by an ultrasound, from pelvis and abdomen.

Question 4
Why do some patients have an indolent course and a long life even with distant metastasis?

ANSWER 4
There is no known explanation for this. Some try to explain according to immune-host response, but this argument is far from convincing as yet.

Question 5
Should a patient that was submitted for the intention of curative resection receive any adjuvant therapy?

ANSWER 5
No. There is no efficient adjuvant therapy of any modality for RCC. These may be used only in the conditions of a clinical trial.

CONTRIBUTORS
Fred F Ferri, MD, FACP
Otavio A Clark, MD
Dinesh S Rao, MD

SPINAL TUMORS

SUMMARY INFORMATION

DESCRIPTION

- Primary tumors of the spinal cord are rare. They constitute between 10% and 19% of all primary central nervous system neoplasia, with approx. 5000 cases diagnosed annually
- Most common primary spinal cord tumors are meningioma and schwannoma, both of which are usually benign
- Clinical signs and symptoms reflect sequelae of spinal cord compression, edema, ischemia, and infarction with resultant motor and sensory deficits
- Magnetic resonance imaging is the radiographic diagnostic procedure of choice
- Prognosis varies from excellent (e.g. meningioma) to dismal (e.g. glioblastoma multiforme), and treatment is primarily surgical with radiotherapy and chemotherapy reserved for incompletely resected or malignant lesions

URGENT ACTION

- Spinal cord compression is a medical emergency; immediate hospitalization, intravenous steroids, and neurosurgical/radiation-oncologist consultation are needed
- Evidence of spinal cord compression and fever with a history of infection, surgery, instrumentation, or intravenous drug abuse may be indicative of epidural abscess and mandates emergent neurosurgical consultation
- Evidence of deep vein thrombosis requires anticoagulation

KEY! DON'T MISS!

- Spinal cord compression is a medical emergency; immediate hospitalization, intravenous steroids, and neurosurgical/radiation-oncologist consultation is needed
- Evidence of deep vein thrombosis requires anticoagulation
- Foramen magnum tumors can be misdiagnosed as amyotrophic lateral sclerosis, cervical disk herniation, and multiple sclerosis
- Intramedullary cervical tumors can be misdiagnosed as syringomyelia
- These tumors are rare and patients with suspicion of spinal tumors should be evaluated by a specialized team

ICD9 CODE

- 170.2 Spine, spinal column
- 191.7 Spine, bulb
- 170.6 Spine, coccyx
- 191.2 Spine, cord
- 192.3 Spine, dura matter
- 170.2 Spine, lumbosacral
- 192.3 Spine, membrane
- 192.3 Spine, meninges
- 171.9 Spine, nerve (root)
- 192.3 Spine, pia mater
- 171.9 Spine, root
- 170.6 Spine, sacrum

CARDINAL FEATURES

- Initial treatment goal is to determine if emergency intervention, such as neurosurgery or radiotherapy, is required
- It is imperative that a patient with a potential spinal cord lesion obtains timely evaluation, diagnosis, and appropriate intervention to prevent permanent/ progressive neurologic dysfunction
- Ideally, patients should undergo radiation or surgery when minimally symptomatic as the more advanced/profound the lesion, the less chance there is of neurologic recovery
- Primary tumors of the spinal cord constitute 10–19% of all primary central nervous system (CNS) neoplasia
- Approx. 5000 cases of primary spinal cord tumor are diagnosed annually
- Bimodal age distribution with first peak at 0–4 years of age, declining between 15 and 24 years, then steadily rising until age 65–79, when incidence levels off
- Different tumor types predominate at different ages
- Approx. half of spinal cord tumors are primary, the other half are metastatic
- Seeding of the spinal cord can occur from cranial or spinal axis tumors through the subarachnoid space
- Anatomically, spinal tumors are classified as extradural and intradural; intradural tumors comprise two types: intramedullary and extramedullary
- Intradural intramedullary tumors account for 4–16% of CNS tumors and often contain cystic structures called syrinxes. Ependymoma is the most common, followed by ependyma; the others are oligodendroglioma, ganglioglioma, medulloblastoma, and various hemangiomas and hemangioblastomas
- Intradural extramedullary neurilemmomas and meningiomas are the most common. Other intradural extramedullary tumors are chordomas and epidermoids
- 50% occur in thoracic region, 30% in lumbosacral region, and 20% in cervical region
- Most extradural tumors represent either metastasis or primary bone tumors
- The most common primary spinal cord tumors are meningioma and schwannoma, both of which are usually benign
- Clinical signs and symptoms reflect sequelae of spinal cord compression, edema, ischemia, and infarction with resultant motor and sensory deficits
- Magnetic resonance imaging (MRI) is the radiographic diagnostic procedure of choice; lumbar puncture may also be indicated
- Usually these tumors are classified according to the degree of differentiation. Those with low grade are more differentiated and some are considered to have a benign histology
- Some of these with benign histology are considered to have malignant behavior due to the severity of the disease that they cause

Specific spinal tumor types

- Most common primary spinal cord tumors are schwannoma, meningioma, and glioma
- Gliomas include astrocytomas, ependymomas, and oligodendrogliomas
- Ependymomas constitute approx. 60% of primary spinal gliomas

Ependymomas:

- Ependymomas constitute 12.8–15.1% of primary spinal cord tumors, <2% of all CNS tumors, are intramedullary, and more common in adults
- Graded histologically with grade having prognostic significance
- Ependymomas most commonly present near the fourth ventricle in children; however, in adults they are usually present in the central cord, especially the cauda equina and the conus medullaris
- >50% of ependymomas occur in the caudal cord
- Given their proximity to the ventricular system, ependymomas can disseminate through the cerebrospinal fluid (CSF)
- Myxopapillary ependymomas most commonly occur in the filum terminale and can invade bone and involve nerve roots
- Total curative resection is often not feasible with postoperative radiotherapy indicated

Astrocytomas:

- Astrocytomas constitute 6.5–11.2% of primary spinal cord tumors, are intramedullary, of variable malignancy, and are graded from low to high
- Astrocytomas include anaplastic astrocytoma, fibrillary astrocytoma, glioblastoma multiforme, pilocytic astrocytoma, and pleomorphic xanthoastrocytoma
- Astrocytomas occur throughout the cord but have a predilection for the thoracic cord
- Most astrocytomas are benign; however, anaplastic astrocytoma and glioblastoma are malignant, representing 10% of astrocytomas
- Glioblastoma multiforme, a kind of malignant CNS primary tumor, constitutes 1.5% of all spinal cord tumors and 1–5% of all glioblastomas

Oligodendrogliomas:

- Oligodendrogliomas constitute 1.9% of primary spinal cord tumors and most commonly occur in the thoracic cord
- Oligodendrogliomas are low-grade lesions but approx. 20% are considered to be malignant

Meningiomas:

- Meningiomas constitute 25.5–42% of primary spinal cord tumors, are usually extramedullary intradural tumors, can be extradural, can rarely be both intradural and extradural, and are usually benign
- Meningiomas arise from the meninges and are attached to the dura, tend to be slow-growing, are more common in women, usually occur in people older than 40, and compress but do not invade the cord; however, they may rarely extend into bone
- Meningiomas are found throughout the cord, 80% are located in the thoracic spine
- Meningiomas are the most common neoplasm of the foramen magnum
- Meningiomas are usually solitary, multiple lesions suggest neurofibromatosis type 2
- May spread to extradural or extraspinal space by local extension, most meningiomas are found anterior or posterior to the cord
- Malignant meningiomas are rare and can invade CNS structures

Schwannomas:

- Schwannomas constitute 22–29% of primary spinal cord tumors, are usually extramedullary intradural tumors, can be extradural, are rarely both intradural and extradural, are rarely intramedullary, and can grow to 10cm in size
- Schwannomas usually involve dorsal sensory nerves but can involve motor nerves, especially when tumor is extradural

- Usually occur between the ages of 20 and 50 years
- Found throughout the spine, schwannomas are most frequent in the thoracic spine
- Most schwannomas are solitary; however, multiple schwannomas can occur in von Recklinghausen's disease
- May spread to extradural and extraspinal space by local extension (i.e. through intervertebral foramen)

Neuronal tumors:
- Neuronal tumors are rare and include gangliocytomas and ganglioglioma
- Gangliogliomas have low metastatic potential with good prognosis but frequently recur
- Gangliogliomas tend to occur in children, involve the cervical cord, and usually exhibit less mass effect and edema when compared to other primary spinal cord tumors

Metastatic disease:
- Most common primaries for metastatic disease are: lung, breast, gastrointestinal, kidney, and melanoma
- Most metastatic disease is extradural
- Epidural metastatic disease occurs in approx. 5% of those with malignancy
- Choriocarcinoma also has a high propensity for CNS metastasis
- Metastasis to the extradural space can rarely occur from spread of tumor through intervertebral foramina
- Metastasis may rarely present as an intramedullary lesion with breast and lung cancer being the most common intramedullary metastatic lesions
- Adenocarcinoma, lymphoma, and melanoma have also been reported as intramedullary metastatic lesions
- The thoracic cord is most commonly involved by intramedullary metastatic disease
- Intracranial tumors (e.g. ependymomas, medulloblastomas) may also spread to the spinal cord usually by CSF seeding
- Approx. 1.2% of cerebral glioblastomas and 1.5% of anaplastic gliomas metastasize to the spinal cord
- Radiographically can present as a space-occupying mass lesion (e.g. enhancing intramedullary lesion)
- If a mass effect is present, it can result in sensory, motor, or autonomic dysfunction with a subacute or acute course
- Can cause edema, infarction, ischemia, spinal cord vascular thrombosis/compromise, and vertebral body collapse
- Metastatic lesions range in size from several millimeters to several centimeters and are solitary or multiple
- May involve the central canal, spinal cord tracts/parenchyma, nerve roots, vertebra, and intradural and epidural spaces
- Occasionally present with spinal cord compression with sudden neurologic dysfunction that mandates emergent neurosurgical intervention/consultation
- Diagnosis usually made through MRI and CSF examination
- Unlike primary cord tumor there is usually evidence of a primary neoplasm (e.g. breast, lung, brain)
- Meningeal carcinomatosis can occur with multiple lesions studding the spinal cord and nerve roots

Poorly differentiated tumors are probably of neuroectodermal origin but have lost most of their phenotypic features.

Medulloblastoma is highly malignant, usually occurs in children, found primarily in the cerebellum, and is extremely radiosensitive.

Other rare primary spinal cord tumors:

- Sarcomas constitute 11.9% of primary spinal cord tumors
- Vascular tumors constitute 6.2% of primary spinal cord tumors and are usually extramedullary and intradural
- Chordomas constitute 4.0% of primary spinal cord tumors, are usually extramedullary and intradural, and occur in the sacral spine
- Epidermoids constitute 1.4% of primary spinal cord tumors and are usually extramedullary and intradural
- Primary CNS lymphoma is very rare and accounts for <1% of all CNS lymphomas
- Ganglioglioma, ganglioneuroblastoma, hemangioblastoma, and neuroblastoma are primary spinal cord tumors that are usually intramedullary
- Hemangioblastomas constitute 3% of spinal cord tumors, are more common in men in the third to fifth decades of life, and 25–30% are associated with the von Hippel-Lindau disease
- Most common in the cervical-thoracic cord, hemangioblastomas can also be associated with posterior fossa hemangioblastomas
- Hemangioblastomas are usually solitary lesions; however, 20% are multiple

CAUSES

Common causes

Spinal tumors are of many different types and we cannot expect to determine one unique cause for them.

Contributory or predisposing factors

- Electromagnetism, fertilizers, herbicides, pesticides, petrochemicals, trauma, viruses, craniospinal irradiation, and participation in the health care profession are suspected predisposing factors for CNS tumors; however, studies have not been able to establish a definitive association
- Immunosuppression may predispose to primary CNS lymphoma as patients with acquired immunodeficiency syndrome and transplant recipients on immunosuppressive therapy have a higher incidence of primary CNS lymphoma; however, this association has not been established

EPIDEMIOLOGY

Incidence and prevalence

INCIDENCE

- Approximate incidence: 0.01–0.02/1000 people
- Incidence is dependent on age

Demographics

AGE

- Bimodal distribution
- First peak: 0–4 years
- Steady increase after 24 years of age reaching a plateau between 65 and 79 years of age
- Low-grade astrocytomas are more common in children
- In adults, gliomas most commonly occur between the fourth and sixth decades of life
- Schwannomas and meningiomas are more common in adults
- Meningiomas usually occur after the age of 40
- Schwannomas usually occur from 20 to 50 years of age
- Hemangioblastomas most commonly occur in men in their third to fifth decade of life

GENDER

- Spinal meningioma female:male ratio 10:1
- Spinal ependymoma male:female ratio 1.8:1
- 58% of primary spinal cord tumors in women are meningiomas
- Gliomas are more common in men

GENETICS

Gliomas:

- Multiple genetic insults are observed and correlate with progression from low- to high-grade
- p53 inactivation and overexpression of platelet-derived growth factor-alpha are found in low-grade astrocytomas
- Transition to high-grade astrocytoma characterized by alterations in the RB and p16/CDKNZA tumor suppressor genes
- p53 alterations and amplification of epidermal growth factor receptor gene are found in glioblastomas as well as alterations of KI-67

Meningiomas:

Loss of chromosome 22q long arm and NF2 gene mutations are described.

DIAGNOSIS

DIFFERENTIAL DIAGNOSIS

Multiple neoplastic and non-neoplastic processes can involve the spinal cord, resulting in a spinal cord mass/cyst and presenting with any combination of sensory, motor, and autonomic dysfunction.

Osteoarthritis

Osteoarthritis is a polyarticular or monoarticular disease characterized by degeneration of joint cartilage and narrowing of the joint space that, in the spine, can lead to nerve root impingement.

FEATURES

- Like primary spinal cord tumors, can present with sensory, motor, and autonomic dysfunction usually from spinal root impingement
- Like primary spinal cord tumors, symptoms can be progressive over several months
- Unlike primary spinal cord tumors, patients usually complain of back and joint (e.g. knee) pain of several years' duration with typical osteoarthritis symptoms (e.g. gelling)
- Unlike primary spinal cord tumors, X-ray/magnetic resonance imaging (MRI) can demonstrate foramina narrowing, joint-space narrowing, and osteophyte impingement on nerve roots without spinal cord mass

Vertebral disc disease

Herniation of intervertebral disc that can impinge on spinal cord or nerve roots.

FEATURES

- Like primary spinal cord tumors, can present with sensory, motor, and autonomic dysfunction from impingement of spinal roots or cord
- Like primary spinal cord tumors, symptoms can be progressive over several months or acute over several weeks/days
- Like primary spinal cord tumors, can present as acute/hyperacute spinal cord compression from sudden disc herniation with profound motor, sensory, and autonomic dysfunction mandating immediate neurosurgical intervention
- Unlike primary spinal cord tumors, patients usually relate a precipitating event prior to acute/hyperacute cord/nerve root compression
- Unlike primary spinal cord tumors, most patients complain of back and joint pain of several years' duration
- Unlike primary spinal cord tumors, MRI demonstrates herniation of intervertebral disc with variable cord/nerve root impingement without a spinal cord mass

Spinal stenosis

Progressive narrowing of spinal canal with gradual impingement of cord/nerve roots.

FEATURES

- Like primary spinal cord tumors, can present with sensory, motor, and autonomic dysfunction
- Unlike primary spinal cord tumors, symptoms are slowly progressive over many years
- Unlike primary spinal cord tumors, patients usually complain of back pain of many years duration with typical spinal stenosis symptoms (e.g. worse when walking down hill, better when sitting and leaning forward)
- Unlike primary spinal cord tumors, X-ray/MRI demonstrates narrowing of the spinal canal without cord mass

Infectious disease

Bacterial, fungal, and parasitic infections can involve any part of the spinal cord/axis (e.g. cord, meninges, paraspinal structures) and damage the cord through abscess, atrophy, compression, cyst formation, demyelination, edema, fibrosis, infarction, inflammation, mass effect, meningitis, myelitis, necrosis, pachymeningitis, syringomyelia, or vascular compromise (e.g. thrombosis, congestion, arteritis, insufficiency). Infection usually occurs through hematogenous spread from a distant site, but can also result from direct extension (e.g. vertebral osteitis) and through cerebrospinal fluid (CSF) seeding. Infections involving the cord/spinal axis include but are not limited to: aspergillosis, blastomycosis, brucellosis, coccidioidomycosis, cryptococcosis, cysticercosis, echinococcosis, epidural abscess, gnathostomiasis, histoplasmosis, neurosyphilis, paracoccidioidomycosis, paragonimiasis, protozoal (e.g. *Toxoplasma gondii*), pyogenic abscess, schistosomiasis, subdural abscess, trichinosis, tuberculosis (Pott's disease), vertebral osteomyelitis.

FEATURES

- Like primary cord tumors, can present radiographically as a space-occupying lesion (e.g. enhancing intramedullary lesion) or meningioma that can result in sensory, motor, or autonomic dysfunction with a subacute or acute course
- Like primary cord tumors, can cause edema, infarction, ischemia, spinal cord vascular thrombosis/compromise, and vertebral body collapse
- Like primary cord tumors, can cause lesions that range in size from several millimeters to several centimeters that are solitary or multiple
- Like primary cord tumors, can involve the central canal, spinal cord tracts/parenchyma, nerve roots, vertebra, and intradural and epidural spaces
- Like primary cord tumors, can occasionally present with spinal cord compression with sudden neurologic dysfunction that mandates emergent neurosurgical intervention/consultation
- Like primary cord tumors, diagnosis is usually made through MRI and CSF examination
- Unlike primary cord tumors, CSF can show neutrophils and low glucose
- Unlike primary cord tumors, there is usually evidence of distant infection that can be characterized by fever, positive blood cultures, and an identifiable source (e.g. pneumonia, urinary tract, osteomyelitis, abscess)
- Unlike primary cord tumors, there may be a history of instrumentation, penetrating injury, intravenous drug abuse, or surgery
- Sometimes the differential diagnosis is difficult

Vertebral osseous tumors

Rare, account for 3.4–9% of all primary skeletal neoplasms. Usually present as a solitary lesion in a patient with back pain. Benign lesions include: aneurysmal bone cyst, enostosis, giant cell tumor, hemangioma, osteoblastoma, osteochondroma, and osteoid osteoma. Malignant lesions include: chondrosarcoma, chordoma, Ewing's tumor, and osteosarcoma. Advanced lesions with spinal cord involvement may be radiographically similar to primary cord lesions with bone involvement.

FEATURES

- Like primary cord tumors, can involve any part of the spine
- Like primary cord tumors, can present with back pain of several weeks/months duration with neurologic signs and symptoms
- Like primary cord tumors, can present with sensory, motor, or autonomic dysfunction with a subacute or acute course
- Like primary cord tumors, can cause lesions that range in size from several millimeters to several centimeters and can be benign or malignant
- Like primary cord tumors, can occasionally present with spinal cord compression with sudden neurologic dysfunction that mandates emergent neurosurgical intervention/consultation
- Unlike primary spinal cord tumors, X-ray shows typical radiographic features of primary bone tumor (e.g. 'moth eaten' appearance, speculated periosteal reaction)
- Unlike primary cord tumors, these lesions arise in bone

Multiple sclerosis

Multiple sclerosis (MS) is a demyelinating disease that affects the CNS and may clinically involve only the cord. Acute necrotizing myelopathy is considered a variant of MS and can present as an acute or subacute necrotizing myelopathy.

FEATURES

- Like primary spinal cord tumors, can present with sensory, motor, and autonomic dysfunction
- Like primary spinal cord tumors, can occur throughout the cord; however, the cervical cord is most often involved
- Like primary spinal cord tumors, can produce atrophy and edema with solitary or multiple lesions
- Like primary spinal cord tumors, clinical course can be subacute or acute
- Like primary spinal cord tumors, MRI is the principle diagnostic modality
- Like primary spinal cord tumors, active MS can radiologically present as a spinal cord mass with a high-signal enhancing lesion
- Unlike primary spinal cord tumors, most patients have intracranial plaques on MRI; however, approx. 12% have disease limited to the cord

Devic's disease (neuromyelitis optica)

Demyelinating lesion involving the cord and optic chiasm/nerves.

FEATURES

- Like primary spinal cord tumors, can cause atrophy, edema, and necrosis of the cord
- Like primary spinal cord tumors, can occur throughout the cord causing sensory, motor, and autonomic dysfunction
- Unlike primary spinal cord tumors, symptoms are usually acute and severe and are either followed by or antedated by bilateral optic nerve involvement; interval between spinal cord and optic nerve symptoms can range from weeks to months
- Unlike primary spinal cord tumors, CSF shows neutrophils and markedly increased protein

Sarcoidosis

Sarcoidosis is a systemic inflammatory disease characterized by noncaseating granulomata. Most commonly involves the cervical-thoracic cord.

FEATURES

- Like primary spinal cord tumors, can affect any part of the cord or its coverings; however, the cervical-thoracic cord is most commonly affected
- Like primary spinal cord tumors, can present as a intramedullary lesion
- Like primary spinal cord tumors, MRI and lumbar puncture are initial diagnostic modalities; however, CSF findings are frequently normal or nonspecific
- Like primary spinal cord tumors, biopsy is needed for definitive diagnosis; however, biopsy should be performed on organs with high probable diagnostic yield (e.g. lung, skin, conjunctiva)
- Unlike primary spinal cord tumors, there is usually evidence of sarcoidosis involving other organs; however, isolated spinal sarcoidosis has been reported

Malignant schwannoma

Malignant tumor that can occur anywhere along a peripheral nerve.

FEATURES

- Like some primary spinal tumors, can involve the nerve roots, resulting in sensory, motor, and autonomic dysfunction
- Like some primary spinal cord tumors, can be locally invasive
- Unlike primary spinal cord tumors, originate in the nerve, not the spinal cord, and have high metastatic potential
- Unlike primary spinal cord tumors, is associated with neurofibromatosis type 1

Neurofibromatosis

Neurofibromatosis is a benign nerve root tumor. Spinal cord involvement usually results from local extramedullary extension.

FEATURES

- Like some primary spinal tumors, can involve the nerve roots, resulting in sensory, motor, and autonomic dysfunction
- Like schwannomas, can be associated with von Recklinghausen's disease
- Like some primary spinal cord tumors, solitary neurofibromas are often completely resectable with minimal if any morbidity
- Unlike schwannomas that are usually solitary, neurofibromas are often multiple

Plexiform neurofibroma

Can occur anywhere along a peripheral nerve.

FEATURES

- Like primary spinal cord tumors, can be intradural or extradural, and can clinically present as a myelopathy and radiculopathy with sensory, motor, and autonomic dysfunction
- Like some primary spinal cord tumors, there is potential malignant transformation to a malignant schwannoma
- Like primary spinal cord tumors, can cause cord compression and spinal deformity
- Unlike primary spinal cord tumors, originate in the nerve, not the spinal cord
- Unlike primary spinal cord tumors, are associated with neurofibromatosis type 1
- Unlike primary spinal cord tumors, are frequently multiple
- Unlike many primary spinal cord tumors, often invade surrounding structures making complete resection technically unfeasible with significant potential morbidity

Inflammatory disease

Several inflammatory diseases can involve the spinal cord and include Behçet's disease, rheumatoid arthritis, systemic lupus erythematosus, and vasculitis.

FEATURES

- Like primary spinal cord tumors, can occur throughout the cord or its coverings resulting in an intramedullary lesion with cord damage secondary to inflammation/vasculitis
- Like primary spinal cord tumors, can produce infarction and necrosis with sensory, motor, and autonomic dysfunction

Micellaneous conditions

FEATURES

- Dermoid cysts, epidermoid cysts, and lipomas can occur in the spinal cord and are usually extramedullary
- Several conditions can cause acute necrosis of the spinal cord and include encephalomyelitis, hemorrhagic leukoencephalopathy, lymphoproliferative disease, and viral infection
- Hemangiopericytoma are rare, usually solitary and attached to the dura
- Paragangliomas are spinal intradural tumors that usually present in the filum terminale and cauda equina
- NonHodgkin's lymphoma can have malignant cells in the CSF and involve the intradural nerve roots and spinal cord
- Germ cell tumors mostly involve the pineal and suprasellar region; however, they can spread to the cord through the CSF
- Pineocytomas and pineoblastomas involve the pineal gland and can spread through the CSF to involve the cord
- Schwannosis is associated with neurofibromatosis type 2, and is characterized by a benign ingrowth of Schwann cells into the spinal cord and can present as a cord mass

- Syringomyelia can result in sensory loss, weakness, arm/hand-wasting, long tract signs and can present similar to a cervical intramedullary tumor; MRI is the diagnostic procedure of choice
- Von Hippel-Lindau (VHL) disease is an autosomal dominant disease characterized by capillary hemangioblastomas of the CNS including the spinal cord; 25–30% of spinal hemangioblastomas are associated with VHL disease
- Vascular disease can result in venous thrombosis with subsequent spinal cord infarction resulting in a wide range of neurologic sequelae
- Other rare tumors/lesions/vascular lesions of the spinal axis are amyloid angiopathy, aneurysmal bone cysts, arteriovenous malformations, cavernous hemangiomas, chordomas, cryptic vascular lesions, epidural hematoma, Foix-Alajouanine syndrome, hemorrhage, infarction, interosseous schwannomas, lipoma, meningeal cysts, neuroblastoma, spinal dural arteriovenous fistulas, synovial cysts, teratomas, venous angiomas, and vertebral arteriovenous fistulas
- Rare cystic lesions that can involve the cord include endodermal cysts, ependymal cysts, extradural cysts, inflammatory cysts, meningeal cysts, neoplastic cysts, subarachnoid cysts, and syringomyelia-hydromyelia

SIGNS & SYMPTOMS

Signs

- Signs and symptoms of primary spinal cord tumors can be divided into three distinct syndromes: sensory/motor, radicular, and syringomyelic
- Sensory/motor clinical presentation usually related to spinal cord compression with asymmetric motor complaints predominating that progress over a period of weeks to months
- Radicular syndromes result from compression and involvement of spinal roots with pain following a sensory nerve root distribution
- Radicular pain may be dull/achy or sharp/stabbing, and is increased by actions that elevate intracranial pressure (i.e. cough/sneeze)
- Radicular pain may also present with sensory deficits (impaired pain/touch), paraesthesia, or motor deficits (muscle atrophy/weakness)
- Radicular signs usually precede spinal cord compression by several months
- Syringomyelic syndromes usually result from intramedullary tumors that cause cavitation of the central gray matter and can cause combined motor and sensory defects
- Motor defects result from lower motor neurons involvement and are characterized by loss of reflexes and muscle weakness/wasting
- Sensory defects can include impaired pain and temperature sensation
- Touch is usually spared; however, significant cavitation can result in impaired position sense, touch, and vibration sense
- Motor signs predominate
- Signs of extramedullary tumors result from spinal cord compression and ischemia
- Signs of intramedullary tumors result from destruction of spinal cord tissue
- Signs of spinal cord compression depend on tumor location and can be local or distal
- Local signs reflect lesion's location along spinal axis
- Distal signs reflect involvement of spinal cord motor and sensory long tracts
- Ultimately all spinal tumors will manifest remote signs with symptoms and signs involving structures innervated below the level of the cord lesion
- Sensory impairment is common, usually beginning in feet but depends on tumor location
- Muscular atrophy and weakness can occur and depend on tumor location
- Segmental sensory and motor loss can result from gray matter compression
- Brown-Sequard's syndrome (cord hemisection) can rarely occur
- Tumors located above the conus medullarus are characterized by weakness and spasticity
- Tumors located below the conus medullarus are characterized by weakness and flaccidity
- Bladder dysfunction is a late finding for tumors located above the conus medullarus and an early finding for tumors located at or below the conus

Signs specific to tumor location:
- Foramen magnum – cerebellar ataxia; cranial nerve XI and XII palsy
- Cervical spine – fibrillation of ipsilateral arm, neck, and shoulder girdle musculature; wasting of ipsilateral arm, neck and shoulder girdle musculature
- Thoracic spine – abdominal muscle weakness; upper extremities are spared
- Lumbosacral spine – ankle jerk brisk; bladder dysfunction/paralysis; knee jerk decreased; pelvic muscle weakness
- Cauda equina – bladder dysfunction/paralysis; bowel dysfunction/paralysis

Symptoms
- Symptoms related to spinal cord compression and tumor edema
- Symptoms dependent on tumor location and rate of growth
- Motor and sensory symptoms predominate and tend to be slowly progressive
- Schwannoma symptoms tend to be referred to the involved nerve
- Symptoms may be nonlocalizing or localize to a specific cord region
- Symptoms are initially usually unilateral but will often progress to bilateral
- Extradural tumors tend to manifest symptoms from days to weeks
- Intradural tumors tend to manifest symptoms over a period of months
- Back pain, especially with metastatic disease or primary spinal cord disease invading bone

Spinal root involvement can cause:
- Atrophy
- Pain (e.g. sharp, stabbing, burning)
- Numbness
- Weakness
- Sensory loss (e.g. pain, temperature)

Symptoms specific to tumor location:
- Foramen magnum – neck pain
- Cervical spine – cervical pain; wasting of ipsilateral arm, neck, and shoulder girdle musculature
- Thoracic spine – abdominal muscle weakness
- Lumbosacral spine – bladder dysfunction/paralysis; impotence; pelvic muscle weakness
- Cauda equina – back pain, unilateral or bilateral; urine/bowel retention/incontinence

ASSOCIATED DISORDERS
- Neurofibromatosis type 2 is associated with meningioma, glioma, ependymoma, and schwannoma
- Hemangioblastoma is associated with VHL disease and posterior fossa hemangioblastomas
- Von Recklinghausen's disease is associated with multiple schwannoma

KEY! DON'T MISS!
- Spinal cord compression is a medical emergency; immediate hospitalization, intravenous steroids, and neurosurgical/radiation-oncologist consultation is needed
- Evidence of deep vein thrombosis requires anticoagulation
- Foramen magnum tumors can be misdiagnosed as amyotrophic lateral sclerosis, cervical disk herniation, and multiple sclerosis
- Intramedullary cervical tumors can be misdiagnosed as syringomyelia
- These tumors are rare and patients with suspicion of spinal tumors should be evaluated by a specialized team

CONSIDER CONSULT

- Refer to an experienced team for evaluation as soon as possible
- When symptoms of compression are present, it is an emergency situation and referral should be immediate
- Refer to a radiation-oncologist and/or oncologist for partially resected or malignant tumors

INVESTIGATION OF THE PATIENT

Direct questions to patient

- Q **When did your symptoms begin?** Most spinal cord tumors are slow-growing and cause symptoms that progress over weeks to months. However, acute onset of motor, sensory, or autonomic dysfunction can occur over a course of days
- Q **Do you have back pain?** Spinal tumors or metastatic disease to the spine can invade vertebra, causing pain. Tumors may also involve nerve roots resulting in neuropathic back pain
- Q **Do you have any trouble moving part of your body or have you noticed any part of your body becoming weak?** Spinal tumors can cause motor weakness that is dependent on the level of cord involvement
- Q **Is any part of your body numb or feeling different?** Spinal tumors can cause sensory dysfunction resulting in sensory deficits, paresthesia, or pain
- Q **Do you have any problems with urination such as losing urine or urinary retention?** Spinal tumors, especially those of the lumbosacral area, may cause bladder dysfunction
- Q **Do you have any problems with your bowel movements such as losing bowel control or constipation?** Spinal tumors, especially those of the lumbosacral area, may cause bowel dysfunction
- Q **Do you have any problems with balance or walking?** Tumors of the foramen magnum may present with cerebellar ataxia
- Q **Do you have any problems talking?** Tumors of the foramen magnum may have cranial nerve XII palsy
- Q **Do you have any problems maintaining an erection?** Tumors of the lumbosacral spine may be associated with impotence

Contributory or predisposing factors

- Q **Has the patient been exposed to vinyl chloride?** Vinyl chloride is associated with gliomas
- Q **Does the patient have a history of lung, breast, skin, kidney, or other types of cancer?** Spinal metastasis is common for some cancers

Family history

- Q **Does anyone in your family have a history of neurofibromatosis type 2 or von Hippel-Lindau disease?** Both of these disorders are inherited autosomal disorders that are associated with spinal cord lesions.

Examination

- **Is the patient ataxic?** Ataxia can be found in foramen magnum tumors
- **Is there weakness of the trapezius or steromastoid muscles?** Foramen magnum tumors can result in cranial nerve XI palsy
- **Does the patient garble his/her words?** Cranial nerve XII palsy can be found in foramen magnum tumors
- **Does the patient have motor weakness?** Involvement of the motor nerve roots and cord can result in motor weakness; site of motor weakness depends on level of cord/root involvement
- **Does the patient exhibit a sensory deficit?** Involvement of the spinal nerve roots or cord can cause sensory dysfunction with loss of pain, temperature, or touch sensation; site of sensory deficit depends on level of cord/root involvement
- **Is there evidence of muscle atrophy?** Involvement of motor nerve roots can cause atrophy; site of muscle atrophy depends on level of cord/root involvement

- **Is the ankle jerk brisk?** Tumors of the thoracic spine can result in a brisk ankle jerk
- **Is the knee jerk decreased?** Tumors of the thoracic spine can result in a decreased knee jerk

Summary of investigative tests

Initial studies to document disease:

- MRI of the spinal axis/cord is the usual initial test of choice to demonstrate a spinal lesion
- An initial computed tomography (CT) scan can be ordered in the initial evaluation of patients with suspicion of spinal tumors and can be useful in the diagnosis. A negative CT does not rule out a spinal tumor
- Spinal X-ray may be also used to identify vertebral/spinal disease

Once a spinal lesion is identified, the following tests are used to determine if the lesion is neoplastic or non-neoplastic:

- Diffusion-perfusion MRI, dynamic contrast-enhanced MRI, functional MRI, and MR spectroscopy may be used to evaluate the tumor and are normally ordered by a specialist
- MR spectroscopy can help differentiate high-grade from low-grade lesions and identify necrosis, and is ordered by a specialist
- Lumbar puncture may be used to rule out other disease and for cytological CSF examination
- Radionuclide bone scan may also be indicated to evaluate bony malignancy and is ordered by a specialist
- Angiography may help determine if a spinal lesion is an aneurysm, a vascular malformation, or a vascular tumor (i.e. hemangioblastoma), and is ordered by a specialist
- Angiography may also be used preoperatively to define tumor vascular supply and potential for embolization, and is usually ordered by a specialist
- Myelography may be used to further characterize tumor location and is usually ordered by a specialist
- Those with a diagnosis of probable metastatic spinal cord tumor should have a complete history and physical examination, chest X-ray, and mammogram if female

If the clinical index of suspicion remains high for a neoplastic spinal cord/column lesion, the following tests/procedures are usually performed:

- Laminectomy is usually performed to obtain tissue for histologic examination, usually using frozen section
- Biopsy with histologic review is the only way to make a definitive diagnosis
- Surgical resection is indicated if frozen section reveals neoplasia

DIAGNOSTIC DECISION

- History and physical examination establish a clinical index of suspicion for spinal pathology
- Initial diagnostic decision in any process that potentially involves the cord is to determine if cord compression/disease exists that may necessitate immediate specialized intervention/consultation from an experienced team
- Early clinical presentation may be vague and nonspecific; however, most patients will experience neurologic deficits as lesion progresses
- Always consider the possibility of a spinal tumor in patients with symptoms referable to the cord or nerve roots
- MRI is an appropriate diagnostic modality for infectious disease-related, oncologically related, painful, slowly progressive, stepwise progressive, sudden onset, and traumatic myelopathy
- MRI with gadolinium is an appropriate diagnostic modality for infectious disease-related, slowly progressive, and stepwise progressive myelopathy
- Plain radiograph (i.e. spinal radiograph) is an appropriate diagnostic modality for infectious disease-related, oncologically related, painful, slowly progressive, sudden onset, and traumatic myelopathy

- Laboratory testing cannot establish or exclude a diagnosis of spinal cord cancer; definitive diagnosis requires biopsy
- There are no serologic markers that have demonstrated adequate sensitivity of specificity to encourage use
- If clinical index of suspicion is high for spinal tumor with other causes of spinal pathology ruled out and if radiographic findings are suggestive of spinal tumor, many surgeons will proceed directly to laminectomy with intraoperative biopsy for frozen section histopathological review
- If frozen section demonstrates neoplasia surgical resection of tumor is usually attempted
- Definitive tissue diagnosis should be obtained prior to surgery, radiotherapy, or chemotherapy, and is usually obtained through biopsy
- Positron emission tomography may help differentiate radiation necrosis from tumor recurrence and is ordered by a specialist

CLINICAL PEARLS

The use of corticosteroids can improve the initial symptoms and signs of compression as well as prevent later complications, but the patient still needs to be referred quickly.

THE TESTS

Body fluids

CEREBROSPINAL FLUID

Description

- Collection of CSF by insertion of needle in subarachnoid space
- Cytological examination of CSF for neoplastic cells, protein, and glucose

Advantages/Disadvantages

Advantages:

- Can help determine etiology of spinal cord lesion (e.g. meningitis, multiple sclerosis, syphilis serology)
- Cytological examination of CSF may demonstrate neoplastic cells
- Elevated protein and normal glucose may be suggestive of spinal neoplasia but is not diagnostic
- Relatively safe, simple, and inexpensive
- Minimal risk of infection

Disadvantages:

- Negative cytology does not rule out spinal cord tumor
- Xanthochromic CSF without red blood cells (RBCs) may be suggestive of spinal neoplasia but is not diagnostic
- If intracranial lesion is present, can cause cerebellar or temporal lobe herniation; hence, computed tomography or MRI is indicated prior to lumbar puncture
- Not sensitive or specific for spinal tumor unless cytology definitively identifies neoplastic cells
- Contraindicated in those with increased intracranial pressure, ongoing infection at needle insertion site, and severe degenerative joint disease
- Complications include back pain, bleeding, CSF leak, headache, herniation, infection, paraesthesia, severe hemorrhage (i.e. aortic/vena cava puncture), spinal cord trauma

Normal

- Color: clear and colorless
- Pressure: $<200cmH_2O$
- Glucose: 50–75mg/dL or 60–70% serum glucose
- Protein: 15–45mg/dL (may be as high as 70mg/dL in children and the elderly)

Abnormal

- Spinal cord tumors typically have normal glucose and negative cytology with elevated protein
- Xanthochromic CSF without RBCs may be indicative of a spinal cord tumor that obstructs the subarachnoid space

Cause of abnormal result

- Abnormal cytology can result from free floating tumor cells in the CSF
- Elevated protein results from disruption of blood-brain barrier permitting large protein molecules to enter CSF

Drugs, disorders and other factors that may alter results

Disorders that can cause abnormal CSF findings include:

- Abscess
- Autoimmune disease
- Bleeding
- Brain cancer
- Cerebral hemorrhage
- Coma
- Spinal/cerebral degeneration
- Demyelination
- Encephalitis
- Hepatic encephalopathy
- Meningitis (e.g. bacterial, tubercular, viral)
- Multiple sclerosis
- Myelitis
- Neurosyphilis
- Reye's syndrome
- Spinal tumor

Biopsy

FROZEN SECTION

Description

- Tumor tissue obtained for histopathological examination
- Usually performed intraoperatively with frozen section
- Patients suspected of having a spinal tumor should undergo laminectomy with tissue obtained for histological examination

Advantages/Disadvantages

Advantages:

- Invasive diagnostic procedure of choice
- Provides tissue for definitive diagnosis of spinal tumor

Disadvantages:

- Complications include bleeding, edema, and neurologic compromise
- General anesthesia is needed

Normal

- No spinal lesion identified
- No abnormal histology

Abnormal

- Spinal lesion identified
- Abnormal histology identified

Cause of abnormal result

Numerous conditions can result in a spinal cord lesion, including:

- Astrocytoma
- Chordomas
- Dermoid cysts
- Devic's disease
- Ependymomas
- Epidermoids
- Ganglioglioma
- Ganglioneuroblastoma
- Hemangioblastoma
- Infections (e.g. bacterial, fungal, parasitic)
- Inflammatory disease (e.g. lupus, rheumatoid arthritis)
- Lipoma
- Lymphoma
- Metastatic disease (e.g. breast, lung)
- Meningioma
- Medulloblastoma
- Multiple sclerosis
- Neurofibroma
- Oligodendroglioma
- Sarcoidosis
- Sarcoma
- Schwannoma
- Vascular tumors

Imaging

MAGNETIC RESONANCE IMAGING

Description

- MRI of the spinal axis used to determine if spinal lesion is present, extent of cord and nerve root compromise, and respectability, and to rule out metastasis
- Radiographic procedure of choice, usually done with gadolinium-diethylenetriaminepenta-acetic acid contrast

Advantages/Disadvantages

Advantages:

- Initial noninvasive imaging procedure of choice used to identify spinal lesion
- Superior to CT, offering higher resolution without bone artifact with scan data acquired from any spinal plane
- Can also be used to guide radiotherapy

Disadvantage: MRI can only identify lesion, cannot determine etiology; however, spinal tumors have characteristic radiographic findings and special MRI imaging can be performed to better categorize lesion

Normal

No spinal lesion identified.

Abnormal

- Spinal lesion identified
- Astrocytoma average lesion length: four vertebral bodies
- Ependymoma average lesion length: four vertebral bodies
- Gangliogliomas average lesion length: eight vertebral bodies

- Ependymomas tend to be centrally located in the cord
- Astrocytomas and gangliogliomas tend to be eccentrically located in the cord

Cause of abnormal result

Numerous conditions can result in a spinal cord lesion, including:

- Astrocytoma
- Chordomas
- Dermoid cysts
- Devic's disease
- Ependymomas
- Epidermoids
- Ganglioglioma
- Ganglioneuroblastoma
- Hemangioblastoma
- Infections (e.g. bacterial, fungal, parasitic)
- Inflammatory disease (e.g. lupus, rheumatoid arthritis)
- Lipoma
- Lymphoma
- Metastatic disease (e.g. breast, lung)
- Meningioma
- Medulloblastoma
- Multiple sclerosis
- Neurofibroma
- Oligodendroglioma
- Sarcoidosis
- Sarcoma
- Schwannoma
- Vascular tumors

X-RAY, SPINE

Description

X-ray of spine, usually of a specific region (i.e. cervical, lumbosacral).

Advantages/Disadvantages

Advantages:

- Can help identify bony disease of the vertebra (i.e. osteoarthritis, compression fracture, bony metastasis)
- May also help identify bony erosion, neural foramina enlargement, and interpeduncular widening
- Noninvasive, safe, and relatively inexpensive

Disadvantage: extremely limited value in identifying cord/nerve root lesions

Normal

No spinal/vertebral lesion identified.

Abnormal

Spinal/vertebral lesion identified.

Cause of abnormal result

- Metastatic vertebral lesions (e.g. prostate cancer)
- Osteoarthritis
- Primary bony vertebral tumors
- Spondyloarthropathies
- Vertebral compression/fracture

TREATMENT

CONSIDER CONSULT

- Multidisciplinary team approach enhances patient satisfaction and may improve recovery, rehabilitation, and survival
- Refer to a radiation oncologist if radiotherapy is indicated
- Refer to an oncologist if chemotherapy is indicated
- Referral to a clinical trial may be appropriate for malignant disease
- Refer to a physical/occupational therapist postresection

IMMEDIATE ACTION

- Spinal cord compression is a medical emergency; immediate hospitalization, intravenous steroids, and neurosurgical/radiation-oncologist consultation are needed
- Evidence of spinal cord compression and fever with a history of infection, surgery, instrumentation, or intravenous drug abuse may be indicative of epidural abscess and mandates emergent neurosurgical consultation
- Evidence of deep vein thrombosis requires anticoagulation

PATIENT AND CAREGIVER ISSUES

Forensic and legal issues

- Most patients will be able to consent for treatment
- If patient cannot give consent, determine who has authority to consent
- With the exception of a life-threatening complication or potential severe irreversible neurologic compromise that necessitates immediate intervention, the treatment of spinal cord tumors can be delayed until consent is obtained

Impact on career, dependants, family, friends

- Most spinal tumors are benign and most patients can expect to return to careers and family
- Depending on amount of residual neurologic compromise postresection, physical rehabilitation may be necessary and may delay a return to full activity
- Many patients with benign totally resected tumors who do not experience any permanent neurologic compromise can expect a cure and complete recovery
- Some patients will have permanent neurologic compromise postresection that may limit their ability to pursue a career or return to a level of activity previously enjoyed
- Some spinal cord tumors have a poor prognosis and some patients, family, and friends will have to deal with end-of-life issues
- For patients with tumors that carry a poor prognosis, there can be significant impact on career given the physical and psychological demands of diagnosis/treatment, potentially severe and debilitating neurologic compromise, and poor overall prognosis
- Psychological impact of cancer diagnosis is profound with patients, families, and friends experiencing a variety of emotions, including but not limited to anger, anxiety, bereavement, denial, depression, and grief

MANAGEMENT ISSUES

Goals

- Initiate evaluation for surgical intervention
- Initiate evaluation for chemotherapy/radiotherapy if indicated
- Achieve complete curative resection if possible
- Prevent spread of disease
- Enhance survival and quality of life
- Achieve adequate pain control
- Insure adequate nutrition
- Evaluate rehabilitation potential
- Evaluate social support

- Determine desire for resuscitation
- Determine attitudes toward hospice if indicated
- Prepare patient for end-of-life, if indicated

Management in special circumstances

COEXISTING DISEASE

- Control hypertension, as elevated blood pressure can increase tumor-related edema
- Aggressively treat any infection because fever and infection are likely to increase neurologic sequelae of spinal cord tumor; most common infections include pneumonia and urinary tract infection
- Patients with comorbidities tend to have a longer recovery and may have less rehabilitation potential
- For malignant disease, patients with comorbidities tend to have a worse prognosis

SPECIAL PATIENT GROUPS

Rehabilitation should be tailored to appreciate patient's previous level of activity, expectations, neurologic status postresection, and any comorbidities.

PATIENT SATISFACTION/LIFESTYLE PRIORITIES

- Patients will have questions regarding treatment and prognosis
- Patients will be concerned about pain control and quality of life
- Patients will be concerned about their own rehabilitation potential
- Patients with malignant/metastatic disease will need assistance with end-of-life issues
- Side-effects of chemoradiotherapy may negatively impact patient's quality of life
- Severe disability can result from neurologic compromise that may be irreversible
- Severe disability can result from terminal disease

SUMMARY OF THERAPEUTIC OPTIONS

Choices

Initial treatment:

- Initial treatment goal is to determine if emergency exists and to maximally preserve neurologic function
- It is imperative that a patient with a potential spinal cord lesion obtains timely evaluation, diagnosis, and intervention to prevent permanent/progressive neurologic dysfunction
- Ideally patients should undergo treatment when minimally symptomatic as the more advanced/profound the lesion, the less chance of neurologic recovery
- Glucocorticoids are indicated for spinal cord compression
- Spinal cord compression is an emergency. Retrospective studies suggest that early radiotherapy preserves function. One small randomized controlled trial (RCT) suggests that adding high-dose steroids improves the chances of walking 6 months after radiotherapy for spinal cord compression

Surgery:

- First choice is complete macroscopic and microscopic cytoreductive surgical resection usually through laminectomy
- Glucocorticoids (i.e. dexamethasone) are usually indicated preoperatively, perioperatively, and postoperatively

Surgical palliation, chemoradiotherapy, and supportive care:

- Given poor prognosis of some spinal tumors, the primary goal may be palliation, and in advanced disease palliation is often the primary goal
- Radiotherapy and chemotherapy are reserved for tumors that are unresectable, partially resected, or found to be malignant
- Address lifestyle issues in all patients

Clinical pearls

Patients with spinal tumors and symptoms of spinal compression that are submitted to radiation can have a remission of symptoms if treated in a timely manner.

FOLLOW UP

- Follow up primarily to evaluate treatment efficacy, manage complications, and evaluate rehabilitation needs
- Specific areas of investigation include evaluation of recurrence/spread and surgical- or chemoradiotherapy-related complications

Plan for review

- Following treatment, evaluate symptom relief and disease recurrence/spread
- Evaluate patient for signs and symptoms of postoperative complications
- Evaluate patient for signs and symptoms of chemotherapeutic toxicity
- Evaluate patient for signs and symptoms of radiation toxicity
- Evaluate patient for neurologic deterioration or improvement
- Evaluate patient for response to physical rehabilitation
- Spinal MRI may be indicated to evaluate treatment efficacy and to rule out metastasis

Information for patient or caregiver

- Patients need to know that most spinal tumors can be cured; however, some spinal tumors can carry a poor prognosis
- Patients need to know that prompt evaluation and treatment are necessary to prevent further neurologic deterioration
- Patients need to know that postresection physical rehabilitation will probably be necessary
- Patients should understand that only hope for cure is curative resection
- Some patients will have to decide on end-of-life issues and be educated regarding options
- Appropriate hospice, skilled nursing facility, or home health care referral may be needed depending on the patient's medical condition, personal preference, and social/financial support

DRUGS AND OTHER THERAPIES: DETAILS

Drugs

GLUCOCORTICOIDS

- Glucocorticoids are used to reduce tumor/radiation/surgery-related edema and inflammation to preserve neurologic function and relieve symptoms
- Several glucocorticoids are used and include dexamethasone

Dose

- Dose varies according to clinical response; lowest dose possible should be used
- Loading dose is usually given prior to establishing a maintenance dose

Efficacy

- Can effectively relieve tumor/radiation/surgery-related edema and improve neurologic function
- Spinal cord compression is an emergency. Retrospective studies suggest that early radiotherapy preserves function. One small RCT suggests that adding high-dose steroids improves the chances of walking 6 months after radiotherapy for spinal cord compression

Risks/Benefits

Risks:

- False-negative skin allergy tests. Overwhelming septicemia if patient has an infection
- Loss of control of blood glucose in those with diabetes
- Use caution in the elderly due to risk of diabetes and osteoporosis
- Use caution in patients with psychosis, seizure disorders, or myasthenia gravis

- Use caution in congestive heart failure, hypertension
- Use caution in ulcerative colitis, peptic ulcer, or esophagitis

Side-effects and adverse reactions
- Side-effects are minimized by short duration of therapy
- Cardiovascular system: hypertension, thromboembolism
- Central nervous system: insomnia, euphoria, depression, psychosis, seizures
- Endocrine: adrenal suppression, impaired glucose tolerance, growth suppression in children
- Eyes, ears, nose, and throat: cataract, glaucoma, blurred vision
- Gastrointestinal: dyspepsia, peptic ulceration, esophagitis, oral candidiasis, nausea, vomiting
- Musculoskeletal: proximal myopathy, osteoporosis
- Skin: delayed healing, acne, striae

Interactions (other drugs)

■ Adrenergic neurone blockers, alpha-blockers, beta-blockers, beta-2-agonists ■ Vaccines ■ Aminoglutethamide ■ Anticonvulsants (carbamazepine, phenytoin, barbiturates) ■ Rifampin ■ Antidiabetics ■ Antidysrhythmics (calcium channel blockers, cardiac glycosides) ■ Nitrates ■ Nonsteroidal anti-inflammatory drugs (NSAIDs) ■ Antifungals (amphotericin, ketoconazole) ■ Cyclosporine ■ Erythromycin ■ Methotrexate ■ Nitroprusside ■ Oral contraceptives ■ Ritonavir ■ Somatropin ■ Antihypertensives (ACE inhibitors, diuretics: loop and thiazide, acetazolamide; angiotensin II receptor antagonists, clonidine, diazoxide, hydralazine, methyldopa, minoxidil)

Contraindications

■ Systemic infection ■ Avoid live virus vaccines in those receiving immunosuppressive doses

Surgical therapy
- Complete tumor resection with microscopically negative resection margins offer only hope for cure
- Most resections are performed through an operating microscope
- Goal of surgical intervention is curative resection with preservation of neurologic function
- Because spinal tumors are rare, one of the most important predictors of successful resection is the experience of the surgical team
- Ultrasound, CO_2 laser ablation, and Cavitron ultrasonic aspirator (CUSA) may also be used intraoperatively
- Astrocytoma, ependymoma, and hemangioblastoma can usually be resected through a laminectomy/myelotomy with the tumor bulk removed by CO_2 laser or CUSA
- Glucocorticoids are indicated preoperatively, perioperatively, and postoperatively
- Decompression of the spinal cord through debulking is second option if complete resection not feasible
- Surgical resection is the treatment of choice for primary spinal tumors
- Frozen section of tumor is usually obtained intraoperatively prior to surgical resection; if malignant tumor is found, surgical resection is abandoned in favor of radiotherapy
- Surgical technique is variable and depends on surgeon, medical center, and patient
- Patients with positive resection margins should be offered chemotherapy and/or radiotherapy
- Routine preoperative evaluation includes history and physical, chest X-ray, serum electrolytes, complete blood count, and coagulations studies
- Patients with unrespectable disease or malignant disease should be offered supportive care, surgical debulking for palliation, chemotherapy/radiotherapy, and entry into a clinical trial

LAMINECTOMY/CYTOREDUCTION
- Standard surgical approach offering best exposure of cord and surrounding structures
- Spinal cord is exposed through laminectomy; in post-tumor resection the vertebra are fused in their former location

- Monitoring of spinal cord sensory and motor tracts by a neurophysiologist is usually used intraoperatively to limit iatrogenic spinal cord dysfunction
- Ultrasound is often used intraoperatively to determine adequacy of surgical exposure
- Surgical resection may utilize coagulation, lasers, suction, and ultrasonic dissection
- Surgical resection may be indicated for tumor recurrence

Efficacy
- Meningiomas and schwannomas ca usually be completely resected through laminectomy and cure should be expected for most patients
- Astrocytoma, ependymoma, and hemangioblastoma can usually be resected through laminectomy/myelotomy
- Ependymomas usually have distinct cleavage planes that separate tumor tissue from normal spinal tissue that enhance respectability; however, only approx. 60% of ependymomas are amendable to complete resection
- Completely resectable ependymomas tend to be low-grade and confined to the cauda equina
- Surgical technique for ependymomas varies from total reliance on cytoreductive surgery vs radical irradiation vs a combination of surgery and radiotherapy
- Astrocytomas usually do not have distinct cleavage planes that separate tumor tissue from normal spinal tissue, and hence are more difficult to completely resect; however, debulking provides palliation

Risks/Benefits

Risks:
- Complications include bleeding, infection, wound infection, and cord damage resulting in permanent neurologic dysfunction
- In general, the more aggressive the resection attempt, the greater the risk for significant morbidity
- Temporary spinal cord dysfunction is common postresection
- Morbidity and mortality are surgeon-, tumor-, and patient-dependent
- Major complication is neurologic deficit (i.e. paralysis) secondary to intraoperative spinal cord manipulation; neurophysiologist monitors spinal cord pathways intraoperatively with feedback on cord status to surgeon
- Laminectomy with subsequent spinal fusion can result in variable degrees of spinal disability depending on the extent of vertebral resection/fusion
- Age, comorbid medical conditions, and poor performance status increase risk of perioperative morbidity and mortality

Benefit: surgical excision with negative resection margins offers only hope for cure and preservation of neurologic function

Acceptability to patient

Though associated with some morbidity, the prospect for the preservation and return of normal neurologic function coupled to the high probability of curative resection make laminectomy acceptable to most patients.

Follow up plan
- Follow up should include complete history and physical with special attention to resolution/emergence of neurologic defects
- Follow up magnetic resonance imaging (MRI) of the spine may be indicated
- Ensure adequate postoperative pain control
- Observe for bleeding, meningitis, wound infection, neurologic deterioration, and other postoperative complications

- Most patients will need to be followed by neurologists, neurosurgeons, and orthopedic surgeons postoperatively, especially children who may develop spinal deformity that should be aggressively managed

Patient and caregiver information
- Patients and caregivers need to be able to recognize major postoperative complications like bleeding and wound infection
- Warn patient and caregivers that the patient may feel weak postoperatively with temporary spinal cord dysfunction

Radiation therapy

RADIOTHERAPY
- Radiotherapy has an important role in the palliative treatment of spinal tumors
- Even in patients with metastatic disease in the spine, radiation should be offered as soon as possible when compression symptoms appear
- Radiotherapy reserved for tumors that are unresectable, partially resected, or malignant
- Normal spinal cord tissue is radiosensitive and limits radiation dosage
- Goal of radiotherapy is to reduce tumor size, pain, and neurologic sequelae
- Radiotherapy is used primarily for palliation
- Glucocorticoids are often indicated during and after radiotherapy
- Normal spinal cord tissue is radiosensitive and limits radiation dosage
- Radiation dose and target volume depend on type, size, and location of tumor
- Radiation therapy recommended for ependymomas that cannot be completely resected en bloc, incompletely resected, or resected 'piecemeal'
- Radiation therapy not recommended for ependymomas that have been resected en bloc
- Radiotherapy has limited efficacy in treating malignant disease
- There is no evidence that radiotherapy improves survival
- Radiotherapy usually not indicated for low-grade tumors

Efficacy
- Radiotherapy can improve survival in patients with low-grade astrocytomas and unresectable/partially resected ependymomas
- Radiotherapy can provide significant palliation for unresectable or partially resectable disease
- Postoperative radiotherapy can improve local control, disease-free survival, and overall survival in those with partially resected ependymomas
- Postoperative radiotherapy may improve survival in low-grade astrocytoma
- No dose-response relationship for radiotherapy and ependymoma/astrocytoma has been established
- Spinal cord compression is an emergency, even in patients with metastatic disease. Retrospective studies suggest that early radiotherapy preserves function. One small RCT suggests that adding high-dose steroids improves the chances of walking 6 months after radiotherapy for spinal cord compression

Risks/Benefits

Risks:
- Radiation therapy may cause increased tumor-related edema or demyelination, resulting in temporary neurologic deterioration lasting approx. 6–16 weeks
- Radiation-related necrosis may result in neurologic deterioration and can occur from 3 months to 10 years or more postradiation
- Transient (early delayed) radiation myelopathy (i.e. paresthesia with neck flexion) can occur 3–4 months postradiation and usually resolves without therapy in 3–6 months
- Late delayed radiation myelopathy, occurs at 12–14 and 24–28 months postradiation, and carries a 50% mortality rate usually from complications

- Late delayed radiation myelopathy is irreversible and is often characterized by progressive loss of motor function and rarely para- or quadriplegia that develops over hours to days
- Complications primarily from radiation exposure/damage to surrounding spinal cord and structures

Acceptability to patient

Warn patient about potential skin irritation over radiated site and to the possibility of delayed symptoms such as radiation myelopathy.

Follow up plan

- Follow up should include complete history and physical with special attention to neurologic examination
- Evaluate patient for tumor burden reduction
- Follow up spinal MRI may be indicated

Chemotherapy

CHEMOTHERAPY

- Chemotherapy reserved for tumors that are unresectable, partially resected, or malignant
- Chemotherapy is used primarily for palliation
- Goal of chemotherapy is to reduce tumor size, pain, and neurologic sequelae
- Consider entry into clinical trial
- Multiple chemotherapeutic agents are in use and depend on tumor type
- No single agent or combination of agents has been shown to be superior
- Regional drug delivery is used in conjunction to systemic chemotherapy or alone
- Some authors recommend nitrosourea-based chemotherapy for astrocytomas but the evidence is weak
- Intrathecal and intraventricular chemotherapy is limited to treatment of micrometastasis from leptomeningeal spread; lesions >5mm are not likely to benefit
- Multiple clinical trials are presently underway
- Chemotherapy has limited efficacy in treating malignant disease; no particular chemotherapeutic agent has demonstrated superior efficacy in treating malignant spinal cord lesions
- There is no evidence that chemotherapy improves survival
- Chemotherapy usually not indicated for low-grade tumors
- Not all chemotherapeutic agents can penetrate the central nervous system barrier

Efficacy

- Efficacy is limited by systemic toxicity, direct toxicity to spinal tissue, and the ability of the chemotherapeutic agent to penetrate the blood-brain barrier
- Palliation may last from weeks to months
- The vasculature supplying extramedullary spinal tumors is usually more permeable to chemotherapeutic agents than the vasculature supplying intramedullary spinal tumors

Risks/Benefits

Risks:

- May result in temporary clinical deterioration secondary to edema and tumor cell death
- All chemotherapy is limited by systemic and local effects
- Intra-cerebrospinal fluid with a significant risk of neurotoxicity
- Depending on agent used, may have high side-effect profile that includes myelosuppression, nausea, vomiting, nephrotoxicity, neuropathy, and ototoxicity

Acceptability to patient

Side-effect profile dependent on agents used and compliance may be influenced by side-effects.

Follow up plan

- Follow up should include history and physical, complete blood count, and serum electrolytes
- Follow up spinal MRI may be indicated
- Additional follow up studies may be indicated depending on agents used
- Aggressively manage nausea, vomiting, and diarrhea
- Nausea/vomiting can be controlled with 5-HT3 antagonist with glucocorticoid
- Monitor fluid status in patients with profound diarrhea/vomiting

Patient and caregiver information

Warn patient about side-effects; however, emphasize that these problems can be managed.

OUTCOMES

EFFICACY OF THERAPIES

- Surgery with complete microscopic and macroscopic tumor resection offers the only chance for cure
- Recurrence is a significant problem for some spinal cord tumors, occurring up to >12 years postresection
- Patients with benign resectable disease can expect cure with variable return of normal neurologic function
- Chemotherapy and radiotherapy are primarily for palliation with modest impact on survival for malignant or unresectable disease
- The rates of cure and the length of survival depend on the histology, location, and spread of the tumor

PROGNOSIS

- Prognosis depends on tumor type, extent of invasion, extent of feasible surgical resection, and histology
- For patients with signs of compression, timing of the beginning of therapy is an important prognostic factor
- Several grading systems are used for astrocytomas and can help determine prognosis; in general astrocytomas are graded from low-grade to high-grade
- Meningiomas and schwannomas have an excellent prognosis with most of these tumors amendable to complete resection and cure
- Gangliogliomas have a good prognosis
- Ependymomas usually have a better prognosis than astrocytomas but frequently recur and often cannot be totally resected

Astrocytomas:

- Low-grade astrocytomas may not be amendable to complete resection; however, debulking does provide palliation
- 5-year survival for low-grade astrocytomas postirradiation: 60–90%
- 10-year survival for low-grade astrocytomas postirradiation: 40–90%
- Astrocytomas tend to recur within 3 years postresection
- 5-year recurrence-free survival for irradiated low-grade astrocytoma: 66–83%
- 10-year recurrence-free survival for irradiated low-grade astrocytoma: 53–83%

Ependymomas:

- Prognosis for ependymomas depends on completeness of resection and tumor grade
- Relative risk for death is 9 for grades II–IV when compared to grade I
- Survival is enhanced by complete resection
- 5-year survival for irradiated ependymomas: 60–100%
- 10-year survival for irradiated ependymomas: 68–95%
- 5-year survival for well-differentiated ependymoma: 97%
- 5-year survival for intermediate/poorly differentiated ependymoma: 71%
- Myxopapillary ependymomas localized to the conus medullaris have a better prognosis than cellular ependymomas found in the spinal cord
- Ependymomas can recur up to 12 years postresection; recurrence is usually local
- Ependymomas removed 'piecemeal' have high recurrence rates, up to 43%
- 10-year recurrence-free survival for irradiated ependymomas: 43–61%
- Recurrence rate for irradiated ependymomas: 25%

- High-grade and myxopapillary ependymomas tend to recur in the thecal sac
- Anaplastic astrocytoma and glioblastoma multiforme have extremely poor prognosis of <8 months
- Gangliogliomas have a high rate of recurrence but low metastatic potential
- Consider entry into clinical trial should be strongly considered
- Pain control and quality of life should be a priority

Clinical pearls

The outcomes of the therapy are closely related to the degree of neurologic impairment before therapy. A prompt start can offer a better prognosis.

Therapeutic failure

- Consider entry into clinical trial
- Pain control and quality of life should be a priority

Recurrence

- Recurrence is likely with many spinal tumors given the difficulty achieving complete surgical resection
- Surgical resection may be indicated for recurrence
- Chemotherapy, radiotherapy, and entry into clinical trial should also be considered for recurrence

Deterioration

- Deterioration may result from increase in tumor size, tumor recurrence, or treatment-related complications
- Surgical resection, chemotherapy, or radiotherapy may be indicated for deterioration
- Entry into clinical trial should be strongly considered
- Pain control and quality of life should be a priority

Terminal illness

- Pain control and quality of life should be a priority
- Assist patient and family in dealing with end-of-life issues
- Have patient evaluated for hospice or home health care

COMPLICATIONS

- Hemorrhage is a potential complication of primary spinal cord tumors, with oligodendrogliomas and glioblastoma having a predilection toward hemorrhage
- Hyponatremia may result from central nervous system tumors
- Hyponatremia may also result from hypotonic intravenous fluid administration
- Seizures may indicate intracranial spread of primary spinal cord tumor
- Pain may be severe and should be managed aggressively
- Deep vein thrombosis is a recognized complication of malignancy
- Paralysis can be a complication of the tumor or surgery

CONSIDER CONSULT

- Refer to hospice for treatment failure, clinical deterioration, or terminal disease
- Refer to a psychiatrist/psychologist for emotional support and insight
- Refer to a pain specialist for intractable pain

PREVENTION

There is no known intervention that can prevent primary spinal cord tumors.

RISK FACTORS

Vinyl chloride has been associated with gliomas.

MODIFY RISK FACTORS

Lifestyle and wellness

ENVIRONMENT

Avoid vinyl chloride, which has been associated with gliomas.

SCREENING

There are no screening recommendations regarding spinal cord tumors.

PREVENT RECURRENCE

Recurrence can be prevented by adequate surgical resection with microscopic and macroscopic free resection margins, and radiotherapy when indicated.

Reassess coexisting disease

PATIENT SATISFACTION/LIFESTYLE PRIORITIES

- Most patients with recurrence will be concerned about resection of recurrence
- If recurrence cannot be adequately resected, many patients will be concerned with quality-of-life and end-of-life issues
- Pain control and patient comfort should be a priority

ASSOCIATIONS

American Cancer Society
1599 Clifton Road NE
Atlanta, GA 30329
Tel: (800) 227-2345 (800) ACS-2345)
www.cancer.org

Cancer Hope Network
Two North Road
Chester, NJ 07930
Tel: (877) 467-3638 (877) HOPENET)
E-mail: info@cancerhopenetwork.org
www.cancerhopenetwork.org

Cancer Links USA
9737 N.W. 41st Street, Suite 183
Miami, FL 33178
E-mail: lynx@cancerlinks.com
www.cancerlinksusa.com

National Brain Tumor Foundation
785 Market Street, Suite 1600
San Francisco, CA 94103
Tel: (800) 934-CURE (415) 284-0208)
www.braintumor.org/

National Cancer Institute
Public Inquires Office
Building 31, Room 10A03
31 Center Drive, MSC 2580
Tel: (800) 422-6237 (800) 4-CANCER)
E-mail: cancermail@cips.nci.nih.gov
www.cancer.gov/

National Coalition for Cancer Survivorship
1010 Wayne Avenue, Suite 505
Silver Springs, MD 20910–5600
Tel: (800) 622-7337
E-mail: info@cansearch.org
www.cansearch.org

National Comprehensive Cancer Network
50 Huntington Pike, Suite 200
Rockledge, PA 19046
Tel: (215) 728-3877 or
Tel: (888) 909-6226 (888) 909-NCCN)
E-mail: information@nccn.org
www.nccn.org

National Hospice and Palliative Care Organization
1700 Diagonal Road, Suite 300
Alexandria, VA 22314
Tel: (800) 658-8898
email: helpline@nhpco.org
www.nhpco.org

KEY REFERENCES

- Cotran RS, Kumar V, Collins T. Robbins pathological basis of disease. 6th edn. Philadelphia: WB Saunders, 1999, p1343–57
- DeVita VT, Hellman S, Rosenberg SA. Cancer: principles and practice of oncology. 6th edn. New York: Lippincott-Raven, 2001, p2100–60
- American College of Radiology. ACR appropriateness criteria for myelopathy. Radiology 2000;215(Suppl):494–505
- Arce D, Sass P, Abul-Khoudoud H. Recognizing spinal cord emergencies. Am Fam Physician 2001;15:64:631–8
- Waldron JN, Laperriere NJ, Jaakkimainen L, et al. Spinal cord ependymomas: a retrospetive analysis of 59 cases. Int J Radiat Oncol Biol Phys 1993;27:223–9
- Wen BC, Hussey DH, Hitchon PW, et al. The role of radiation therapy in the management of ependymomas of the spinal cord. Int J Radiat Oncol Biol Phys 1991;20:781–6

FAQS

Question 1

Should patients with advanced neoplasms and signs of spinal compression be referred as quickly as those with primary spinal tumors?

ANSWER 1

Yes. They should be referred as soon as possible, regardless of the primary site of the tumor. If the treatment is initiated fast, there is a better chance of recovery.

Question 2

If magnetic resonance imaging is not available for the initial evaluation of patients with possible spinal tumors, can a computed tomography (CT) scan help?

ANSWER 2

Yes. A CT can detect extramedullary lesions and some intramedullary tumors. Be aware that a negative CT does not exclude the diagnosis of spinal tumors.

Question 3

Why are some spinal tumors with benign histology considered malignant?

ANSWER 3

Because they have a malignant behavior. They do not appear to cause distant metastasis but the local growth can be lethal or very severe.

Question 4

When should corticotherapy begin in patients with possible spinal tumors?

ANSWER 4

If there is no contraindication, immediately. It can help in diminishing the edema and symptoms. Corticoids can also prevent late complications.

CONTRIBUTORS

Gordon H Baustian, MD
Otavio A Clark, MD
Sandeep Garg, MD

THALASSEMIA

SUMMARY INFORMATION

DESCRIPTION

- Congenital disorders of hemoglobin synthesis
- Characterized by deficient synthesis of one or more hemoglobin polypeptide chains
- Beta-thalassemia results in an excess of alfa-globins, leading to the formation of alfa-globin tetramers that accumulate in the erythroblast
- Alfa-thalassemia results in an excess of beta-globins, which leads to the formation of beta-globin tetramers called hemoglobin H
- Hemoglobin H can precipitate, causing damage to the red blood cell membrane and leading to red cell breakage
- Clinical classification is by phenotype: thalassemia may be major, intermedia, minor, or silent
- Genotypes are far more complex and determine the clinical picture, which is of a spectrum of disease

URGENT ACTION

Transfusion is required in thalassemia major.

ICD9 CODE

282.4 Thalassemia.

SYNONYMS

- Cooley's anemia
- Mediterranean anemia

CARDINAL FEATURES

- Congenital disorders of hemoglobin
- Characterized by deficient synthesis of one or more hemoglobin polypeptide chains, leading to an imbalance in numbers of alfa and beta chains
- The interaction of alfa- and beta-thalassemia gives rise to a less severe hemolytic anemia
- In most thalassemias, globin chains are reduced but are structurally normal
- Some structural hemoglobin variants produce thalassemic syndromes; interactions of the different forms of thalassemia and other hemoglobinopathies is common
- Clinical classification is by phenotype: thalassemia may be classified as major, intermedia, minor, or silent
- Genotypes are far more complex and the clinical disease ranges along a continuous spectrum
- Prevalent in the Mediterranean region, Middle East, and southeast Asia
- Both alfa- and beta-thalassemia traits are frequent in African-Americans, but symptomatic thalassemia is rare
- Microcytic anemia is characteristic
- Hemoglobin electrophoresis is usually abnormal, with increased HbA2 and sometimes fetal hemoglobin (HbF)
- Major forms may benefit from splenectomy
- Allogeneic bone marrow transplant is potentially curative if an HLA (human leukocyte antigen) match is available

CAUSES

Common causes

Genetic:

- Most of the alfa-thalassemia syndromes result from gene deletions
- Most of the beta-thalassemia syndromes result from nucleotide substitutions or deletions in genes that are otherwise intact
- The clinical heterogeneity of the thalassemia syndromes is a reflection of the great heterogeneity of mutations that affect the globin genes
- Thalassemia intermedia may be produced by a great variety of genotypes

Normal hemoglobin:

- Adults have mainly hemoglobin A, made up of two alfa and two beta chains, together with HbA2 $<2\%$ (two alfa and two delta chains), and no HbF (two alfa and two gamma-globin chains)
- There are four alfa genes (located on chromosome 16) and two beta genes (on chromosome 11)
- At birth, HbF accounts for 70–90% in normal individuals, and gamma-chain synthesis is only replaced by beta chains gradually
- Impairment of beta synthesis leads to the patient being asymptomatic at birth

Alfa-thalassemias:

- The alfa-thalassemias result from mutations that cause decreased synthesis of structurally normal globin
- Two alfa-thalassemia phenotypes are recognized, and are referred to as follows: alfa-thalassemia 1 and alfa-thalassemia 2 (alfa+ thalassemia – low level of alfa chains)

- Hydrops fetalis has no alfa-globin gene (alfa0 thalassemia- no alfa chains)
- Hemoglobin H disease has one alfa-globin gene

Beta-thalassemias:

- There is only one beta-globin gene, of which there are two alleles (paternal and maternal)
- Globin chain synthesis in the homozygous state reveals two major types of beta-thalassemia: beta+ type (suboptimal beta chains present) and beta0 type (total absence of beta chains)
- The beta-thalassemia syndromes are caused by mutations of the expressed beta+ allele and nonexpressed beta-0 alleles
- The mutations affect gene regulation or expression rather than gene deletion, and can result in decreased synthesis of structurally normal globin
- In individuals with beta+ thalassemia, the amount of beta-globin messenger RNA in reticulocytes and bone marrow normoblasts is decreased 3- to 10-fold
- In patients with homozygous beta0 thalassemia, beta-globin synthesis is absent

Deltabeta-thalassemia:

- This disorder is characterized by decreased or absent synthesis of both delta- and beta-globin chains
- Most of the deltabeta-thalassemias result from gene deletions

Gammadeltabeta-thalassemia:

- This rare form of thalassemia is characterized by deletion or inactivation of the entire beta gene complex
- The homozygous state has not been encountered

Hereditary persistence of fetal hemoglobin (HPFH):

- As in deltabeta-thalassemia, delta and beta chain synthesis is decreased or absent in patients with HPFH
- Unlike deltabeta-thalassemia, the increase in gamma chain synthesis is sufficient to almost balance alfa chain synthesis
- Both deletion and nondeletion forms of HPFH have been characterized

Pathophysiology of thalassemia: how does defective hemoglobin cause disease?

- Selective deficiency of one or more polypeptide chains causes decreased hemoglobin synthesis and imbalance between alfa and nonalfa chain production
- In the absence of complementary globin chains with which to bind, chains with normal synthesis form aggregates, precipitate within the cytoplasm, damage cell membranes, and lead to premature cell destruction
- In patients with alfa-thalassemia, the defect in alfa chain synthesis results in an accumulation of gamma chains in the fetal and neonatal periods and of beta chains thereafter
- The excess of beta chains oxidize and precipitate with cell aging
- In homozygous beta-thalassemia, a deficiency of beta chain synthesis results in an accumulation of alfa chains
- The free alfa chains aggregate to form insoluble inclusions in bone marrow erythroid precursors
- In thalassemia syndromes there is often ineffective erythropoiesis and hemolysis, which lead to anemia

Contributory or predisposing factors

Genetic.

EPIDEMIOLOGY

Incidence and prevalence

Most common genetic disorder worldwide.

PREVALENCE

- Currently, there are approximately 1000 patients with severe thalassemia in the US
- The incidence of thalassemia trait within the ethnic groups involved ranges from 3% to 5%
- 50–100 per 1000 in southeast Asia
- 30 per 1000 worldwide
- 50 per 1000 in African-Americans
- 150–300 per 1000 in Italy, Greece, and among Americans of Italian or Greek descent

Demographics

AGE

- Congenital condition
- Beta-thalassemia major causes severe anemia and jaundice from age 3–6 months
- Alfa-thalassemia causes intrauterine death if all four chains are affected; other forms may not present until later life
- Beta-thalassemia minor is usually asymptomatic

GENDER

Male=female.

RACE

- 50–100 per 1000 in southeast Asia
- 50 per 1000 in African-Americans
- 150–300 per 1000 in Italy, Greece, and among Americans of Italian or Greek descent

GENETICS

- Inherited in an autosomal recessive pattern
- Inheritance of one defective gene causes the mild type of thalassemia; inheritance of two defective genes causes the severe type of thalassemia
- Two alfa-thalassemia phenotypes are recognized; one is characterized by thalassemia minor in the heterozygous state and the other is marked by no clinical or hematologic abnormality in the heterozygous state
- There are also two major types of beta-thalassemia: one with some residual beta chains (beta+ type) and another with no beta chains (beta0 type)
- 92% of the beta-thalassemia genes in Italians and Greeks are accounted for by six mutations, more than 90% of those in Sicilians by three alleles, 96% of those in Sardinians by two alleles, and 91% of those in south Chinese and southeast Asians by four alleles

GEOGRAPHY

- The distribution of the thalassemias is similar to that of malaria
- The purported advantage afforded the thalassemic red cell has been attributed to its low concentration of hemoglobin, an essential nutrient for the malaria parasite
- Most common in the Mediterranean and the Middle East, particularly Greece
- Hemoglobin H (HbH) disease affects individuals throughout southeast Asia, the Mediterranean islands, and parts of the Middle East; it occurs rarely in populations of African descent
- The highest concentration of alfa-thalassemia genes is found in southeast Asia and among those populations who have their origin along the west coast of Africa
- In the eastern oases of Saudi Arabia, more than 50% of the population appears to have a clinically silent form of alfa-thalassemia, and HbH disease is recognized with increasing frequency
- In African-Americans, alfa-thalassemia is relatively common, but rarely is it of clinical significance. Of African-American infants born in Philadelphia, 3% were found to have the electrophoretic and hematologic characteristics
- Two million refugees from Cambodia, Laos, and Vietnam during 1970–80 led to symptomatic alfa-thalassemia syndromes increasing throughout North America and Europe

DIAGNOSIS

DIFFERENTIAL DIAGNOSIS

Iron deficiency

Anemia secondary to inadequate iron supplementation or excessive blood loss.

FEATURES

- Usually normal on examination
- Skin pallor may be present
- Hypochromic microcyctic anemia
- Red blood cells (RBCs) with central pallor, anisocytosis, and poikilocytosis
- Elevated RBC distribution width
- Elevated reticulocyte count
- Absent iron marrow stores
- Decreased serum ferritin
- Decreased serum iron and increased total iron-binding capacity

Other hemoglobinopathies

Inherited disorders of hemoglobin structure or production. The most common is sickle cell anemia. Sickle cell trait may occur in combination with thalassemia, and the degree to which the patient is affected depends on the thalassemia gene present (i.e. whether there are any normal beta chains present). There are many other hemoglobin variants caused by structural globin chain defects (e.g. hemoglobin E disease, the most common variant in southeast Asia, which causes a mild microcytic anemia). The hemoglobin variants may occur in combination with thalassemia.

FEATURES

- Diagnosed on electrophoresis
- Family studies may be needed to identify genotype of heterozygous forms

Other hemolytic anemias

Hemolysis is premature lysis of RBCs: the normal lifespan of 120 days may be reduced to <5 days. Hemolytic anemia may be inherited or acquired.

Inherited types:

- Enzyme deficiencies (e.g. glucose-6-phosphate dehydrogenase (G6PD) deficiency, pyruvate kinase deficiency)
- Hemoglobinopathies (e.g. sickle cell disease, thalassemia)
- Disorders of the red cell membrane (e.g. congenital spherocytosis, congenital elliptocytosis)

Acquired types:

- Immune: alloimmune (e.g. rhesus incompatibility, ABO incompatibility)
- Nonimmune: infection (especially falciparum malaria, *Clostridium welchii*), drugs, burns, valve prosthesis, and other causes of hypersplenism

FEATURES

- Apart from in hemoglobinopathies, hemoglobin electrophoresis is normal
- Peripheral blood film may reveal abnormal cell forms
- G6PD deficiency: episodic hemolysis, laboratory testing for G6PD assay is low
- Pyruvate kinase deficiency is much rarer, causes chronic hemolytic anemia, and the specific enzyme assay is diagnostic

SIGNS & SYMPTOMS

Signs

Thalassemia trait has no signs or symptoms. Other forms of thalassemia may be associated with the following signs:

- Pallor
- Poor growth
- Inadequate food intake
- Splenomegaly
- Jaundice
- Maxillary hyperplasia
- Dental malocclusion
- Cholelithiasis
- Systolic ejection murmur in the presence of severe anemia
- Pathologic fractures

Symptoms

- Symptoms of anemia: tiredness, breathlessness, poor exercise tolerance
- Abdominal pain due to hypersplenism and splenic infarction may occur
- Right upper quadrant pain caused by gallstones may occur

ASSOCIATED DISORDERS

Sickle cell anemia trait may be inherited in conjunction with one thalassemia gene.

CONSIDER CONSULT

- All patients with transfusion-dependent thalassemia or thalassemia intermedia should be under the care of a hematologist
- All patients with minor thalassemia should be referred for genetic counseling if they are contemplating pregnancy

INVESTIGATION OF THE PATIENT

Direct questions to patient

Exclude sickle cell disease and heterozygosity with beta-thalassemia:

Q **Do you ever have pains in your stomach or joints?** Look for evidence of sickle cell crises

Q **Have you ever had swelling of your hands or feet?** Have you ever suffered from priapism? Have you suffered from gallstones? Have you ever had leg ulcers? All these may be symptoms of sickle cell disease

In beta-thalassemia the major presentation is at age 3–6 months:

Q **How long has your baby been unwell for?** Intercurrent infection is a common cause of hemolysis in babies, particularly those with G6PD

Q **Was your baby jaundiced at birth?** May indicate G6PD deficiency or red cell membrane disorders such as sperocytosis

Q **Did your baby have any bleeding at birth or from the cord stump?** Consider coagulation disorders

Q **Has your baby passed any blood or dark stools?** Consider blood loss from the gut (e.g. intussusception, Meckel's diverticulum)

Q **Has your baby ingested anything unusual?** Drugs are a common cause of hemolysis in babies, particularly those with G6PD deficiency

Q **Has your baby been growing well?** Thalassemia major often presents with failure to thrive with severe anemia and jaundice at around 6 months

Q **Have you ever lost a baby in pregnancy?** Fetal hydrops caused by complete failure to synthesis alfa chains leads to death in utero

In thalassemia intermedia, signs and symptoms are comparable to those of thalassemia major but of lesser magnitude; presentation may be much later

- Q **Have you/your child ever required a transfusion?** Although chronically anemic, individuals with thalassemia intermedia do not require transfusions, except in association with intercurrent illness
- Q **Has your child's growth always been satisfactory?** Growth and development during childhood is relatively uncompromised in nonmajor thalassemias, pubescence takes place normally, and fertility is preserved
- Q **Do you think your child's face has changed?** Facial bony changes similar to those of thalassemia major are observed regularly in thalassemia intermedia
- Q **Have you/your child always been pale? Have you been anemic? Have you ever been jaundiced?** Pallor, intermittent icterus, and splenomegaly are common in thalassemia intermedia

In thalassemia minor, there may be no symptoms other than slight anemia:

- Q **Have you been anemic before?** Thalassemia minor leads to chronic anemia, which may only be discovered incidentally
- Q **Were you anemic in pregnancy?** Anemia usually worsens in pregnancy
- Q **Have you been given iron therapy for anemia in the past?** This is a clue that there has been a hypochromic microcytic anemia in the past, misdiagnosed as iron deficiency
- Q **Did the iron therapy work?** In thalassemia it would not
- Q **Have you ever been jaundiced?** Mild jaundice may be a sign of hemolysis

Family history

- Q **Has anyone in your family had anemia before?** A detailed family tree of affected members will be helpful. It can also be useful to know the ages of onset of anemia in family members
- Q **Has any member of your family ever had a bleeding problem?** Consider coagulation disorders
- Q **Has anyone in your family had thalassemia, sickle cell disease, or any other blood problem?**
- Q **Were your parents related before they married?** Consanguinity increases the chance that homozygosity will result in the children of the union
- Q **Do your parents or your families come originally from the same part of the world? Where is that?** This again looks for the possibility of homozygosity
- Q **Do you know if any of your family or your ancestors were from southern Europe, the Middle East, Africa, or Asia?** Look for links to areas where thalassemias are more prevalent

Examination

- **Is the patient pale? Are the conjunctiva pale?** Anemia usually produces pall, as it does when the hemoglobin is much below 8g/dL (80g/L). It can be harder to detect in African-American patients
- **Is the patient jaundiced?** Look at the sclera. Hemolysis often produces mild but clinically detectable jaundice, especially in intermedia (and major) thalassemias
- **Is the patient jumpy or do they appear unwell?** Consider intercurrent infection, bone marrow failure
- **Is the patient facially dysmorphic?** Look particularly for maxillary overgrowth and frontal bossing. This syndrome is still sometimes seen in thalassemia intermedia
- **Is the patient's liver or spleen enlarged?** This suggests thalassemia major or intermedia, but an enlarged spleen is also seen in congenital spherocytosis
- **Is the heart clinically enlarged?** Suggests thalassemia major or intermedia
- **Is there a systolic ejection murmur?** Suggests thalassemia major or intermedia with severe anemia

Summary of investigative tests

The symptomatic thalassemia syndromes rarely pose problems in diagnosis. The hematologic features of the asymptomatic syndromes are subtle, but the following tests should be performed:

- Complete blood count (CBC)
- Hemoglobin electrophoresis permits differentiation of the alfa- and beta-thalassemias
- Peripheral blood smear: changes in red cell morphology and in the relative amounts of hemoglobin fractions are sufficiently great as to be distinctive and in themselves diagnostic
- Hematocrit may be helpful and is part of the standard workup to assess anemia
- Serum ferritin, transferrin, and iron-binding capacity help to distinguish thalassemia from iron deficiency
- Serum bilirubin may be raised in hemolysis
- Urine urobilin and urobilinogen may be present
- Globin gene analysis may be performed by a specialist if other tests and family history do not fully explain genotype
- Bone marrow aspiration may be performed by a specialist

DIAGNOSTIC DECISION

Symptomatic thalassemia syndromes:
In major thalassemia, diagnosis is obvious from hemoglobin electrophoresis. The symptomatic thalassemia syndromes rarely pose problems in diagnosis.

(Alfa-thalassemia major syndromes)
Electrophoresis is normal in the absence of hemoglobin H disease.

(Hemoglobin H disease)

- Patients with this condition have a severe anemia, and often require blood transfusions to survive
- The diagnosis is confirmed by hemoglobin electrophoresis showing the presence of hemoglobin H
- At birth, 20–40% Hb Bart's is found (Hb Bart's is deletion of all four alfa-globin genes)
- The level of HbA2 is decreased (average 1.55%)
- A hemoglobin band migrating more slowly than HbA2 is seen in individuals with hemoglobin Constant Spring

(Beta-thalassemia major (Cooley's anemia))

- Anemia and morphologic alterations of circulating erythrocytes are first detected at 6 weeks and splenomegaly at 8 weeks of age
- In the absence of transfusion therapy, the hemoglobin concentration slowly falls to 3–5g/dL (30–50g/L)
- The reticulocyte count is elevated (5–15%)
- HbA2 is increased variably
- Absent or reduced hemoglobin
- Increased fetal hemoglobin (HbF)

(Thalassemia intermedia)

- Signs and symptoms of thalassemia intermedia are comparable to those of thalassemia major but of lesser magnitude
- The hemoglobin concentration is maintained in the range 6–9g/dL (60–90g/L) without transfusion
- The hemoglobin electrophoretic pattern is highly variable – a reflection of the heterogeneity of genotypes that produce this clinical syndrome

Asymptomatic thalassemia syndromes:
(Alfa-thalassemia minor)

- This disorder is suspected in the newborn on the basis of a low mean corpuscular volume (less than 94fL) and an increase in Hb Bart's
- Failure to detect Hb Bart's does not exclude alfa-thalassemia
- Confirmation of the diagnosis of alfa-thalassemia minor is possible through family studies
- In the absence of a specific screening test, a definitive diagnosis can be made only by demonstrating a reduced rate of alfa chain synthesis in reticulocytes

(Beta-thalassemia minor)

- The diagnosis of heterozygous beta-thalassemia is confirmed by the following: increase in HbA2, red cell microcytosis, hypochromia, target cells, and basophilic stippling
- 50% of patients have a mild elevation in HbF of 1–3%
- Hemoglobin electrophoresis demonstrates a predominance of HbA, increased levels of HbA2 (3.5–8%), and normal or minimally increased levels of HbF

CLINICAL PEARLS

- Iron deficiency is the most common form of anemia and may present similarly to beta-thalassemia
- Iron deficiency causes reduced levels of HbA2 in thalassemic patients; elevated levels cannot be demonstrated until the iron deficiency is corrected
- The diagnosis of transient aplastic crisis due to parvovirus B19 is often presumptive, based on a falling hemoglobin and a low reticulocyte count in a patient with a hemolytic anemia

THE TESTS

Body fluids

COMPLETE BLOOD COUNT

Description

Blood test.

Advantages/Disadvantages

Advantages: easy, quick, and cheap routine blood test

Normal

- Hemoglobin: female 12–15g/dL (120–150g/L); male 13.6–17.7g/dL (136–177g/L)
- Mean corpuscular volume (MCV): 80–100mcm^3 (80–100fL)
- Mean corpuscular hemoglobin (MCHC): 32–36mg/dL
- Reticulocyte count: 0–1%
- Note: in neonate normal reticulocyte count is 1.5–7%, hemoglobin 14.5–23g/dL (145–230g/L), MCV 98–119mcm^3 (98–119fL)
- RBC count: male 4.3–5.9x10^6/mm^3; female 3.5–5x10^6/mm^3
- RBC distribution width (RDW): 11.5–14.5

Abnormal

- In symptomatic thalassemias, hemoglobin is markedly reduced, MCV and MCHC are reduced, and reticulocyte count is raised
- In thalassemia minor, hemoglobin is variably reduced, and MCV and MCHC are reduced
- In hereditary persistence of fetal hemoglobin, hemoglobin may be increased
- RBC count is normal or may be increased in alfa-thalassemia (despite a reduced hematocrit/hemoglobin value)
- RDW may be normal or elevated in thalassemias
- Reticulocytes are elevated in hemolysis generally, but often not as elevated in thalassemia as one would expect on the basis of other indices

Cause of abnormal result

Thalassemia major:

- Anemia usually is pronounced when first documented at age 3–6 months
- Before transfusion, the hemoglobin concentration is 2.5–6.5g/dL (25–65g/L) and the packed cell volume is 0.11–0.24L/L
- The anemia is microcytic (MCV 48–72fL) and hypochromic (MCHC 23–32g/dL)
- Leukocytes characteristically are increased in number and platelet numbers are normal
- In the absence of transfusion therapy, the hemoglobin concentration slowly falls to 3–5g/dL (30–50g/L)
- The reticulocyte count is elevated (5–15%)

Thalassemia intermedia:

The hemoglobin concentration is maintained in the range of 6–9g/dL (60–90g/L) without transfusion.

Thalassemia minor:

- Anemia is mild or absent
- The RBC count is elevated, and the MCV and MCHC values are reduced; the degree of reduction in the MCV is directly related to the degree of reduction in beta-globin production
- The MCHC is normal or only slightly decreased

Iron deficiency:

- Also causes microcytic hypochromic anemia
- Iron deficiency causes reduced levels of HbA2 in thalassemic patients; elevated levels cannot be demonstrated until the iron deficiency is corrected
- Iron deficiency also lowers serum ferritin
- Iron deficiency is easily confused with thalassemia minor

Drugs, disorders and other factors that may alter results

- Parvovirus B19 infection may produce 'aplastic crisis' and severe reticulocytopenia in thalassemia
- Iron deficiency causes reduced levels of HbA2 in thalassemic patients; elevated levels cannot be demonstrated until the iron deficiency is corrected; iron deficiency also lowers serum ferritin

HEMATOCRIT

Description

Blood test.

Advantages/Disadvantages

Advantages: easy, quick, and cheap routine blood test

Normal

- Male 39–49%
- Female 33–43%

Abnormal

- Values below the normal ranges
- Keep in mind the possibility of a falsely abnormal result

Cause of abnormal result

- 28–40% in alfa-thalassemia trait and beta-thalassemia trait
- May fall to less than 10% in beta-thalassemia major
- Reduced in iron deficiency, hemoglobinopathies, and any blood loss (acute or chronic)

Drugs, disorders and other factors that may alter results
Parvovirus B19 infection may produce 'aplastic crisis' and severe reticulocytopenia in thalassemia.

PERIPHERAL BLOOD FILM SMEAR
Description
- Blood test: sample is placed on slide and examined under medium and high-power field
- The appearance of RBCs on smears of the peripheral blood is both striking and characteristic

Advantages/Disadvantages
Advantages:
- Easy and quick to perform
- Will produce diagnostic picture of thalassemia major if present

Normal
Normal morphology without basophilic stippling, distortion, or target cells.

Abnormal
Abnormal forms.

Cause of abnormal result
Alfa-thalassemia minor:
- Red cell morphology is abnormal with microcytosis, hypochromia, and slight anisopoikilocytosis
- Punctate basophilic stippling
- High percentage of target cells

Beta-thalassemia major:
- Anisocytosis is significant, with cells ranging from 3 to 15mm in diameter. They contain little pigment and may be so distorted in shape that they appear to be composed almost exclusively of a thin, nearly colorless membrane
- Target cells are numerous, many of them having a bridge joining the central and peripheral zones of pigment
- Few cells are fully pigmented. Basophilic stippling is prominent
- Poorly pigmented normoblasts are regularly present, their number ranging from 10 per 100 leukocytes to several times the number of leukocytes
- Morphologic alterations of circulating erythrocytes are first detected at 6 weeks and splenomegaly at 8 weeks of age

In thalassemia intermedia, peripheral blood erythrocytes show changes comparable to those of thalassemia major:
- Significant anisocytosis
- Hypochromia
- Target cells
- Basophilic stippling
- Numerous nucleated forms

Thalassemia minor:
- Morphologic alterations of peripheral blood erythrocytes are prominent. These changes include microcytosis, hypochromia, anisocytosis, poikilocytosis, target cells, and basophilic stippling
- Nucleated red cells are not present

Hereditary persistence of fetal hemoglobin (HPHF):
- Minor abnormalities of red cell morphology may be seen, including microcytosis (MCV 68–84fL), anisocytosis, and target cells

HEMOGLOBIN ELECTROPHORESIS

Description

Electrophoretic examination of peripheral blood sample.

Advantages/Disadvantages

Advantages:

- Easy to perform as part of standard workup for unexplained hemolytic anemia
- Allows diagnosis of major and intermedia forms and identifies fetal hemoglobin (HbF) and concurrent presence of HbS (sickle cell hemoglobin)

Normal

- In the normal adult, hemoglobin A, which is composed of two alfa- and two beta-globins (a2b2), is the most prevalent, comprising about 95% of all hemoglobin
- Two minor hemoglobins also occur: hemoglobin A2, composed of two alfa- and two delta-globins (a2d2), comprises 2–3.5% of hemoglobin; whereas HbF is composed of two alfa- and two gamma-globins (a2g2), and comprises less than 2% hemoglobin
- HbF is the dominant hemoglobin in the fetus, and begins to decrease after gestational week 30

Abnormal

General:

In addition to the more detailed findings given below, the following general features may be observed:

- Elevated HbA2 levels in beta-thalassemia trait
- Elevated HbA2, elevated HbF, reduced or absent HbA1 in beta-thalassemia major or intermedia

Alfa-thalassemias:

Normal except for the presence of hemoglobin H (HbH) in HbH disease.

(HgH disease)

- At birth, 20–40% Hb Bart's is found. Hb Bart's is replaced gradually during the first months of life by HbH, which stabilizes at a level between 5 and 40%
- The level of HbA2 is decreased (average 1.55%)
- A hemoglobin band migrating more slowly than HbA2 is seen in individuals with Hb Constant Spring

Beta-thalassemias:

(Beta-thalassemia major)

- Absent or reduced HbA
- Increased HbF
- Variable increase in HbA2

(Thalassemia intermedia)

The hemoglobin electrophoretic pattern is highly variable – a reflection of the heterogeneity of genotypes producing this clinical syndrome.

(Thalassemia minor)

- Hemoglobin electrophoresis demonstrates a predominance of HbA, increased levels of HbA2 (3.5–8%), and normal or minimally increased levels of HbF
- In Hemoglobin Lepore the concentration of HbA2 is normal or reduced, and that of HbF is normal or elevated. Hemoglobin Lepore is produced at a reduced rate, accounting for only 5–15% of the total concentration of hemoglobin
- The most consistent feature of thalassemia minor is an increase in HbA2
- HbA2 levels in persons with heterozygous beta+ thalassemia are lower than those in persons with beta0 thalassemia, and may fall to within the normal range

(Thalassemia minima)
The hemoglobin pattern is normal.

Silent carrier state:
Hematologically normal.

(Alfa-thalassemias in association with structural variants)
- The beta chain variants noted in association with alfa-thalassemia include HbS (sickle cell hemoglobin), HbC, HbE, and HbJ Bangkok
- The interaction of alfa-thalassemia and HbS trait produces a variable amount of HbS

(HgH disease)
- At birth, 20–40% Hb Bart's is found
- Hb Bart's is replaced gradually during the first months of life by HbH, which stabilizes at a level between 5 and 40%
- The level of HbA2 is decreased (average 1.55%)

Herediary persistence of fetal hemoglobin:
- Persistence of HbF into adult life
- In the homozygous state HbF constitutes 100% of the hemoglobin concentration; HbA and HbA2 are absent
- In the African-American variant the level of HbA2 is low (1.6–2.2%), and HbF is increased to 10–36% (mean 26%)
- In the Greek variant the relative concentration of HbF in the heterozygous state is lower (15–25%) than that associated with African-American HPFH
- Levels of HbF are lower in association with iron deficiency
- Greek HPFH in association with heterozygous beta-thalassemia: the major hemoglobin is HbA, and both HbA2 (3.6–5.2%) and HbF (20–40%) levels are increased

Cause of abnormal result
Thalassemias.

Drugs, disorders and other factors that may alter results
- There are a large number of nonthalassemic hematologic disorders that are often associated with an increase in HbF
- These include juvenile chronic myelocytic leukemia, the Di Guglielmo syndrome, sideroblastic anemia, pernicious anemia, myelofibrosis, aplastic anemia, the Diamond-Blackfan syndrome, and paroxysmal nocturnal hemoglobinuria

SERUM FERRITIN, TRANSFERRIN, AND IRON-BINDING CAPACITY
Description
Blood test.

Advantages/Disadvantages
Advantages:
- Easily performed with other standard tests
- Helps distinguish iron-deficiency anemia from thalassemia minor

Normal
- Ferritin: 18–300ng/mL (18–300mcg/L)
- Transferrin: 170–370mg/dL (1.7–3.7g/L)
- Serum iron-binding capacity 250–460mcg/dL (45–82mcmol/L)

Abnormal

- Plasma iron turnover is increased out of proportion with the increase in erythrocyte iron turnover
- Serum iron levels are increased, serum transferrin is often fully saturated, and a nontransferrin-bound iron fraction may be present
- Serum iron-binding capacity is decreased in hemolytic anemias

Cause of abnormal result

- Transferrin is elevated and ferritin is decreased in iron deficiency
- Transferrin is decreased in hemolytic anemias
- Ferritin is increased in iron replacement therapy
- Serum iron-binding capacity is elevated in iron deficiency and decreased in hemolysis

Drugs, disorders and other factors that may alter results

- Iron therapy will normalize ferritin levels in iron deficiency
- Transfusion will raise ferritin levels in thalassemias

SERUM BILIRUBIN (INDIRECT)

Description

Blood test.

Advantages/Disadvantages

Advantage: easy, standard test

Normal

0–1.0mg/dL (2–18mcmol/L).

Abnormal

Increased unconjugated bilirubin levels.

Cause of abnormal result

Elevated in hemolysis, liver disease, hepatic congestion secondary to congestive heart failure, Gilbert's disease, Crigler-Najjar syndrome, hyperthyroidism (rarely).

URINE UROBILIN AND UROBILINOGEN

Description

Urine test.

Advantages/Disadvantages

Advantage: easy and quick

Normal

Absence of urobilin or urobilinogen.

Abnormal

Urobilin or urobilinogen present.

Cause of abnormal result

- In thalassemia and other causes of hemolysis, the urine often contains increased quantities of urobilin or urobilinogen, and may be dark brown because of the presence of dipyrroles and mesobilifuscin
- Urobilin or urobilinogen also raised in hepatitis and liver cell dysfunction

TREATMENT

CONSIDER CONSULT

Worsening of clinical condition.

IMMEDIATE ACTION

Transfusion in acute anemia. Criteria for transfusion in the emergent setting are based on clinical symptoms of anemia.

PATIENT AND CAREGIVER ISSUES

Forensic and legal issues

- Jehovah's Witnesses will not always consent to receiving blood or blood products
- Where life is at risk, children can be transfused without parental consent
- Where life is not imminently at risk, the consent of the courts must be sought
- In adults who are able to give informed consent, transfusion cannot be given if consent is withheld

Impact on career, dependants, family, friends

- Thalassemia major is a severe illness that shortens life expectancy dramatically
- The psychological consequences can be immense, both for the child and for parents; feelings of guilt and distress are common
- The same is true for thalassemia intermedia
- Further distress will arise where puberty is delayed, where fertility is an issue, and where the typical facies are present and are viewed as stigmatous
- It is still not uncommon, particularly among recent immigrant populations, for thalassemia minor to present in pregnancy. Where this is the case, urgent testing of the father of the pregnancy is obviously important, and genetic counseling should be extended to the whole family. Antenatal testing should be offered if appropriate to parental genotypes
- Different illness beliefs and translation difficulties may cause great difficulties in these populations

MANAGEMENT ISSUES

Goals

- Offer genetic counseling and information to whole family to minimize impact of disease on future generations
- Minimize impact of disease on life
- Minimize impact of disease on growth, development, puberty, and fertility
- Minimize impact of transfusion therapy on health
- Treat infections promptly and protect against bloodborne diseases
- Maintain adequate hemoglobin concentration and suppress erythropoietic response
- Avoidance of iron therapy unless iron deficiency is documented biochemically

Management in special circumstances

COEXISTING DISEASE

Parvovirus B19:

- The most important etiologic agent in transient aplastic crisis is parvovirus B19
- The virus commonly causes the childhood illness 'Fifth disease', which is usually a minor ailment
- Malaise, low-grade fever, arthralgias, and a skin rash (often manifested as red, 'slapped' cheeks) are hallmarks of the condition. Parvovirus B19 infections in adults are frequently associated with transient arthropathy

- In patients with hemolytic anemia, parvovirus B19 suppresses bone marrow erythropoietic activity, leading to transient aplastic crisis
- The virus integrates into a specific site in the human genome. The infected cells fail to divide, impairing the production of new erythrocytes
- Reticulocyte counts often fall to as low as 0.1–0.5% from the routine values of 6–20% in patients with hemolytic anemias
- Hemolytic anemias per se do not predispose patients to infection with parvovirus B19
- The diagnosis of transient aplastic crisis due to parvovirus B19 is often presumptive, based on a falling hemoglobin and a low reticulocyte count in a patient with a hemolytic anemia
- A rising IgM antibody to the virus is another means of diagnosing parvovirus B19 infection; polymerase chain reaction test to detect virus may be more sensitive and faster to obtain
- Transient aplastic crisis is usually self-limiting and requires only supportive measures
- Physicians should warn patients with hemolytic disorders and their parents of the signs and symptoms of Fifth disease

COEXISTING MEDICATION

Instruct patients to avoid any complementary therapies or vitamin supplements that might contain iron.

SPECIAL PATIENT GROUPS

Genetic counseling is advisable for parents or other relatives of a child with thalassemia, and for any individual with beta-thalassemia minor.

Fertility in the individual with thalassemia:
Reduced fertility is common among individuals with transfusion-dependent thalassemia, such as beta-thalassemia major.

Causes of reduced fertility include the following:
- Some women with beta-thalassemia have primary amenorrhea; this must be corrected and menstruation initiated in order for such a woman to conceive and carry a pregnancy
- Reduced fertility in the individual with thalassemia is mainly attributable to iron overload in the pituitary gland

Management to prevent reduced fertility or infertility:
- The best approach to prevent reduced fertility or infertility is to control iron levels
- Studies suggest that effective use of deferoxamine can lead to normal sexual maturation
- Patients fare better if treatment is started early, before iron levels become high, as indicated by increased ferritin levels
- Those that maintain their iron at low levels throughout treatment also appear to have a better chance to preserve their fertility
- However, even those with very high ferritin levels over a long period of time can experience normal sexual maturation, although rarely

Pregnancy in patients with transfusion-dependent thalassemia:
- Although fertility is reduced, pregnancy may be possible for some
- Pregnancy in a handful of women has been reported in the medical literature, most having beta-thalassemia intermedia and a few having beta-thalassemia major
- The woman with transfusion-dependent thalassemia who is pregnant or considering becoming so should seek the advice of a hematologist, perinatologist, genetic counselor, and other specialists
- The hematologist is integral to monitoring the transfusion regimen, which tends to increase in pregnancy, as well as the administration and dosages of iron-chelating agents and other medications

- A high-risk obstetrician or perinatologist is also needed to monitor the health of the expectant mother, as well as that of the fetus
- Removing excess iron through the use of chelating medication is critical to the health and longevity of women with thalassemia. Increased transfusion requirements during pregnancy may increase the need for chelation therapy

SUMMARY OF THERAPEUTIC OPTIONS

Choices

Primary management of patients with transfusion-dependent thalassemia falls under four major headings: transfusion therapy, splenectomy, iron chelation, and bone marrow transplantation. Also, several therapeutic strategies are in the developmental stages, including pharmacologic activation of gamma-globin synthesis, gene therapy, and bone marrow stem-cell transplantation.

Patients with thalassemia intermedia and others who are able to maintain a hemoglobin concentration in excess of 7.5g/dL (75g/L) usually do not require chronic transfusion therapy. In general, mild cases should be treated on an outpatient basis, whereas inpatient treatment may be required for transfusion therapy.

General measures:

- Mild cases require no therapy
- Certain lifestyle measures can be instituted to prevent traumatic damage to the spleen prior to splenectomy, and to help reduce and maintain a low level of iron
- Avoid iron therapy: the sole therapeutic precaution for alfa- and beta-thalassemia minor is the avoidance of therapeutic iron supplementation unless iron deficiency is documented biochemically
- Thalassemia intermedia: normally no therapy is necessary, unless hemoglobin levels fall to a dangerous level; the patient may then need transfusion therapy
- Patients with severe thalassemia: maintain a mean hemoglobin level of at least 9.3g/dL (93g/L) with a regular transfusion schedule (transfusions of approximately 15mL/kg at 3- to 5- week intervals)
- Folate supplementation. In association with other chronic hemolytic anemias, folate supplementation may be necessary during pregnancy and periods of marginal food consumption to prevent megaloblastic arrest of erythropoiesis
- Iron overload: patients receiving transfusion therapy increase total body iron four times over the normal amount, and iron chelation therapy may be required
- Iron chelation therapy with deferoxamine. Continuous subcutaneous or intravenous infusion with a small infusion pump 40mg/kg/day (about a 10-h period); usually started before 5–8 years of age
- In pregnant women undergoing iron chelation therapy, vitamin C (ascorbic acid) is administered to enhance removal of iron
- In those patients in whom deferoxamine is contraindicated or who cannot tolerate the required doses, an alternative agent is deferiprone (however, this is still at the experimental stage).
- Antibiotics for infection: infectious illnesses require prompt attention, especially in children who have undergone splenectomy

Surgical measures:

- Splenectomy may be needed if hypersplenism causes a marked increase in the transfusion requirement. The recommendation is to defer surgery until the patient is 4–6 years of age (because of increased infection risk at younger ages)
- Severe facial deformities resulting from unchecked erythroid hyperplasia may require surgical and orthodontic correction

Preventive measures:
- Administer polyvalent pneumococcal vaccine one month before splenectomy
- Prophylaxis with a daily regimen of penicillin
- Hepatitis B vaccine is recommended for all patients before starting transfusion therapy. Also, another major concern in this regard is hepatitis C, which was frequently transmitted by blood transfusions in the past (one study estimated the proportion of transfusion-dependent thalassemia patients with hepatitis C as high as 50%)
- The toxic effect of iron on endocrine glands may necessitate hormone replacement therapy for delayed sexual maturation or for growth disturbances related to growth hormone deficiency

Bone marrow transplantation (BMT)
- BMT is available for selected patients with a matched sibling or unrelated donor
- Cures the disease, but may be associated with significant mortality and morbidity

Clinical pearls
Do not administer high-dose (>200mg/day) vitamin C (ascorbic acid) in iron-loaded patients because it can lead to increased absorption of iron (and may precipitate cardiac failure). Do not administer vitamin C without iron-chelation treatment (e.g. deferoxamine).

Never
- The sole therapeutic precaution for alfa- and beta-thalassemia minor is the avoidance of therapeutic iron supplementation unless iron deficiency is documented biochemically
- Both of these thalassemia syndromes are associated with increased iron absorption. Iron therapy is without effect on hematologic values or cell morphology, and contributes to a tendency toward excessive iron accumulation in adult life
- The symptomatic thalassemia syndromes are predictably complicated by tissue iron toxicity. Avoidance of unnecessary iron exposure is of paramount importance

FOLLOW UP
Plan for review
- Thalassemia major and intermedia: lifelong monitoring is necessary because both the therapy and disease progression have numerous possible complications
- Thalassemia minor and minima: no follow up is usually necessary

Information for patient or caregiver
- There are a number of ongoing trials that are recruiting patients at present
- Patients who are interested in joining trials for iron chelation or gene therapy should investigate the Cooley's Anemia Foundation website

DRUGS AND OTHER THERAPIES: DETAILS
Drugs
IRON CHELATION THERAPY
- Most patients with thalassemia major die from complications of iron overload
- At a total body iron burden of 40g, organ function begins to fail, and at 60g or more, intractable cardiac failure has its onset
- The most effective iron-chelating agent widely available is deferoxamine
- It is recommended that deferoxamine be started after the first 10–20 transfusions, or when the serum ferritin reaches 1000ng/mL
- In general these criteria are reached at about 3 years of age. Infusions started at this age can maintain iron balance

Dose

- When given before 3 years of age, deferoxamine must be given at a reduced dose (20–30mg/kg/day) to prevent the drug's adverse effect on linear growth
- After 3 years of age, the dose of deferoxamine may be increased to 40–50mg/kg/day
- The total daily dose is infused over an 8–12h period at night, with a small portable infusion pump
- Limited experience with high-dose deferoxamine (6–12g/day) given intravenously suggests that it may be superior to conventional subcutaneous therapy in heavily iron overloaded patients
- It is recommended that deferoxamine be started after the first 10–20 transfusions, or when the serum ferritin reaches 1000ng/mL

Efficacy

- Chronic chelation therapy begun during the first decade of life reduces hepatic iron levels, retards the progression of hepatic fibrosis, and facilitates continued growth
- Heart failure, diabetes mellitus, and early death are prevented when deferoxamine is begun at an early age and is given in amounts that are proportional to the transfusion-related iron load
- Iron excretion after the administration of deferoxamine is proportional to body iron stores
- In patients with thalassemia major who are begun on regular transfusions during the first year of life, mobilization of clinically significant amounts of iron cannot be achieved with daily intramuscular injections of deferoxamine until 5–10 years of age, and negative iron balance is achieved infrequently at any age
- Nevertheless, chronic chelation therapy begun during the first decade of life reduces hepatic iron levels, retards the progression of hepatic fibrosis, and facilitates continued growth
- Chronic deferoxamine infusions appear to prevent or delay the development of heart disease in heavily transfused patients

Risks/Benefits

Risks:

- Deferoxamine in excessive dosages may result in growth retardation, sensorineural ototoxicity, and ocular toxicity, as well as bone deformities
- Compliance with constant parenteral administration is an issue with many patients
- Elimination of iron is increased by forming an inactive water-soluble compound, ferrioxamine. In anuric patients it cannot be excreted without dialysis
- Small risk of mucormycosis
- Impaired cardiac function with concomitant use of high-dose vitamin C supplements

Side-effects and adverse reactions

- Cardiovascular system: palpitations, tachycardia, hypotension, shock
- Central nervous system: anxiety, confusion, dizziness, drowsiness, fatigue, neuritis, paresthesia, poor circulation
- Gastrointestinal: anorexia, constipation, diarrhea, dry mouth, nausea, vomiting, abdominal discomfort
- Genitourinary: dysuria, frequency, impotence, retention
- Hematologic: rare blood dyscrasias, bone marrow suppression, hemolytic anemia
- Respiratory: acute respiratory distress syndrome

Interactions (other drugs)

- Vitamin C
- Prochlorperazine
- Gallium-67
- Anticholinergics

Contraindications

- Narrow-angle glaucoma
- Bladder neck obstruction
- Severe renal disease or anuria

Acceptability to patient
Because this is a therapy that requires daily administration of a parenteral drug, it can be quite difficult for the patient and/or caregivers. Proper counseling and instructions must be given, especially to parents of a child with thalassemia requiring iron-chelation therapy.

Follow up plan
As for underlying condition.

ASCORBIC ACID

- The net amount of iron excreted by iron-overloaded subjects receiving deferoxamine is increased 2-fold by the daily oral administration of 200–500mg ascorbic acid
- Vitamin C administration should not exceed a daily dose of 200mg, and should not be given without iron chelation
- Unfortunately, ascorbate also increases the toxicity of tissue iron
- For this reason, ascorbic acid probably should be reserved for use in individuals who are not severely iron overloaded

Dose
200–500mg ascorbic acid daily.

Efficacy
Ascorbic acid appears to render tissue iron more accessible to deferoxamine, thereby enhancing total iron excretion without increasing iron absorption.

Risks/Benefits
Risks:

- Excessive doses for prolonged periods should not be taken by diabetics, patients with renal calculi, patients undergoing anticoagulant therapy, or those with a history of gout
- Increases the toxicity of tissue iron

Benefit: enhances the amount of iron excreted by iron-overloaded subjects receiving deferoxamine

Side-effects and adverse reactions

- Central nervous system: dizziness, fatigue, flushing, headache, insomnia
- Gastrointestinal: anorexia, cramps, diarrhea, heartburn, nausea, vomiting
- Genitourinary: crystalluria, oxalate or urate renal stones, polyuria, urine acidification
- Hematologic: hemolysis (after large doses in patients with glucose-6-phosphate (G6PD) deficiency), sickle cell crisis

Interactions (other drugs)
Antacids.

Contraindications
■ Pregnancy category A if doses do not exceed the recommended daily allowance ■ Pregnancy category C if doses exceed the recommended daily allowance ■ Tartrazine sensitivity ■ Sulfite sensitivity ■ G6PD deficiency ■ Excessive doses for prolonged periods of time should not be taken by diabetics, patients with renal calculi, patients undergoing anticoagulant therapy, or those with a history of gout

Acceptability to patient
Usually acceptable.

Follow up plan

As for underlying condition.

FOLATE SUPPLEMENTS

- Enhanced production of red cells associated with hemolytic anemias requires a large amount of folic acid
- Folate deficiency in these patients can impair erythropoiesis, with consequent exacerbation of anemia
- Although this complication is not common, most patients with hemolytic anemias are maintained with supplements of folic acid

Dose

5mg/day.

Efficacy

Given for presumed benefit; evidence for efficacy not found.

Risks/Benefits

- Risk: use caution in patients with undiagnosed anemia
- Benefits: low cost, no side-effects, easy to take

Side-effects and adverse reactions

- Respiratory: bronchospasm (rare)
- Skin: itching and rash

Interactions (other drugs)

■ Anticonvulsants ■ Cholestyramine ■ Colestipol ■ Colchicine ■ Fluoxetine ■ Lithium ■ Lometrexol ■ Metformin ■ Methotrexate ■ Nonsteroidal anti-inflammatory drugs (NSAIDs) ■ Phenobarbital ■ Phenytoin ■ Pyrimethamine ■ Sulfasalazine

Contraindications

Hypersensitivity to folate.

Acceptability to patient

Usually problem-free and highly acceptable.

Follow up plan

As appropriate to underlying clinical condition.

EXPERIMENTAL THERAPIES

- 5-Azacytidine is a cytidine analog that, when incorporated into newly synthesized DNA, leads to extensive demethylation. This drug was found to reactivate repressed genes in tissue culture cells and to induce a striking increase in gamma-globin synthesis in baboons, the globin gene organization of which is similar to that in humans
- Several other cell cycle-specific agents, including hydroxyurea, cytarabine, and vinblastine, as well as erythropoietin, butyric acid, and other short-chain fatty acids, were demonstrated to upregulate gamma-globin synthesis and HbF production
- Another treatment strategy, also in the experimental stages, involves bone marrow stem-cell transplantation. This will be more widely applicable than allogeneic bone marrow transplantation

Efficacy

In general, the responses to these agents by patients with both thalassemia major and thalassemia intermedia have been variable and disappointing, although some patients have benefited.

Follow up plan

As per trial protocols and as appropriate to underlying disease.

Surgical therapy

SPLENECTOMY

- Splenomegaly is a problem for patients with thalassemia major who have not had optimal transfusion therapy, and for many patients with thalassemia intermedia and HbH disease, syndromes for which transfusions are given infrequently
- Progressive splenomegaly expands the blood volume, shortens red cell survival, increases the transfusion requirement, and accelerates iron loading. Splenic trapping of platelets and leukocytes can produce thrombocytopenia and leukopenia
- The main indication for splenectomy is an increasing transfusion requirement
- If the actual blood requirement is 50% greater than that predicted from the standard curve, then surgical removal of the organ is recommended
- Findings of recent studies have prompted the recommendation to remove the spleen when the red cell transfusion requirement exceeds 200–250mL packed red cells/kg/year
- The procedure should be postponed until late childhood or adolescence if possible because of the exaggerated risk of fatal sepsis in thalassemic children whose spleens have been removed during the first years of life
- Splenectomy is often required in adults with HbH disease and thalassemia intermedia to correct symptoms resulting from mechanical pressure or to ameliorate worsening anemia

Efficacy

Return of the blood requirement to the expected range occurs promptly after splenectomy.

Risks/Benefits

Risks:

- Those of major surgery
- Exaggerated risk of fatal sepsis in thalassemic children whose spleens have been removed during the first years of life

Benefit: improves clinical condition

Acceptability to patient

- Depends on patient's attitude to surgery
- Clearly a major undertaking for the patient

Follow up plan

A normal surgical follow up, and follow up as appropriate to the underlying clinical condition.

Patient and caregiver information

- Advise patients regarding immunizations: pneumococcal, meningococcal
- In the UK annual influenza vaccination is recommended for all patients with chronic disease and for all patients with splenectomy

Other therapies

BLOOD TRANSFUSION

- Most patients with more severe grades of anemia require regular blood transfusions in order to facilitate growth and permit participation in normal activities
- Transfusion regimens where pretransfusion hemoglobin is <9.5g/dL (95g/L) are currently the standard of care. Chronic transfusions should generally not be carried out when hemoglobin levels are above this because there is a risk of iron loading

- Goals of transfusion therapy are correction of anemia, suppression of erythropoiesis, and inhibition of increased gastrointestinal absorption of iron
- Currently there is a debate as to the use of hyper- and supertransfusion as therapeutic approaches. These approaches decrease erythropoiesis but may cause iron loading, which is the main transfusion-related complication
- Regular transfusions should be started when the hemoglobin concentration falls below 7g/dL (70g/L) or when there is impaired growth

Efficacy
- Moderate transfusion protocols (i.e. restricting the start of regular transfusions to patients with a pretransfusion hemoglobin of 9.5g/dL (95g/L) or lower) have been shown to reduce iron loading substantially, without a large expansion in endogenous erythropoiesis
- Hypertransfusion programs effectively suppress erythroid activity and prevent the unlimited bone marrow expansion that underlies the skeletal pathology of thalassemia major, but may contribute to iron loading. Within 1–4 months of raising the minimum hemoglobin value to 12g/dL (120g/L), the transfusion requirement returns to that necessary to maintain a minimum level of 9g/dL (90g/L)
- Supertransfusion: maintenance of a mean hemoglobin value of 14–15g/dL (140–150g/L) almost completely suppresses endogenous erythropoiesis

Risks/Benefits
- Risks: this is a life-saving treatment, but it ultimately leads to death in thalassemia major due to iron loading

- Benefits: hypertransfusion and supertransfusion have some benefits in terms of decreased endogenous erythropoiesis and decreased iron absorption. However, the risk of substantial iron loading has been documented, although it remains controversial

Acceptability to patient

This treatment is difficult for patients, who will often regard transfusion as a very mixed blessing.

Follow up plan

Review regularly depending on patient's clinical condition.

Patient and caregiver information
- Patients need to receive information on the risks and benefits of transfusion in thalassemia
- Each transfusion should only be given if the benefits are greater than the risks

ALLOGENEIC BONE MARROW TRANSPLANTATION
- The high probability of cure, with potentially acceptable morbidity or mortality, supports the recommendation that patients with thalassemia major who have HLA-identical family members be offered BMT
- Unfortunately, less than 20% of patients meet these criteria

Efficacy

High probability of cure if tissue match is available, and patient and family are willing.

Risks/Benefits
- Risk: morbidity and mortality low, but nevertheless significant
- Benefit: the best success rate is in young patients who are more well, and who may therefore feel they have more to lose

Acceptability to patient

- Each patient or family must weigh the emotional and financial costs of chronic transfusion therapy and daily chelation therapy against the risks of early death and chronic graft-versus-host disease associated with BMT
- It is usually highly acceptable because it offers the prospect of a cure, and therefore greatly increased life expectancy

Follow up plan

- Intensive at first with regular review
- If patient remains clinically well once the procedure is concluded then follow up is as appropriate to the clinical condition: lifelong occasional review

GENE THERAPY

- The hemoglobinopathies are ideal candidates for gene therapy in that the tissue to be treated can be removed, treated, and reinfused with relative ease
- At present, no means are known whereby globin genes can be introduced into bone marrow stem cells and their expression regulated
- Great ethical issues surround the application of genetic engineering to the prevention and treatment of human disease

Efficacy

- Not yet known – early experimental stage
- Retrovirus-mediated gene transfer is a technique that holds greater promise. It takes advantage of the synthesis by the retrovirus of a copy of its genome, which is then inserted into the DNA of the host cells
- Insertion of retroviral vectors into stem cell progenitors and expression of the cloned genes might permit repopulation of the bone marrow with cells in which the genetic defect is corrected by genes carried by the vector
- Nevertheless, formidable problems remain unresolved, particularly those that involve increasing the frequency with which genes can be introduced successfully into foreign cells, developing the means for enriching the target cells and amplifying, and at the same time regulating gene expression
- Such amplification and regulation are particularly important to avoid the thalassemia phenotype

LIFESTYLE

- Avoid strenuous activities (e.g. football, soccer), particularly prior to splenectomy when there is increased risk of traumatic splenic rupture due to the spleen being large, soft, and relatively unprotected by the rib cage
- Acceptable activity levels will need to be determined on an individual basis depending on severity of disorder
- Avoid iron-rich foods (meats such as liver, and some cereals)
- Drinking tea may possibly help reduce iron

ACCEPTABILITY TO PATIENT

Young patients may find any lifestyle restrictions difficult to accept.

FOLLOW UP PLAN

Regular review in major thalassemia is essential to spot problems before they arise, particularly psychological problems in young people and their families living with chronic genetic disease.

PATIENT AND CAREGIVER INFORMATION

- Genetic counseling
- Teach parents the signs of hepatitis, iron overload
- Printed patient information is available from the Cooley's Anemia Foundation website

OUTCOMES

EFFICACY OF THERAPIES

People with the condition live far longer than the 5–10 years that was common when Thomas Cooley first described it.

The treatment mainstays in thalassemia major are transfusion, iron chelation, splenectomy, and marrow transplantation. Attention to intercurrent infection, protection against blood-borne diseases, and management of the endocrine and cardiac complications of hemosiderosis are essential as disease progresses.

Transfusion:

- Blood transfusions have greatly improved the duration and quality of life for patients with thalassemia major. The bone and facial deformities that Cooley noted are now uncommon in most countries
- The main complications for patients are iron overload and hepatitis
- Regular transfusions should be started when the hemoglobin concentration falls below 7g/dL (70g/L) or when there is impaired growth. When begun early in life, transfusions prevent the facial stigmata of thalassemia and facilitate normal growth, prevent congestive splenomegaly, lead to fewer severe infectious illnesses, and improve cardiac reserve

Iron chelation:

- The most effective iron-chelating agent widely available is deferoxamine
- Heart failure, diabetes mellitus, and early death are prevented when deferoxamine is begun at an early age in amounts proportional to the transfusion-related iron load

Ascorbic acid:

- Appears to render tissue iron more accessible to deferoxamine, thereby enhancing total iron excretion without increasing iron absorption
- Unfortunately, ascorbate also increases the toxicity of tissue iron

New agents:

- Deferiprone may not provide the needed control of body iron in a significant proportion of chronically transfused patients, but it is an oral medication that may be more practical in developing countries and is the most promising so far
- 5-Azacytidine was found to reactivate repressed genes in tissue culture cells and to induce a striking increase in gamma-globin synthesis in baboons
- Several other cell cycle-specific agents were demonstrated to upregulate gamma-globin synthesis and fetal hemoglobin production

Splenectomy:

- Splenectomy is recommended when the red cell transfusion requirement exceeds 200–250mL packed red cells/kg/year
- Return of the blood requirement to the expected range occurs promptly after splenectomy
- The procedure should be postponed until late childhood or adolescence if possible because of the exaggerated risk of fatal sepsis in thalassemic children whose spleens have been removed during the first years of life
- Pneumococcal immunization is recommended before splenectomy

Bone marrow transplantation:

- In Italian studies, patients younger than 16 years of age with none of the adverse risk factors (class I) have an event-free survival of 90% following HLA-matched allografting. Those in the same age group with extensive liver damage related to iron overload (class III) have a high transplant mortality rate and an event-free survival of only 50%
- The results obtained by the Italian group have not been matched by others

Gene therapy:
Although it is still experimental and at present no means are known to introduce globin genes into bone marrow stem cells and regulate their expression, there is cautious optimism that gene therapy may offer promise for the future.

Review period

- Thalassemia major and intermedia: lifelong monitoring necessary because both the therapy and disease progression have numerous possible complications
- Thalassemia minor and minima: no follow up is usually necessary

PROGNOSIS

Outlook varies depending on type.

Thalassemia minor:
Patients have a normal lifespan.

Thalassemia intermedia:

- Growth and development during childhood is relatively uncompromised, pubescence takes place normally, and fertility is preserved
- Survival into adulthood is the rule, and patients typically enjoy a full lifespan

Thalassemia major:

- Effective iron chelation improves longevity
- The most important factors associated with survival are the age at which chelation therapy was introduced and the success with which serum ferritin was maintained below 2500ng/mL
- The natural course of untransfused thalassemia major is of recurrent infections, progressive cachexia, and death by 5 years of age
- Aggressive transfusion therapy permits near-normal growth and development in childhood, but itself produces progressive organ damage, with death from iron overload in adolescence or early adult life
- Transfusional iron overload is compounded by increased intestinal absorption of iron
- The introduction of iron chelation therapy in the 1970s constituted a further therapeutic advance. In the US the mean age of patients with thalassemia major increased from approximately 11 years in 1973 by 80% to a median age of 23 years by 1994. In one series, the median age of survival was 31 years

Clinical pearls

Initiation of iron chelation therapy in a timely manner is key to improving prognosis in patients with thalassemia major and thalassemia intermedia. Liver biopsy with quantitative determination of iron provides crucial information, and cannot be replaced with noninvasive imaging studies.

Deterioration

- Full diabetes care is required in patients who develop diabetes mellitus
- Full supportive care for liver disease is required in patients with hepatic fibrosis or hepatitis, and cirrhosis
- Full supportive medical treatment is required for patients with cardiac hemosiderosis leading to congestive cardiac failure

Terminal illness

- Most patients with thalassemia major die from complications of iron overload and cardiac hemosiderosis leading to congestive cardiac failure
- At a total body iron burden of 40g, organ function begins to fail, and at 60g or more, intractable cardiac failure has its onset
- Supportive care should be offered, with symptomatic treatment

COMPLICATIONS

Beta-thalassemia major:

(General)

- Susceptibility to infections after splenectomy
- Infections from blood transfusion
- Intercurrent infections
- Worsening of anemia during infections
- Jaundice
- Leg ulcers
- Cholelithiasis
- Pathologic fractures
- Impaired growth rate
- Delayed or absent puberty
- Hepatic siderosis
- Hemolytic anemia
- Splenomegaly
- Cardiac disease from iron overload
- Aplastic and megaloblastic crises

(Skeletal abnormalities)

- Changes to the skull and facial bones. The outer and inner tables are thin, and perpendicular striations appear between the tables, resulting in an X-ray appearance suggestive of hair standing erect on the scalp
- Pneumatization of the sinuses is delayed
- Severe malocclusion
- Pathologic fractures
- Compression fractures of the vertebrae
- Premature fusion of a segment of the epiphysis of the proximal end of the humerus or the distal end of the femur is relatively common
- The ribs are broad, especially at their sites of articulation with the transverse processes of the vertebrae
- Erosion of the marrow through the cortex at this site produces a paravertebral mass, which rarely extends into the spinal column to produce cord compression
- In portions of the skeleton where red marrow normally is replaced by fat, lesions produced by thalassemia undergo regression; in portions supporting active erythropoiesis into adulthood, thalassemic changes progress with time

(Effects on growth and endocrine system)

- Growth retardation in early childhood is a consequence of severe anemia
- It can be prevented (although not corrected) by an aggressive blood transfusion program
- Even in children optimally transfused the preadolescent and adolescent growth spurt is delayed and curtailed, so that full potential stature is rarely realized
- Pubescence is delayed and often is incomplete
- In 250 adolescents who had had the benefit of both transfusion and chelation therapy, pubescence was lacking completely in 38% of girls and 67% of boys of age 12–18 years. Only 19% of the girls experienced menarche, and secondary amenorrhea intervened in one-third of this group
- Boys may have active spermatogenesis but lack libido
- Pituitary response to provocative stimulation is described as normal or deficient, suggesting a failure either of hypothalamic maturation or pituitary function
- Overt diabetes mellitus and hypoparathyroidism are well documented
- Insulin resistance and increased insulin secretion precede the development of diabetes
- Most endocrine abnormalities are noted only in older, chronically transfused patients

(Cardiopulmonary complications)
- After the first decade, many patients experience one or more episodes of sterile pericarditis, characterized by pain, friction rub, and pericardial effusion without tamponade. The illness is self-limited
- Both pericardial iron deposits and infection with rheumatogenic strains of streptococci have been invoked as possible causative factors
- Myocardial hemosiderosis is the leading cause of death in transfused patients
- Congestive heart failure and arrhythmias may be noted as early as age 6, but these conditions do not usually have their onset until the middle of the second decade
- Despite careful medical management, most patients with symptomatic heart disease do not survive more than a few months
- Echocardiography and radionuclide cineangiography permit detection of myocardial dysfunction before the development of overt disease

(Hepatobiliary disease)
- Liver enlargement in early life is related to extramedullary hematopoiesis, but later results from extensive cirrhosis
- Iron deposits produce pathologic findings indistinguishable from those of idiopathic hemochromatosis
- The incidence of gallstones is determined in large part by the aggressiveness of transfusion therapy. Recent estimates based on ultrasonographic evaluation place the incidence at between 2 and 4%

(Hepatitis)
- Patients with thalassemia acquire hepatitis most often from viruses contracted with blood transfusions
- Advances in detection of blood-borne viruses has greatly diminished the risk of infection with blood transfusion
- Patients who have substantial iron overload (ferritin levels >3000) have a much greater incidence of active liver injury than those with lesser iron burdens

Thalassemia intermedia:
- Complications in adult life include pathologic fractures, cholelithiasis, and thoracic masses composed of hematopoietic tissue
- The primary cause of premature death is myocardial hemosiderosis
- Iron overload is more the result of augmented gastrointestinal iron absorption than of transfusional iron loading
- The estimated amount of iron that subjects with thalassemia intermedia absorb on a standard diet is 3–10 times more than normal, and is attributed to a greatly expanded erythropoietic effort
- By the third or fourth decades, the iron load may be similar in magnitude to that of transfusion-dependent thalassemic patients in their teens

CONSIDER CONSULT
- Any patients who develop endocrine, hepatobiliary, or cardiac complications of disease
- Any patients with psychological problems arising from their disease
- Any patients who may be suitable for bone marrow allografting
- All transfusion-dependent patients should be under specialist care
- All patients needing occasional transfusion should be referred at least for occasional specialist review

PREVENTION

Prenatal information:

- Genetic counseling
- Prenatal diagnosis: study of globin genes performed on fetal cell DNA obtained by amniocentesis after 14 weeks

Complication prevention:

- Evaluation for thalassemia by one year of age for offspring of adult thalassemia patients
- Avoidance of infections
- Prompt treatment of infections (after splenectomy, patients should have a supply of ampicillin to take if symptoms of infection appear)
- Periodic dental checkups
- Avoidance of activities that could result in bone fractures

Prenatal diagnosis and carrier detection:

- Family history is critical to detect thalassemia prenatally
- Initial attempts to identify fetuses at risk for thalassemia major depended on fetal blood sampling during the second trimester
- The application of recombinant DNA technology to carrier detection and prenatal diagnosis greatly enhanced its accuracy and availability
- These approaches require that the specific mutation sought first is determined from a study of family members or from population surveys
- The spectrum of beta-thalassemia mutations has been determined for most of the world's population at greatest risk, including the Italians, Sicilians, Greeks, Spaniards, Turks, Lebanese, Indians, Chinese, and Melanesians
- The global development of prenatal screening programs in the early 1980s was monitored by the World Health Organization's International Registry for Prenatal Monitoring of Hereditary Anemias, providing a mechanism for the rapid dissemination of new knowledge

SCREENING

Published guidelines on Screening for hemoglobinopathies are available from National Guideline Clearinghouse [1].

Major recommendations:

- Screening newborn infants for hemoglobinopathies with hemoglobin electrophoresis or other tests of comparable accuracy on umbilical cord, or heelstick blood specimens is recommended ('A' recommendation). In geographic areas with a very low incidence of hemoglobin disorders, selective screening of newborns may be more efficient than universal screening. Infants with sickle cell disease must receive prompt follow up, including oral penicillin prophylaxis, diagnostic testing, immunizations, and regular evaluations of growth and nutritional status. Their families should receive genetic counseling regarding testing of family members and risks to future offspring, information about the disease, education about early warning signs of serious complications, and referrals for peer support groups and sources of medical and mental health services
- Offering screening for hemoglobinopathies with hemoglobin electrophoresis or other tests of comparable accuracy to pregnant women at the first prenatal visit is recommended

('B' recommendation), especially for those who are members of racial and ethnic groups with a high incidence of hemoglobinopathies (e.g. individuals of African, Caribbean, Latin-American, Mediterranean, Middle Eastern, or southeast Asian descent). Carriers identified through testing should be urged to have the father tested and should receive information on the availability of prenatal diagnosis if the father is positive and the fetus is at risk of having a clinically significant hemoglobinopathy

- There is insufficient evidence for or against screening for hemoglobinopathies in adolescents and young adults from ethnic and racial groups that are known to be at increased risk for sickle cell disease, thalassemias, and other hemoglobinopathies, in order for them to make informed reproductive choices ('C' recommendation). Recommendations to offer such testing may be made on other grounds, including burden of suffering and patient preference. If provided, testing should be accompanied by counseling, which should include a description of the significance of the disease, how it is inherited, the availability of a screening test, and the implications to individuals and their offspring of a positive result

PRENANTAL DIAGNOSIS AND CARRIER DETECTION

- The application of recombinant DNA technology to carrier detection and prenatal diagnosis has greatly enhanced its accuracy and availability
- Fetal DNA is prepared from amniocytes obtained at 15–17 weeks of gestation or from chorionic villus sampling at 9–11 weeks. Fetal loss after the latter procedure (1–3%) is similar to natural wastage for pregnancies of this duration
- Fetal DNA may be amplified enzymatically by polymerase chain reaction (PCR), making it possible to provide specific diagnoses within 1–3 days
- These approaches require that the specific mutation sought first is determined from a study of family members or from population surveys
- The spectrum of beta-thalassemia mutations has been determined for most of the world's population at greatest risk, including Italians, Sicilians, Greeks, Spaniards, Turks, Lebanese, Indians, Chinese, and Melanesians

Cost/efficacy

- These programs have had a major impact on the incidence of thalassemia major in parts of the world where its prevalence has exceeded available resources
- The combined efforts of screening couples at risk and prenatal diagnosis have reduced the birth rate of children with thalassemia major by 70–90% in Sardinia, Greece, Cyprus, and Ferrara. Among patients with thalassemia living in Connecticut, the relative number of children younger than 5 years dropped from 34% to 4% between 1973 and 1985
- A corollary of the decline in the birth rate of affected infants is an increase in the reproductive experiences of couples at risk of having children with thalassemia major. For example, Greek Cypriots with thalassemia minor in London, most of whom elected not to have children before the availability of prenatal testing, had children at the same rate as other London Cypriots after the introduction of prenatal diagnosis programs

HIGH-PRESSURE LIQUID CHROMATOGRAPHY AND POLYMERASE CHAIN REACTION

Some recent studies have reported on the use of newer technologies for screening large populations. These include:

- High-performance liquid chromatography (HPLC) to detect abnormal hemoglobins [2]
- PCR for detecting abnormal alfa and beta-globin genes [3]

RESOURCES

ASSOCIATIONS

Northern California Comprehensive Thalassemia Center
747 52nd Street
Oakland, CA 94609
Tel: (510) 428-3885, x 4398
www.thalassemia.com

Cooley's Anemia Foundation
(National Office)
129–09 26th Avenue – #203
Flushing, NY 11354
Tel: (800) 522-7222
Fax: (718) 321-3340
E-mail: info@cooleysanemia.org
www.thalassemia.org

KEY REFERENCES

- Lukens JN. The thalassemias and related disorders: quantitative disorders of hemoglobin synthesis. In Lee GR, ed. Wintrobe's Clinical Hematology, 10th edn. Philadelphia: Lippincott Williams & Wilkins, 1998
- Cao A, Gabutti V, Masera G, et al. Management Protocol for the Treatment of Thalassemia Patients. New York: Cooley's Anemia Foundation, 1992
- Collins AF, Pearson HA, Giardina P, et al. Oral sodium phenylbutyrate therapy in homozygous beta-thalassemia: a clinical trial. Blood 1995;85:43–9
- Fucharoen S, Siritanaratkul N, Winichagoon P, et al. Hydroxyurea increases hemoglobin F levels and improves the effectiveness of erythropoiesis in beta-thalassemia/hemoglobin E disease. Blood 1996;87:887–92
- Giardina PJ, Grady RW. Chelation therapy in beta-thalassemia: the benefits and limitations of desferrioxamine. Semin Hematol 1995;32:304–12
- Issaragrisil S, Visuthisakchai S, Suvatte V, et al. Brief report: transplantation of cord-blood stem cells into a patient with severe thalassemia. N Engl J Med 1995;332:367–9
- Lucarelli G, Clift RA, Galimberti M. Marrow transplantation for patients with thalassemia: results in class 3 patients. Blood 1996;87:2082–8
- Olivieri NF, Brittenham GM. Review: iron-chelating therapy and the treatment of thalassemia. Blood 1997;89:739–61
- Hoffbrand AV. Oral iron chelation. Semin Hematol 1996;33:1–8
- Prati D, Zanella A, Bosoni P, et al. The incidence and natural course of transfusion-associated GB virus C/hepatitis G virus infection in a cohort of thalassemic patients. The Cooleycare Cooperative Group. Blood 1998;91:774–7

Evidence references and guidelines

1 Guide to Clinical Preventive Services, 2nd edn. Baltimore: Williams & Wilkins, 1996, p485–94
2 Lorey F, Cunningham G, Shafer F, et al. Universal screening for hemoglobinopathies using high-performance liquid chromatography: clinical results of 2.2 million screens. Eur J Hum Genet 1994;2:262–71
3 Old JM, Varawalla NY, Weatherall DJ. Rapid detection and prenatal diagnosis of beta-thalassemia: studies in Indian and Cypriot populations in the UK. Lancet 1990;336:834–7

FAQS

Question 1

How does hematologic/clinical presentation vary as a function of the number of alfa-gene deletions?

ANSWER 1

Patients with one gene deletion (- alfa/alfa alfa) are clinically silent; those with two gene deletions ((- -/alfa alfa) or (alfa -/alfa -)) present with a low mean corpuscular volume (MCV) with or without mild anemia. Those with three gene deletions (- -/- alfa) present with hemolysis and splenomegaly. Those with four gene deletion have a condition incompatible with life (Hb Bart, $gamma_4$).

Question 2

What is hereditary persistence of fetal hemoglobin (HPFH), and how dangerous is this condition?

ANSWER 2

This is an hereditary condition, usually presenting with increased red blood cell (RBC) count and 70–100% HbF on hemoglobin electropheresis. It is a benign condition.

Question 3

What is a typical complete blood (RBC) count finding in beta-thalassemia?

ANSWER 3

Mean corpuscular volume <80 with increased RBC count is said to be 75% sensitive and 97% specific for thalassemia syndromes.

Question 4

What happens in patients with iron overload?

ANSWER 4

In patients with high iron overload (i.e. those with hepatic iron exceeding 15mg/g liver), there is a high risk of early death due to cardiac disease.

Question 5

The patient who is on chronic subcutaneous continuous infusion of deferoxamine presents with severe abdominal pain, fever, and diarrhea. What should I do?

ANSWER 5

The patient with iron overload, particularly if they are on iron-chelation treatment, is susceptible to *Yersinia* infection. The iron-chelation should be stopped and appropriate stool and blood cultures and serologic testing should be obtained.

CONTRIBUTORS

Gordon H Baustian, MD
Benjamin Djulbegovic, MD, PhD
Dinesh S Rao, MD